D1517023

SECOND EDITION

EXERCISE
IN HEALTH and
DISEASE

Evaluation and Prescription
for Prevention and Rehabilitation

Michael L. Pollock, Ph.D.

Professor
Departments of Medicine, Physiology and
Exercise and Sport Sciences
University of Florida
Gainesville, Florida

Jack H. Wilmore, Ph.D.

Margie Gurley Seay Centennial Professor
Department of Kinesiology & Health Education
The University of Texas at Austin
Austin, Texas

W.B. SAUNDERS COMPANY
A Division of Harcourt Brace & Company

Philadelphia   London   Toronto   Montreal   Sydney   Tokyo

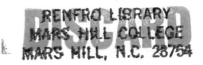
W.B. SAUNDERS COMPANY
A Division of
Harcourt Brace & Company

The Curtis Center
Independence Square West
Philadelphia, Pennsylvania 19106

Library of Congress Cataloging-in-Publication Data

Pollock, Michael L.
    Exercise in health and disease: evaluation and prescription for
prevention and rehabilitation/Michael L. Pollock, Jack H. Wilmore.—
2nd ed.

    p. cm.

    Includes bibliographical references.

1. Exercise therapy.   I. Wilmore, Jack H., 1938–   II.
    Exercise in Health and Disease: Evaluation and Prescription for
    Prevention and Rehabilitation.

RM725.P64   1990 613.7′1–dc20   89–37393
                                                             CIP

ISBN 0–7216–2948–2

Editor: William Lamsback
Designer: Terri Siegel
Production Manager: Linda R. Turner
Manuscript Editor: David Indest
Mechanical Artist: Karen Giacomucci
Illustration Coordinator: Walt Verbitski
Indexer: Nancy Weaver

Exercise in Health and Disease: Evaluation and
Prescription for Prevention and Rehabilitation   ISBN   0–7216–2948–2

Printed in the United States of America.

Last digit is the print number: 9   8   7   6   5   4   3

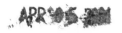

This book is dedicated to our wives, Rhonda and Dottie, and our children, Jonathan and Lauren Pollock and Wendy, Kristi, and Melissa Wilmore, for their love, support, and understanding. Further, we would both like to dedicate this book to Jesus Christ, our Savior and Lord, from whom we receive the ability, strength, and stamina to undertake the task of writing such a book.

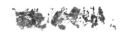

Acknowledgments

We wish to express a special acknowledgment to our secretaries, Ms. Linda LeGrand and Ms. Kristi Wilmore, for their diligent typing, proofreading, and general administrative skills, which assisted us greatly in manuscript preparation; and to Ms. Cathy Rapinett and Ms. Kelleigh Jacobs for their help in proofreading the final manuscript.

Contents

SECTION B

PHYSIOLOGY OF EXERCISE RELATED TO

PHYSICAL ACTIVITY IN HEALTH AND DISEASE

Since the time of the Industrial Revolution, technology has advanced at an astounding rate. From that time to today, there has been a remarkable transformation of a basically hard-working, physically active, rural-based society into a population of anxious and troubled city dwellers and suburbanites with little or no opportunity for physical activity. These advances in modern technology have enabled our present-day society to live a life of relative comfort. Hand or push lawn mowers have been replaced by power lawn mowers, the most advanced having seats to support the person's body weight. Even grass itself is being replaced by synthetic turf! Elevators and escalators have replaced stairs—just try to find an open stairway in a modern high rise. The walk to the corner market has been replaced by a short drive to the supermarket in the neighborhood shopping center. Life *is* getting easier—easier, that is, from the viewpoint of conserving effort and human energy. But can "easier" be equated with a better and more productive life? In short, do we profit from this newly acquired sedentary existence, or does the sedentary lifestyle contribute in its own way to a totally new set of problems?

To answer this last question, it is necessary only to reflect on the simple but intricate manner in which the body functions and the delicate manner in which the body systems are so consistently in perfect harmony. Disrupt that harmony in even a simple way (e.g., the common cold or the tension headache), and the whole person suffers. There is a growing body of evidence that is beginning to demonstrate without question that physical inactivity and the increased sedentary nature of our daily living habits pose a serious threat to the body, causing major deterioration in normal body function. Such common and serious medical problems as coronary artery disease, hypertension, obesity, anxiety and depression, and lower back problems have been either directly or indirectly linked with a lack of physical activity. In addition to physical inactivity, a number of other factors are associated with these diseases or medical problems, including smoking, overeating, improper diet, excessive alcohol consumption, and emotional stress. These factors are all complications of the modern lifestyle, and they are interactive. Thus, to make the most significant impact on improving general health and reducing the risk of disease and disability, it is imperative to deal with the total person, altering the total lifestyle to achieve good health habits.

The first two chapters of this book discuss those diseases and associated health problems that are attributable, at least in part, to physical inactivity, with the major focus on cardiovascular disease and obesity. After a brief introduction, each chapter will focus on the pathophysiology of the disease or condition, discuss the associated risk factors, and then summarize the current knowledge concerning the role of physical activity in the prevention and treatment of that disease or condition. The underlying theme of both chapters is that physical fitness is more than the absence of disease. Rather, physical fitness represents a means to attain optimal health.

1

CARDIOVASCULAR DISEASE

INTRODUCTION

Since the early 1900's, cardiovascular disease has been the leading cause of death in the United States across all age groups. As recently as 1981, over half of all deaths in this country were the result of cardiovascular disease. Or, stated more dramatically, the sum total of all other forms of death combined did not equal the number of deaths from cardiovascular disease alone. Cardiovascular disease continues to be the leading cause of death in the United States. Cardiovascular diseases accounted for almost 978,500 deaths in 1986, which represented about 47 percent of the total annual mortality rate.[1] Cardiovascular diseases include coronary artery disease, hypertension, stroke, congestive heart failure, peripheral vascular disease, congenital heart defects, valvular heart disease, and rheumatic heart disease. Figure 1–1 illustrates the leading causes of death in the United States. These figures are estimates for 1986, the most recent year for which complete data are available.

Coronary artery disease (CAD), also referred to as coronary heart disease (CHD), was the major cause of cardiovascular disease deaths (heart attacks) in 1986.[1] The three major cardiovascular diseases and their associated mortality rates are illustrated in Figure 1–2. More than one out of every four deaths was the result of CAD, maintaining CAD as the single leading cause of death in the United States. Coronary artery disease is almost always the result of atherosclerosis, which is a narrowing of the coronary arteries, the arteries that supply the heart muscle, or myocardium (Fig. 1–3). The actual process of atherosclerosis is discussed in detail in the following section.

As the coronary arteries become narrowed and hardened, an imbalance between oxygen demand and delivery can develop. This is most likely to occur during periods of emotional stress or during

3

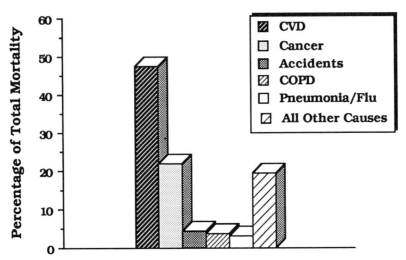

Figure 1–1. Leading causes of death in the United States: 1986 estimate. CVD = cardiovascular disease, COPD = chronic obstructive pulmonary disease. (Data from the National Center for Health Statistics, U.S. Public Health Service, Department of Health and Human Services.)

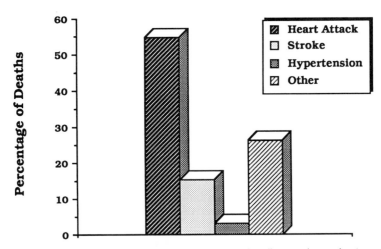

Figure 1–2. Estimated deaths due to cardiovascular disease by major type of disorder: 1986 estimate. (Data from the National Center for Health Statistics, U.S. Public Health Service, Department of Health and Human Services.)

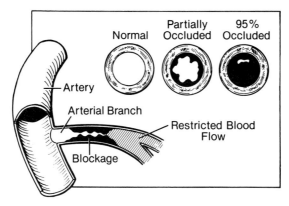

Figure 1–3. Gradual narrrowing of a coronary artery through the progression of atherosclerosis.

exercise, when the heart is beating at a rate well above resting levels. The oxygen and energy demands of the heart are highly related to the heart rate alone and even more highly related to the product of heart rate and systolic blood pressure ($r = 0.88$ and $r = 0.90$, respectively).[2] The latter index, heart rate times systolic blood pressure, is referred to as the double product or the rate-pressure product. The higher the heart rate or the double product, the higher the oxygen and energy demands of the heart. When the coronary arteries become narrowed to a certain critical point, it is no longer possible to supply sufficient oxygen to the heart at the higher heart rates; thus, the demand exceeds the supply. Figure 1–4 illustrates the relationship between the double product and myocardial blood flow, and how this relationship changes with increased narrowing of the coronary vessels.

When coronary blood flow is unable to meet the myocardial oxygen demands, the individual typically feels chest pressure, an intense pain, or a dull ache, sometimes radiating up into the neck, jaw, or left shoulder or down the left arm. This transient chest discomfort is referred to as angina pectoris and is the result of localized ischemia, lack of adequate blood flow, in that section of the myocardium distal to the narrowed section of the coronary artery. This narrowed section of the coronary artery may close or become totally occluded; a spasm of the coronary artery may occur; or a blood clot may lodge in this area, resulting in a myocardial infarction (MI) or heart attack. Another form of heart attack that frequently leads to death is caused by a disturbance in the heart's rhythm (an arrhythmia). A fatal arrhythmia can occur in the presence of normal coronary arteries. This is one of the more common forms of heart attack death in young adults, particularly

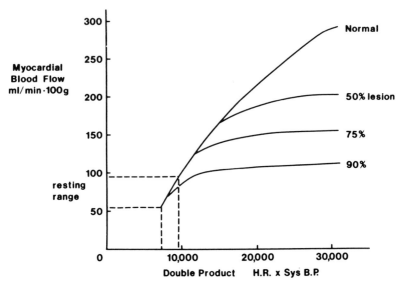

Figure 1–4. Illustration of the relationship between increases in the double product and increases in myocardial blood flow. The family of curves illustrates how the blood supply to the heart is limited as the degree of luminal narrowing increases from 50 to 90% occlusion. At 90% occlusion, there is barely sufficient blood flow potential to meet the heart's needs at rest.

in young athletes.[3] In these deaths the arrhythmia is typically secondary to a congenital abnormality.

Hypertension is the most prevalent of the cardiovascular diseases. Over 60 million American adults and children were estimated to have hypertension in 1986.[1] Hypertension is simply a condition in which the blood pressure is chronically elevated above levels considered desirable or healthy for the person's age and size. For the adult, a systolic blood pressure between 140 and 159 mmHg or a diastolic pressure between 90 and 95 mmHg is considered to be borderline hypertension. A systolic pressure of 160 mmHg or greater or a diastolic pressure of 96 mmHg or greater is considered to be absolute hypertension.[4] More recently, the Joint National Committee on Detection, Evaluation, and Treatment of High Blood Pressure revised these standards.[5] The new standards are as follows:

Classification	Systolic Pressure mmHg	Diastolic Pressure mmHg
Normal	<140	<85
High Normal		85–89
Mild Hypertension	140–159	90–104
Moderate Hypertension		105–114
Severe Hypertension	≥160	≥115

These standards are reduced in the pediatric population, with the absolute standard traditionally defined as the 95th percentile of the normative data for a specific age.[6] For a 10-year-old boy, the 95th percentile would be 130 mmHg for systolic and 85 mmHg for diastolic blood pressure.[7]

Stroke is the result of obstructions in or hemorrhages of blood vessels in and around the brain, which lead to the death of brain tissue.[8] The most common cause of stroke leading to the death of brain tissue is cerebral infarction resulting from atherosclerosis of the cerebral vessels. Cerebral infarction can also result from a cerebral embolism, in which an embolus or blood clot breaks loose from another site in the body and lodges in a cerebral artery, reducing or restricting blood flow distal to the clot. Cerebral hemorrhage is the other principal cause of stroke and is the result of a ruptured artery that bleeds into the substance of the brain or into the fluid-filled spaces over the surface of the brain. Approximately 500,000 people suffer strokes each year, resulting in nearly 150,000 deaths per year.[1]

Congestive heart failure describes the situation in which the heart is physically unable to deliver adequate blood to satisfy the oxygen and nutritional needs of the body at rest and during normal physical activity.[8] With chronically reduced blood delivery (reduced cardiac output), there is an excessive accumulation of fluids in the body. The excess fluid retention combined with failure of the heart is called congestive heart failure. Three kinds of impairment of heart function can lead to congestive heart failure: a diminished force of contraction of the ventricles, a mechanical failure in filling of the ventricles during diastole, and an overloading of the ventricles during systole.[8]

Peripheral vascular diseases involve both the systemic arterial and venous blood vessels. Peripheral arterial diseases are primarily of four kinds: occlusive, in which blood flow is blocked; vasospastic, in which small arteries constrict or go into spasm; functional, in which the small arteries dilate; and aneurysmal, in which the arterial wall balloons or bulges because of wall weaknesses.[8] Arteriosclerosis obliterans, a chronic, progressive arterial disease, is one of the major peripheral artery diseases and includes intermittent claudication, which is an ischemic pain in the lower extremities that results from narrowed arteries. Of the peripheral venous diseases, varicose veins and phlebitis are the most common. In varicose veins, the wall of the vein weakens and may become dilated, or the valves in the vein that prevent backward flow fail to function normally. This results in venous pooling and a discoloration of the vessels from the stagnating blood. With phlebitis, a clot or thrombus forms in the vein, partially or completely stopping the flow of blood. This can be fatal if the clot dislodges and travels to the lungs, i.e., pulmonary embolus.

Congenital heart defects occur in approximately one out of every 100 births, and the cause can be determined in only about 3 percent of the cases.[8] These defects can include narrowed heart valves (stenosis), constriction of the aorta (coarctation), septal defects, and abnormal shunts of blood.

Valvular heart disease involves one or more of the four valves that control the direction of blood flow from each of the four chambers of the heart. Valvular disease has numerous causes, but in all cases the heart is forced to do more work to deliver the same amount of blood, which can lead to serious cardiac complications. Rheumatic heart disease is the result of rheumatic fever, a disease caused by a streptococcal infection of the upper respiratory tract. Rheumatic fever most frequently strikes children of school age. Patients with rheumatic heart disease are prone to develop infection of the heart valves or the lining of the heart (endocarditis).[8]

The remainder of this chapter focuses on the two major cardiovascular diseases, CAD and hypertension. Although the other cardiovascular diseases are of considerable importance, relatively little is known about the role of physical activity in altering their development.

PATHOPHYSIOLOGY OF CORONARY ARTERY DISEASE AND HYPERTENSION

How do CAD and hypertension develop? What factors predispose one to atherosclerosis and myocardial infarction at an early age? What physiological changes occur that lead to a narrowing of the coronary arteries? What causes blood pressure to increase and to remain elevated throughout one's life? These and similar questions are addressed in this section in an attempt to better explain the mechanisms underlying CAD and hypertension.

Coronary Artery Disease

Coronary artery disease is now recognized as a pediatric disease, even though the clinical manifestations of the disease appear much later in life.[9] It is now recognized that there are three basic periods of disease development.[10] First, the incubation period occurs between infancy and adolescence. During this period, mesenchymal cushions form on the intima, or inner layer, of the arterial wall, particularly at points of bifurcation. These consist of a meshwork of embryonic connective tissue, with an increase in ground substance, disordered elastic fibers, and possibly some lipid deposits. In the second phase of this period, fatty flecks or streaks begin to appear. There is a slight focal thickening of the intima, an increased number of fibroblasts, and possible precursors of smooth muscle cells. The end result is a small round or oval plaque that is visible to the naked eye. Fatty streaks are found in the aorta in the first years of life and almost universally by the age of 3 years.[10] Second, the latent period occurs between adolescence and early adulthood. During this period, the fatty streaks are found in the coronary arteries. Although these are considered to be the precursors of the atherosclerotic lesions, they are certainly reversible at this stage.[10] Likewise, the presence of fatty streaks in children or adolescents is not a good forecaster of adult lesions. The fatty streak, however, does precede the fibrous plaque, which is generally considered irreversible, and leads to a complicated lesion. The final period is referred to as the clinical period, in which the clinical manifestations of the disease become apparent: angina pectoris, myocardial infarction, cerebral infarction, peripheral vascular disease, and sudden death. The fibrous plaque progresses to produce a substantial narrowing of the coronary artery lumen, thus reducing the coronary flow reserve.

The normal artery is composed of three distinct layers: the intima, or inner layer; the media, or middle layer; and the adventitia, or outer layer (Fig. 1–5). The media is composed of large numbers of smooth muscle cells, each surrounded by small amounts of collagen, small elastic fibers, and other connective tissue matrix components. The adventitia consists mainly of fibroblasts and loosely arranged collagen. The intima is the layer critical to the formation of atherosclerotic lesions.

The intima, although the innermost layer of the arterial wall, is protected from the blood and its constituents by a layer of endothelial cells. The endothelium normally provides a barrier to the passage of plasma proteins from the blood to the intima.[11] Local injury to the endothelium increases the concentration of plasma proteins in the intima at the point of injury, which can eventually lead to the migration of smooth muscle cells from the media into the intima. At this point, the smooth muscle cells can either proliferate or undergo cellular destruction, depending on the internal environment. Within a favorable environment, the smooth muscle cells undergo destruction and the affected area is repaired. Within an unfavorable environment (e.g., in the presence of hyper-

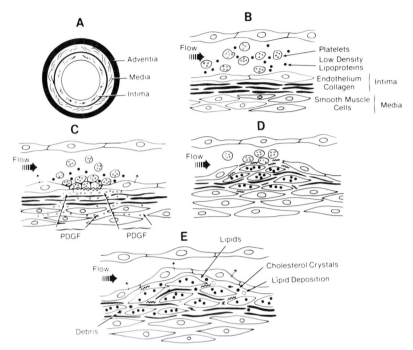

Figure 1–5. Changes in the arterial wall with injury, illustrating the disruption of the endothelium and the subsequent alterations. PDGF = platelet-derived growth factor. *A* through *E* represents the order of progression.

tension, increased blood lipid concentration, and hormonal imbalances), the smooth muscle cells proliferate and the newly formed plaque increases in size.[11]

In a review of the genesis of atherosclerosis, Ross[11] provides an excellent summary of research supporting his current theory on plaque formation. Findings of both experimental research and autopsy studies show that atherosclerotic plaques are the result of proliferated smooth muscle cells in the intima, not lipid degeneration and accumulation as had previously been thought. It is now recognized that three cellular changes are involved in this process. First, smooth muscle cells proliferate or multiply within the intima. Second, smooth muscle cells synthesize and release substances associated with connective tissue, including collagen, elastic fibers, and carbohydrate-containing proteins. Last, there is a deposition of lipids within the proliferated smooth muscle cells. Thus, the plaque is not a mass of fat, but a mass of smooth muscle cells that provide a repository for fats (see Fig. 1–5).

With this current theory, it is necessary to explain how the smooth muscle cells migrate from the media to the intima and how, once in the intima, they are able to continue to proliferate. As was stated earlier, injury to the endothelium appears to be the necessary first step. Endothelial cells at the site of the injury are shed into the blood stream, exposing subendothelial connective tissue. Blood platelets adhere to the arterial wall and to each other at the site of the injury. These platelets degranulate and release a mixture of products that interact to promote the migration and proliferation of smooth muscle cells to the damaged portion of the arterial wall. One of these products is a mitogen, a substance essential for growth, that is referred to as platelet-derived growth factor (PDGF) and is known to induce smooth muscle cell proliferation.

Ross[12] has recently added more facts to his original model. Monocytes, effector cells of the immune system, attach between endothelial cells and localize in the subendothelial spaces where they become foam cells, or macrophages, and form fatty streaks. Smooth muscle cells then accumulate under the foam cells. When endothelial cells separate or are sloughed off due to injury, the subendothelium is exposed, and the foam cells are either lost into the circulation or become available for platelet adherence and clumping. This is illustrated in Figure 1–6.

One final aspect of this process that needs to be better defined is the actual mechanism by which the arterial wall is injured. Texon[13] has proposed a hemodynamic basis for arterial wall injury. Applying the laws of fluid mechanics, he has demonstrated that atherosclerosis may be considered the reactive biological response of blood vessels to the effects of the mechanics of fluid flow, namely diminished lateral pressure that creates a suction or pulling effect in certain areas of vessels, e.g., areas of curvature, branching, bifurcation, and tapering. Ross[11] discusses experiments in which both mechanical injury and diet to increase plasma levels of low-density lipoprotein cholesterol (LDL-C) can induce arterial wall injury to initiate the atherosclerotic process. There may well be multiple factors that initiate or contribute to the injury process. At this point it is important to note that not everyone subscribes to the endothelial injury theory. McGill presents a convincing argument challenging this theory.[14]

One of the major breakthroughs in better understanding the entire process of atherosclerosis has come from the Nobel Prize-winning work of Brown and Goldstein.[15] Recognizing that high levels of LDL-C in the blood are associated with an increased risk for CAD, they found that LDL-C levels are controlled by receptors on cells that are highly specific for LDL-C. When the LDL-C receptor number per cell is high, LDL-C levels remain low. As the LDL-C receptor number decreases, LDL-C levels increase and the

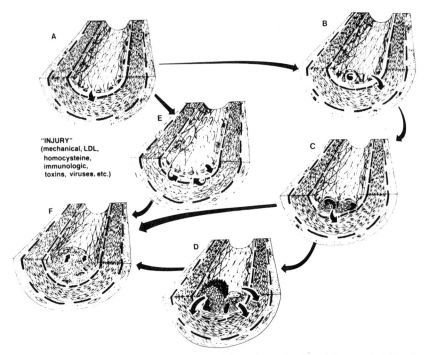

Figure 1–6. The revised response-to-injury hypothesis. Advanced intimal proliferative lesions of atherosclerosis may occur by at least two pathways. The pathway demonstrated by the clockwise (long) arrows to the right has been observed in experimentally induced hypercholesterolemia. Injury to the endothelium (A) may induce growth factor secretion (short arrow). Monocytes attach to the endothelium (B), which may continue to secrete growth factors (short arrow). Subendothelial migration of monocytes (C) may lead to fatty-streak formation and release of growth factors such as platelet-derived growth factor (PDGF) (short arrow). Fatty streaks may become directly converted to fibrous plaques (long arrow from C to F) through release of growth factors from macrophages or endothelial cells or both. Macrophages may also stimulate or injure the overlying endothelium. In some cases, macrophages may lose their endothelial cover, and platelet attachment may occur (D), providing three possible sources of growth factors—platelets, macrophages, and the endothelium (short arrows). Some of the smooth-muscle cells in the proliferative lesion itself (F) may form and secrete factors such as PDGF (short arrows).

An alternative pathway for development of advanced lesions of atherosclerosis is shown by the arrows from A to E to F. In this case, the endothelium may be injured but remains intact. Increased endothelial turnover may result in growth-factor formation by endothelial cells (A). This may stimulate migration of smooth-muscle cells from the media into the intima, accompanied by endogenous production of PDGF by smooth muscle as well as growth factor secretion from the "injured" endothelial cells (E). These interactions could then lead to fibrous plaque formation and further lesion progression (F). (From Ross, R.: The pathogenesis of atherosclerosis—an update. **N. Engl. J. Med.** 314:488–500, 1986.)

atherosclerotic process is accelerated. A high-fat diet or a diet high in cholesterol leads to a reduction in LDL-C receptor number.

As was discussed earlier in this section on the pathophysiology of atherosclerosis, the disease process begins at an early age. The actual pathological changes begin in infancy and progress during childhood.[9] This is confirmed in the work of Enos and associates,[16] who demonstrated that 70 percent of autopsied American soldiers killed in Korean War combat, with an average age of 22.1 years, already had at least moderately advanced coronary atherosclerosis. Korean soldiers killed in combat did not demonstrate early signs of coronary atherosclerosis. In a later study, McNamara and colleagues[17] found evidence of atherosclerosis in 45 percent of Vietnam War casualties, with 5 percent demonstrating severe coronary atherosclerosis. Mason[18] and Rigal and associates[19] reported similar findings in groups of young men. It is important to recognize the early onset of this disease, for prevention is preferable to rehabilitation and must be initiated at an early age. Later in this chapter, it becomes evident that risk factors associated with the premature development of CAD are already present in children.

Hypertension

The pathophysiology of hypertension is not nearly as well defined. In fact, Kaplan[20] has stated that the overwhelming majority of all hypertensive cases are idiopathic, i.e., of unknown origin. In a randomly chosen group of 689 hypertensive men between 47 and 54 years of age in Göteborg, Sweden, the disease was found to be idiopathic in nearly 95 percent of the cases. Secondary causes of hypertension were chronic renal disease (4%), renovascular disease (1%), coarctation of the aorta (0.1%), and primary aldosteronism (0.1%).[21] Idiopathic hypertension, sometimes referred to as essential hypertension, may be the result of genetic factors, high levels of sodium in the diet, obesity, physical inactivity, psychological stress, a combination of these factors, or other factors yet to be substantiated or determined.

CORONARY ARTERY DISEASE AND HYPERTENSION: AN EPIDEMIOLOGIC APPROACH

While the pathophysiology of CAD and hypertension has been studied by direct experimental research and autopsy studies, another branch of medicine has been actively investigating the disease through observation of large population samples. Epidemiology is that branch of medicine that studies the relationships of various factors that determine frequencies and distributions of a disease. With respect to CAD and hypertension, epidemiology has attempted to identify those factors that are *associated* with the disease. These identified factors, when present, place that particular individual at an increased risk for the premature or early development and subsequent manifestation of the disease.

Epidemiological studies can be either *retrospective*, i.e., looking back on data previously collected to observe relationships, or *prospective*, i.e., planned well in advance of the period of data collection with well-defined objectives and a comprehensive experimental design. The Framingham Study exemplifies the prospective epidemiological approach to the study of CAD.

In 1948, the United States Public Health Service began to initiate plans for a major prospective epidemiological study of cardiovascular disease, with the focus on atherosclerosis and hypertension. Framingham, Massachusetts, a small community 21 miles west of Boston, was selected for this monumental study. Framingham had also been selected in the first community study of tuberculosis in 1917. After several years of preparing the community and the staff for such a major undertaking, the study was begun in 1952. From the age group of 30 to 59 years, 6,600 individuals were randomly selected from a potential population of approximately 10,000, of which 5,209 were actually enrolled in the study. It was anticipated that this would yield approximately 2,150 new cases of cardiovascular disease by the end of the 20th year of the study. Periodically, those who were selected and who elected to participate in the study were given extensive medical examinations, and their medical histories were recorded. This study has become one of the most productive of its kind in the history of medicine. As individuals developed cardiovascular disease, it was possible to group those individuals by disease and determine what factors they shared in common. These became recognized as CAD and hypertensive disease risk factors.

At the present, CAD risk factors are classified into two categories, primary risk factors and secondary, or contributing, risk factors. The primary risk factors are those that have been shown without question to be implicated in the genesis of atherosclerosis. The secondary risk factors are not necessarily of any lesser importance but may simply need additional research support to elevate them to the level of being primary factors. To date, hypertension, cigarette smoking, and elevated blood cholesterol levels have been identified as the primary risk factors for CAD. Secondary risk factors include those that can be controlled or altered, i.e., emotional stress, obesity, diabetes, and physical inactivity. Unalterable contributing risk factors include age, sex, and family history.[1] These risk factors are summarized in Table 1–1. Since hypertension can be diagnosed rather simply with multiple blood pressure determinations, little attention has been given to the concept of risk factors for hypertensive disease. However, overweight and diet, particularly a diet high in sodium intake, appear to be the major factors, but age, race, and family history are also important.

Primary Risk Factors

According to the United States National Health and Nutrition Examination Survey (NHANES I) of 1971 to 1974, 18 percent of the adult population in the United States were hypertensive.[22] Data from 1976 to 1980, reported in NHANES II, estimated that 39 percent and 38 percent of the black female and male populations, respectively, are hypertensive compared with 25 percent and 33 percent of the white female and male adult populations.[1] Although hypertension can be identified by blood pressure screening, it is important to recognize that multiple determinations of blood pressure should be taken and that care should be used in the selection of the proper blood pressure cuff. Frequently, individuals are misdiagnosed as hypertensive on the basis of only a single blood pressure measurement or the selection of a cuff that is too short or too narrow for that particular individual.[23] This is discussed in further detail in Chapter 6.

Hypertension has become one of the most powerful predictors of CAD, and the risk increases markedly when hypertension is coupled with other risk factors. Studies have demonstrated the following:

- The risk of premature cardiovascular disease and death rises

Table 1–1. Coronary Heart Disease Risk Factors

Primary Risk Factors	Secondary Risk Factors
Alterable	*Alterable*
Hypertension	Diabetes
Blood Lipids	Stress
Elevated LDL-C	Physical Inactivity
Elevated Triglycerides	Obesity
Decreased HDL-C	*Unalterable*
Smoking	Age
	Male Gender
	Heredity

sharply with increased resting levels of systolic or diastolic blood pressure (Fig. 1–7).[24]

- Even within the "statistically normal" level of blood pressure, there are a greater number of heart attacks and strokes among the so-called high normal than in persons with lower blood pressure readings.
- There are indications that the incidence of strokes and heart failure can be reduced in groups of patients whose high blood pressure is lowered by medication.[25]

Cigarette smoking is undoubtedly the single most important health hazard in the United States today. The total mortality rate from all causes combined is nearly twice as high in heavy smokers as in nonsmokers. Of this excess mortality, 19 percent is due to lung cancer and 37 percent to CAD. Cardiovascular mortality rate is also doubled in heavy smokers compared with nonsmokers. The Surgeon General's report on smoking and health, issued in 1964, addressed the issue of cigarette smoking, disease, and death. This report contributed to a general reduction in the prevalence of cigarette smokers in the total population. Subsequent statements issued by the Surgeon General have had considerable impact on reducing the number of smokers in the United States. For example,

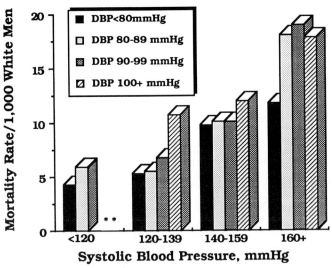

Figure 1–7. Increased risk for coronary artery disease with increased levels of blood pressure. DBP = diastolic blood pressure. (Data from Rutan, G.H., et al.: Mortality associated with diastolic hypertension and isolated systolic hypertension among men screened for the Multiple Risk Factor Intervention Trial. **Circulation** 77:504–514, 1988.)

the prevalence of cigarette smokers among adult men declined from 51 percent in 1965 to 34 percent in 1982.[26] However, during that same period the overall percentage of adult female smokers has decreased only slightly from 33 percent in 1965 to 29 percent in 1982.

The research literature concerning smoking and increased risk for CAD is quite clear (Fig. 1–8). The evidence includes the following:

- The risk and frequency of heart attacks are greater in persons who smoke, and increase according to the number of cigarettes smoked.[27]
- The rate of heart attacks is lower among those who have given up smoking as compared with current smokers.[27]
- Mechanisms have been identified linking the components of tobacco smoking with arterial damage and the subsequent development of arteriosclerosis.[28, 29]

Of recent concern has been the effect of tobacco smoke on the nonsmoker. The passive or involuntary smoker is one who is exposed to the smoke of others. An excellent study by White and Froeb[30] concluded that chronic exposure to tobacco smoke in the workplace is deleterious to the nonsmoker and significantly reduces

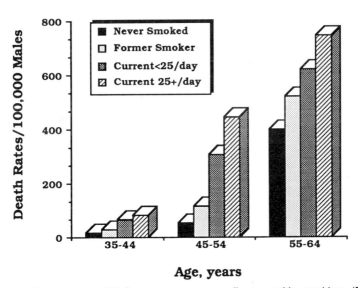

Age, years

Figure 1–8. Increased risk for coronary artery disease with smoking. (Data from Mattson, M.E., Pollack, E.S., and Cullen, J.W.: What are the odds that smoking will kill you? **Am. J. Publ. Health** 77:425–431, 1987.)

small-airways function. Spirometry tests showed the passive smoker to have the same profile as smokers who do not inhale or light smokers. Matsukura and associates[31] reported that cotinine, the major metabolite of nicotine found in the urine, was elevated in nonsmokers who lived or worked with others who smoked, and that the cotinine levels were directly proportional to the extent of exposure to tobacco smoke. More recent studies have now demonstrated that passive smoking does increase the nonsmoker's risk of death and heart disease.[32, 33]

Increased levels of blood cholesterol have been linked with a substantial increase in risk for CAD, particularly for those under the age of 50 years.[34] For a number of years, it was recognized that CAD is low in populations that subsist on low-fat, low-cholesterol diets or diets that are low in saturated fats and is high in populations consuming high saturated fat or high-cholesterol diets.[8] However, it is now acknowledged that the relationship of cholesterol to CAD is not simple, but very complex. Lipids, being insoluble in the blood plasma, must be packaged or combined with protein molecules. This combination of lipid with protein is termed a lipoprotein. Lipoprotein molecules are of different sizes and densities but are generally classified into one of four major categories: chylomicrons, very low-density lipoproteins (VLDL), low-density lipoproteins (LDL), and high-density lipoproteins (HDL). Figure 1–9 illustrates the relationship between the various lipoprotein carriers as cholesterol and triglycerides are transported throughout the body. High-density lipoprotein cholesterol (HDL-C) contains the highest proportion of protein and carries approximately 20 percent of the plasma cholesterol; it is thought to be responsible for carrying cholesterol away from the arterial wall back to the liver, where it is metabolized and excreted. High levels of HDL-C have been associated with a low risk for CAD, which would be expected on the basis of its proposed function. On the other hand, LDL-C is associated with a high risk for CAD when present in high concentrations.[35] Low-density lipoprotein is responsible for transporting approximately 65 percent of the plasma cholesterol. Monkeys subjected to a diet high in cholesterol leading to increased LDL-C levels have been shown to develop atherosclerosis within a period of 2 years.[11]

The Framingham Study and other epidemiological studies have presented rather convincing evidence that both elevated total cholesterol and LDL-C levels place the individual at increased risk for CAD.[36] Conversely, these studies and others have shown that elevated levels of HDL-C provide some degree of protection from CAD.[36] The relationship of both total cholesterol and HDL-C to

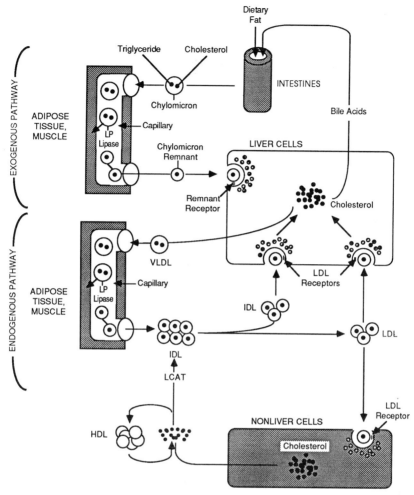

Figure 1–9. The exogenous and endogenous pathways for the transport of fat. Dietary cholesterol is absorbed through the wall of the intestine and is transported, along with triglycerides, in chylomicrons. In the capillaries of both fat and muscle, the lipoprotein (LP) lipase cleaves the triglyceride molecule, and fatty acids are removed. The chylomicron remnant, which is cholesterol rich, goes to the liver, where it binds to special receptors, and is taken up by the liver. Cholesterol is then either secreted into the intestine as bile acids, or is repackaged with triglycerides in very low-density lipoprotein (VLDL) particles and secreted into the circulation. As the VLDL particles pass through the adipose and muscle tissue, LP lipase again removes the triglycerides, leaving a cholesterol-rich intermediate density lipoprotein (IDL). IDL either binds to the liver, where it is taken up, or it remains in the circulation, where it is converted to low-density lipoprotein (LDL). Cholesterol that leaches from cells binds to high-density lipoprotein (HDL) and is esterified by the enzyme LCAT. HDL esters are transferred to IDL and then LDL and are eventually taken up by cells. (Adapted from Brown, M.S., and Goldstein, J.L.: How LDL receptors influence cholesterol and atherosclerosis. **Sci. Amer.** 251:58–66, 1984.)

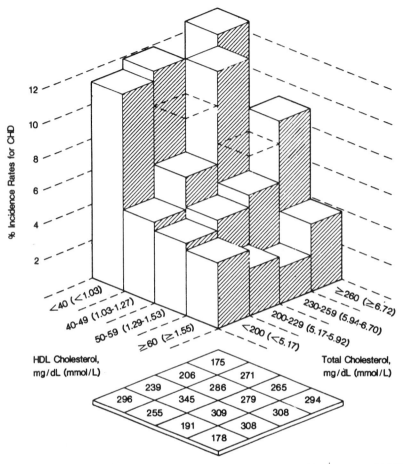

Figure 1–10. Increased risk for coronary artery disease with decreased HDL cholesterol and increased total cholesterol. (From Castelli, W.P., et al.: Incidence of coronary heart disease and lipoprotein cholesterol levels. **JAMA** 256:2835–2838, 1986.)

CAD is illustrated in Figure 1–10. Recently, clinicians have expressed HDL-C relative to total cholesterol, i.e., total cholesterol/ HDL-C, with a ratio of 5.0 or higher indicating high risk and a ratio of 3.5 or lower indicating low risk for CAD (see Table 6–1, Chapter 6).

An additional factor should be noted. The only way to produce atherosclerosis in animals is to feed them diets high in cholesterol. Also, cholesterol is predominant in the atherosclerotic plaques. Reducing cholesterol in the diet has led to a reduction in the degree of atherosclerosis in animals and reduces the risk of death from CAD in human populations.[37] In 1984, the Lipid Research Clinics'

Coronary Primary Prevention Trial results were announced. They found that the lowering of plasma cholesterol levels with bile acid sequestrants reduced the frequency of several manifestations of CAD, including myocardial infarction.[38]

Secondary, or Contributing, Risk Factors

With respect to the unalterable risk factors, it is obvious that the older the individual, the greater the risk of death from CAD.[40] Race also appears to be a distinct factor. With respect to hypertension, the black population is at substantially greater risk than the white population, although this is not the case with CAD.[41] Family history, or the genetic component, is much more difficult to quantify. It is nearly impossible to divorce the influence of environment from family history. A family typically eats together, is exposed to similar stresses in the home, and shares many common experiences that may either increase or decrease the risk for CAD. Still, it is fairly clear that if CAD manifests itself at an early age in one or two close relatives, the individual is placed in an elevated risk category. Investigators are now attempting to determine if this increase in risk associated with family history is an independent risk factor or if the increase in risk is due to the other risk factors that are heavily influenced by genetic factors.[42–45]

Finally, men appear to be at a substantially increased risk compared with women.[46] The gap tends to diminish during the later years coincident with the attainment of menopause. It was at one time thought that hormonal differences were the major cause of the reduced risk for women. Studies investigating this possibility showed just the opposite of what was expected. Men given female hormones were actually found to have an increased risk for CAD.[8] Thus, this difference in rates of CAD between men and premenopausal women has yet to be adequately explained.

With respect to the alterable secondary risk factors, obesity is one risk factor that has been quite controversial. Keys and associates[47] investigated the relationship of relative weight and of skinfold thickness to the 5-year incidence of CAD in men 40 through 59 years of age. When the other risk factors were disregarded, an excessive incidence of CAD was associated with overweight and obesity. However, when the influence of the other risk factors was factored out, overweight and obesity were found to be unrelated to future CAD. Gordon and Kannel,[48] however, reporting data from the Framingham Study, demonstrated that a higher relative weight was associated with an increased risk for CAD. At 35 percent above ideal weight, the odds of CAD were 1.6 and 1.4 times greater for men and women, respectively, compared with those who were at their ideal weight. More recent data from Framingham over a longer period of follow-up indicate that without question overweight or obesity is a distinct risk factor, independent of the other risk factors for both men and women. Also, weight gain after age 25 years resulted in increased risk of CAD in both sexes, independent of initial weight or other risk factors.[49] The relationship between overweight and CAD is shown in Figure 1–11. Also of concern is the change in weight one experiences with age. Figure 1–12 illustrates from the same Framingham data that weight gain with age is also a risk factor for CAD.

Diabetes has been moved from the list of secondary risk factors to the list of primary risk factors and then back again.[1] It is now recognized that diabetes doubles the risk for cardiovascular mortality, and the risk is substantially greater in women.[39] Unfortunately, the pathogenesis of CAD in the diabetic is not well understood, but there does appear to be something unique about the diabetic that accelerates the atherosclerotic process.

Emotional stress has been suggested as a possible risk factor for CAD. This would appear obvious, but the relationship is not so simple. As an example, corporate executives have a relatively low

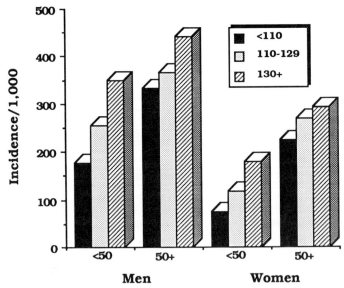

Figure 1–11. Role of being overweight in increasing risk for coronary artery disease. (Data from Hubert, H.A., et al.: Obesity as an independent risk factor for cardiovascular disease. A 26-year follow-up of participants in the Framingham heart study. **Circulation** 67:968–977, 1983.)

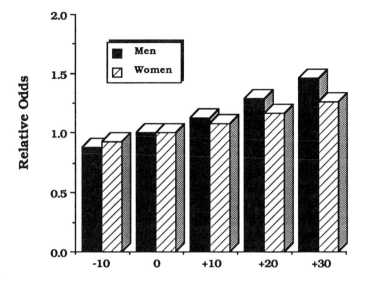

Unit Change in Metropolitan Relative Weight, %

Figure 1–12. Role of the change in relative weight in increasing the risk for coronary artery disease. (Data from Hubert, H.A., et al.: Obesity as an independent risk factor for cardiovascular disease. A 26-year follow-up of participants in the Framingham heart study. **Circulation** 67:968–977, 1983.)

incidence of CAD, whereas those who are on their way up the ladder have a relatively high incidence. Also, the prevalence of CAD decreased considerably in those individuals who were held prisoner in German World War II concentration camps, yet the stress levels had to be very high.

Another area that has received considerable attention over the past 10 years is the coronary-prone behavior pattern. Pioneered by Friedman and Rosenman,[50] the coronary-prone behavior pattern is characterized by excesses of aggression, hurrying, and competition; such individuals are often deeply committed to their vocation or profession to the exclusion of other aspects of their lives and have a sense of restlessness and guilt during leisure hours or periods of relaxation. Although there is a growing body of research to support the concept of the coronary-prone behavior pattern, or the Type-A behavior,[51] the concept is not without its critics.[52] Alteration of Type-A behavior in patients who have had myocardial infarction has been shown to reduce the risk of subsequent nonfatal myocardial infarction.[53] Some feel that to try to classify all individuals into either a coronary-prone (Type-A) or non–coronary-prone (Type-B) behavior pattern is a great oversimplification. More recent research is demonstrating that the anger and hostility characteristics may account for the increased risk for CAD associated with the more global Type-A behavior pattern.[54] The inhibited expression of hostility and anger may represent the toxic component of the Type-A pattern.[55]

Physical inactivity as a risk factor for CAD is discussed in considerable detail in the following section. Other factors have been proposed as risk factors, with little or no supporting evidence. At one time, coffee drinking was considered to be a risk factor, but subsequent studies were unable to confirm this.[8] Soft water has also been proposed as a risk factor, but the evidence is not conclusive.[8]

As was mentioned earlier in this chapter, risk factors for CAD are already present in children. In two studies conducted by Wilmore and his associates, it has been clearly demonstrated that between 8 and 12 years of age and between 13 and 15 years of age, a significant percentage of normal, randomly selected male children demonstrate risk factors for CAD.[56, 57] These are illustrated in Table 1–2. Gilliam and his colleagues,[58] Lauer and his colleagues with the Muscatine Study,[59] and Berenson and his colleagues with the Bogalusa Heart Study[60] have likewise found risk factors to be present in children at relatively early ages. Importantly, there appears to be a reasonable degree of tracking of at least lipoproteins[61] and blood pressure[62] as these children age, i.e., those with "at risk" values remain at risk as they age. Further, the Bogalusa Heart Study has demonstrated a relationship between early atherosclerotic lesions in the aorta and coronary arteries in young people at autopsy, who had been a part of this study before death, and serum lipoprotein levels and systolic blood pressure measurements taken before death.[63]

PHYSICAL ACTIVITY, CORONARY ARTERY DISEASE, AND HYPERTENSION

It is extremely difficult to ascertain directly the role of physical activity in the prevention of CAD and hypertension. The ideal study would necessitate a large population of infants randomly assigned to either a sedentary or an active lifestyle. After 60 years or more of close and detailed observation, accurate conclusions could, ideally, be drawn. Obviously, such a study will never be conducted. Thus, to gain some insight into the basic relationship between physical activity, CAD, and hypertension, it has become necessary to accept indirect lines of inquiry into this problem.

Table 1–2. Coronary Heart Disease Risk Factor Prevalence in Boys,
8 through 15 Years of Age

Risk Factor	8- to 12-Year-Olds (n = 96) (Percent)	13- to 15-Year-Olds (n = 308) (Percent)
Blood Lipids		
Total Cholesterol	20.0	11.0
≥ 200 mg/100 ml		
HDL-C	—	14.6
≤ 36 mg/100 ml		
Triglycerides	8.4	25.0
≥ 100 mg/100 ml		
Blood Pressure		
Systolic	0.0	13.0
> 90th percentile		
Diastolic	0.0	4.9
> 90th percentile		
Smoking	0.0	0.0
≥ 10 cigarettes/day		
Diabetic	0.0	1.3
Abnormal ECG	4.5	6.5
Relative Body Fat	12.6	14.9
≥ 25% fat		
Maximum Oxygen Uptake	3.2	18.8
≤ 42 ml • kg $^{-1}$ • min $^{-1}$		
Family History	33.7	30.9
MI ≤ 60 years of age		
Presence of Risk Factors		
None	36.0	29.9
One	46.0	35.4
Two	14.0	22.1
Three	3.0	10.7
Four	1.0	1.9

Several indirect approaches have been used. First, epidemiologists have investigated the prevalence of CAD in active versus inactive populations, predominantly using occupation or leisure time as the index of activity level. Second, epidemiologists have compared the prevalence of CAD in former athletes versus that in nonathletes. Third, researchers have observed the influence of physical training, usually of a cardiorespiratory endurance nature, on the reduction of certain CAD risk factors. Fourth, researchers have attempted to use animal models to investigate physical activity, CAD, and hypertension. Last, several studies have attempted to determine the influence of physical activity on the long-term outlook of those patients who have documented CAD, i.e., angina pectoris, myocardial infarction, and coronary artery bypass surgery. Each of these five areas is discussed separately to determine if a consistent pattern emerges across all lines of evidence.

Epidemiological Studies

ACTIVE VERSUS SEDENTARY POPULATIONS

A number of studies have been published in which the prevalence of CAD has been compared between active and sedentary populations. The first of these, conducted by Morris and associates[64] and published in 1953, compared "sedentary" bus drivers with "active" conductors who worked on double-decked buses for the London Transport Executive. They found the more physically active conductors to have a 30 percent lesser occurrence of all manifestations of CAD and 50 percent fewer myocardial infarctions. Mortality from CAD was less than half as frequent in the conductors. A similar finding was reported by the same investigators in a companion study of postal workers, comparing active mail carriers with less active postal service clerks.[64] Interestingly, and difficult to explain, the more active populations in these studies, i.e., the conductors and the mail carriers, had approximately twice the frequency of angina pectoris.

Morris and his associates followed their initial publication with a 1956 report entitled "Physique of London Busmen: The Epidemiology of Uniforms." [65] For any given height, the drivers, upon entry into the Transport Executive, were fitted with trousers that had at least a 1-inch greater waist circumference than those of the conductors, and the drivers had higher serum cholesterol and blood pressure levels.[66] Because the groups were already different upon entry into the Transport Executive, it is difficult to determine if the greater physical activity of the conductors helped lower their CAD risk or if the conductors were simply different, even before entry into the Transport Executive.

These initial studies by Morris and his colleagues led to a number of similar studies, most confirming their early work. These studies were summarized in 1986 in a comprehensive review by Shephard.[67] With only several exceptions, most of these observational studies showed a lower age-specific rate of CAD in the more active groups. The disease, when present, was found to be less severe in the more active groups, and the mortality rate was also lower. In most cases, there was approximately a two- to threefold greater risk associated with a sedentary lifestyle.

These earlier studies suggested several interesting points. First, it does not appear to require considerable amounts or high intensities of exercise in order to achieve some degree of protection from CAD. Second, the protection gained from an active lifestyle appears to be transient, unless the activity is a lifelong pursuit.

The results from several studies dealing with these specific issues is briefly reviewed.

Zukel and coworkers[68] demonstrated a significant relationship between the incidence of CAD and hours of heavy labor. Their data revealed that people who engaged in from one to two hours of heavy physical labor per day had less than one fifth the incidence of coronary events as those whose life pattern included no heavy work. Unfortunately, these data did not permit an analysis for heavy work of less than one hour per day. Frank and associates,[69] in their report of the large (55,000 men) study of the Health Insurance Program of urban New York, found that the main difference in the incidence of heart attack deaths occurred between the least active and the moderately active groups. The few extra blocks of walking, extra stair climbing, and other activities of the moderately active group appeared to help protect them from heart attack deaths, which suggests potential benefits for "useful" increased activity without a great change in lifestyle.

It has been proposed by Bassler that the marathon runner's lifestyle is necessary to provide immunity from CAD.[70] However, only a relatively small percentage of the population of the United States could rise to the level of commitment necessary to complete a 26.2-mile race. Further, this theory has not been substantiated and, in fact, has been refuted.[71] Skinner and colleagues[72] have calculated that daily caloric expenditure increases of only 400 to 500 kcal above the normal sedentary level were associated with a significantly lower prevalence of CAD in the multiracial communities of Evans County, Georgia. Rose[73] reported that just walking 20 minutes or more to work was associated with a one-third lower incidence of ischemic-type electrocardiographic abnormalities.

Most recently, LaPorte and his colleagues[74] have raised the question as to whether distinctions should be made between those activity levels needed to increase "physical fitness" versus those necessary to provide protection from CAD. They believe that it is quite possible, even probable, that the intensity of activity to provide the health-related benefits of exercise does not have to be of that intensity necessary to obtain gains in physical fitness. This is an interesting concept that has some support from the epidemiologic research literature. However, the concept has not been directly tested.

The benefits of an active lifestyle appear to be related to lifetime activity levels. Brown and associates[75] found the manifestations of coronary disease in men over 65 years of age to be fewer among those whose lifetime activity patterns placed them in a relatively more active group as compared with their more sedentary colleagues. With respect to the transient nature of the protection afforded by an active lifestyle, Kahn's review of postal workers in Washington, D.C., suggests that the difference in the incidence of CAD became indistinguishable within 5 years after an individual left the physically more active occupational status.[76] Thus, it appears that the potential benefits from physical activity cannot be stored, to be drawn from throughout the remainder of one's life. Rather, exercise habits should be continued regularly if the benefits are to be retained.

Almost all of the early studies concentrated on defining a physically active or sedentary group solely on the basis of occupation. However, it is important to recognize that many very active individuals are employed in sedentary jobs. For example, from mid-1970 to the present, thousands of individuals have been attracted to participate in marathon races. However, by occupation, most of these individuals would have to be classified as sedentary. Recognizing this inherent weakness of previous study designs and realizing that work in advanced societies is increasingly light and sedentary, Morris and coworkers[77] attempted to study leisure-time activity and the incidence of CAD in a group of executive-grade civil servants, thus holding occupation constant. They studied the leisure activity patterns of 16,882 men over a Friday and Saturday, between the years 1968 and 1970. In their first follow-up report of 1973,[77] they found that men who had reported vigorous exercise during this 2-day period had a relative risk of developing CAD that was approximately 33 percent of that in comparable men who did not record vigorous exercise. In a more recent follow-up, Morris and coworkers[78] reported that they had observed 1,138 first clinical episodes of CAD in their original sample. They concluded that men who engaged in vigorous sports and kept fit in the initial survey in 1968 to 1970 had an incidence of CAD in the next 8½ years that was somewhat less than half that of their colleagues who recorded no vigorous exercise. They concluded that "the generality of the advantage suggests that vigorous exercise is a natural defense of the body, with a protective effect on the aging heart against ischemia and its consequences."

Holme and colleagues[79] studied the association between physical activity at work and leisure, coronary risk factors, social class, and mortality in approximately 15,000 Oslo men, 40 to 49 years of age. The 4-year total mortality rate and CAD mortality rate showed a decrease in risk with an increasing degree of *leisure* activity but an increase in risk with an increasing *work* activity. There was no immediate explanation for this apparent paradox.

Paffenbarger and his associates have studied San Francisco

Bay area longshoremen and Harvard and University of Pennsylvania alumni in a series of studies considered to be among the most definitive in the literature. In 1977, they reported on a 22-year follow-up of 3,686 San Francisco longshoremen.[80] They found that higher energy output on the job reduced the risk of fatal heart attack, especially sudden death, in the two younger age groups, with the less active workers at a threefold increased risk. They estimated that combined low-energy output, heavy smoking, and high blood pressure increased risk by as much as 20 times. Most important, they indicated that by the elimination of these three adverse influences, the population under study might have had an 88 percent reduction in its rate of fatal heart attack during the 22 years. In their study of 16,936 Harvard male alumni, 35 to 74 years of age, Paffenbarger and colleagues[81] reported that men with an index above 2,000 kcal per week of physical activity were at 39 percent lower risk for developing CAD than their less active classmates. Exercise remained a significant risk factor even when other risk factors were controlled statistically (Fig. 1–13).[82] There were, however, no differences in sudden death. With respect to mortality from all causes, Paffenbarger and associates[83] concluded that this level of activity, compared with a sedentary lifestyle, by the age of 80 years would result in an additional one to two years, or more, of life.

Powell and his colleagues at the Centers for Disease Control in Atlanta have conducted an extensive analysis of the research literature to identify all of those studies that have investigated the relationship between physical inactivity and CAD.[84] A total of 43 studies were selected for an in-depth analysis on the basis of strict selection criteria. They concluded that the observations reported in the literature support the inference that physical activity is inversely and causally related to the incidence of CAD. In a published comment on this research,[85] it was stated that physical inactivity is a far more important risk factor than elevated serum cholesterol, smoking, and hypertension, the three major risk factors. This statement was based on the fact that the strength of physical inactivity's association with CAD is equal to that of the three major risk factors and on the fact that there are far more people who are physically inactive than those who smoke, have elevated cholesterol levels, or have high blood pressure. These relationships are illustrated in Table 1–3 and Figure 1–14.

FORMER ATHLETES VERSUS NONATHLETES

Numerous studies have observed differences in life expectancy between former athletes and nonathletes. These studies have been

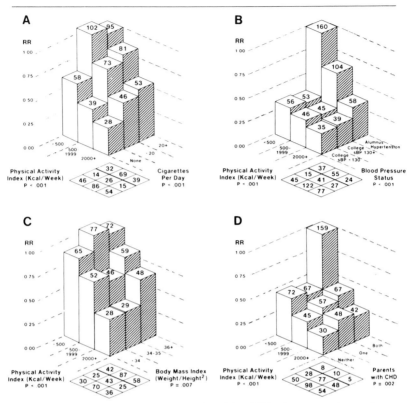

Figure 1–13. Incidence rates and relative risks (RR) of coronary heart disease (CHD) by cross-tabulations of physical activity index and *(A)* cigarette smoking habits, *(B)* student or alumnus blood pressure status, *(C)* body mass index, and *(D)* history of parental CHD. Numbers atop bars represent incidence rates per 10,000 man-years of observation. Rates in back corner bars establish the RR of 1.00. Significance probabilities are based on trends of incidence rates adjusted for differences in age and the paired characteristic. Numbers of CHD cases are given in the corresponding diamond key below each figure. (Data from Paffenbarger, R.S., et al.: Physical activity, other life-style patterns, cardiovascular disease and longevity. **Acta Med. Scand.** (Suppl)711:85–91, 1986.)

Table 1–3. Physical Inactivity and Coronary Heart Disease

CHD Risk Factor	Relative Risk
Smoking ($\geq$ 1 pack/day vs. none)	2.5
Cholesterol ($\geq$ 268 vs. $\leq$ 218 mg/dl)	2.4
Hypertension (SBP $\geq$ 150 vs. $\leq$ 130 mmHg)	2.1
Physical Inactivity (sedentary vs. active)	1.9

Protective effect of physical activity on coronary heart disease. *Morbidity and Mortality Weekly Report* Centers for Disease Control U.S. Department of Health and Human Services 36(#26):426–430, 1987.

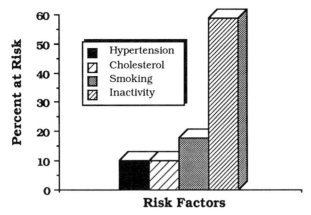

Figure 1–14. U.S. population at risk for physical inactivity compared with the three major risk factors. (Adapted from Caspersen, C.J.: Physical inactivity and coronary heart disease. **Physician Sportsmed.** 15:43–44, 1987.)

adequately summarized by Shephard,[67] Yamaji and Shephard,[86] and by Olson and associates.[87] Generally, little difference has been found between former athletic versus nonathletic populations relative to total mortality as well as to mortality from CAD. Olson and associates have concluded that there is no clear evidence for a long-term protective effect of athletics on health (Fig. 1–15).[87] As Yamaji and Shephard[86] have noted, athletic competition occupies too short a portion of the total life span to have a significant effect on longevity. They believe that the important question may well be *not* which kind of sport was pursued or what was the intensity of activity during the required training, but whether the activity was continued to an advanced age. The data on Harvard graduates support this finding.[81–83] As was stated earlier, the benefits of physical activity are transient and are lost rapidly once the individual assumes a sedentary lifestyle. Whether one was active as a youngster, teenager, or young man or woman probably plays far less a role in disease protection than the present lifestyle of that individual. Optimally, however, an active lifestyle would start early, i.e., during early childhood, and continue through old age.

Physical Activity and Coronary Artery Disease Risk Factors

The specific physiological changes that result from physical training are covered in considerable detail in Section B. However,

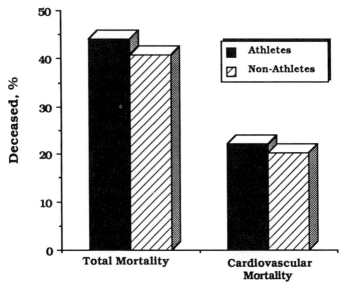

Figure 1–15. Comparison of percentages of deceased athletes and nonathletes. (Data from Olson, H.W., et al.: The longevity and morbidity of college athletes. **Physician Sportsmed.** 6:62–65, 1978.)

because of the importance of many of these changes to the CAD risk profile of the individual, several of the more important studies are discussed. These studies fall into one of two major categories: cross-sectional or longitudinal. In cross-sectional studies, a large number of individuals are usually observed only once, and comparisons are made between those considered to be physically fit and those considered to be unfit. Fitness is typically determined on the basis of the individual's actual or predicted maximal oxygen uptake ($\dot{V}O_2$max). In longitudinal studies, individuals are assessed initially, placed on a physical training program for a certain interval, and then reevaluated at the conclusion of the training period. For a number of reasons, longitudinal studies are to be preferred. However, they are expensive and usually involve small numbers of subjects. With cross-sectional studies, large numbers of individuals can be observed in a relatively short period.

Cooper and associates[88] observed the relationship between physical fitness, as determined by the length of time the subject could remain on the treadmill using the Balke protocol, and various CAD risk factors. They reported a consistent inverse relationship between physical fitness and resting heart rate; body weight; percent body fat; serum levels of cholesterol, triglycerides, and glucose; and systolic blood pressure. They interpreted their results to imply that higher levels of fitness are related to a lower coronary risk profile. This study was cross-sectional in nature, with approximately 3,000 men constituting the data base, numbers that would have been clearly impossible to obtain with a longitudinal format. Similar findings have been shown with more than 3,900 adult women.[89]

With respect to the major risk factors, numerous studies have been conducted. Cardiorespiratory endurance training is known to have a rather profound influence on plasma lipids and lipoproteins. Athletes who participate in cardiorespiratory endurance sports such as cross-country skiing and long-distance running have a very characteristic plasma lipid and lipoprotein pattern. Further, endurance training of nonathletes leads to the same characteristic profile. In 1979, Wood and Haskell published a comprehensive review addressing the issue of lipid and lipoprotein alterations with endurance activity.[90] This was updated by reviews by Dufaux and coworkers[91] and Haskell.[92]

Both cross-sectional studies of endurance-trained individuals and longitudinal studies of individuals before and after an extended period of endurance training suggest that endurance training results in modest reductions in total cholesterol and VLDL-C, relatively small reductions in LDL-C, and relatively large increases in HDL-C. In addition, plasma triglyceride concentrations are typically reduced. The ratio of total cholesterol to HDL-C is reduced considerably, an alteration that is associated with a reduction in risk for CAD.[90, 93]

Although these represent impressive alterations in lipid and lipoprotein profiles and present a solid link between endurance activity and reduced risk for CAD, the data must be interpreted cautiously. First, not all studies have been able to demonstrate these changes. Second, it is not clear whether these changes are directly the result of the exercise or the physiological concomitants of an active lifestyle. Leanness, or reduction in body fat, has been suggested as a potential mechanism leading to these alterations in plasma lipids and lipoproteins. Third, a certain minimal training threshold may be necessary for changes to occur. Williams and colleagues[94] have shown that running approximately 10 miles a week may be a minimum threshold at which to expect changes in HDL-C.

Hypertension, the second of the three major risk factors, also appears to respond positively to chronic physical activity of an endurance nature. Much of the early work in this area was confounded by the use of subjects with normal blood pressure. Endurance training of individuals with normal blood pressure failed to reduce that pressure to lower, or subnormal, levels. In retrospect, a reduction in pressure below normal should not have been expected. Endurance training of hypertensive individuals does appear to result in moderate reductions in both systolic and diastolic blood pressure of about 10 mmHg.[95–97] Again, as with the area of blood lipids and lipoproteins, there have been studies that have failed to demonstrate blood pressure reductions in hypertensive patients with endurance exercise. The bulk of evidence, however, appears to favor endurance exercise as an effective intervention for reducing blood pressure, particularly when combined with reductions in total body weight and salt intake. The mechanisms by which chronic endurance training lowers blood pressure are not clear at present, but they could include any one or more of the following: reductions in resting sympathetic tone; decreases in baroreceptor sensitivity; changes in myogenic structures, tone, or relationships; and decreases in resting cardiac output.[95]

With respect to cigarette smoking, the third of the three primary risk factors, exercise, may play a significant role. First, those who adopt an active lifestyle soon find that cigarette smoking is not compatible with their new goals and priorities, and many are able to withdraw from their dependency on tobacco. Second, and somewhat related, several of the more popular smoking control or cessation programs are using endurance activity, e.g., long brisk walks or jogging, as a substitute behavior for smoking. Unfortunately, the literature in this area is not extensive. In one of the few studies conducted, Hill[98] randomly assigned 36 smokers who wished to quit to one of two groups that differed only in their level of physical activity. Both groups participated twice weekly in a standard group counseling smoking cessation program for 5 weeks, and the experimental group also participated twice weekly in an aerobic exercise program. The experimental group was able to achieve a lower smoking behavior score at the termination of the treatment compared with that of the control group. However, the overall results were not all that impressive.

An active lifestyle has also been shown to be important for those predisposed to diabetes as well as for the diabetic patient. Frisch and her colleagues[99] reported that long-term training is associated with a lower risk for the development of diabetes in women 20 to 70 years of age. The role of physical activity in the Type-I, or insulin-dependent, diabetic is not well understood. Activity may have a limited positive effect, but this is relatively minor when seen with the total picture of glycemic or blood sugar control in the Type-I patient.[100, 101] For the Type-II, or late-onset, diabetic, physical activity plays a major role in the treatment plan. Physical training appears to increase insulin sensitivity and decrease insulin release. This results in decreased plasma insulin levels but has little or no effect on glucose tolerance.[100, 102]

Endurance activity is an important component of any weight loss program, for exercise combined with modest reductions in the total number of calories consumed results in substantial decreases in total body fat and prevents the losses in lean body mass that usually accompany weight loss through low-calorie diets.[103, 104] In their comprehensive review, Brownell and Stunkard conclude that physical inactivity is associated with an increased risk for obesity and CAD and that physical activity is an important component of any weight reduction program.[105] Hagan and his colleagues,[106] however, have demonstrated that exercise alone, in the absence of diet, has little effect on body weight and body fat over a period of 12 weeks. The topic of body composition alterations with physical conditioning is extensively reviewed in Chapter 4. With respect to emotional factors, endurance activity appears to have a mediating effect, increasing self-esteem, reducing stress and anxiety, and facilitating recovery from episodes of depression.[107] There are also many changes in cardiorespiratory function resulting from endurance training that would lead to a more favorable CAD risk profile. These are not discussed here, as that is the focus of Chapter 3.

Thus, with respect to CAD risk factors, physical activity of a cardiorespiratory endurance nature does facilitate positive changes in the CAD risk profile, apparently reducing the overall risk for heart attack, stroke, and hypertension. Although there are isolated reports to the contrary,[108] the evidence overwhelmingly supports the prophylactic benefits of chronic endurance activity.

ANIMAL STUDIES

Animal models have become quite popular in the study of many diseases. However, considerable care must be taken when translating results from the animal models to humans. Some results and concepts obtained from animal work are directly transferable to humans, but others need considerable interpretation and possible modification before they are applied to man.

Several excellent review articles[109–112] have summarized the knowledge in this area through the early 1980's. The animal research has demonstrated a number of physiological and morphological alterations with exercise training that would imply a general reduction in risk for CAD. First, numerous animal studies have demonstrated cardiac hypertrophy induced by vigorous endurance exercise. This enlarged heart is typically the result of increases in chamber size, predominantly in the left ventricle, although more recent studies have also demonstrated changes in left ventricular wall thickness. This adaptation is considered important to improved myocardial contractility and increased cardiac work capacity. Within the myocardium, there appears to be a hyperplasia and lengthening of muscle fibers, without fiber thickening. Also, there is consistent evidence that endurance training leads to an increased capillary-to-fiber ratio. When infarction is induced experimentally, there is a decrease in myocardial infarct size in the exercised animal.

Changes in the coronary circulation with chronic endurance exercise have also been demonstrated in animals. Corrosion-cast techniques have been used to determine the size of the coronary arterial tree, and several studies have demonstrated increased coronary tree size and increased luminal cross-sectional area of the main coronary arteries. These alterations would lead to an increased capacity for myocardial blood flow, even in the presence of atherosclerosis of the coronary arteries.

The collateral circulation has also been studied, the theory being that as the major coronary arteries become narrowed as a result of atherosclerosis, chronic endurance exercise would facilitate the development of the coronary collateral circulation. In one of the earliest studies, Eckstein[113] studied the effects of exercise and artificial coronary artery narrowing on coronary collateral flow. He surgically induced a constriction in the circumflex artery of approximately 100 dogs. Various degrees of narrowing were induced, and only dogs that developed abnormal changes in their electrocardiogram were included in the study. The dogs were divided into two groups, one receiving regular exercise on the treadmill and the other remaining sedentary. The study demonstrated that moderate and severe arterial narrowing resulted in collateral flow proportional to the degree of narrowing and that exercise led to even greater collateral flow. More recent studies have confirmed these initial results of Eckstein.[113]

Several animal studies have observed mechanical and metabolic performance changes of the heart with chronic endurance activity. Trained animals demonstrate higher levels of cardiac work and cardiac output. In addition, they have a greater myocardial oxygen uptake at or near maximal capacity and produce less lactate and pyruvate. In short, the heart of the trained animal is a more efficient pump.

Finally, several studies have attempted to induce atherosclerosis in experimental animals through atherogenic diets, observing the effects of chronic endurance exercise on the subsequent arterial narrowing and plaque formation. Although many of the initial studies were equivocal, a classic study by Kramsch and coworkers[114] demonstrated rather remarkable differences between an exercise group and a sedentary control group. They studied the effect of moderate conditioning with treadmill exercise on the development of CAD in monkeys on an atherogenic diet. Although the total serum cholesterol level was the same in the exercising and nonexercising monkeys, the exercise group had significantly higher HDL-C levels and much lower levels of triglycerides, LDL-triglycerides, and VLDL-triglyceride. Ischemic changes in the electrocardiogram and sudden death attributable to CAD were observed only in the nonexercising group. Exercise was associated with substantially reduced overall atherosclerotic involvement, lesion size, and collagen accumulation. It also produced larger hearts and wider coronary arteries (Fig. 1–16), further reducing the degree of luminal narrow-

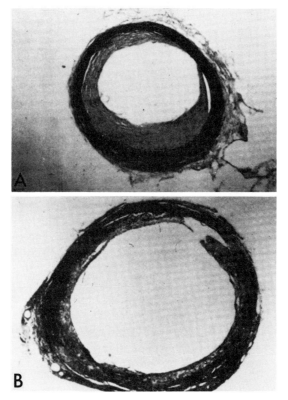

Figure 1–16. Comparison of the left main coronary artery in sedentary *(A)* vs. exercising *(B)* monkeys. (From Kramsch, D.M., et al.: Reduction of coronary atherosclerosis by moderate conditioning exercise in monkeys on an atherogenic diet. **N. Engl. J. Med.** 305:1483–1489, 1981.)

ing. Kramsch and associates concluded that moderate exercise may prevent or retard CAD in primates.

Secondary and Tertiary Prevention: The Role of Physical Activity

Finally, chronic endurance activity has been prescribed for those individuals who are symptomatic for CAD or who have sustained a myocardial infarction, to determine if an active lifestyle will improve their general prognosis. Although this has classically been referred to as secondary prevention, Froelicher and Brown[115] have redefined this terminology. By their new definition, tertiary prevention is now the area that deals with the minimization of disability, morbidity, and mortality once the disease is clinically manifest.

With respect to cardiac morphology, little or no change has been demonstrated in left ventricular mass and volume after 6 months of exercise training. Similarly, coronary angiography has not been able to demonstrate significant changes in atherosclerotic lesions or collateral vessels. However, studies have indicated that certain patients show considerable improvement in left ventricular function and in indices of myocardial blood flow with training, but when these patients are averaged in with those who demonstrate no improvement or who actually have decreased capacity, the positive results are masked.[116, 117]

The work of Ehsani and his colleagues at Washington University (St. Louis, Missouri) deserves special recognition. They have trained patients with coronary artery disease for periods of 12 months and longer. Further, they have taken a relatively aggressive approach to the training of these patients. In one of their studies,[118] they trained 25 patients for a period of 12 months, three times a week for the first 3 months, and five times per week thereafter. They started training these patients 40 to 45 minutes per exercise session for the first 3 months, increasing to 50 to 60 minutes the next 3 months. Exercise intensity was increased from 60 to 70 percent of $\dot{V}O_2$max for the first 3 months to 70 to 90 percent over the next 6 months. The patients averaged 18 miles of running per week during the last 3 months of the study, at an intensity that averaged 89.4 percent of their $\dot{V}O_2$max. $\dot{V}O_2$max increased by 37 percent, and maximal supine ejection fraction increased from 52 to 58 percent. Systolic blood pressure and the rate-pressure product during maximal exercise were higher after training. The systolic blood pressure–end-systolic volume relationship was shifted upward and to the left, with an increase in maximal systolic blood pressure and a smaller end-systolic volume. This suggested an improvement in the contractile state after training. Markers of myocardial ischemia also showed improvement after training, i.e., reduced S-T–segment depression at maximal effort and significantly less angina. No changes were found in a control group. Ehsani has conducted an extensive review of the existing literature and has concluded that high-intensity exercise training is associated with an improvement in left ventricular function, largely independent of cardiac loading conditions, and a reduction in myocardial ischemia that cannot be attributed solely to the lower myocardial oxygen demand in the trained state.[119]

Several studies have attempted to observe morbidity and mortality in CAD patients, comparing those who exercise with those who remain sedentary. Although some of the early studies showed marked differences in both CAD morbidity and mortality favoring the exercising groups, the results must be viewed with caution, because those patients too sick to exercise were often the patients who were assigned to the sedentary control group. In more recent, highly controlled studies, in which all patients included in the study were considered to be fit enough to exercise, the patient population was randomly assigned to either the exercise or sedentary control group. Although the results of these studies have not demonstrated dramatic differences between the exercise and control groups, the trend indicates that a substantial differential in both morbidity and mortality may be evident over a longer period of follow-up and with a larger patient population.[120] Pollock has summarized the nine randomized clinical trials that have evaluated the effect of exercise, or a combination of exercise and other lifestyle modifications, on mortality from CAD.[120] These trials have been summarized in Table 1–4. There are major problems associated with most of these studies; as the number of subjects has been too small to achieve statistical significance, there have been a large number of dropouts, there frequently is an insufficient training stimulus because improved fitness is seldom documented, and the control group oftentimes will start exercising on its own. Thus, pooling data from several studies has provided useful insight into this area. May and coworkers,[121] and more recently Oldridge and coworkers[122] and Kent and Pollock,[123] have pooled the data from these studies and found that there was a significant reduction in mortality from CAD in the exercise intervention groups.

Table 1–4. Mortality Results from Randomized Controlled Trials of Cardiac Rehabilitation after Myocardial Infarction

Trial (yr)	Follow-up (yr)	Control		Rehabilitation		p-Value
		n	*death*	*n*	*death*	
Kentala (1972)	1.0	146	21.9	152	17.1	NS
Wilhemsen (1975)	4.0	157	22.3	158	17.7	NS
Palatsi (1976)	3.2 (C) 3.7 (R)	200	14.0	180	10.0	NS
Kallio (1979)	3.0	187	29.9	188	21.8	SIG
Shaw (1981)	3.0	328	7.3	323	4.6	NS
Vermueulen (1983)	5.0	51	14.5	47	11.6	SIG
Carson (1983)	2.1	152	14.0	151	8.0	NS
Roman (1983)	3.6	100	24.0	93	14.0	NS
Rechnitzer (1983)	4.0	354	7.3	379	9.5	NS

R = rehabilitation group; C = control group; NS = nonsignificant; SIG = significant mortality differences between control and rehabilitation groups.

(From Pollock, M. L.: Benefits of exercise: effect on mortality and physiological function. In Kappagoda, C. T. (ed.): **Long Term Management of Patients After Myocardial Infarction.** Boston, Martinus Nijhoff Publishers, 1988.)

SUMMARY

For more than 30 years, CAD has been the single greatest cause of death in the United States. More than one of every four deaths is the result of CAD. However, death rates for CAD reached their peak during the mid-1960's and have steadily declined since then, for a total reduction that has exceeded 30 percent (Fig. 1–17).[124] The reasons for this decrease are not totally clear, but it does seem evident that an increasing concern for disease prevention and the subsequent modification of unhealthy lifestyles have made a major contribution to this decline. Although a significant portion of this decrease has resulted from better treatment, e.g., pharmacological intervention and coronary artery bypass surgery, treatment is very expensive and represents a substantial portion of total health care costs. Thus, the major thrust for combating CAD must be focused on the area of primary prevention, an area in which exercise must play a significant part.

Does exercise prevent or reduce the risk for CAD? The review presented in this chapter, although not conclusive, provides strong evidence for the importance of exercise. The "Statement on Exer-

Percent Decline from 1968 Rates

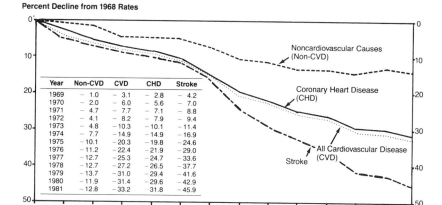

Year	Non-CVD	CVD	CHD	Stroke
1969	- 1.0	- 3.1	- 2.8	- 4.2
1970	- 2.0	- 6.0	- 5.6	- 7.0
1971	- 4.7	- 7.7	- 7.1	- 8.8
1972	- 4.1	- 8.2	- 7.9	- 9.4
1973	- 4.8	-10.3	-10.1	-11.4
1974	- 7.7	-14.9	-14.9	-16.9
1975	-10.1	-20.3	-19.8	-24.6
1976	-11.2	-22.4	-21.9	-29.0
1977	-12.7	-25.3	-24.7	-33.6
1978	-12.7	-27.2	-26.5	-37.7
1979	-13.7	-31.0	-29.4	-41.6
1980	-11.9	-31.4	-29.6	-42.9
1981	-12.8	-33.2	-31.8	-45.9

Figure 1–17. Trends in mortality for cardiovascular disease and noncardiovascular causes of death: decline by age-adjusted death rates, U.S., 1968–1981. (From Kannel, W.B., et al.: Report of Inter-Society Commission for Heart Disease Resources. **Circulation** 70:158A, 1984.)

cise," prepared by the American Heart Association's Subcommittee on Exercise/Cardiac Rehabilitation, and published in 1981, states our present knowledge in this area most succinctly:

Exercise training can increase cardiovascular functional capacity and decrease myocardial oxygen demand for any given level of physical activity in normal persons as well as most cardiac patients. Regular physical activity is required to maintain the training effects. The potential risk of vigorous physical activity can be reduced by appropriate medical clearance, education, and guidance. Exercise may aid efforts to control cigarette smoking, hypertension, lipid abnormalities, diabetes, obesity, and emotional stress. Evidence suggests that activity may protect against coronary heart disease and may improve the likelihood of survival from a heart attack.[125]

References

1. American Heart Association: **1989 Heart Facts**. Dallas, TX, American Heart Association, 1989.
2. Kitamura, K., Jorgensen, C.R., Gobel, F.L., Taylor, H.L., and Wang, Y.: Hemodynamic correlates of myocardial oxygen consumption during upright exercise. **J. Appl. Physiol.** 32:516–522, 1972.
3. Van Camp, S.P.: Exercise-related sudden death: risks and causes. **Physician Sportsmed.** 16:97–112, 1988.
4. Kannel, W.B., Sorlie, P., Castelli, W.P., and McGee, D.: Blood pressure and survival after myocardial infarction: the Framingham Study. **Am. J. Cardiol.** 45:326–330, 1980.
5. National Institutes of Health: The 1984 report of the Joint National Committee on Detection, Evaluation, and Treatment of High Blood Pressure. **Arch. Int. Med.** 144:1045–1047, 1984.

6. Lauer, R.M., and Shekelle, R.B., (eds.): **Childhood Prevention of Athero-sclerosis and Hypertension**. New York, Raven Press, 1980.
7. American Academy of Pediatrics: Report of the task force on blood pressure control in children. **Pediatrics** 59:802–803, 1977.
8. American Heart Association: **Heart Book: A Guide to and Treatment of Cardiovascular Disease**. New York, E.P. Dutton, 1980.
9. Kannel, W.B., and Dawber, T.R.: Atherosclerosis as a pediatric problem. **J. Pediatr**. 80:544–554, 1972.
10. McMillan, G.C.: Development of arteriosclerosis. **Am. J. Cardiol**. 31:542–546, 1973.
11. Ross, R.: The genesis of atherosclerosis. In **National Research Council: 1980 Issues and Current Studies**. Washington, D.C., National Academy of Sciences, 1981.
12. Ross, R.: The pathogenesis of atherosclerosis—an update. **N. Engl. J. Med**. 314:488–500, 1986.
13. Texon, M.: The hemodynamic basis of atherosclerosis. **Bull. N.Y. Acad. Med**. 52:187–200, 1976.
14. McGill, H.C., Jr.: Persistent problems in the pathogenesis of atherosclerosis. **Arteriosclerosis** 4:443–451, 1984.
15. Brown, M.S., and Goldstein, J.L.: How LDL receptors influence cholesterol and atherosclerosis. **Sci. Am**. 251:58–66, 1984.
16. Enos, W.F., Holmes, R.H., and Beyer, J.: Coronary disease among United States soldiers killed in action in Korea. **JAMA** 152:1090–1093, 1953.
17. McNamara, J.J., Molot, M.A., Stremple, J.F., and Cutting, R.T.: Coronary artery disease in combat casualties in Vietnam. **JAMA** 216:1185–1187, 1971.
18. Mason, J.K.: Asymptomatic disease of coronary arteries in young men. **Br. Med. J**. 2:1234–1237, 1963.
19. Rigal, R.D., Lovell, F.W., and Townsend, F.M.: Pathologic finds in the cardiovascular systems of military flying personnel. **Am. J. Cardiol**. 6:19–25, 1963.
20. Kaplan, N.M.: The control of hypertension: a therapeutic breakthrough. **Am. Sci**. 68:537–545, 1980.
21. Berglund, G., Anderson, O., and Wilhelmsen, L.: Prevalence of primary and secondary hypertension: studies in a random population sample. **Br. Med. J**. 2:554–556, 1976.
22. U.S. Department of Health and Human Services, Public Health Service, National Center for Health Statistics: **Hypertension in Adults 25–74 Years of Age: United States, 1971–75**. Vital and Health Statistics. Series 11—No. 221. DHHS Pub. No. (PHS)81-1971. Washington, D.C., U.S. Government Printing Office, April 1981.
23. Dischinger, P., and DuChene, A.G.: Quality control aspects of blood pressure measurements in the multiple risk factor intervention trial. **Controlled Clinical Trials** 7:137S–157S, 1986.
24. Rutan, G.H., Kuller, L.H., Neaton, J.D., Wentworth, D.N., McDonald, R.H., and Smith, W.M.: Mortality associated with diastolic hypertension and isolated systolic hypertension among men screened for the Multiple Risk Factor Intervention Trial. **Circulation** 77:504–514, 1988.
25. U.S. Department of Health and Human Services: **The 1984 Report of the Joint National Committee on Detection, Evaluation, and Treatment of High Blood Pressure**. Public Health Service, National Institutes of Health. NIH Publication No. 84-1088, 1984.
26. Remington, P.L., Forman, M.R., Gentry, E.M., Marks, J.S., Hogelin, G.C., and Trowbridge, F.L.: Current smoking trends in the United States: the 1981–1983 behavioral risk factor surveys. **JAMA** 253:2975–2978, 1985.
27. Mattson, M.E., Pollack, E.S., and Cullen, J.W.: What are the odds that smoking will kill you? **Am. J. Public Health** 77:425–431, 1987.
28. McGill, H.C.: The cardiovascular pathology of smoking. **Am. Heart J**. 115:250–257, 1988.
29. Caro, C.G., Lever, M.J., Parker, K.H., and Fish, P.J.: Effect of cigarette smoking

on the pattern of arterial blood flow: possible insight into mechanisms underlying the development of arteriosclerosis. **Lancet** 2:11–13, 1987.

30. White, J.R., and Froeb, H.F.: Small-airways dysfunction in nonsmokers chronically exposed to tobacco smoke. **N. Engl. J. Med.** 302:720–723, 1980.

31. Matsukura, S., Taminato, T., Kitano, N., Seino, Y., Hamada, H., Uchihashi, M., Nakajima, H., and Hirata, Y.: Effects of environmental tobacco smoke on urinary cotinine excretion in nonsmokers: evidence for passive smoking. **N. Engl. J. Med.** 311:828–832, 1984.

32. Svendsen, K.H., Kuller, L.H., Martin, M.J., and Ockene, J.K.: Effects of passive smoking in the multiple risk factor intervention trial. **Am. J. Epidemiol.** 126:783–795, 1987.

33. Helsing, K.J., Sandler, D.P., Comstock, G.W., and Chee, E.: Heart disease mortality in nonsmokers living with smokers. **Am. J. Epidemiol.** 127:915–922, 1988.

34. Anderson, K.M., Castelli, W.P., and Levy, D.: Cholesterol and mortality. **JAMA** 257:2176–2180, 1987.

35. Grundy, S.M.: Cholesterol and coronary heart disease. **JAMA** 256:2849–2858, 1986.

36. Castelli, W.P., Garrison, R.J., Wilson, P.W.F., Abbott, R.D., Kalousdian, S., and Kannel, W.B.: Incidence of coronary heart disease and lipoprotein cholesterol levels. **JAMA** 256:2835–2838, 1986.

37. Tyroler, H.A.: Review of lipid-lowering clinical trials in relation to observational epidemiologic studies. **Circulation** 76:515–522, 1987.

38. Lipid Research Clinics Program: The Lipid Research Clinics Coronary Primary Prevention Trial results: I. Reduction in incidence of coronary heart disease. **JAMA** 251:351–364, 1984.

39. Kannel, W.B., and McGee, D.L.: Diabetes and cardiovascular risk factors: the Framingham Study. **Circulation** 59:8–13, 1979.

40. Leon, A.S.: Age and other predictors of coronary heart disease. **Med. Sci. Sports Exerc.** 19:159–167, 1987.

41. Neaton, J.D., Kuller, L.H., Wentworth, D., and Borhani, N.O.: Total and cardiovascular mortality in relation to cigarette smoking, serum cholesterol concentration, and diastolic blood pressure among black and white males followed up for five years. **Am. Heart J.** 108:759–770, 1984.

42. Perkins, K.A.: Family history of coronary heart disease: Is it an independent risk factor? **Am. J. Epidemiol.** 124:182–194, 1986.

43. Austin, M.A., King, M.C., Bawol, R.D., Hulley, S.B., and Friedman, G.D.: Risk factors for coronary heart disease in adult female twins. **Am. J. Epidemiol.** 125:308–318, 1987.

44. Khaw, K.T., and Barrett-Connor, E.: Family history of heart attack: a modifiable risk factor? **Circulation** 74:239–244, 1986.

45. Barrett-Connor, E., and Khaw, K.T.: Family history of heart attack as an independent predictor of death due to cardiovascular disease. **Circulation** 69:1065–1069, 1984.

46. Lerner, D.J., and Kannel, W.B.: Patterns of coronary heart disease morbidity and mortality in the sexes: a 26-year follow-up of the Framingham population. **Am. Heart J.** 111:383–390, 1986.

47. Keys, A., Aravanis, C., Blackburn, H., VanBuchem, F.S.P., Buzine, R., Djordjevic, B.S., Fidanza, F., Karvonen, M.J., Menotti, A., Puddu, V., and Taylor, H.L.: Coronary heart disease: overweight and obesity as risk factors. **Ann. Intern. Med.** 77:15–27, 1972.

48. Gordon, T., and Kannel, W.B.: The effects of overweight on cardiovascular disease. **Geriatrics** 28:80–88, 1973.

49. Hubert, H.A., Feinleib, M., McNamara, P.M., and Castelli, W.P.: Obesity as an independent risk factor for cardiovascular disease. A 26-year follow-up of participants in the Framingham heart study. **Circulation** 67:968–977, 1983.

50. Friedman, M., and Rosenman, R.H.: **Type A Behavior and Your Heart.** Greenwich, CT, Fawcett Publications, Inc., 1974.

51. Matthews, K.A., and Haynes, S.G.: Type A behavior pattern and coronary disease risk: update and critical evaluation. **Am. J. Epidemiol.** 123:923–960, 1986.
52. Shekelle, R.B., Hulley, S.B., Neaton, J.D., Billings, J.H., Borhani, N.O., Gerace, T.A., Jacobs, D.R., Lasser, N.L., Mittlemark, M.B., and Stamler, J.: The MRFIT behavior pattern study: II. Type A behavior and incidence of coronary heart disease. **Am. J. Epidemiol.** 122:559–570, 1985.
53. Friedman, M., Thoresen, C.E., Gill, J.J., Ulmer, D., Powell, L.H., Price, V.A., Brown, B., Thompson, L., Rabin, D.D., Breall, W.S., Bourg, E., Levy, R., and Dixon, T.: Alteration of type A behavior and its effect on cardiac recurrences in post myocardial infarction patients: summary results of the recurrent coronary prevention project. **Am. Heart J.** 112:653–665, 1986.
54. Williams, R.B., Jr.: Psychological factors in coronary artery disease: epidemiologic evidence. **Circulation** 76(Suppl. I):117–123, 1987.
55. Manuck, S.B., Kaplan, J.R., and Matthews, K.A.: Behavioral antecedents of coronary heart disease and atherosclerosis. **Arteriosclerosis** 6:2–14, 1986.
56. Wilmore, J.H., and McNamara, J.J.: Prevalence of coronary heart disease risk factors in boys, 8 to 12 years of age. **J. Pediatr.** 84:527–533, 1974.
57. Wilmore, J.H., Constable, S.H., Stanforth, P.R., Tsao, W.Y., Rotkis, T.C., Paicius, R.M., Mattern, C.M., and Ewy, G.A.: Prevalence of coronary heart disease risk factors in 13- to 15-year-old boys. **J. Cardiac Rehabil.** 2:223–233, 1982.
58. Gilliam, T.B., Katch, V.L., Thorland, W., and Weltman, A.: Prevalence of coronary heart disease risk factors in active children, 7 to 12 years of age. **Med. Sci. Sports** 9:21–25, 1977.
59. Lauer, R.M., Connor, W.E., Leaverton, P.E., Reiter, M.A., and Clarke, W.R.: Coronary heart disease risk factors in school children: The Muscatine Study. **J. Pediatr.** 86:697–706, 1975.
60. Berenson, G.S., Foster, T.A., Frank, G.C., Frerichs, R.R., Srinivasan, S.R., Voors, A.W., and Webber, L.S.: Cardiovascular disease risk factor variables at the preschool age: The Bogalusa Heart Study. **Circulation** 57:603–612, 1978.
61. Mellies, M.J., Laskarzewski, P.M., Tracy, T., and Glueck, C.J.: Tracking of high- and low-density-lipoprotein cholesterol from childhood to young adulthood in a single large kindred with familial hypercholesterolemia. **Metabolism** 34:747–753, 1985.
62. Woynarowska, B., Mukherjee, D., Roche, A.F., and Siervogel, R.M.: Blood pressure changes during adolescence and subsequent adult blood pressure level. **Hypertension** 7:695–701, 1985.
63. Newman, W.P., Freedman, D.S., Voors, A.W., Gard, P.D., Srinivasan, S.R., Cresanta, J.L., Williamson, G.D., Webber, L.S., and Berenson, G.S.: Relation of serum lipoprotein levels and systolic blood pressure to early atherosclerosis. **N. Engl. J. Med.** 314:138–144, 1986.
64. Morris, J.N., Heady, J.A., Raffle, P.A.B., Roberts, C.G., and Parks, J.W.: Coronary heart-disease and physical activity of work. **Lancet** 2:1053–1057, 1111–1120, 1953.
65. Morris, J.N., Heady, J., and Raffle, P.A.B.: Physique of London busmen: the epidemiology of uniforms. **Lancet** 2:569–570, 1956.
66. Morris, J.N., Kagan, A., Pattison, D.C., Gardner, M., and Raffle, P.: Incidence and prediction of ischemic heart disease in London busmen. **Lancet** 2:553–559, 1966.
67. Shephard, R.J.: Exercise in coronary heart disease. **Sports Med.** 3:26–49, 1986.
68. Zukel, W.J., Lewis, R., Enterline, P., Painter, R.C., Ralston, L.S., Fawcett, R.M., Meredith, A.P., and Peterson, B.: A short-term community study of the epidemiology of coronary heart disease. **Am. J. Public Health** 49:1630–1639, 1959.
69. Frank, C.W., Weinblatt, E., Shapiro, S., and Sager, R.V.: Physical inactivity as a lethal factor in myocardial infarction among men. **Circulation** 34:1022–1033, 1960.

70. Bassler, T.J.: Marathon running and immunity to heart disease. **Physician Sportsmed**. 3:77–80, 1975.
71. Noakes, T.D., Opie, L.H., Rose, A.G., and Kleynhans, P.H.T.: Autopsy-proved coronary atherosclerosis in marathon runners. **N. Engl. J. Med**. 301:86–89, 1979.
72. Skinner, J.S., Benson, H., McDonough, J.R., and Hames, C.G.: Social status, physical activity and coronary proneness. **J. Chronic Dis**. 19:773–783, 1966.
73. Rose, G.: Physical activity and coronary heart disease. **Proc. R. Soc. Med**. 62:1183–1187, 1969.
74. LaPorte, R.E., Adams, L.L., Savage, D.D., Brenes, G., Dearwater, S., and Cook, T.: The spectrum of physical activity, cardiovascular disease and health: an epidemiologic perspective. **Am. J. Epidemiol**. 120:507–517, 1984.
75. Brown, R.G., Davidson, A.G., McKeown, T., and Whitfield, A.G.W.: Coronary artery disease: influences affecting its incidence in males in the seventh decade. **Lancet** 2:1073–1077, 1957.
76. Kahn, H.A.: The relationship of reported coronary heart disease mortality to physical activity of work. **Am. J. Public Health** 53:1058–1067, 1963.
77. Morris, J.N., Adam, C., Chave, S.P.W., Sirey, C., Epstein, L., and Sheehan, D.J.: Vigorous exercise in leisure-time and the incidence of coronary heart-disease. **Lancet** 1:333–339, 1973.
78. Morris, J.N.N., Pollard, P., Everitt, M.G., Chave, S.P.W., and Semmence, A.M.: Vigorous exercise in leisure-time: protection against coronary disease. **Lancet** 2:1207–1210, 1980.
79. Holme, I., Helgeland, A., Hjermann, I., Leren, P., and Lund-Larson, P.G.: Physical activity at work and at leisure in relation to coronary risk factors and social class. **Acta Med. Scand**. 209:277–283, 1981.
80. Paffenbarger, R.S., Hale, W.E., Brand, R.J., and Hyde, R.T.: Work-energy level, personal characteristics, and fatal heart attack: a birth cohort effect. **Am. J. Epidemiol**. 105:200–213, 1977.
81. Paffenbarger, R.S., Jr., Hyde, R.T., Wing, A.L., and Steinmetz, C.H.: A natural history of athleticism and cardiovascular health. **JAMA** 252:491–495, 1984.
82. Paffenbarger, R.S., Hyde, R.T., Hsieh, C.C., and Wing, A.L.: Physical activity, other life-style patterns, cardiovascular disease and longevity. **Acta Med. Scand**. (Suppl.)711:85–91, 1986.
83. Paffenbarger, R.S., Hyde, R.T., Wing, A.L., and Hsieh, C.C.: Physical activity, all-cause mortality, and longevity of college alumni. **N. Engl. J. Med**. 314:605–613, 1986.
84. Powell, K.E., Thompson, P.D., Caspersen, C.J., and Kendrick, J.S.: Physical activity and the incidence of coronary heart disease. **Ann. Rev. Public Health** 8:253–287, 1987.
85. Caspersen, C.J.: Physical inactivity and coronary heart disease. **Physician Sportsmed**. 15:43–44, 1987.
86. Yamaji, K., and Shephard, R.J.: Longevity and cause of death of athletes. **J. Hum. Ergol**. 6:15–27, 1977.
87. Olson, H.W., Montoye, H.J., Sprague, H., Stephens, K., and Van Huss, W.D.: The longevity and morbidity of college athletes. **Physician Sportsmed**. 6:62–65, 1978.
88. Cooper, K.H., Pollock, M.L., Martin, R.P., White, S.R., Linnerud, A.C., and Jackson, A.: Physical fitness levels vs. selected coronary risk factors: a cross-sectional study. **JAMA** 236:166–169, 1976.
89. Gibbons, L.W., Blair, S.N., Cooper, K.H., and Smith, M.: Association between coronary heart disease risk factors and physical fitness in healthy adult women. **Circulation** 67:977–983, 1983.
90. Wood, P.D., and Haskell, W.L.: The effect of exercise on plasma high density lipoproteins. **Lipids** 14:417–427, 1979.
91. Dufaux, B., Assmann, G., and Hollmann, W.: Plasma lipoproteins and physical activity: a review. **Int. J. Sports Med**. 3:123–136, 1982.
92. Haskell, W.L.: The influence of exercise training on plasma lipids and lipoproteins in health and disease. **Acta Med. Scan**. (Suppl.)711:25–37, 1986.

93. Kannel, W.B.: High-density lipoproteins: epidemiologic profile and risks of coronary artery disease. **Am. J. Cardiol.** 52:98–128, 1983.

94. Williams, P.T., Wood, P.D., Haskell, W.L., and Vranizan, K.: The effects of running mileage and duration on plasma lipoprotein levels. **JAMA** 247:2674–2679, 1982.

95. Tipton, C.M., Matthes, R.D., Bedford, T.B., Leininger, J.R., Oppliger, R.A., and Miller, L.J.: Exercise, hypertension, and animal models. In Lowenthal, D.T., Bharadwaja, K., and Oaks, W.W., (eds.): **Therapeutics through Exercise**. New York, Grune & Stratton, 1979.

96. Seals, D.R., and Hagberg, J.M.: The effect of exercise training on human hypertension: a review. **Med. Sci. Sports Exerc.** 16:207–215, 1984.

97. Hagberg, J.M., and Seals, D.R.: Exercise training and hypertension. **Acta Med. Scand.** (Suppl.)711:131–136, 1986.

98. Hill, J.S.: Effect of a program of aerobic exercise on the smoking behaviour of a group of adult volunteers. **Can. J. Public Health** 76:183–186, 1985.

99. Frisch, R.E., Wyshak, G., Albright, T.E., Albright, N.L., and Schiff, I.: Lower prevalence of diabetes in female former college athletes compared with non-athletes. **Diabetes** 35:1101–1105, 1986.

100. Bjorntorp, P., and Krotkiewski, M.: Exercise treatment in diabetes mellitus. **Acta Med. Scand.** 217:3–7, 1985.

101. Kemmer, F.W., and Berger, M.: Exercise in therapy and the life of diabetic patients. **Clin. Sci.** 67:279–283, 1984.

102. Koivisto, V.A., and DeFronzo, R.A.: Exercise in the treatment of type II diabetes. **Acta Endocrinol.** (Suppl.) 262:107–111, 1984.

103. Zuti, W.B., and Golding, L.A.: Comparing diet and exercise as weight reduction tools. **Physician Sportsmed.** 4:49–53, 1976.

104. Pavlou, K.N., Steffee, W.P., Lerman, R.H., and Burrows, B.A.: Effects of dieting and exercise on lean body mass, oxygen uptake and strength. **Med. Sci. Sports Exerc.** 17:466–471, 1985.

105. Brownell, K.D., and Stunkard, A.J.: Physical activity in the development and control of obesity. In Stunkard, A.J., (ed.): **Obesity**. Philadelphia, W.B. Saunders Co., 1980.

106. Hagan, R.D., Upton, S.J., Wong, L., and Whittam, J.: The effects of aerobic conditioning and/or caloric restriction in overweight men and women. **Med. Sci. Sports Exerc.** 18:87–94, 1986.

107. Morgan, W.P.: Affective beneficence of vigorous physical activity. **Med. Sci. Sport Exerc.** 17:94–100, 1985.

108. Sedgwick, A.W., Brotherhood, J.R., Harris-Davidson, A., Taplin, R.E., and Thomas, D.W.: Long-term effects of physical training programme on risk factors for coronary heart disease in otherwise sedentary men. **Br. Med. J.** 2:7–10, 1980.

109. Froelicher, V.F.: Animal studies of effect of chronic exercise on the heart and atherosclerosis: a review. **Am. Heart J.** 84:496–506, 1972.

110. Froelicher, V., Battler, A., and McKirnan, M.D.: Physical activity and coronary heart disease. **Cardiology** 65:153–190, 1980.

111. Cohen, M.V.: Coronary and collateral blood flows during exercise and myocardial vascular adaptations to training. **Exerc. Sport Sci. Rev.** 11:55–98, 1983.

112. Dowell, R.T.: Cardiac adaptations to exercise. **Exerc. Sport Sci. Rev.** 11:99–117, 1983.

113. Eckstein, R.W.: Effect of exercise and coronary artery narrowing on coronary collateral circulation. **Circ. Res.** 5:230–235, 1957.

114. Kramsch, D.M., Aspen, A.J., Abramowitz, B.M., Kreimendahl, T., and Hood, W.B.: Reduction of coronary atherosclerosis by moderate conditioning exercise in monkeys on an atherogenic diet. **N. Engl. J. Med.** 305:1483–1489, 1981.

115. Froelicher, V.F., and Brown, P.: Exercise and coronary heart disease. **J. Cardiac Rehabil.** 1:277–288, 1981.

116. Jensen, D., Atwood, J.E., Froelicher, V., McKirnan, M.D., Battler, A., Ashburn, W., and Ross, J.: Improvement in ventricular function during exercise studied

with radionuclide ventriculography after cardiac rehabilitation. **Am. J. Cardiol.** 46:770–777, 1980.

117. Froelicher, V., Jensen, D., Atwood, J.E., McKirnan, D., Gerber, K., Slutsky, R., Battler, A., Ashburn, W., and Ross, J.: Cardiac rehabilitation: evidence for improvement in myocardial perfusion and function. **Arch. Phys. Med. Rehabil.** 61:517–522, 1980.

118. Ehsani, A.A., Biello, D.R., Schultz, J., Sobel, B.E., and Holloszy, J.O.: Improvement of left ventricular contractile function by exercise training in patients with coronary artery disease. **Circulation** 74:350–358, 1986.

119. Ehsani, A.A.: Cardiovascular adaptations to endurance exercise training in ischemic heart disease. **Exerc. Sport Sci. Rev.** 15:53–66, 1987.

120. Pollock, M.L.: Benefits of exercise: effect on mortality and physiological function. In Kappagoda, C.T. (ed.): **Long Term Management of Patients After Myocardial Infarction**. Boston, Martinus Nijhoff Publishers, 1988.

121. May, G.S., Eberlein, K.A., Furberg, C.D., Passamani, E.R., and DeMets, D.L.: Secondary prevention after myocardial infarction: a review of long-term trials. **Progr. Cardiovasc. Dis.** 24:331–352, 1982.

122. Oldridge, N.B., Guyatt, G.H., Fischer, M.E., and Rimm, A.A.: Cardiac rehabilitation after myocardial infarction: combined experience of randomized clinical trials. **JAMA** 260:945–950, 1988.

123. Kent, L.K., and Pollock, M.L.: Cardiac rehabilitation services: a scientific evaluation. **J. Cardiopulmonary Rehabil.** in press, 1989.

124. Kannel, W.B., Doyle, J.T., Ostfeld, A.M., Jenkins, C.D., Kuller, L., Podell, R.N., and Stamler, J.: Optimal resources for primary prevention of atherosclerotic diseases. **Circulation** 70:157A–205A, 1984.

125. American Heart Association, Subcommittee on Exercise/Cardiac Rehabilitation: Statement on Exercise. **Circulation** 64:1302–1304, 1981.

2

OBESITY AND WEIGHT CONTROL

INTRODUCTION

Overweight and obesity, as a single disease entity, constitute one of the most serious health problems in the United States today.[1] Both are either directly or indirectly associated with a wide variety of diseases that collectively account for a significant percentage of the annual United States mortality. Further, the most recent data from the second cycle of the National Health and Nutrition Examination Survey (NHANES II) indicate that between 6 and 61 percent of the adult population are overweight, depending on gender, age, and race, with evidence that the prevalence is increasing.[1] Before beginning a detailed discussion of prevalence data, it is first important to define the terms overweight and obesity, since they are often used incorrectly.

Overweight is simply defined as that condition where an individual's weight exceeds the population norm or average, as determined on the basis of gender, height, and frame size (Tables 2–1 and 2–2). The standardized height and weight tables had their genesis in the 1912 publication of the "Medico-Actuarial Mortality Investigation," by the Association of Life Insurance Medical Directors and the Actuarial Society of America.[2] The original tables gave the average values for men and women of specific ages who obtained life insurance policies between the years of 1888 and 1905. The data were obtained mostly from urban centers on the Eastern seaboard, and heights and weights were recorded with shoes and clothing. In the early 1940's, the Metropolitan Life Insurance Company developed tables of "desirable weight" from this original data. These tables were subsequently revised in 1959, with the data placed into a format that provided weight ranges for each of three frame sizes according to each 1-inch increment in height.[3, 4] As an example, a 6-foot 2-inch man with a "large" frame size would be allowed to weigh between 173 and 194 pounds (see Table 2–1).

Table 2–1. Standard Table for Men's Weight (in Indoor Clothing)* for Height and Frame Size

Desirable Weights for Men Aged 25 Years and Over				
Height with Shoes 1-inch Heels		*Small Frame*	*Medium Frame*	*Large Frame*
Feet	Inches			
5	2	112–120	118–129	126–141
5	3	115–123	121–133	129–144
5	4	118–126	124–136	132–148
5	5	121–129	127–139	135–152
5	6	124–133	130–143	138–156
5	7	128–137	134–147	142–161
5	8	132–141	138–152	147–166
5	9	136–145	142–156	151–170
5	10	140–150	146–160	155–174
5	11	144–154	150–165	159–179
6	0	148–158	154–170	164–184
6	1	152–162	158–175	168–189
6	2	156–167	162–180	173–194
6	3	160–171	167–185	178–199
6	4	164–175	172–190	182–204

*For nude weight, deduct 5 to 7 lb.

(Prepared by Metropolitan Life Insurance Company. Derived primarily from data of the Build and Blood Pressure Study, Society of Actuaries, 1959.)

Table 2–2. Standard Table for Women's Weight (in Indoor Clothing)* for Height and Frame Size

Desirable Weights for Women Aged 25 Years and Over				
Height with Shoes 2-inch Heels		*Small Frame*	*Medium Frame*	*Large Frame*
Feet	Inches			
4	10	92–98	96–107	104–119
4	11	94–101	98–110	106–122
5	0	96–104	101–113	109–125
5	1	99–107	104–116	112–128
5	2	102–110	107–119	115–131
5	3	105–113	110–122	118–134
5	4	108–116	113–126	121–138
5	5	111–119	116–130	125–142
5	6	114–123	120–135	129–146
5	7	118–127	124–139	133–150
5	8	122–131	128–143	137–154
5	9	126–135	132–147	141–158
5	10	130–140	136–151	145–163
5	11	134–144	140–155	149–168
6	0	138–148	144–159	153–173

*For nude weight, deduct 2 to 4 lb.

(Prepared by Metropolitan Life Insurance Company. Derived primarily from data of the Build and Blood Pressure Study, Society of Actuaries, 1959.)

Any weight below 173 pounds would be classified as underweight, and any weight over 194 pounds would be considered overweight.

The 1959 tables looked very scientific and accurate, but they contained basically the same data that was published in 1912, with the categorization into frame size done in a rather arbitrary manner.[2] In fact, no directions were given as to how to estimate frame size when using these 1959 tables. Many determined their frame size on the basis of the column in which they found their weight! In 1983, the revised Metropolitan Life Insurance tables were published, reflecting data from the 1979 Build Study.[3] Although these tables included directions for determining frame size, both the method of frame size determination[5] and the new more liberal weight ranges[6] came under heavy criticism. The American Heart Association has recommended the continued use of the 1959 tables, because the new tables list average weight range increases of 13 pounds for short men and 10 pounds for short women, with lesser increases for medium-height men and women and insignificant increases for tall men and women, increases which they do not consider healthy or justified.[6]

The problem of using standard normative data for determining one's desired or ideal weight were illustrated by Welham and Behnke in 1942.[7] In a study of professional football players, they found that these athletes were grossly overweight, yet they had very high specific gravities, indicating low levels of body fat and high levels of fat-free tissue, i.e., muscle and bone. Of the 25 men studied, 17 would have been considered unfit for military service and would not have qualified for first-class life insurance because they would have been considered overweight. The mean specific gravity for the group was equivalent to a relative fat value of 9.3 percent. Converting specific gravity to relative body fat, two of these athletes were 23.5 percent fat, one was 19 percent fat, two were 17 percent fat, one was 16 percent fat, and the remaining 19 athletes were less than 14 percent fat. By present day criteria, three of these athletes would be considered overfat, three would be borderline overfat, and the remaining 19 would be considered to have desirable body composition values. Thus, it is possible to be overweight but of normal or below normal levels of body fat. Likewise, it is also possible to be excessively fat, yet to fall within the normal weight range for height and frame size. Since the original work of Welham and Behnke, many other studies have confirmed the fact that the standard tables do not provide accurate estimates of ideal or desirable weight for a large segment of the population.[8]

Body Composition Assessment

The major problem associated with the use of the standard tables is that these tables do not take into consideration the composition of the body. Although the body is composed of numerous elements, scientists have categorized the total body mass into various compartments on the basis of either a chemical or anatomical classification scheme. These are illustrated in Table 2–3, as adapted from Lohman.[9] Most typically, scientists have used the four component model: the adipose tissue or fat mass; the bone mass; the muscle mass; the organs and the remainder. To simplify this categorization even further, two component parts have been identified: the fat mass and the fat-free mass. Procedures have been developed that allow for a relatively accurate fractionization of the total body weight into its two component parts.

The most accurate of these procedures involves weighing the individual while submerged underwater. The difference between scale weight and the underwater weight, when corrected for trapped air volumes, is equal to the volume of the body.[10] This is illustrated in Figure 2–1. Dividing the body mass or weight by the body volume provides an accurate estimate of the density of the body,

Table 2–3. The Chemical and Anatomical Composition of the Body

Chemical	Anatomical	Behnke	Brožek, Siri	Von Dobeln
Fat	Adipose Tissue	Excess Fat	Fat	Adipose
Protein		↑ Essential Lipids		
Carbohydrate	Muscle			Muscle
Water	Organs	Lean Body Mass	Fat-Free Body	
	Other			Muscle Free Lean
Mineral	Bone			

(Adapted from Lohman, T. G.: Applicability of body composition techniques and constants for children and youths. **Exerc. Sport Sci. Rev.** 14:325–357, 1986. Copyright American College of Sports Medicine, 1986.)

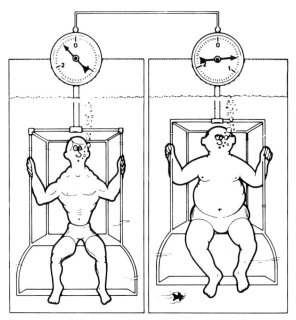

Figure 2–1. Illustration of the underwater weighing technique to determine body density, from which total body fat can be determined. The two individuals have the same total body weight, but the individual on the left weighs more underwater because of a higher percentage of lean tissue and a lower percentage of fat tissue.

i.e., M/V = density. The density of fat has been determined to be approximately 0.900 g/ml, and it varies little between and within individuals. The density of the lean tissue is much more variable, but the constant of 1.100 g/ml is typically used in most equations that provide an estimate of relative body fat from body density. Further methodological considerations are discussed in Chapter 6.

The underwater weighing technique is the most accurate laboratory test available to determine the total density of the body and its subsequent composition, i.e., fat and fat-free weights. However, it does have its limitations. For those individuals undergoing changes in bone mineral, i.e., increasing bone mineral in children as they mature or decreasing bone mineral in aging individuals, particularly postmenopausal women, the equations used to estimate relative fat from body density will be inaccurate, providing an overestimation of the actual fat concentration. Lohman[9] has estimated the changes in the fat-free body composition, i.e., water, minerals, and potassium, and their effect on the density of the fat-free body of men and women between the ages of 7 and 25 years. These are illustrated in Figure 2–2. For those individuals with a larger preponderance of bone or with bone that is denser than the

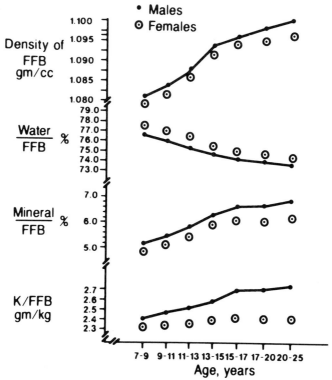

Figure 2-2. Estimated changes in fat-free body (FFB) composition as a function of age. (From Lohman, T.G.: Applicability of body composition techniques and constants for children and youths. **Exercise Sport Sci. Rev.** 14:325–327, 1986, with permission. Copyright American College of Sports Medicine, 1986.)

population average, the estimate of relative fat will also be inaccurate, with an underestimation of the actual fat concentration. The authors of this book have observed this phenomenon in children, adolescents, and senior or master athletes, who are all overestimated, and in young male athletes with large bone structure, who are estimated to be 3 percent body fat or less, values that are physiologically impossible. Fortunately, these inaccuracies occur infrequently, but the fact that they do occur should be recognized.

For a given total body density, the use of the appropriate density of the fat-free body can make a considerable difference. Table 2–4 illustrates this for two individuals, an 8-year-old boy and a chemically mature, 25-year-old male black athlete. The density of the fat-free body used for the boy, i.e., 1.085, was taken from the data of Lohman,[9] whereas that used for the black male athlete (1.113) was taken from Schutte and associates.[11]

Table 2–4. Calculation of Body Composition in an 8-Year-Old Boy and a Mature Black Athlete Using Standard and Specific Densities of the Fat-Free Mass

Basic Equation to Compute Relative Fat (RF) from Total Body Density (Db)

$$RF, \% = \frac{Dffw \cdot Dfw}{Db} \times \frac{1}{(Dffw \times Dfw)} \times \frac{Dfw}{(Dffw - Dfw)}$$

where, Dffw = density of the fat-free mass; Dfw = density of the fat mass; and Db = total body density.

8-Year-Old Boy

Using Dffw = 1.085 and Dfw = 0.901

$$RF, \% = \frac{1.085 \cdot 0.901}{Db} \times \frac{1}{(1.085 - 0.901)} \times \frac{0.901}{(1.085 - 0.901)} = \frac{531.3}{Db} - 489.7$$

With a Db of 1.060, the Siri equation,* which uses a Dffw = 1.100, estimates RF = 17.0%, whereas the new equation provides an estimate of RF = 11.5%.

20-Year-Old Black Athlete

Using Dffw = 1.113 and Dfw = 0.901

$$RF, \% = \frac{1.113 \cdot 0.901}{Db} \times \frac{1}{(1.113 - 0.901)} \times \frac{0.901}{(1.113 - 0.901)} = \frac{473.0}{Db} - 425.0$$

With a Db of 1.075 the Siri equation,* which uses a Dffw = 1.100, estimates RF = 10.5%, whereas the new equation provides an estimate of RF = 15.0%.

$$*\text{Siri equation} = \frac{495.0}{Db} - 450$$

Other techniques have been used to estimate body composition in living animals and humans. These are outlined in Table 2–5. For a brief description of each of these, please refer to Lohman.[12]

Densitometry, despite its limitations, is considered the "gold standard" for evaluating body composition. The procedure, however,

Table 2–5. Available Techniques for the Assessment of Body Composition

Fat and Fat-Free Body	Muscle	Bone
Densitometry	Spectrometry (^{40}K)	Photon absorptiometry
Hydrometry	Ultrasonics	Radiographics
Spectrometry (^{40}K)	Radiographics	Neutron activation
Ultrasonics	Neutron activation	NMR
Radiographics	NMR	
Electrical conductivity	Creatinine excretion	
Neutron activation	Serum creatinine	
NMR	Urinary 3-methylhistidine	

(Adapted from Lohman, T. G.: Research progress in validation of laboratory methods of assessing body composition. **Med. Sci. Sports Exerc.** 16:596–603, 1984.)

is time consuming, requires considerable space and equipment, and must be conducted by someone who is highly trained in body composition assessment. As a result, most body composition evaluations, particularly in nonresearch clinical settings, are derived through anthropometric techniques. Using skinfold thickness measurements, girths, and diameters, either singly or in combination, it is possible to derive accurate estimates of body composition.[13] For many years it was assumed that the equations to predict the various components of body composition—fat-free weight, fat weight, and relative fat—were population specific, i.e., that they were accurate only for a population similar to the population from which the equations were derived. Recently, Jackson and Pollock[14] and Jackson, Pollock, and Ward[15] have derived a series of equations for men and women, respectively, that are generalized equations applicable for men and women of varying age and body composition. The actual application of these equations is discussed in Chapter 6.

Prevalence of Obesity

Understanding that there is a definite distinction between overweight and obesity, it is possible to better understand the data now available regarding the prevalence of overweight and obesity in the United States. According to the U.S. Public Health Service, obesity has become a health problem of epidemic proportions, with approximately 20 percent of the adult population overweight to a degree that may interfere with optimal health and longevity. After age 40, this figure increases to 35 percent.[16] These figures are impressive, but they are derived on the basis of variations in weight from the standard height and weight table. Thus, they reflect only the extent of the problem relative to overweight and not obesity.

More recent surveys have attempted to differentiate between overweight and obesity by using skinfold measurements in addition to total body weight. The Ten-State Nutrition Survey, conducted between 1968 and 1970, identified between 9 and 25 percent of the black and white male and female teenage population evaluated as exceeding an established criterion for obesity based on triceps skinfold thickness.[17] The U.S. Health and Nutrition Examination Survey (HANES), conducted between 1971 and 1974, evaluated 12,900 individuals in the 20- to 74-year-old age range and found the following. With respect to the appropriate weight for height, 18 percent of men and 13 percent of women were from 10 to 19 percent in excess of their desired values, and an additional 14 percent of men and 24 percent of women were 20 percent or more

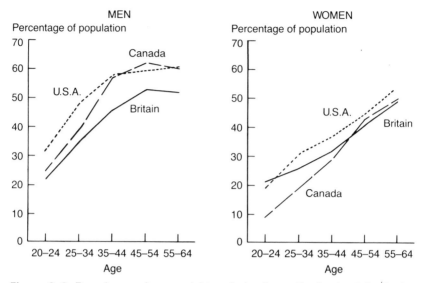

Figure 2–3. Prevalence of overweight and obesity on the basis of the body mass index for populations in Britain, Canada, and the United States. (Adapted from Millar, W.J., and Stephens, T.: The prevalence of overweight and obesity in Britain, Canada, and United States. **Am. J. Public Health** 77:38–41, 1987.)

above their desired values. It was also found that overweight increases sharply beyond 30 years of age, with the highest values reaching 39 percent for men and 50 percent for women who are 10 percent or more overweight. Using skinfold fat values and projecting to the total population, the study estimated that 10 to 50 million Americans are overweight or obese, and 2.8 million men and 4.5 million women are severely obese.[18]

Frustrated by the lack of actual body composition data on a large population base, scientists have been in a constant search for a simple ratio of height and weight that will more accurately reflect the body composition of the individual. Most recently, Quetelet's index has been generally accepted as being most representative. Also referred to as the Body Mass Index (BMI), the index is determined as the ratio of weight to height squared, or BMI = weight/height^2 (kg/m^2). When the BMI is used, underweight is defined as a value of 20 or less, normal weight as a value between 20.1 and 25.0, overweight as a value between 25.1 and 30.0, and obesity as a value of 30.0 or more.[19] Using these criteria, Millar and Stephens[19] determined the prevalence of overweight and obesity in Britain, Canada, and the United States using data obtained from large population surveys between the years of 1976 and 1981. The results of their analysis are presented in Figure 2–3.

Economic Consequences of Overweight and Obesity

The problems associated with obesity are considerable. In 1973, it was estimated that 10 billion dollars per year were invested in the diet industry. Of this total, it was estimated that 14.9 million dollars went to Weight Watchers International, 220 million dollars to health spas and reducing salons, 100 million dollars to exercise equipment, 54 million dollars to the "legal" diet pill market, and 1 billion dollars to the diet food market.[20] One can only guess how these numbers have been multiplied into the 1980's and 1990's! In addition, it is not unusual to find at least one diet book on the list of the top ten selling books in the United States at any one time.

Hannon and Lohman[21] speculated on the economic costs of obesity in a totally different manner. Using the data from the National Health Survey for 18- to 79-year-olds,[22] in which skinfold fat data were available, they calculated the body composition and the excess body fat for the adult United States population, assuming a population data base of 146.8 million people in 1975. They calculated 377 million kg of excess fat in men and 667 million kg of excess fat in women, for a total excess fat in the adult population of the United States of 1.04 billion kg, or 2.3 billion pounds! The energy saved by dieting to achieve desirable weight in these individuals would be equal to 1.3 billion gallons of gasoline. The savings accrued from the fact that persons would eat less to maintain this new weight would equal 750 million gallons of gasoline per year, or enough to fuel 900,000 average American autos at 12,000 miles per year at 14 miles per gallon! Similarly, such savings would provide the total electrical demands of the cities of Boston, Chicago, San Francisco, and Washington, D.C., for one full year. The economic consequences of obesity are truly staggering.

Medical Consequences of Overweight and Obesity

There are also a series of medical problems that are associated with obesity. These have been reviewed by Van Itallie[1] and Frankle and Yang.[23] As was discussed in the previous chapter, obesity is a risk factor for cardiovascular disease, particularly coronary artery disease (CAD) and hypertension. With respect to CAD, the data was once considered equivocal. The seven-country study reported by Keys and colleagues[24] indicated that overweight and obesity were unrelated to CAD risk when all other CAD risk factors were statistically controlled. However, the Framingham data, reported by Hubert and associates,[25] indicate that obesity is a discrete risk factor independent of the other CAD risk factors (see Figs. 1–11 and 1–12). Thus, obesity may be a primary risk factor for CAD, or it may exert its influence through the other known risk factors, such as hypertension, diabetes, reduced plasma high-density lipoprotein cholesterol concentrations, and hypercholesterolemia. Hypertension, on the other hand, is clearly related to obesity in a causal manner, imparting considerable risk for stroke and congestive heart failure. Among overweight Americans aged 20 to 44 years, they have a 5.6 times greater risk for hypertension compared with normal weight Americans of the same age.[1] Weight reduction has been demonstrated to be one of the most effective measures for reducing and controlling high blood pressure.[26]

Obesity is a major factor for diabetes, particularly late-onset diabetes. Overweight Americans aged 20 to 44 years have a 3.8 times greater risk for diabetes compared with normal weight Americans of the same age.[1] With obesity, there appears to be an increase in insulin secretion of well over 100 to 200 percent, and yet there is still a relative insulin deficiency, as indicated by elevated blood glucose levels.[27] It appears that as one becomes obese, there is a reduction in insulin receptor sites, a reduced receptor sensitivity, or both. This leads to an overproduction of insulin in an attempt to control blood glucose levels. As the obese individual undergoes weight loss, there is a subsequent return of receptor sites, sensitivity, or both, and blood glucose levels are brought under control. Whether receptor sites are actually increased or decreased, whether they become active or inactive, or whether receptor sensitivity increases or decreases is not well understood.

Abnormal plasma lipid and lipoprotein concentrations are commonly associated with obesity.[1] Most common are elevated levels of plasma triglycerides, usually due to increased rates of production of very low-density lipoproteins by the liver. Total cholesterol and low-density lipoprotein cholesterol are typically elevated, and high-density lipoprotein cholesterol is reduced in the obese patient. This lipid and lipoprotein profile is characteristic of the individual at high risk for CAD; however, weight reduction does tend to normalize these abnormal values.

Gallstones, gout, and carcinoma have also been associated with obesity.[28] Other diseases and disorders associated with obesity include respiratory insufficiency, thromboembolic disease, congestive heart failure, and increased risk from surgery.[29] Obesity also has potential social and psychological consequences.[30] The obese population is a prime target group of the mass media, which promote the image of thinness and the undesirability of being fat. The cosmetic and clothing industries also perpetuate this image.[20] Society frequently looks on the obese individual as lacking self-control and practicing overindulgence. They see obesity as a self-inflicted disability. Obesity may actually be the cause of downward mobility in society, and it may adversely influence acceptance into college, job hiring, and promotion.[20, 31] There are also practical considerations, such as impaired sexual relations, the fact that a higher percentage of one's income must go for food and clothing, and even the fact that most seats are too small to accommodate the obese individual comfortably. Despite these potential problems, the obese remain emotionally stable when compared with the general population at large.[30]

Van Itallie[1] has raised an important point in his review of the health implications of overweight and obesity in the United States. He has conducted an analysis of the independent risk associated with being overweight versus being obese. Figure 2–4 illustrates his classification system that allows the differentiation between overweight and obesity. Using this system, he has demonstrated that there are health risks associated with being overweight, even

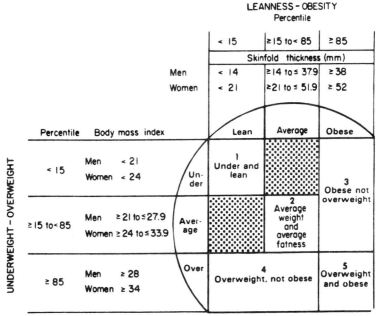

Figure 2–4. Cross-classification of the distribution of body mass index and triceps plus subscapular skinfold measurements. (From Van Itallie, T.B.: Health implications of overweight and obesity in the United States. **Ann. Int. Med.** 103:983–988, 1985.)

when the individual is not obese. Bray[32] also makes an important point that the risk associated with overweight/obesity is curvilinear. This is demonstrated in Figure 2–5 in reference to the BMI. Finally, Bjorntorp[33] has summarized a series of studies that suggests that the regional patterns of fat distribution are the most critical factors in assessing disease risk. Hypertension, CAD, diabetes, and lipid abnormalities have been closely linked with the android or male pattern of fat distribution, i.e., abdominal obesity. The risk for these diseases increases sharply when the waist to hip ratio exceeds 1.0 in men and 0.8 in women.[33]

The above discussion implies serious consequences for those who become obese. The most serious would appear to come in the area of increased morbidity and mortality from various diseases. However, there have been challenges to this assumption. Andres, after an extensive review of epidemiological studies, concluded that the major population studies of obesity and mortality fail to show that, overall, obesity leads to a greater risk. He even suggests that new research be initiated to look into the possible benefits of moderate obesity![34] Fitzgerald,[35] in a 1981 review article, presents three theses for consideration. First, obesity may be more an aesthetic and moral problem than one of physical health. Second, the therapy for obesity may be, in some circumstances, more detrimental than the degree of fatness. Finally, there may be some

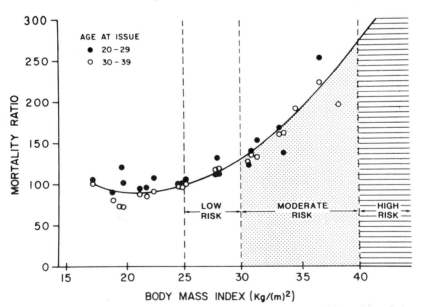

Figure 2–5. Relation of body mass index to excess mortality. (From Bray G.A.: Obesity: definition, diagnosis and disadvantages. **Med. J. Australia** 142:S2–S8, 1985.)

advantages, in medical and other senses, to being fat. She contends that when such a high percentage of the population is overweight, or exceeds the normal values, then the standards should be raised so that "normal" truly reflects normal. Finally, in a tribute to the obese, she states:

> **A well-adapted animal has the ability to store fat during periods of abundant food supply in preparation for the inevitable intervals of famine. It may be, then, that the prevalence of obesity in the United States is due to the conjunction of millions of years of evolutionary thrust with a remarkable sufficiency of food available at minimal exertion. The fat may be the most highly evolved among us. And should food become scarce through natural disaster, war, or shortages of energy, the fat may be the most likely survivors.[35]**

These views, however, appear to represent only a minority opinion.

PATHOPHYSIOLOGY OF OBESITY

To understand the pathophysiology of obesity, it is necessary to review first the morphology of adipose tissue and then the various factors that lead to the obese state, i.e., the etiology of obesity. With a basic appreciation for both the morphology of adipose tissue and the etiology of obesity, the roles of physical inactivity as a contributing factor and of physical activity as a means of dealing with the problem can be more clearly delineated.

First, what is adipose tissue? It is a form of connective tissue composed of cells (adipocytes) that are separated from each other by a matrix of collagenous fibers and yellow elastic fibers. Fat accumulates by the filling of existing adipocytes (hypertrophy) and by the formation of new fat cells (hyperplasia). The normal, nonobese individual increases fat stores from birth to maturity by a combination of hypertrophy and hyperplasia. At maturity, the obese individual has 60 to 100 billion fat cells, compared with 30 to 50 billion for the nonobese, or about two times more. Obese individuals also typically have more fat per cell.

Development of Fat Stores

How does the obese individual become obese? This may vary, depending on whether the obesity was of early or late onset. Knittle,[36] in an article reviewing much of the initial work in this area, proposed several possibilities in the genesis of obesity. Early work suggested that fat stores increased steadily for the first 9 months of life and then leveled off or increased slightly until the age of 7 years, when they once again increased. A final spurt of fat deposition supposedly occurred during adolescence. Using the needle biopsy technique, Knittle and his associates were able to determine the actual changes in fat cell size and number during these critical periods of fat deposition. In their studies, they were able to obtain samples of subcutaneous fat from obese and nonobese subjects between 2 and 26 years of age. At all age levels studied, the obese children had larger fat cells, attaining adult size by the age of 11 years, and a greater number of fat cells, often attaining the adult cell number at an early age. They concluded that it is reasonable to assume that subjects who have exceeded normal adult values for cellularity will most likely retain their obesity, whereas those who are within the normal range or below may outgrow their "baby fat."

Much of the early work indicated that fat cell number increased markedly during the first year of life, increased gradually until puberty, and then increased markedly again for a period of several years, with the maximal number of fat cells becoming stabilized or fixed by the late teens or early twenties.[36] Apparently, according to this theory, adult-onset obesity could only be the result of hypertrophy, since fat cell number became fixed before adulthood was reached. These findings seemed to be at odds with both clinical observation and subsequent scientific studies. Clinicians reported increases in total body fat in patients who were lean in early adulthood—increases that could not be accounted for only on the basis of an increase in the size of the existing cells, for adipocytes are known to have a maximal size that cannot be exceeded.[37] In a fascinating study of piglets, Widdowson and Shaw[38] took litters of pigs with a normal complement of fat cells at 10 days of age and fed half of the pigs a normal diet while starving the other half. At the end of the first year, those pigs that had been starved weighed only 5 to 6 kg, compared with a weight of 200 kg for the control group. The starved pigs had no detectable fat cells at the end of one year, although they had possessed a normal complement at 10 days of age. At the end of the first year, the starved pigs were allowed to eat freely, and were soon of normal or above normal body fat. This study and others raised serious questions regarding the stability of fat cell number at a specific age and cast doubts on the methodology that had been used to assess fat cell number.[37, 39]

The potential problem of methodological error in fat cell counting is an important issue. If fat cell number is increased only to a certain age, i.e., maturity, at which point it becomes fixed, then the first 20 years of one's life are extremely critical with respect to preventing or controlling obesity. Entering adulthood with a low number of fat cells should ensure one a life free of extreme obesity, since the existing fat cells cannot enlarge beyond a certain size. On the other hand, those who enter adulthood with an elevated number of cells will be doomed to a life of obesity. It has been suggested that the initial methods used to determine fat cell number may have, in fact, underestimated the true number of fat cells.[37] Using an automated cell counter for counting osmium-fixed fat cells, the early studies most likely were not able to measure cells with a diameter of less than 25 microns. Also, early studies were unable to detect preadipocytes and undifferentiated cells that were destined to become adipocytes. Sjostrom[37] provides an excellent discussion of these methodological considerations in his review. A more accurate technique involves taking a frozen slice of adipose tissue and calculating a mean cell diameter from individual measurements of 100 or more adipocytes. Mean cell volume can be calculated from the mean cell diameter, and this value is then used to determine the mean fat cell weight. Dividing total body fat by mean fat cell weight then provides an estimate of total fat cell number.[37]

Current evidence suggests that fat cells can be increased throughout life and that the achievement of some mean adipocyte size triggers the events that culminate in an increase in the number of adipocytes.[40] Whether this increase in cell number is the result of newly formed cells or simply the use of existing preadipocytes or undifferentiated cells has yet to be resolved.

With respect to the developmental aspects of adipose tissue, Sjostrom and his colleagues conducted a longitudinal study on 16 healthy, nonobese infants from the first through the eighteenth month of life.[37] Six biopsies from gluteal adipose depots were taken throughout this 18-month period. Fat weight increased from 0.7 to 2.8 kg during the first 12 months, an increase that was primarily the result of increases in fat cell size, with little increase in fat cell number. Fat weight increased another 0.5 kg during the next 6 months, with cell size remaining constant and cell number increasing. By 12 months of age, the existing fat cells had reached adult size. This would tend to confirm the hypothesis that increases in cell number are triggered by the attainment of a certain maximal cell size.

Alterations in Fat Cell Size and Number

A number of studies have been conducted in an attempt to manipulate fat cell size and number. Faust and coworkers[41] placed newborn rat pups into either small litters (4 pups/litter) or large litters (20 pups/litter). After weaning, half of the rats from the small litters and half from the large litters were placed on ordinary stock diets for nearly a year, while the remaining halves of the large and small litters were placed on the stock diet for the first 6 months and then switched to a highly palatable high-fat diet for the remaining 6 months. The average body weights of the four groups at the end of the experiment were 704 versus 956 g for the large and small litter rats fed the high-fat diet, and 584 versus 749 g for the large and small litter rats fed the stock diet throughout the study. Fat cell size was not influenced by the size of the litters, but fat cell number was greater in rats raised in small litters. The high-fat diet resulted in increases in both cell size and cell number. The authors pointed to the importance of early nutrition in establishing a basis for obesity later in life. This is certainly true with respect to fat cell number, as fat cell number apparently can only increase, never decrease. Fat cell size, however, is much more amenable to change.[42]

Studies have also been conducted on experimental obesity in humans. Sims[43] has conducted several studies on experimental weight gains in both college students and inmates from a state prison. First, he found that it was difficult to add even 10 percent to the normal body weight when the activity of the subject was not restricted. He reported data on 22 volunteers with restricted activity who achieved a weight gain of 20 percent or more of their initial weight.[43] He found that once a desired experimental level of overweight was achieved, it took the consumption of a considerable number of calories to maintain that weight, i.e., 3,100 kcal maintained the subjects' initial weight, but 5,100 kcal were necessary to maintain their experimental overweight. He found that the initial weight gain and the subsequent weight loss back to the original weight were accomplished without a change in the number of fat cells, i.e., fat cell number did not increase with weight gain or decrease with weight loss. Salens and associates[44] reported similar results with a 3- to 4-month period of weight gain. Their six subjects had a mean gain of 16.2 kg, 10.4 kg being fat. This gain in fat and the subsequent reductions back to normal values were not accompanied by changes in fat cell number, just changes in fat cell size.

From the preceding discussion, it appears that fat cell size can vary throughout life, but only up to a certain maximal dimension. Fat cell number also appears to vary throughout life, although it is relatively stable once maturity is reached. Increases in cell number are probably the result of the existing fat cells attaining a certain maximal cell size, which then acts to trigger an increase in cell number. Hypercellularity leads to a permanently elevated cellular mass, making weight loss in the obese an extremely difficult task. This possibly, at least partially, explains the high rate of failure of obese subjects on weight reduction programs. In fact, there is evidence that women with hyperplastic obesity (elevated cell number) have a much more difficult time with weight reduction[45] in that they appear to be more resistant to weight loss and regain weight rapidly after weight loss. Once fat cells reach a certain minimal size, they appear to be resistant to further weight or fat losses.

Distribution of Body Fat

The manner in which the body makes decisions on where to store fat is now much better understood. Triglycerides, being insoluble in the blood, are transported in the circulation by chylomicrons, one of several lipid protein carriers. The enzyme lipoprotein lipase is produced in the chylomicrons but works on the surface of the adjacent capillary endothelium (inner lining of the capillary). Where lipoprotein lipase is heavily concentrated, and thus has high activity in the tissue capillaries, the adipocytes are trapped, and the triglyceride is hydrolyzed and transported into the adipocyte. Thus, lipoprotein lipase acts as a "gatekeeper" controlling the distribution of triglyceride in the various storage depots. This explains, in part, the differences in fat patterning between men and women. Women who are normally menstruating have very high lipoprotein lipase levels and activity in the hip and thigh regions compared with the abdominal region. Lipolytic activity (breaking down of fat stores) is also very low in the hip and thigh regions. With high lipoprotein lipase activity and low lipolytic activity in the hip and thigh regions, it is understandable that women would pattern fat selectively in these regions. This preferential selection of the hip and thigh regions for fat deposition appears to be related to reproductive function in that these depots are active fuel reserves during the last trimester of pregnancy and throughout the period of lactation. The reader is referred to an excellent summary of the research in this area by Bjorntorp.[46] This predictable pattern of fat distribution between sexes should relate in some manner to the higher health risk associated with upper body (male) versus lower body (female) obesity.

Set-Point Theory of Weight Control

During the past 20 years, there have been a growing number of scientists who are turning to the set-point theory of weight regulation, a theory that explains, at least in part, the resistance of both humans and animals to weight gains and losses. When animals and humans are either overfed to promote weight gains or underfed to induce weight losses, once the animal or human returns to ad libitum feeding or eating, normal weight is quickly reestablished. There is now considerable evidence to support the set-point theory.[47]

With periods of overeating the body increases its metabolic rate, a phenomenon that is referred to as the thermogenic response to food, or dietary-induced thermogenesis (DIT). The normal, non-obese individual increases his or her resting metabolic rate by 15 to 25 percent or more in response to a 750 to 1,000 kcal dietary intake.[23] The obese individual, however, appears to have a blunted DIT response to the same standardized dietary intake.[23] Obese individuals also appear to attenuate their thermogenic response to a cold stress, i.e., they have a smaller increment in resting metabolic rate in response to the cold stress.

With dietary restriction, there is generally a reduction in the resting metabolic rate (RMR) and in voluntary physical activity.[23] This reduction in RMR can be of the magnitude of 20 percent or higher, with several studies reporting decreases of 30 percent.[48] This would indicate that the body is attempting to protect or defend its weight. Thus, the body is able to achieve some stability in weight even with extended periods of overfeeding or underfeeding through alterations in RMR, DIT, and physical activity. This is illustrated as follows:

	Overfeeding	**Underfeeding**
Resting Metabolic Rate	increased	decreased
Dietary-Induced Thermogenesis	increased	decreased
Voluntary Physical Activity	increased	decreased

The degree of control exerted by these mechanisms to defend body weight is rather remarkable. An imbalance of 10 kcal per day, or approximately one potato chip, will lead to an approximate weight gain of one pound per year (10 kcal × 365 days/year = 3,650 kcals/year). With an average caloric intake of 2,500 kcal per day, this would be an error of only 0.4 percent! A 100 kcal error, i.e., intake greater than expenditure by 100 kcal/day, would lead to a 10 pound weight gain per year. Yet, this would be only a 4.0 percent error in metabolism.

How is weight set-point controlled? There does appear to be a center in the hypothalamus responsible for controlling food intake.[47] The lateral hypothalamus is postulated to contain the feeding center. Lesions to this center reduce the drive to eat, whereas stimulation of this center increases the drive to eat. The ventral medial hypothalamus is postulated to contain the satiety center. Lesions to this center increase the drive to eat, and stimulation of this center reduces the drive to eat.[47] Keesey[47] has conducted a number of studies with animals, observing their eating behavior in response to hypothalamic lesions and stimulation. Figure 2–6 illustrates a series of experiments conducted on rats that had received lateral hypothalamic lesions during periods of ad libitum and restricted feeding. Keesey's experiments provide convincing evidence for the existence of a set-point for body weight. The reader is referred to Keesey's excellent summary of the research on set-point theory for additional information in this area.[47]

Can set-point be altered? There is now evidence that indicates that set-point can be altered.[47] Long-term exposure to weight-promoting diets appears to alter set-point to allow a greater body weight. Anoretic drugs and hormones also appear to alter the body's

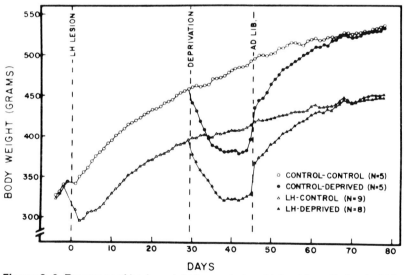

Figure 2–6. Recovery of body weight by control and lateral hypothalamic (LH)-lesioned rats after a period of food restriction. The body weights of both deprived groups were first reduced to 80% of the weight maintained by the nondeprived control and LH-lesioned animals. The deprived groups were then returned to an ad libitum feeding schedule. (From Mitchel, J.S., and Keesey, R.E.: Defense of a lowered weight maintenance level by lateral hypothalamically lesioned rats: evidence from a restriction-refeeding regimen. **Physiol. Behavior** 18:1123, 1977.)

set-point. Cessation of smoking may alter set-point upward, and increased physical activity may lower set-point. Aging may also alter set-point, allowing increases in weight with age.[47]

The final question to be asked with respect to set-point theory is one that is still being debated. Is obesity the result of a regulatory failure, i.e., inability to regulate at the appropriate set-point, or is obesity the result of an elevated set-point? The limited evidence to date would suggest that there may be, in fact, two forms of obesity: regulatory failure and elevated set-point.[47] If this is true, this would have important implications with respect to the treatment of obesity and expected outcomes.

Metabolic Efficiency

During the 1980's, investigators became interested in a concept that they feel might explain not only why individuals become obese but also why those who are obese have difficulty losing weight and maintaining their new weight once weight loss has occurred. The concept of metabolic or energy efficiency is closely related to set-point theory as discussed in the previous section. The body appears to adjust its metabolic rate in an attempt to maintain a given weight. As an example, studies of both nonobese men[48, 49] and obese men and women[50–53] have shown that RMR is reduced with caloric restriction and weight loss. Bray[51] fed his subjects a 3,500 kcal diet for a period of 7 days followed by a 450 kcal diet for 24 days. Resting oxygen consumption decreased by 15 percent (Fig. 2–7). The body appears to be sensing a crisis and reduces the rate of energy expenditure to conserve energy stores.

A similar phenomenon has been reported with individuals who undergo what has been termed "weight cycling." These individuals go on and off of diets repeatedly throughout their lives, a sequence that has been referred to as "yo-yo" dieting.[54] With each dieting cycle, there appears to be a slower rate of weight loss and a faster rate of weight regain. Brownell and colleagues[54] have studied this in rats. They took rats through two cycles of weight loss and weight gain through refeeding. During the second cycle, the rate of weight loss was decreased to only half of that for the first cycle, and the rate of regain was increased by a factor of three. To lose the same amount of weight (131 g), it took the rats 46 days in the second cycle and only 21 days in the first. During the period of refeeding, to regain the weight lost during the period of food restriction, it took 46 days for the first cycle and only 14 days for the second. This study is illustrated in Figure 2–8. Steen and associates[55]

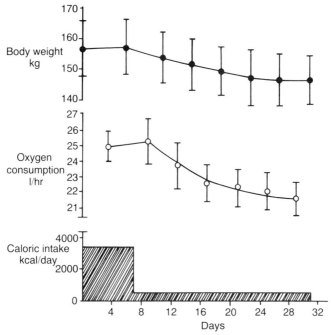

Figure 2–7. Reduction in energy expenditure during a caloric restriction diet from 3,500 to 450 kcal per day. (Adapted from Bray, G.A.: Effect of caloric restriction on energy expenditure in obese patients. **Lancet** 2:397–398, 1969.)

observed lower mean RMR in wrestlers who went through repeated cycles of weight loss and weight regain when compared with wrestlers who maintained relatively stable body weights during the competitive season. Gray and coworkers,[56] however, were not able to confirm a similar metabolic efficiency in obese rats who went through two successive periods of weight loss and weight regain.

Thus, it appears that the body makes constant adaptations to protect its energy stores and that the more these energy stores are challenged, the more the body adapts to prevent further insults. This promises to be an exciting area for future research.

ETIOLOGY OF OBESITY: RISK FACTORS

How does obesity develop? What factors contribute to its development? Society has been both kind and cruel in its perception of the obese individual, swinging like a pendulum from the one extreme of "glandular problems" to the other extreme of gluttony.

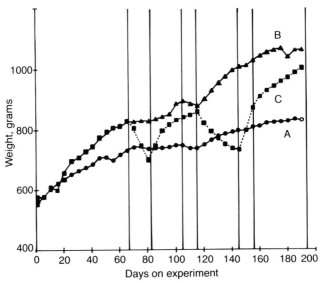

Figure 2–8. Variation in body weight in rats eating normal rat chow (A), rats eating a high-fat diet throughout the experiment (B), and rats fed a high-fat diet who went through two cycles of weight loss and regain (C). (Adapted from Brownell, K.D., et al.: The effects of repeated cycles of weight loss and regain in rats. **Physiol. Behavior** 38:459–464, 1986.)

In the first, all blame is removed from the individual; in the second, the individual must accept full responsibility. Fox, in his classic article entitled "The Enigma of Mass Regulation," states that to dispose of obesity as being due to overeating is about as helpful as attributing alcoholism to the consumption of too much alcohol.[57] It is now clear that obesity is the result of a number of causes, an observation that has led to the formation of several classification systems for obesity.

One of the first classification systems was proposed by von Noorden in the early 1900's.[27] He classified obesity into two major types: endogenous (including metabolic abnormalities, endocrine abnormalities, and brain lesions) and exogenous, which comprised basically everything from outside the body (including overeating and physical inactivity). Bray proposed an anatomical classification, i.e., hypertrophic versus hyperplastic, or obesity due to increases in cell size versus increases in cell number,[58] as well as an etiological classification.[59] In his etiological classification, Bray lists the following factors: genetics, nutrition, inactivity, endocrine function, hypothalamic function, and drugs.[59] Five of these six factors are discussed briefly here. Drugs are not reviewed.

Genetics

The genetic aspects of obesity are difficult to discern. There are certain genetic disorders that predispose one to obesity, such as the Laurence-Moon-Bardet-Biedl syndrome, Alstrom's syndrome, and Morgagni's syndrome.[59] Of greater concern, however, is the familial aspect of obesity. Is there a genetic link between the obese parent and the obese child, or is the obesity the result of their eating at the same table and living under the same environmental conditions? These are not easy questions to answer. Foch and McClearn[60] have published a review of the literature in this area. They reported that studies on various species of animals indicate that there is a definite genetic component to obesity. With humans, investigations are much more difficult to control, and the results are not as definitive. Typical models used include observing identical twins raised in the same or in different environments and observing adopted children compared with their biological parents (genetic) and their adoptive parents (environmental). Foch and McClearn concluded that twin studies and family studies implicate a heritable component in the development of obesity, but the evidence is far from clear.[60] The magnitude of the genetic contribution varied considerably with the criterion of obesity, e.g., weight versus skinfolds, and depended on age and sex.

Most recently, Stunkard and colleagues[61, 62] have provided convincing evidence for a strong genetic component in human obesity. In a sample of 540 adult Danish adoptees, there was a strong relation between the weight class of the adoptees and the BMI of their biological parents, but there was no relation with the BMI of their adoptive parents. This is illustrated in Figure 2–9. In a second study of 1,974 monozygotic and 2,097 dizygotic male twin pairs, concordance rates for different degrees of overweight were twice as high for monozygotic twins as for dizygotic twins, with approximately 80 percent of the variance in BMI accounted for by genetic factors. Garn[63] makes a plea for caution in interpreting studies such as these. He feels that the statistical procedures may be leading to overestimates and that both genetic and social factors interact to create the obese state.

Nutrition

In the previous sections on the morphology of adipose tissue and set-point theory, a number of studies were cited that supported the importance of nutritional factors in the development of obesity.

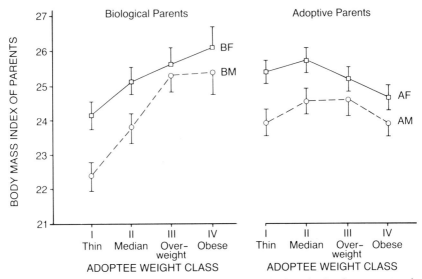

Figure 2–9. The mean body mass index of biological and adoptive parents of 4 weight classes of adoptees. F = father, M = mother. (From Stunkard, A.J., Foch, T.T., and Hrubec, Z.: A twin study of human obesity. **JAMA** 256:51–54, 1986.)

Overfeeding, as demonstrated by the rats raised in small litters and by the overfeeding studies in humans, leads to major increases in total body fat.[41, 43] Rats placed on high-fat diets also gain substantially more body fat than similar rats fed standard stock diets.[41] The cafeteria or supermarket diet, a diet with a great variety of highly palatable foods with a high percentage of fat and simple sugars, has been repeatedly demonstrated to produce marked obesity in animal models.[64] This diet was patterned after the typical American diet. The size and number of meals per day also influence the development of obesity, with frequent small meals resulting in smaller gains in adipose tissue.[57] Thus, total calories, the composition and palatability of the diet, the variety of foods available, and meal size and frequency are all factors that appear to be linked to obesity.

Inactivity

Many of the early studies that are reviewed in this section suggest that childhood obesity is associated more with physical inactivity than with overeating. Jean Mayer, world-famous nutritionist, has stated, "I am convinced that inactivity is the most important factor in explaining the frequency of 'creeping' overweight in modern Western societies."[65] Bruch studied a group of 160 obese children and found that 76 percent of the boys and 68 percent of the girls were abnormally inactive, whereas only 8 percent of the boys and 22 percent of the girls fell within what would be considered to be a normal range of activity.[66] Rony,[67] Bronstein and coworkers,[68] Graham,[69] Tolstrup,[70] and Juel-Nielsen[71] observed similar results. Fry[72] found obese children to have average caloric intakes comparable with those of nonobese children of the same age, but a much higher proportion of the obese were labeled as only moderately active or as inactive. Johnson and associates[73] observed two groups of high school girls—28 obese and 28 nonobese of similar height, age, and grade—with respect to maturation, food intake, and physical activity. The obese girls showed advanced development, with an earlier deceleration of growth in height and an earlier menarche. The caloric intake of the obese group was significantly lower than that of the nonobese group, and although both groups were found to be relatively inactive, the obese girls were significantly more so.

Stefanik and colleagues[74] studied food intake and energy expenditure patterns of 14 obese adolescent boys in relation to a paired control group of nonobese boys during summer camp. The energy intake of the obese boys was significantly less than that of the nonobese boys. In addition, although little difference was noted in the amount of time scheduled for light, moderate, and very active exercise, the degree of participation in active exercise was generally less for the obese. Bullen and associates[75] employed a motion picture technique for comparing activity levels of obese and nonobese adolescent girls while they engaged in three sports at a summer camp. Three-second shots were taken at regular intervals and were analyzed for the time spent motionless and for energy expenditure calculated on the basis of type and speed of locomotion and intensity of movement. On the basis of nearly 30,000 observations, it was concluded that the obese girls were far less active than the nonobese girls. Corbin and Pletcher[76] observed the caloric intake and physical activity patterns of obese and nonobese elementary school children; they found the groups to have similar energy intakes, but the obese had significantly lower activity levels.

However, to the contrary, Durnin[77] observed energy intake and expenditure in approximately 100 boys and girls, 13 to 15 years of age. Although energy intake was not specified by classification of obesity, he found that there was no difference in the number of minutes per day spent in moderate or heavy physical activity between lean, normal, and obese subjects. Watson and O'Donovan[78] studied 85 17- to 18-year-old school boys and found no relationship between relative leanness and fatness and the level of habitual physical activity. Wilkinson and coworkers[79] reported on the energy intake and physical activity levels of obese and matched nonobese 10-year-old boys and girls and found no significant differences between the groups for energy intake or expenditure. Bradfield and colleagues[80] reported no significant differences in energy expenditure between nonobese and obese girls during physical education classes, school classroom activities, and afterschool work or play. Three-day activity assessments showed that both groups were very inactive, 70 percent of their time being spent either in sleep or in very light activities. Waxman and Stunkard[81] converted measures of activity into caloric expenditure by measuring oxygen consumption and found that obese boys actually expended more calories through activity than did nonobese boys.

In the adult population, Brownell and Stunkard[82] conclude that obese adults are less active than are those of normal weight, on the basis of studies that have used self-report, pedometers, spontaneous use of stairs in place of escalators in public places, and a device that discriminates standing from sitting. In a classic study, Brownell and associates observed the use of stairs versus escalators in several locations where the stairs and escalators were adjacent to each other, i.e., shopping mall, train station, and bus terminal.[83] Initial observations showed 1.5 percent of the obese and 6.7 percent of the nonobese to use the stairway in one study, and 6.6 percent and 11.8 percent in a second study. When cartoon sketches of a heart using the stairs with the message "Your heart needs exercise" were placed in front of the stairway, twice as many nonobese individuals used the stairways in both studies, whereas 7.8 percent of the obese responded by using the stairs in the first study, but there was no increase in the second study! They suggest that caution be used in interpreting these data, since lower levels of activity may not represent lower levels of energy expenditure because of the greater cost of activities for the obese person. Also, it is not clear whether the inactivity is a cause of obesity or the result of it.

Thus, for the population of both children and adults, the role of physical inactivity in predisposing one to obesity is still not resolved. Additional research is needed. Such research must approach this problem from a fresh perspective, using tight controls and taking advantage of recent developments in monitoring equipment. It is becoming clear, however, that there are increasing levels of obesity in the pediatric population. Gortmaker and colleagues[84] have reported that over an approximate 10- to 15-year span, obesity in 6- to 11-year-olds and 12- to 17-year-olds had increased by 54 percent and 39 percent, respectively, while superobesity increased by 98 percent and 64 percent, respectively. This increase may or may not be the direct result of the observed decreases in physical activity.

Endocrine Function

Three different endocrine manipulations can produce obesity: administration of insulin, administration of glucocorticoids, and castration.[58] Also, approximately 12 substances, which either are hormones or have hormone-like activity, have been identified as being involved in stimulating lipogenesis, and an additional nine stimulate lipolysis.[57] Thus, it is not surprising that the endocrine system is implicated in weight control and obesity. With respect to the three endocrine manipulations, experimental elevation of insulin produces hyperphagia, or overeating. This hyperphagia is in response either to lowered blood glucose levels or to the direct effect of insulin on the brain. Glucocorticoids administered experimentally to animals often result in increases in body fat with little or no increase in body weight. Evidently, steroid administration modifies the metabolism of adipose tissue toward increased fat storage.[58] Castration of animals results in substantial redistributions of body fat, undoubtedly mediated through altered estrogen and testosterone levels in the blood plasma.

Hypothalamic Function

The hypothalamus is implicated in obesity primarily through lesions in specific areas of the lower anterior portion of the ventromedial nucleus. Most lesions are experimentally induced in animals to determine changes in feeding behavior. This was discussed earlier in this chapter under set-point theory. Although this information is important in trying to better understand what controls eating behavior, actual lesions of the hypothalamus in the human population are extremely rare.

PREVENTION AND TREATMENT OF OBESITY

Ideally, obesity should be prevented. However, realistically, millions of Americans are obese, and many are desperately seeking help. Although prevention is basically a matter of balancing caloric expenditure with caloric intake, treatment of the obese person involves a much more complex plan of action. For those who are moderately obese (no more than 20 to 30 pounds above ideal weight as determined by body composition assessment), a modest reduction in caloric intake of approximately 250 kcal per day and an equally modest increase in activity level of 250 kcal per day (e.g., 2.5 miles of walking) should result in a 1-pound weight loss per week. This 500 kcal deficit per day would total 3,500 kcal per week, which is approximately the energy equivalent of a pound of adipose tissue. Over a 20- to 30-week period, weight would return to desirable levels. For those who are grossly obese, more drastic measures are often taken. The forms of treatment generally used include diet; drugs; surgery; behavioral modification, self-help groups, psychoanalysis, and psychotherapy; and physical activity. Several textbooks have reviewed these areas of treatment in considerable detail.[23, 85–90] A very brief review is conducted in this chapter on the areas of diet, drugs, surgery, and the behavioral aspects. Physical activity is discussed in considerable detail in Chapter 4.

Once obesity has been identified, it is important to start treatment as soon as possible. Generally, the greater the degree of obesity, the more difficult it is to treat successfully. Three key factors in any treatment program are motivation, expectation, and self-responsibility. Providing information to the obese individual is not sufficient by itself, as most obese individuals are very well-educated in this area. Motivation can take many forms, but it can be illustrated by the general program used in behavior modification, in which a system of goals and rewards is established. There must also be a well-defined reason for the weight loss, one that will truly be motivational for the individual. For many, the reason may be cosmetic, i.e., they want to look better. For others, health may be the reason, e.g., the hypertensive or diabetic patient. Regarding expectations, the obese person must have established a realistic weight goal. When this goal is a considerable distance from the present weight, intermediate goals must be set, along with designated times for accomplishing them. If weight loss does not follow the patient's expectation, he or she will typically become discouraged and discontinue the treatment program. The patient should also be warned about plateaus, or periods of decreased rate of weight loss. If these are expected, they will not produce serious anxiety, guilt, and discouragement when they occur.

In the dietary treatment of obesity, several levels of treatment are possible: starvation and fasting, semistarvation or very low-calorie diets (300 to 600 kcal), and diets that are moderately deficient in calories, i.e., 500 kcal or less below maintenance levels. Starvation and fasting are usually considered to be synonymous terms, but with starvation, vitamins and minerals are not typically supplemented. In total fasting, the amount of glucose stored in the muscles and liver can suffice for only relatively short periods of time, after which amino acids from muscle protein are used for gluconeogenesis. Thus, protein loss does occur, and there are accompanying losses of nitrogen. During fasting, the major fuel for most tissues is derived from free fatty acids, with the release of ketone bodies into the blood. These are referred to as ketoacids and include acetone, which imparts a characteristic odor to the breath. In a 24-hour fast, a normal man lying down uses 1,800 kcal of energy, including 360 kcals from 75 g of protein. The remaining energy comes from triglycerides. The contribution of protein decreases to 18 to 24 g per day with prolonged fasting. The initial loss of 75 g of protein per day can be reduced to 15 g per day by having the subject consume a liter of dextrose water (10 percent solution).[28]

With a total fasting regime, the typical 300-pound patient averages a weight loss of approximately a pound per day for the first 2 months. Up to 46 pounds of this 60-pound weight loss can come from the lean tissues, leaving a loss of body fat of approximately 14 to 16 pounds, or only 23 to 25 percent of the total weight loss. Most of the water loss (67 percent) comes from the extracellular fluid compartment, with a plasma volume loss of from 400 to 700 ml. There are a number of potential complications of total fasting, including nausea, diarrhea, persistent vomiting, postural hypotension, nutritional deficiencies, menstrual irregularities, and sudden death. There is, however, a general loss of appetite within the first 2 days, which remains throughout the period of fasting; this is considered to be a positive aspect of this approach to weight loss.

The long-term benefits of fasting, evaluated on the basis of follow-up studies, are disappointing.[28] The large amounts of weight lost during the fast are quickly regained. It is important to evaluate any treatment regimen on the basis of long-term follow-up studies. Although the immediate results are of interest, the real test is in the follow-up data of 5 years or more.

Semistarvation, or very low-calorie, diets result in changes similar to those seen in total fasting, although to a lesser degree. Water losses are considerable during the first several weeks of dieting, but the protein losses are of a much lower magnitude. In both fasting and semistarvation diets, ketone bodies are formed from the increased metabolism of free fatty acids. High blood and urine levels of ketone bodies (ketosis) may be responsible for loss of appetite, but they may also have undesirable side effects. Thus, many diets suggest monitoring urine on a daily basis for the presence of ketosis, so that modifications can be made if ketone levels are too high.

More recently, traditional very low-calorie diets have been modified to reduce the loss of protein, i.e., protein-sparing modified fasting diets. In addition, supplements have been added to some of these diets to ensure adequate intake levels of the essential vitamins and minerals. Finally, small amounts of glucose have been added to increase even more the protein-sparing aspects of the diet. A fairly standard low-calorie diet includes 15 to 25 g of high biological value protein, such as egg albumin, and 45 g of carbohydrate. The early diets used a low-grade protein source, and approximately 60 deaths were reported associated with the use of these early diets.

Moderate decreases in caloric intake can be achieved without major alterations in the individual's diet. Simply cutting down on portion sizes, reducing the intake of highly calorie-dense foods, and eliminating between-meal snacking can lead to reductions in total caloric intake of 200 to 500 kcal. Although this is a much slower approach, the individual is learning a new pattern of eating that, ideally, will result in a more permanent loss of weight. Also, the losses in lean tissue and body water are much less, resulting in larger percent decreases in body fat, i.e., the percentage of the weight lost from fat is increased.

Although common sense is probably the best guide to dieting for optimal weight loss, many individuals feel that they must follow one or more of the popular diets currently in vogue. Most of these diets have far more similarities than differences, but some can be potentially dangerous. The reader is referred to several excellent reviews of popular diets written by Smoller and colleagues,[91] Hodgson,[92] and Nicholas and Dwyer.[93]

The use of drugs has become a very popular means of treating obesity. Drugs presently used include anorexigenic agents, thyroid preparations, digitalis, diuretics, bulking agents, starch blockers, and human chorionic gonadotropin. Anoretic drugs, by definition, are those agents that act to decrease appetite, and they are usually classified as amphetamines and nonamphetamines.[94] The mechanisms through which these drugs act are quite complex and well beyond the scope of this chapter.[95] The anoretic drugs do appear to result in weight loss, but the loss is usually only temporary, with weight being quickly regained after the cessation of drug therapy. There are moderate to serious side effects associated with anoretic drugs, including the potential for drug abuse or addiction. Thyroid preparations have been used in the treatment of obesity, but this practice is not a very effective form of drug therapy, and it is no longer popular. Similarly, digitalis was at one time a popular drug for the treatment of obesity, but it is seldom used by physicians today. Diuretics have also been popular in weight loss programs in which large weight losses are desired. These lead to major losses in total body water, however, with little loss in body fat. With certain individuals, diuretics may aggravate the loss of electrolytes, which is certainly an undesirable side effect. Bulking agents are usually calorically inert bulk materials that lead to feelings of fullness in the stomach. They have been used with little or no success. Starch blockers, or alpha-amylase inhibitors, supposedly blocked the digestion of starch in meals. Over one million starch-blocker tablets were consumed daily in the United States in the first part of 1982.[96] The Food and Drug Administration removed these from the shelves in stores, and studies were unable to demonstrate any benefits from their use.[96] Finally, about 25 years ago, a new treatment was proposed in which the subject was injected with human chorionic gonadotropin, a compound obtained from the urine of pregnant women. Daily injections coupled with a 500 kcal diet were supposed to lead to major losses of body fat. Controlled studies have failed to demonstrate that these injections are any more effective than the 500 kcal diet alone.[94, 97]

Surgery has become an increasingly popular means of dealing with the grossly obese patient when all other forms of treatment have failed. The first surgical intervention was the jejunoileal bypass surgery, in which the jejunum is connected with the terminal ileum, bypassing a substantial portion of the small intestine. Although this procedure resulted in substantial weight loss for most patients, the side effects were typically major. In addition to a high operative mortality rate (up to 6 percent), complications included pulmonary embolus, serious wound infection, and renal failure. Liver failure is an occasional complication, and persistent diarrhea is almost always present. Gastric bypass surgery has become the more accepted surgical approach in recent years. Referred to as gastric stapling, the stomach is stapled together, dividing it into a proximal and distal portion. The proximal portion is small and becomes the functional portion of the stomach. The distal portion is much larger and becomes nonfunctional. This procedure has resulted in rather marked weight losses, and the complications appear to be far less serious when compared with those of the intestinal bypass procedure.[98] Most recently, gastric balloons have been used to reduce the size of the stomach. The balloon is inserted into the stomach, inflated to a predetermined size, and then left in the stomach. This procedure is sufficiently new that its long-term results are not available. Finally, jaw wiring has drawn considerable attention because of the uniqueness of the procedure. Through the use of mandibular fixation, the jaws are wired together, preventing the ingestion of solid food. Unlike gastric stapling and intestinal bypass surgery, jaw wiring weight losses are transitory, with weight being quickly regained after the removal of the wires.

A great deal of attention has been focused on the behavioral treatment of obesity and eating disorders. Pioneered by Stuart in 1967[99] and made popular by Stuart and Davis's book *Slim Chance in a Fat World: Behavioral Control of Obesity*,[100] this rather practical approach to the treatment of obesity became very popular in the 1970's and 1980's. Based on an approach to weight loss that focused on the patient's feeding behavior, a major goal was to achieve a permanent change in lifestyle patterns. Attention was given to the patient's ingestive behavior by looking at pace or speed of eating, bite size, bite frequency, pause time between bites, and the length of chewing time. Organismic variables such as the state of hunger, mood state, and the physical state were also evaluated. Behavioral factors such as the physical position while eating, the activities associated with eating, and the stimuli preceding or concurrent with eating, were also important input variables associated with the individual's total eating behavior profile. Once these variables were determined, the individual's behavior was "shaped," making gradual changes in eating behavior. Thus, the individual learned those problem areas in his or her eating behavior that were responsible for the weight problem. Then, eating patterns were altered, or shaped, to produce a more favorable eating behavior that would lead to weight loss and control of weight at desirable levels. Although the early research on behavior modification was highly favorable and the technique was considered superior to other treatment modalities, long-term studies have indicated that it too is not immune from a return to prior eating behaviors and, thus, a return to pretreatment body weight.[101] Most recent studies have pointed to the efficacy of combining behavior modification with very low-calorie diets.[102] Brownell has written an excellent text on the applied behavioral therapy approach.[103]

From the above, it appears that all present forms of the treatment of obesity are confronted with either potential major complications associated with the treatment (e.g., surgery) or with problems of poor compliance (e.g., diet and behavior modification). It is evident that far more research effort must go into two major areas: prevention and compliance. First, it is far easier to prevent obesity than to be challenged with its treatment, and it is far easier to treat obesity if it is identified in its early stages. Second, very little is known about how to deal with problems of noncompliance. This is true not only of treatment programs for obesity but also of treatment programs for hypertension, diabetes, or any other diseases that are treated pharmacologically. Research directed toward gaining a better understanding of those factors that influence compliance is essential. This is a problem that is universal in almost all areas of medicine.

SUMMARY

Overweight and obesity constitute serious health problems in the United States. Overweight refers to any weight that exceeds the range of weights for a specific height, frame size, and gender— a range that was determined on the basis of population averages. Obesity refers to being overfat. Although overweight and obesity are related, there is a sizable percentage of individuals who are "overweight" but of normal or below normal body fat, or who are "normal" weight but excessively fat. A body composition assessment is essential to determine obesity and to estimate a reasonable, desirable, or "ideal" body weight.

The average individual gains approximately a pound of weight per year during each year beyond the age of 25. At the same time, there is a loss of approximately one-quarter to one-half pound per year of lean body tissue, predominantly from muscle and bone. The loss in lean tissue is closely associated with reductions in physical activity, i.e., if you do not use it, you will lose it! The net result is a gain of 1.5 pounds per year of fat weight, or a total of 45 pounds of extra body fat by the age of 55 years. To reiterate, these values represent mean values for the United States population. This increase in body fat has economic, medical, social, and psychological consequences. In a single year, billions of dollars are spent, thousands of people die, and millions suffer, all the result of our present epidemic of obesity.

What is the basic cause of obesity? Unfortunately, the answer to this question is complex and undoubtedly involves genetic, nutritional, endocrine, hypothalamic, and pharmacological factors, in addition to physical inactivity. The end result is an increased fat cell size and probably an increased number of fat cells, or adipocytes. Knittle[36] believes that individuals are probably genetically endowed with a certain range of adipose tissue cellularity that can be modified by a variety of environmental influences. The final depot size will in all likelihood depend upon the interaction of a genetic template with all the environmental and hormonal factors that influence number and size. Several newer theories that tie in both genetic and environmental factors have been proposed to explain obesity. Newsholme[104] has proposed disruption of substrate cycling as a potential basis for obesity. Substrate cycling involves an obligatory loss of chemical energy as heat, and it may be important in burning off excess energy. In obesity, hormonal and nervous control of substrate cycles may be impaired. DeLuise and associates[105] have found the number of sodium-potassium pump units in erythrocytes to be reduced by 22 percent in obese persons as compared with nonobese controls. The cation transport activity of the pump was also reduced, and an increased concentration of sodium was found in the red cells. This would be considered a thermogenic defect resulting in a decrease in cellular thermogenesis. More recent studies have been unable to confirm this theory.[106] These and other theories are being explored, and it is hoped that within the near future we will have a better understanding of the etiology of obesity.

The treatment of obesity is equally complex. Present forms of treatment include diet, drugs, surgery, behavior modification, and increased physical activity. With all forms of treatment, the major problem involves a lack of total commitment on the part of the obese patient. Although rather spectacular decreases in weight can occur with just about any form of treatment, the true success of any treatment is in the long-term follow-up. In all cases, with the exception of surgery, the follow-up results are not encouraging. Thus, attention must be given first to the prevention of the problem. Second, for those who become obese, the condition should be diagnosed as soon as possible. Third, once obesity has been diagnosed, an acceptable plan of treatment should be outlined, and considerable effort should be placed on seeing the patient follow through with that plan, including long-term follow-up well beyond the period of treatment.

References

1. Van Itallie, T.B.: Health implications of overweight and obesity in the United States. **Ann. Intern. Med.** 103:983–988, 1985.
2. Grande, F., and Keys, A.: Body weight, body composition and calorie status. In Goodhart, R.S., and Shils, M.E. (eds.): **Modern Nutrition in Health and Disease,** 6th Ed. Philadelphia, Lea & Febiger, 1980.
3. Harrison, G.G.: Height-weight tables. **Ann. Intern. Med.** 103:989–994, 1985.
4. Metropolitan Life Insurance Company: New weight standards for men and women. **Stat. Bull. Metropol. Life Insur. Co.** 40:3, 1959.
5. Himes, J.H., and Bouchard, C.: Do the new Metropolitan Life Insurance weight-

height tables correctly assess body frame and body fat relationships? **Am. J. Public Health** 75:1076–1079, 1985.

6. Moore, M.: New height-weight tables gain pounds, lose status. **Physician Sportsmed.** 11:25, 1983.

7. Welham, W.C., and Behnke, A.R.: The specific gravity of healthy men: body weight divided by volume and other physical characteristics of exceptional athletes and of naval personnel. **JAMA** 118:498–501, 1942.

8. Wilmore, J.H.: Body composition and sports medicine: research considerations. In Roche, A.F. (ed.): **Body-Composition Assessments in Youth and Adults.** Columbus, OH, Ross Laboratories, 1985.

9. Lohman, T.G.: Applicability of body composition techniques and constants for children and youths. **Exerc. Sport Sci. Rev.** 14:325–357, 1986.

10. Behnke, A.R., and Wilmore, J.H.: **Evaluation and Regulation of Body Build and Composition.** Englewood Cliffs, NJ, Prentice-Hall, 1974.

11. Schutte, J.E., Townsend, E.J., Hugg, J., Shoup, R.F., Malina, R.M., and Blomqvist, C.G.: Density of lean body mass is greater in blacks than in whites. **J. Appl. Physiol.** 56:1647–1649, 1984.

12. Lohman, T.G.: Research progress in validation of laboratory methods of assessing body composition. **Med. Sci. Sports Exerc.** 16:596–603, 1984.

13. Pollock, M.L., and Jackson, A.S.: Research progress in validation of clinical methods of assessing body composition. **Med. Sci. Sports Exerc.** 16:606–613, 1984.

14. Jackson, A.S., and Pollock, M.L.: Generalized equations for predicting body density of men. **Br. J. Nutr.** 40:497–504, 1978.

15. Jackson, A.S., Pollock, M.L., and Ward, A.: Generalized equations for predicting body density of women. **Med. Sci. Sports Exerc.** 12:175–182, 1980.

16. U.S. Department of Health, Education, and Welfare, Public Health Service: **Facts About Obesity.** DHEW Pub. No. (NIH) 76-974. Washington, D.C., U.S. Public Health Service, 1976.

17. Centers for Disease Control: **Ten-State Nutrition Survey 1968–70.** DHEW Pub. No. (HSM) 72-8134. Atlanta, Centers for Disease Control, 1972.

18. Abraham, S., and Johnston, C.L.: Prevalence of severe obesity in adults in the United States. **Am. J. Clin. Nutr.** 33:364–369, 1980.

19. Millar, W.J., and Stephens, T.: The prevalence of overweight and obesity in Britain, Canada, and United States. **Am. J. Public Health** 77:38–41, 1987.

20. Allon, N.: The stigma of overweight in everyday life. In Bray, G.A. (ed.): **Obesity in Perspective.** DHEW Pub. No. (NIH) 75-708. Washington, D.C., U.S. Department of Health, Education, and Welfare, 1975.

21. Hannon, B.M., and Lohman, T.G.: The energy cost of overweight in the United States. **Am. J. Public Health** 68:765–767, 1978.

22. Stoudt, H.W., Damon, A., McFarland, R., and Roberts, J.: **Weight, Height, and Selected Body Dimensions of Adults.** Washington, D.C., U.S. Government Printing Office, 1965.

23. Frankle, R.T., and Yang, M.U. (eds.): **Obesity and Weight Control.** Rockville, MD: Aspen Publishers, Inc., 1988.

24. Keys, A., Aravanis, C., Blackburn, H., Van Buchem, F.S.P., Buzine, R., Djordjevic, B.S., Fidanza, F., Karvonen, M.J., Menotti, A., Puddu, V., and Taylor, H.L.: Coronary heart disease: overweight and obesity as risk factors. **Ann. Intern. Med.** 77:15–27, 1972.

25. Hubert, H.B., Feinleib, M., McNamara, R.M., and Castelli, W.P.: Obesity as an independent risk factor for cardiovascular disease: A 26-year follow-up of participants in the Framingham heart study. **Circulation** 67:968–977, 1983.

26. Dustan, H.P.: Obesity and hypertension. **Ann. Intern. Med.** 103:1047–1049, 1985.

27. Sims, E.A.H.: Syndromes of obesity. In DeGroot, L.J. (ed.): **Endocrinology,** Vol. 3. Baltimore, Williams & Wilkins, 1979.

28. Powers, P.S.: **Obesity: The Regulation of Weight.** Baltimore, Williams & Wilkins, 1980.

29. Petit, D.W.: The ills of the obese. In Bray, G.A., and Bethune, J. E. (eds.): **Treatment and Management of Obesity**. New York, Harper and Row, 1974.
30. Wadden, T.A., and Stunkard, A.J.: Social and psychological consequences of obesity. **Ann. Intern. Med.** 103:1062–1067, 1985.
31. Hirsh, J.: The psychological consequences of obesity. In Bray, G.A. (ed.): **Obesity in Perspective**. DHEW Pub. No. (NIH) 75-708. Washington, D.C., U.S. Department of Health, Education, and Welfare, 1975.
32. Bray, G.A.: Obesity: definition, diagnosis and disadvantages. **Med. J. Aust.** 142:S2–S8, 1985.
33. Bjorntorp, P.: Regional patterns of fat distribution. **Ann. Intern. Med.** 103:994–995, 1985.
34. Andres, R.: Effect of obesity on total mortality. **Int. J. Obesity** 4:381–386, 1980.
35. Fitzgerald, F.T.: The problem of obesity. **Annu. Rev. Med.** 32:221–231, 1981.
36. Knittle, J.L.: Obesity in childhood: a problem in adipose tissue cellular development. **J. Pediatr.** 81:1048–1059, 1972.
37. Sjostrom, L.: Fat cells and body weight. In Stunkard, A.J. (ed.): **Obesity**. Philadelphia, W.B. Saunders Co., 1980.
38. Widdowson, E.M., and Shaw, W.T.: Full and empty fat cells. **Lancet** 2:905, 1973.
39. Gurr, M.I., Kirtland, J., Phillip, M., and Robinson, M.P.: The consequences of early overnutrition for fat cell size and number: the pig as an experimental model for human obesity. **Int. J. Obesity** 1:151–170, 1977.
40. Faust, I.M., Johnson, P.R., Stern, J.S., and Hirsch, J.: Diet-induced adipocyte number increase in adult rats. **Am. J. Physiol.** 235:E279–E286, 1978.
41. Faust, I.M., Johnson, P.R., and Hirsch, J.: Long-term effects of early nutritional experiences on the development of obesity in the rat. **J. Nutr.** 110:2027–2034, 1980.
42. Greenwood, M.R.C.: Adipose tissue: cellular morphology and development. **Ann. Intern. Med.** 103:996–999, 1985.
43. Sims, E.A.: Studies in human hyperphagia. In Bray, G.A., and Bethune, J. E. (eds.): **Treatment and Management of Obesity**. New York, Harper and Row, 1974.
44. Salens, L.B., Horton, E.S., and Sims, E.A.H.: Experimental obesity in man: cellular character of the adipose tissue. **J. Clin. Invest.** 50:1005–1011, 1971.
45. Krotkiewski, M., Sjostrom, L., Bjorntorp, P., Carlgren, G., Garellick, G., and Smith, U.: Adipose tissue cellularity in relation to prognosis for weight reduction. **Int. J. Obesity** 1:395–416, 1977.
46. Bjorntorp, P.: Fat cells and obesity. In Brownell, K.D., and Foreyt, J.P. (eds.): **Handbook of Eating Disorders: Physiology, Psychology, and Treatment of Obesity, Anorexia, and Bulimia**. New York, Basic Books, 1986.
47. Keesey, R.E.: A set-point theory of obesity. In Brownell, K.D., and Foreyt, J.P. (eds.): **Handbook of Eating Disorders: Physiology, Psychology, and Treatment of Obesity, Anorexia, and Bulimia**. New York, Basic Books, 1986.
48. Thompson, J.K., and Blanton, P.: Energy conservation and exercise dependence: a sympathetic arousal hypothesis. **Med. Sci. Sports Exerc.** 19:91–99, 1987.
49. Keys, A., Brozek, J., Henschel, A., Mickelson, O., and Taylor, H.L.: **The Biology of Starvation**. Minneapolis, MN, The University of Minnesota Press, 1950.
50. Apfelbaum, M., Bostsarron, J., and Lacatis, D.: Effect of caloric restriction and excessive caloric intake on energy expenditure. **Am. J. Clin. Nutr.** 24:1405–1409, 1971.
51. Bray, G.A.: Effect of caloric restriction on energy expenditure in obese patients. **Lancet** 2:397–398, 1969.
52. Garrow, J.S., Durrant, M.L., Mann, S., Stalley, S.F., and Warwick, P.M.: Factors determining weight loss in obese patients in a metabolic ward. **Int. J. Obesity** 2:441–447, 1978.

53. Garrow, J.S.: Physiological aspects of obesity. In Brownell, K.D., and Foreyt, J.P. (eds.): **Handbook of Eating Disorders: Physiology, Psychology, and Treatment of Obesity, Anorexia, and Bulimia.** New York, Basic Books, 1986.

54. Brownell, K.D., Greenwood, M.R.C., Stellar, E., and Shrager, E.E.: The effects of repeated cycles of weight loss and regain in rats. **Physiol. Behav.** 38:459–464, 1986.

55. Steen, S.N., Oppliger, R.A., and Brownell, K.D.: Metabolic effects of repeated weight loss and regain in adolescent wrestlers. **JAMA** 260:47–50, 1988.

56. Gray, D.S., Fisler, J.S., and Bray, G.A.: Effects of repeated weight loss and regain on body composition in obese rats. **Am. J. Clin. Nutr.** 47:393–399, 1988.

57. Fox, F.W.: The enigma of mass regulation. **S. Afr. Med. J.** 48:287–301, 1974.

58. Bray, G.A.: The varieties of obesity. In Bray, G.A., and Bethune, J.E. (eds.): **Treatment and Management of Obesity.** New York, Harper and Row, 1974.

59. Bray, G.A.: Experimental models for the study of obesity: introductory remarks. **Fed. Proc.** 36:137–138, 1977.

60. Foch, T.T., and McClearn, G.E.: Genetics, body weight, and obesity. In Stunkard, A.J. (ed.): **Obesity.** Philadelphia, W.B. Saunders Co., 1980.

61. Stunkard, A.J., Sørensen, T.I.A., Hanis, C., Teasdale, T.W., Chakraborty, R., Schull, W.J., and Schulsinger, F.: An adoption study of human obesity. **N. Engl. J. Med.** 314:193–198, 1986.

62. Stunkard, A.J., Foch, T.T., and Hrubec, Z.: A twin study of human obesity. **JAMA** 256:51–54, 1986.

63. Garn, S.M.: Family-line and socioeconomic factors in fatness and obesity. **Nutr. Rev.** 44:381–386, 1986.

64. Sclafani, A.: Animal models of obesity: classification and characterization. **Int. J. Obesity** 8:491–508, 1984.

65. Mayer, J.: Exercise and weight control. **Postgrad. Med.** 25:325–332, 1959.

66. Bruch, H.: Obesity in childhood. IV. Energy expenditure of obese children. **Am. J. Dis. Child.** 60:1082–1109, 1940.

67. Rony, H.R.: **Obesity and Leanness.** Philadelphia, Lea & Febiger, 1940.

68. Bronstein, I.P., Wexler, S., Brown, A.W., and Halpern, L.J.: Obesity in childhood. Psychologic studies. **Am. J. Dis. Child.** 63:238–251, 1942.

69. Graham, H.B.: Corpulence in childhood and adolescence: a clinical study. **Med. J. Aust.** 2:649–658, 1947.

70. Tolstrup, K.: On psychogenic obesity in children IV. **Acta Pediatr.** 42:289–303, 1953.

71. Juel-Nielsen, N.: On psychogenic obesity in children II. **Acta Pediatr.** 42:130–145, 1953.

72. Fry, P.C.: A comparative study of "obese" children selected on the basis of fat pads. **Am. J. Clin. Nutr.** 1:453–468, 1953.

73. Johnson, M.L., Burke, B., and Mayer, J.: Relative importance of inactivity and overeating in the energy balance of obese high school girls. **Am. J. Clin. Nutr.** 4:37–44, 1956.

74. Stefanik, P.A., Heald, F.P., and Mayer, J.: Caloric intake in relation to energy output of obese and nonobese adolescent boys. **Am. J. Clin. Nutr.** 7:55–62, 1959.

75. Bullen, B.A., Reed, R.B., and Mayer, J.: Physical activity of obese and nonobese adolescent girls appraised by motion picture sampling. **Am. J. Clin. Nutr.** 14:211–223, 1964.

76. Corbin, C.B., and Pletcher, P.: Diet and physical activity patterns of obese and nonobese elementary school children. **Res. Q.** 39:922–928, 1968.

77. Durnin, J.V.G.A.: Physical activity by adolescents. **Acta Paediatr. Scand.** (Suppl.) 217:133–135, 1971.

78. Watson, A.W.S., and O'Donovan, D.J.: The relationship of level of habitual activity to measures of leanness-fatness, physical working capacity, strength and motor ability in 17- and 18-year-old males. **Eur. J. Appl. Physiol.** 37:93–100, 1977.

79. Wilkinson, P.W., Parklin, J.M., Pearlson, G., Strong, H., and Sykes, P.: Energy intake and physical activity in obese children. **Br. Med. J.** 1:756, 1977.
80. Bradfield, R.B., Paulos, J., and Grossman, L.: Energy expenditure and heart rate of obese high school girls. **Am. J. Clin. Nutr.** 24:1482–1488, 1971.
81. Waxman, M., and Stunkard, A.J.: Caloric intake and expenditure of obese children. **J. Pediatr.** 96:187–193, 1980.
82. Brownell, K.D., and Stunkard, A.J.: Physical activity in the development and control of obesity. In Stunkard, A.J. (ed.): **Obesity**. Philadelphia, W.B. Saunders Co., 1980.
83. Brownell, K.D., Stunkard, A.J., and Albaum, J.M.: Evaluation and modification of exercise patterns in the natural environment. **Am. J. Psychiatry** 137:1540–1545, 1980.
84. Gortmaker, S.L., Diety, W.H., Sobol, A.M., and Wehler, C.A.: Increasing pediatric obesity in the United States. **Am. J. Dis. Child.** 141:535–540, 1987.
85. Stunkard, A.J. (ed.): **Obesity**. Philadelphia, W.B. Saunders Co., 1980.
86. Greenwood, M.R.C. (ed.): **Obesity**. New York, Churchill Livingston, 1983.
87. Storlie, J., and Jordon, H.A. (eds.): **Evaluation and Treatment of Obesity**. New York, Spectrum Publications, 1984.
88. Storlie, J., and Jordon, H.A. (eds.): **Behavioral Management of Obesity**. New York, Spectrum Publications, 1984.
89. Storlie, J., and Jordon, H.A. (eds.): **Nutrition and Exercise in Obesity Management**. New York, Spectrum Publications, 1984.
90. Brownell, K.D., and Foreyt, J.P. (eds.): **Handbook of Eating Disorders: Physiology, Psychology, and Treatment of Obesity, Anorexia, and Bulimia**. New York, Basic Books, 1986.
91. Smoller, J.W., Wadden, T.A., and Brownell, K.D.: Popular and very-low-calorie diets in the treatment of obesity. In Frankle, R.T., and Yang, M.U. (eds.): **Obesity and Weight Control**. Rockville, MD, Aspen Publishers, 1988.
92. Hodgson, P.: Review of popular diets. In Storlie, J., and Jordon, H.A. (eds.): **Nutrition and Exercise in Obesity Management**. New York, Spectrum Publications, 1984.
93. Nicholas, P., and Dwyer, J.: Diets for weight reduction: nutritional considerations. In Brownell, K.D., and Foreyt, J.P. (eds.): **Handbook of Eating Disorders: Physiology, Psychology, and Treatment of Obesity, Anorexia, and Bulimia**. New York, Basic Books, 1986.
94. Lasagna, L.: Drugs in the treatment of obesity. In Stunkard, A.J. (ed.): **Obesity**. Philadelphia, W.B. Saunders Co., 1980.
95. Douglas, J.G., and Munro, J.F.: The role of drugs in the treatment of obesity. **Drugs** 21:362–373, 1981.
96. Bo-Linn, G.W., Santa Ana, C.A., Morawski, S.G., and Fordtran, J.S.: Starch blockers—their effect on calorie absorption from a high-starch meal. **N. Engl. J. Med.** 307:1413–1416, 1982.
97. Blundell, J.E., and Burridge, S.L.: Control of feeding and the psychopharmacology of anorexic drugs. In Munro, J.F. (ed.): **The Treatment of Obesity**. Baltimore, University Park Press, 1979.
98. Blackburn, G.L., and Miller, M.M.: Surgical treatment of obesity. In Conn, H.L., Jr., DeFelice, E.A., and Kuo, P.T. (eds.): **Health and Obesity**. New York, Raven Press, 1983.
99. Stuart, R.B.: Behavioral control of overeating. **Behav. Res. Ther.** 5:357–365, 1967.
100. Stuart, R.B., and Davis, B.: **Slim Chance in a Fat World: Behavioral Control of Obesity**. Champaign, IL, Research Press, 1972.
101. Wilson, G.T.: Behavior modification and the treatment of obesity. In Stunkard, A.J. (ed.): **Obesity**. Philadelphia, W.B. Saunders Co., 1980.
102. Stunkard, A.J.: Behavioural management of obesity. **Med. J. Aust.** 142:S13–S20, 1985.
103. Brownell, K.D.: **The Learn Program for Weight Control**. Philadelphia, University of Pennsylvania School of Medicine, 1987.

104. Newsholme, E.A.: A possible metabolic basis for the control of body weight. **N. Engl. J. Med.** 302:400–405, 1980.
105. DeLuise, M., Blackburn, G.L., and Flier, J.S.: Reduced activity of the red-cell sodium-potassium pump in human obesity. **N. Engl. J. Med.** 303:1017–1022, 1980.
106. Monti, M., and Ikomi-Kumm, J.: Erythrocyte heat production in human obesity: microcalorimetric investigation of sodium-potassium pump and cell metabolism. **Metabolism** 34:183–187, 1985.

PHYSIOLOGY OF EXERCISE RELATED TO FITNESS DEVELOPMENT AND MAINTENANCE

The next three chapters summarize research findings concerning the effects of physical activity on the major components of health-related fitness. Since risk factor reduction has already been covered, this section deals primarily with cardiorespiratory function, body composition, muscular strength and endurance, and flexibility.

Even though the various components of physiological function are discussed as separate entities, it is important to emphasize that the body functions as a whole, and oftentimes something that affects one bodily system has an effect on the whole. For example, a person who is participating in a jogging program generally would be trying to develop or maintain cardiorespiratory fitness. Jogging would also have an effect on the musculoskeletal system of the legs and trunk, i.e., some muscular strength and endurance would be developed in these areas, with a possible reduction in flexibility. Also, body composition would be affected, resulting in weight and fat loss and maintenance or slight increase in fat-free weight. This particular jogging program may stimulate bone development and, if too strenuous, may cause injury. The mind would also be at work during the jog and could perceive the effort in a positive or negative manner. Hence, one can see the complexity involved in trying to quantify the effects of physical activity on the various bodily systems.

CARDIORESPIRATORY FUNCTION

INTRODUCTION

Cardiorespiratory function depends on efficient respiratory and cardiovascular systems, adequate blood components (red blood cell count, hemoglobin, hematocrit, and blood volume), and specific cellular components that help the body utilize oxygen during exercise.[1–4]

The oxygen transport system comprises the lungs, which bring in fresh air from the external environment and permit oxygen to move across a membrane system (by diffusion) into the circulation. When oxygen reaches the blood, it is picked up within the red blood cells and transported through the arterial portion of the circulatory system to the working cells (diffusion and utilization). End products of cellular metabolism (carbon dioxide and lactic acid) are then transported back through the veins of the circulatory system to the heart and lungs. Various buffering and biochemical reactions are also taking place in the liver, kidney, and cells in an attempt to maintain bodily homeostasis and replenish energy supplies for continued work. The heart is the key to the oxygen transport system, since it must continually pump blood to all bodily systems as well as larger quantities to the more active tissues.

Pulmonary factors, such as total lung volume, maximal breathing capacity, pulmonary diffusion capacity, vital capacity, pulmonary ventilation, and breathing rate, do not limit endurance performance unless one has significant pulmonary disease or is exercising at altitude.[1, 4, 5] That is, under most conditions and at sea level, arterial blood leaving the heart is approximately 97 percent saturated with oxygen; therefore, most of the limitation to endurance performance depends on the capacity of the heart and circulation and on cellular function. An exception to this has been found with a few elite endurance athletes at or near maximal exercise.[5A, 5B]

As shown in Table 3–1, important components of the oxygen transport system improve with endurance training. Cardiac output is the amount of blood pumped out of the heart per minute and is determined by multiplying heart rate (HR) by stroke volume (amount of blood pumped out of the heart per beat). The arterio-venous oxygen difference (A-V O_2 difference) represents the amount of oxygen being utilized by the cells from the arterial blood.

Table 3–1. The Effect of Chronic Physical Activity on Cardiovascular Function and Aerobic Fitness in Healthy Adults and Cardiac Patients

Variables	Units	Changes with Endurance Training	
		Healthy Adults	*Cardiac Patients*
Maximal Values			
Oxygen uptake	ml • kg^{-1} • min^{-1}	Increase	Increase
Cardiac output	l/min	Increase	Unchanged*
Heart rate	beats/min	Unchanged–decrease	Unchanged
Stroke volume	ml	Increase	Unchanged–increase*
Arteriovenous oxygen difference	m/100 ml blood	Increase	Increase
Systolic blood pressure	mmHg	Unchanged	Unchanged?*
Rate-pressure product	beats/min × mmHg × 10^3	Unchanged	Unchanged?*
Endurance	sec	Increase†	Increase†
Ejection fraction	%	Increase‡	Unchanged–decrease*‡
Submaximal Values§			
Oxygen uptake	ml • kg^{-1} • min^{-1}	Unchanged–decrease	Unchanged–decrease
Cardiac output	l/min	Unchanged–decrease	Unchanged
Heart rate	beats/min	Decrease	Decrease
Stroke volume	ml	Increase	Increase
Systolic blood pressure	mmHg	Decrease	Decrease
Rate-pressure product	beats/min × mmHg × 10^3	Decrease	Decrease
Resting Values			
Oxygen uptake	ml • kg^{-1} • min^{-1}	Unchanged	Unchanged
Heart rate	beats/min	Decrease	Decrease
Systolic blood pressure	mmHg	Unchanged–decrease	Unchanged–decrease
Diastolic blood pressure	mmHg	Unchanged–decrease	Unchanged–decrease
Rate-pressure product	beats/min × mmHg × 10^3	Decrease	Decrease

*These values may increase in some patients with high-intensity training.
†The performance will improve, i.e., performance at a given distance will decrease, and performance time on a treadmill or cycle ergometer will increase.
‡Ejection fraction determined as a change from rest to exercise.
§Same absolute workload.

Maximal oxygen uptake ($\dot{V}O_2$max), or aerobic capacity, is the largest amount of oxygen that one can utilize under the most strenuous exercise (Fig. 3–1).[1, 4–7] It correlates highly with maximal cardiac output.[1] Because $\dot{V}O_2$max generally summarizes what is going on in the oxygen transport system (including cellular utilization) during maximal or exhaustive exercise and can be measured rather easily, it has been used as the measure most representative of cardiorespiratory fitness.[1, 2, 4–8]

Because a larger person generally has more muscle mass, and thus the capability of burning more oxygen per unit of time, aerobic capacity is often expressed relative to body weight, i.e., milliliters of oxygen per kilogram of body weight per minute (ml • kg^{-1} • min^{-1}). More specifically, if one's efficiency to move the body from one place to another is important, $\dot{V}O_2$max should be expressed as ml • kg^{-1} • min^{-1}, as mentioned previously. If efficiency of the heart and oxygen transport system is more important, $\dot{V}O_2$max should be expressed in milliliters per kilogram of fat-free weight (FFW) per minute (ml • kg^{-1} FFW • min^{-1}).[9] Because most often it is important to evaluate aerobic capacity in respect to moving one's body weight, $\dot{V}O_2$max expressed as ml • kg^{-1} • min^{-1} is preferred. When an individual gains or loses a large amount of body weight by diet, exercise, or some combination thereof, the percent change in $\dot{V}O_2$max expressed as ml • kg^{-1} • min^{-1} will be biased as a result of change in body weight. In this case, looking at the change in

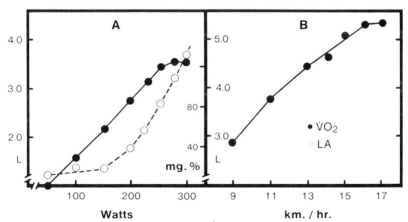

Figure 3–1. Increase in oxygen uptake ($\dot{V}O_2$, continuous line) and blood lactate concentration (hLA, interrupted line) in relation to work load. The subjects were working *(A)* on a cycle ergometer and *(B)* on a treadmill. In both cases a definite plateau for the oxygen uptake was obtained. (Originally published in Åstrand, P. O.: Measurement of maximal aerobic capacity. **Canad. Med. Assoc. J.** 96:732–735, 1967, published with permission.)

$\dot{V}O_2$max expressed as $l \cdot min^{-1}$ would provide better information about the improved aerobic capacity.

The effects of physical training on the cardiorespiratory functions listed in Table 3–1 are based on results from healthy adults who were free from overt signs of heart disease. How these functions may differ in patients with cardiovascular disease is also shown and is discussed later in this chapter and in Chapter 8. Maximal oxygen uptake and cardiac output almost always improve with endurance training. This improvement is most related to increases in stroke volume and A-V O_2 difference.[1–4] Maximal heart rate (HRmax) generally remains constant after training or is reduced by approximately 5 to 7 beats/min.[1, 10]

An indirect measure of coronary blood flow is the rate-pressure product: HR (beats/min) $\times$ systolic blood pressure (mmHg).[11, 12] Thus, since HRmax and maximal systolic blood pressure (BP) are not altered as a result of training, maximal coronary blood flow does not change when ventricular function and the coronary anatomy are normal.

When standard submaximal tests are administered before and after an endurance training regimen, for activities that require little skill, such as walking, running, and bicycling, $\dot{V}O_2$ and cardiac output remain relatively constant, whereas HR and systolic BP are significantly reduced.[1, 13] Stroke volume is increased and is the important factor in maintaining cardiac output or $\dot{V}O_2$ at submaximal levels. The lower HR and systolic BP at a standard submaximal workload indicate lower myocardial blood flow (reduced rate-pressure product) and, thus, improved efficiency of the cardiorespiratory system. For activities that require a lot of skill, such as swimming, rope skipping, and cross-country skiing, $\dot{V}O_2$ and cardiac output will also be reduced at a standard work task as the skill improves.[1]

Increased efficiency of cardiorespiratory fitness is also reflected in a reduced HR and rate-pressure product at rest.[10] In normotensive individuals, blood pressure at rest is usually not affected by aerobic training.[10] However, studies show significant reductions in resting BP with hypertensive patients after both aerobic and weight training.[14–16A] Although most studies concerning exercise training and its effect on BP have been done with adult populations, studies on adolescent hypertensives (above a 95th percentile for their age and sex) show similar results.[16, 17] Usually systolic and diastolic BPs are affected equally.[18, 19] In one review, Hagberg and Seals[19] reported that 11 of 16 studies showed significant reductions in systolic BP and 13 of 16 in diastolic BP at rest with exercise training in essential hypertensives. The average systolic BP was

153 mmHg before training and reduced to 142 mmHg after training. Diastolic BP reduced from 94 mmHg to 86 mmHg during the same time span. Some of this reduction in BP is associated with a concomitant decrease in body weight. Although weight loss by exercise or diet, or both, and other dietary manipulations, such as salt restriction, significantly affect blood pressure, aerobic exercise has been shown to be effective as an independent factor.[18, 19] Although the effect of exercise on BP can be significant with hypertensive patients, most often BP cannot be normalized without the added dietary controls. If diet and exercise do not normalize BP, more aggressive medical management would be recommended. Caution is necessary for persons who are on BP medication and plan to begin an exercise regimen. Once a participant begins a program, the medication may have to be reduced in order to offset the effect of the training program. The above discussion on the effect of exercise training on reduction in BP generalizes to patients with essential hypertension and has not been confirmed with other types of hypertension, such as kidney-mediated forms.[20]

AEROBIC CAPACITY

Because it is easily measured and highly correlated with cardiac output and endurance performance, $\dot{V}O_2$max or its equivalent in multiples of metabolic units above resting (METs) is being used as the "gold standard" for classification of aerobic capacity.[1–8] Oxygen uptake at rest equals approximately 3.5 ml • kg^{-1} • min^{-1}; thus, 1 MET equals 3.5, 2 METs equals 7, and so forth.

Figure 3–2 shows a champion distance runner taking a treadmill test for determination of $\dot{V}O_2$max. More details on treadmill test procedures, protocols, and interpretations are discussed in Chapter 6. Figure 3–3 shows a comparison of $\dot{V}O_2$max values of young and middle-aged men of various fitness levels. The illustration clearly shows the difference in aerobic capacity as related to status of fitness and age. Values for women are approximately 10 to 20 percent lower.[28–30]

Is there a level of aerobic capacity necessary to attain and maintain an optimal level of cardiorespiratory fitness? It is difficult to set a standard for optimal fitness because a specific level of aerobic capacity for optimal health has not been determined. As shown in Figure 3–3, $\dot{V}O_2$max for sedentary middle-aged men characteristically falls below 40 ml • kg^{-1} • min^{-1}. This value drops to 30 ml • kg^{-1} • min^{-1} by age 50 to 60 years. The values of 35 to 50 ml • kg^{-1} • min^{-1} would seem a reasonable estimate for an

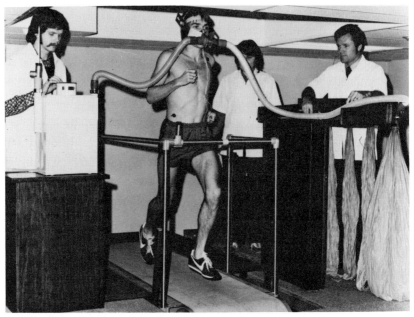

Figure 3–2. The maximum oxygen uptake test is being administered to a premier distance runner, the late Steve Prefontaine. At the time of this test, Prefontaine held 10 American distance running records. His maximum oxygen uptake was 84.4 ml • kg^{-1} • min^{-1}, one of the highest values ever recorded for a runner.[21–23] Breathing valve channels all expired air into a series of bags, which were later analyzed for oxygen and carbon dioxide content. The nose was blocked with a noseclip. Prefontaine was also attached to an electrocardiogram (ECG) machine by a special 20-foot cable lead system. In this way, the electrical action of the heart (ECG) and heart rate could be continually monitored throughout the run. It should be noted that more elaborate automated and computerized breath-by-breath metabolic testing systems are now available and currently in use, as well as 12-lead ECG monitoring systems.[24–26] See Chapter 6 for more details concerning graded exercise testing for functional capacity and for diagnostic purposes. (From Pollock, M. L., Wilmore, J. H., and Fox, S. M.: **Health and Fitness Through Physical Activity.** New York, copyright John Wiley and Sons, 1978, with permission.)

adequate aerobic capacity for ages 20 to 60 years, i.e., values of 45 to 50 ml • kg^{-1} • min^{-1} for the 20-year-old and 35 to 40 ml • kg^{-1} • min^{-1} for the 60-year-old.[1, 2, 27, 31]

Figure 3–4 shows differences in resting HR between sedentary and trained groups of men. This information suggests that the endurance runner has a slower, stronger, and thus more efficient heart.[23] The slower HR is accompanied by a greater stroke volume.[1–4]

A critical exception to the fact that a lower resting HR is characteristic of the trained and healthy heart occurs in the case

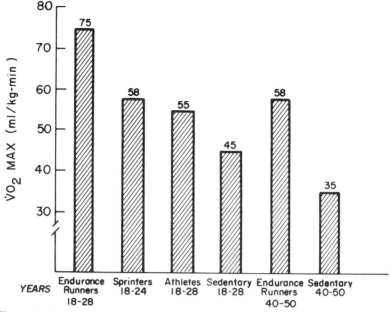

Figure 3–3. Comparison of maximum oxygen uptake of young and middle-aged men of various fitness levels. Values for women average 10 to 20% lower. (From Pollock, M. L., Wilmore, J. H., and Fox, S. M.: **Health and Fitness Through Physical Activity.** New York, copyright John Wiley and Sons, 1978, with permission.)

of certain pathologically diseased hearts. In such cases, the heart may beat more slowly, permitting a decrease in the metabolic needs of the heart muscle.[33] Another problem in using resting HR as a criterion for fitness is its wide variability within the population.[1, 27, 34] For example, Jim Ryun, once world record holder for the one-mile run, had a high resting HR compared with other distance runners (unpublished data: Jack Daniels, University of Texas, Austin, Texas, 1966). Therefore, caution should be taken when using resting HR as a measure of physical fitness. Although women adapt to training in the same manner as men, their resting HRs average 5 to 10 beats/min higher than those in men.[1, 27, 30, 35]

QUANTIFYING THE RESULTS OF ENDURANCE TRAINING PROGRAMS

Improvement in cardiorespiratory fitness is a result of many factors. Generally, providing that a certain minimal threshold of

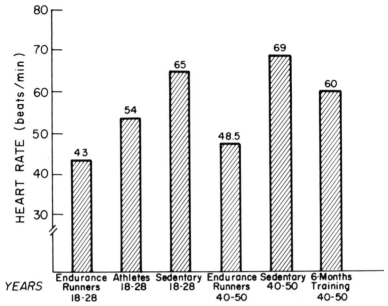

Figure 3–4. Comparison of resting heart rate of young and middle-aged men of various fitness levels. Values for women average 5 to 10 beats/min higher. (From Pollock, M. L., Wilmore, J. H., and Fox, S. M.: **Health and Fitness Through Physical Activity.** New York, copyright John Wiley and Sons, 1978, with permission.)

intensity is achieved, the magnitude of improvement depends on the total work or energy cost of the exercise regimen.[10, 27, 36, 37] Energy cost can be measured by the number of kilocalories expended, and improvement in cardiorespiratory fitness depends on the frequency, intensity, and duration of the exercise program. Improvement is also related to initial status of health and fitness; mode (type) of exercise, such as walking, running, swimming, and cycling; regularity of exercise; and age.[1, 10, 27, 37] These factors, as well as individual interests, should be considered in designing an exercise program to meet the needs and abilities of the person or group involved in the training regimen.

Although many of the data from various training studies and the subsequent recommendations for training programs presented in this chapter—as well as Chapters 4 (body composition) and 5 (muscular strength, endurance, and flexibility)—concern a variety of participants, the main target population is average adults 18 to 70 years of age. More specific information on the training of high-performance athletes can be found elsewhere.[1, 2, 38, 39] Recommendations for cardiac patients and patients with other medical problems are presented in Chapter 8.

Needs and goals differ for elementary school children, athletes, and middle-aged men and women. School children need a broader spectrum of sports and activities to kindle their interests and to provide them with a broad educational experience.[40, 41] The activities of most elementary school programs should provide for physical development, but many existing physical education classes do not. Athletes' programs are geared to competitive situations in which maximum skill and physiological and psychological effort are necessary. Preparing for such events often requires 2 to 3 hours or more of rigorous training daily. Adults generally are concerned with developing and maintaining strength and stamina, avoiding increases in body weight and fat, reducing stress and anxiety, and preventing potential health problems that occur with a sedentary lifestyle. Women often exercise for cosmetic reasons, such as weight and figure control.

CURRENT ACTIVITY LEVEL

An earlier Harris Poll Survey[42] stated that 59 percent of Americans of adult age say they are participating in physical activity programs. Of these, probably no more than 15 to 25 percent were participating in more vigorous fitness programs. Two more recent surveys conducted by the Centers for Disease Control[43] and the National Health Interview Survey[44] show that about 30 to 40 percent of young adults (20 to 30 years of age) meet a minimal standard of 3+ kcal/kg/day of leisure-time activity. This level of activity was achieved by only about 25 percent of 50 year olds and 20 percent of 70 year olds. Data from the Centers for Disease Control suggest that the percentage of individuals involved in vigorous leisure-time activity may be as low as 10 percent.[46] Although the number of people engaging in moderately vigorous physical activity seems low, it has been on the rise.[45] Stephens[45] summarized that adult leisure-time physical activity increased significantly over the last two decades for both men and women, with the largest increase being shown in Americans over 50 years of age.

In 1980, the U.S. Public Health Service[47] published the fitness objectives for the nation in 1990. The report set the goal of 60 percent of adult Americans to participate in exercise involving large muscle groups in dynamic movement for a minimum of 20 minutes, 3 times per week at 60 percent of $\dot{V}O_2$max. An interim report shows that the nation will fall short of its goal of 60 percent; an estimated real figure will be no more than 20 to 30 percent by 1990.[46, 48] It is apparent that great strides have been made in getting North Americans more active physically. It is also apparent that when the goals of the nation concerning how many Americans would be exercising vigorously by 1990 was originally set, the current level (1980) was greatly overestimated. The disparity in some ten surveys taken from 1978 to 1985 (55 to 9 percent) illustrates the problem of estimating and standardizing exercise values.[45, 47] Whether a leveling off of activity patterns has emerged or whether an increased trend will continue is not known. Shephard,[48A] speaking from the Canadian perspective, found that 15 to 20 percent of Canadians in the adult population currently engage in vigorous physical activity. He feels that the rapid growth in active leisure in the 1970's has plateaued in the 1980's. Much of the confusion in determining the physical activity status of populations is due to the fact that the tools of measurement are not standardized and criteria for the proper amount of physical activity and exercise are not clear.

RECOMMENDED DAILY ALLOWANCE (RDA) FOR PHYSICAL ACTIVITY AND EXERCISE

Is there a recommended miminal standard of daily physical activity to meet all our needs? Are physical activity standards for fitness the same as standards for health? In 1978, the American College of Sports Medicine (ACSM) published their position statement (guidelines) on the quantity and quality of exercise needed to develop and maintain fitness in healthy adults.

The ACSM recommendations were

1. **Frequency of training: 3 to 5 days per week.**

2. **Intensity of training: 60 to 90 percent of maximal HR or 50 to 85 percent of $\dot{V}O_2$max or maximal HR reserve.**

3. **Duration of training: 15 to 60 minutes of continuous aerobic activity. Duration depends on the intensity of the activity, thus lower intensity activity should be conducted over a longer period of time. Because of the importance of the "total fitness" effect and the fact that it is more readily attained in longer duration programs and because of the potential hazards and compliance problems associated with high-intensity activity, low- to moderate-intensity activity of longer duration is recommended for the nonathletic adult.**

4. **Mode of activity: Any activity that uses large muscle groups, that**

can be maintained continuously, and is rhythmical and aerobic in nature, e.g., running-jogging, walking-hiking, swimming, skating, bicycling, rowing, cross-country skiing, rope skipping, and various endurance game activities.[37]

The revised statement changes the minimal duration from 15 to 20 minutes of continuous aerobic activity, adds dancing and stair climbing to mode of activity, and lists a fifth statement:

5. **Resistance training: Strength training of a moderate intensity, sufficient to develop and maintain FFW, should be an integral part of an adult fitness program. One set of eight to twelve repetitions of eight to ten exercises that condition the major muscle groups at least 2 days per week is the recommended minimum.**

We are in agreement with these guidelines for healthy adults and their proposed revision. The addition of dancing and stair climbing to mode of activity reflects their current popularity as training programs. The minor change in the recommendation for duration stems from the difficulty to attain 300 kcal of expenditure in 15 minutes of exercise. The addition of resistance training to the statement reflects the importance of having a well-rounded program. The need for a well-rounded program is discussed later in this chapter and in Chapters 7 and 8. The changes from the original position statement have been recommended to the board of trustees of ACSM in an updated version of the stand (if approved by the board at their November 1989 meeting it will be published in *Medicine and Science in Sports and Exercise* in early 1990).

Earlier, the importance of total energy expenditure of a training program was mentioned. It has been estimated that to improve aerobic fitness to the proper level, approximately 300 kcal (based on 70 kg or 154 lb of body weight) should be expended during an exercise session.[27, 31, 36] The proper amount of exercise will usually improve a participant's aerobic capacity 15 to 30 percent over a period of 4 to 6 months.[10, 27] Thus, the proper combination of frequency, intensity, and duration of exercise is important in developing and maintaining the training effect.

The answer to the question whether the standards for the proper amount of physical activity necessary to attain both fitness and health benefits are the same is no. Although it has been recognized for years that health benefits can come from lower intensities of effort than those recommended by ACSM, it has only been emphasized in the last few years.[49–52]

Laporte and associates[49] and Haskell and associates[50, 51] have been helpful in pointing out studies in which subjects conducted their physical activity at lower levels of intensity and attained significant health benefits. For example, Leon and associates[53] reported that in high-risk subjects who were entered into the Multiple Risk Factor Intervention Trial, those who did regular moderate (4.5 kcal/min) exercise during leisure-time activity had a significantly lower rate of coronary heart disease mortality; Smith and colleagues[54] showed significant increases in bone mineral content in elderly women involved in low-level range of motion and calisthenic exercise and walking. These are just a couple of the examples that can be shown that illustrate the general health benefit from low-intensity physical activity. It must be emphasized, though, that usually when studies show significant health benefits from leisure-time physical activity, the duration of activity is also substantial. Thus, the same rationale for regulating the intensity and duration relationship is recommended for both health- and fitness-related goals, i.e., when intensity is lower, the duration is increased. Often, an increased frequency of training would also be recommended.

Most of the criticism of the ACSM guidelines has stemmed from a misinterpretation and lack of understanding of its purpose, intent, and limitations. Often, the guidelines have been taken out of context and overgeneralized to include all conditions or purposes. Because of "the lack of sufficient in-depth and comparative data relative to frequency, intensity, and duration of training," most physiological and health-related variables could not be used as a basis for quantifying the position statement.[37] "Thus, in respect to the above questions, fitness will be limited to changes in $\dot{V}O_2max$, total body mass, fat weight (FW), and lean body weight (LBW) factors."[37] Health changes as related to exercise and physical activity were particularly avoided because of the lack of precise definition and available data.

Another misunderstanding of the ACSM position was the lack of understanding that the guidelines were based on programs that showed improvements in $\dot{V}O_2max$ of 15 to 30 percent. Although it may not have been clearly explained, it was stated that significant improvements in fitness can be attained with lesser amounts of training than that recommended by the guidelines. Although these changes usually do not show a 15 percent improvement in $\dot{V}O_2max$, they are still important. Haskell[51] best states the current feeling on this matter: "Most exercise regimens are evaluated according to their effect on aerobic power or endurance. Health benefits of exercise may occur in conjunction with an improvement in physical performance capacity, but some benefits appear to be achieved by exercise that normally does not lead to improved fitness." Haskell[51] talks about a dose-response or spectrum of exercise and physical activity that encompasses low-intensity, fewer-total-kcal/week training versus moderate- to high-intensity, greater total kcal/week training. Results of these programs generally will be related to the amount of effort accomplished. As discussed in Chapter 1, Paffenbarger and coworkers[55] have shown in their long-term follow-up of Harvard graduates a dose-response relationship between physical activity and mortality for cardiovascular disease and other health factors.

As a result of the ambiguity concerning the guidelines for exercise prescription and fitness versus health benefits from physical activity, the revised ACSM position statement has included a statement recognizing these differences. Although the basic recommendations of the revised ACSM position do not differ much from the 1978 statement, they clearly recognize the dose-response relationship of physical activity and how it affects fitness and health. One final point on this, the ACSM board of trustees has recognized this problem and has appointed a subcommittee to develop a position statement on the quantity and quality of physical activity necessary for improving or maintaining health.

CLASSIFICATION OF WORK AND INTENSITY

The classification of work has traditionally been a grading system used for rating the energy expenditure of industrial tasks (Table 3–2).[56] These tasks were generally based on the average energy expenditure (kcal $\cdot$ min^{-1} $\cdot$ kg^{-1}) for an 8-hour workday. The original data were taken from the steel industry in Sweden.[57] The classification of industrial and leisure-time tasks by using absolute values of energy expenditure has been helpful for industrial medicine, military, nutrition, exercise physiology, and other health professionals in guiding workers into proper job tasks and weight control programs.[58] The energy costs of many leisure-time tasks are listed in Chapter 7. Although grading the intensity of work for industrial tasks has broad application in medicine and in particular in making recommendations for weight control programs, it has little or no meaning for preventive and rehabilitative exercise training programs. To extrapolate absolute values of energy for completing an industrial task based on an 8-hour workday, to a 30- to 60-minute bout of exercise does not make sense. For example, walking and jogging-running can be accomplished at a wide range of speeds; thus, the relative intensity used becomes relevant in these activities.

Because most endurance training regimens are geared for 60 minutes or less of physical activity, a system of classification of

Table 3-2. Work Classification Grading Systems for Industrial Work

Work Category	Men		Women		Activities
	kcal/min/65 kg	METs	kcal/min/55 kg	METs	
Light	2.0–4.9	1.6–3.9	1.5–3.4	1.2–2.7	Walking, reading a book, driving a car, shopping, bowling, fishing, golf, pleasure sailing
Moderate	5.0–7.4	4.0–5.9	3.5–5.4	2.8–4.3	Pleasure cycling, dancing, volleyball, badminton, calisthentics
Heavy	7.5–9.9	6.0–7.9	5.5–7.4	4.4–5.9	Ice skating, water skiing, competitive tennis, novice mountain climbing, jogging
Very heavy	10.0–12.4	8.0–9.9	7.5–9.4	6.0–7.5	Fencing, touch football, scuba diving, basketball, swimming (most strokes)
Unduly heavy	>12.5	>10.0	>9.5	>7.6	Handball, squash, cross-country skiing, paddleball, running (fast pace)

Work classification in kcal/min/kg is from Durnin and Passmore,[56] and estimated METs and activities are from Katch and McArdle.[58]

intensity for this model is necessary. Table 3–3 shows a classification of intensity based on the percent HRmax reserve of exercise conducted over a 30- to 60-minute training period. The use of a realistic period of training common for both cardiac and noncardiac participants and the use of an individual's relative maximal intensity value make this system appropriate for most of the population.

FREQUENCY OF TRAINING

Several studies have placed less importance on frequency of training as a training stimulus than on intensity or duration.[59–63] A couple of these investigations have attempted to evaluate frequency by controlling the total number of training sessions or total work output.[61, 63] These studies generally show no difference in changes in aerobic capacity with frequency of training. For example, a group of men were trained for either 3 or 5 days per week, and at the end of 8 weeks, both groups were re-evaluated. At that time in the experiment, the 5-day-per-week group showed more improvement than the 3-day group. In an attempt to equalize training sessions (total kcal expenditure), the 3-day-per-week group continued to train another 5 weeks. Upon re-evaluation, the improvement of the 3-day-per-week group then equaled that of the 5-day-group.[61] The results of investigations such as this are not surprising, since total energy expenditures were equalized between groups. However, in prescribing exercise, one should not regard frequency of training in this manner because, in reality, training regimens should not terminate after just a few weeks but should continue throughout life.

When weeks of training are held constant instead of total number of training sessions, results generally show frequency to

Table 3–3. Classification of Intensity of Exercise Based on 30 to 60 Minutes of Endurance Training

Relative Intensity		Rating of Perceived Exertion*	Classification of Intensity
HRmax*	$\dot{V}O_2$ max or HRmax Reserve*		
< 35%	<30%	<10	Very light
35–59%	30–49%	10–11	Light
60–79%	50–74%	12–13	Moderate
80–89%	75–84%	14–16	Heavy
≥90%	≥85%	>16	Very heavy

*Calculation of heart rate (HRmax), HRmax reserve, and rating of perceived exertion are discussed in more detail in Chapters 6 and 7.

be a significant factor as a training stimulus.[64–66A] Figure 3–5 shows the results of a training study conducted with men 20 to 35 years of age for a period of 20 weeks.[67] The intensity of training was standardized at 85 to 90 percent of HRmax reserve, with the men participating for 30 minutes in each exercise session. Improvement in $\dot{V}O_2$max was 8, 13, and 17 percent for the 1-, 3-, and 5-day-per-week training groups, respectively.

There are some inconsistencies in the literature related to frequency of training and improvement in aerobic capacity. These experiments have used frequencies of 2,3,4, and 5 days per week for from 5 to 13 weeks of training. Although most of the subjects used were of college age, initially all were generally considered sedentary. In some cases, the investigators found no significant differences in improvement in 2 to 3 days of training per week compared with 5 days per week[62] and in 2 days per week versus 4 days per week.[68] The facts that the subjects used in the investigations were beginners and that the experiments were conducted over such a short time make interpretation of the results difficult. In training experiments with sedentary subjects, it can take several weeks before adaptation to training transpires. In fact, it often takes several weeks for the subject to recover from the initial fatigue and soreness found in the early stages of training. Further, it is certainly possible that the 4- or 5-day-week regimens were too

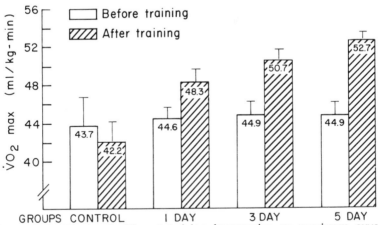

Figure 3–5. Effects of different training frequencies on maximum oxygen uptake ($\dot{V}O_2$max). (Data from Gettman, L. R., et al.: Physiological responses of men to 1, 3, and 5 day per week training programs. **Res. Q.** 47:638–646, 1976. Figure from Pollock, M. L., Wilmore, J. H., and Fox, S. M.: **Health and Fitness Through Physical Activity.** New York, copyright John Wiley and Sons, 1978, with permission.)

frequent for the subjects' initial state of fitness and thus left them partially fatigued during the final test period.

Of the points mentioned previously that can affect the interpretation of training studies, the length of a training experiment appears to be a very critical factor. Pollock and coworkers[64, 65] conducted two training experiments with middle-aged men (30 to 45 years of age) who trained either 2 or 4 days per week; they found both groups improved in $\dot{V}O_2$max, HR response to a standard work task, and other variables related to cardiovascular function. Midtest results of the 16- and 20-week programs showed no differences between groups, but final testing found the 4-day-per-week group to have improved significantly more. Thus, if these experiments would have terminated at their midpoints (8 and 10 weeks), the results would have been similar to those of the short-term studies mentioned earlier.

In two 2-day-per-week experiments conducted with middle-aged men who trained 3 to 4 miles per workout (jogging or running) approximately a 15 percent improvement in $\dot{V}O_2$max was attained.[64, 65] If this is the case, why is a 3-day-per-week minimum recommended? Because in these same 2-day-per-week training studies, the subjects never lost body weight or fat. This fact has been replicated in additional studies in which subjects kept diet relatively constant and did aerobic training 2 days per week.[64-66, 69, 70] The exact mechanism for this is not fully understood, but it appears that training 2 days per week at 4.5 miles per workout (jogging or running) will give approximately the same improvement in aerobic capacity as training 3 days per week at 3 miles, but the latter program will also effect changes in body composition. Thus, when we look at minimal guidelines for exercise prescription, total fitness should be considered. For further discussion concerning changes in body composition with exercise, see Chapter 4.

Two other factors are important to consider when interpreting the improvement in aerobic capacity through training of one or two days per week. First, the studies were jog-run programs of moderate to high intensity (80 to 90 percent of HRmax reserve) and may not be suitable or enjoyable for many adults. Second, research has shown that musculoskeletal injuries to the foot, leg, and knee double when beginners jog-run (even with some walking interspersed) 45 minutes per day compared with 30 minutes (Fig. 3–6).[71]

How about training more than 5 days per week? Training more than 5 days per week is possible, but certain factors should be considered first:

1. It has been estimated that more than 95 percent of the

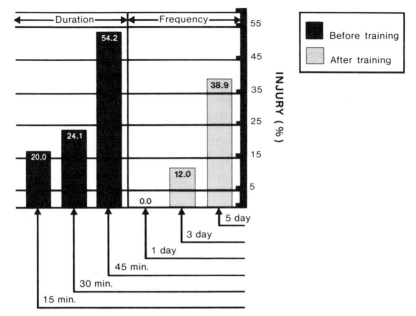

Figure 3–6. Effects of frequency and duration of jog-run training on incidence of injury. Data from Pollock, M. L., et al.: Effects of frequency and duration of training on attrition and incidence of injury. **Med. Sci. Sports** 9:31–36, 1977. From Pollock, M. L.: How much exercise is enough? **Phys. Sportsmed.** 6:50–64, 1978. Reproduced by permission of the **Physician and Sportsmedicine,** McGraw-Hill Publication.

improvement in aerobic capacity can be attained in a jog-run program (or other activities of equivalent intensity) of 4 to 5 days per week.[10] Thus, unless athletic competition is an important factor, added days of training are probably not warranted.

2. Orthopedic injuries appear to increase exponentially with jog-run types of activities in association with increased frequency of training.[71–76] Figure 3–6 shows data from beginning jogger-runners regarding increased injuries with added frequency of training.[71] The data on beginners who trained 30 minutes daily for 1, 3, or 5 days per week strongly suggest that a day's rest between workouts is advisable to prevent injuries. As a participant gets in better shape, frequency can be increased. The injury problem is generally related to the total volume of work done in the program. The greater the frequency of training and number of miles or hours trained per week, the greater the injuries.[71, 73–76] Other aspects of training, e.g., intensity, duration, and mode of activity, as well as age and initial level of fitness, must be considered. Basic anatomical structure is also important, as are proper shoes, texture of training

surface, warm-up, and so on, when discussing the potential of injury. Injury prevention is discussed further in Chapters 7 and 9.

3. The final point regards being realistic. Most adults cannot fit more than 3 to 4 days of training per week into their busy schedules. Although this observation has not been documented, most of us who have been involved in adult fitness programs know it to be true.

There is no question that more research is necessary to better establish and understand the upper-limit guideline. Individual differences certainly dictate how much a participant can accomplish before becoming injured. Figure 3–7 illustrates a U-shaped curve relating frequency of lifting and incidence of low-back injury.[77] There appears to be an optimal amount of lifting at which point participants have the fewest injuries, with the two extremes (those rarely lifting and those frequently lifting) showing significantly higher injury rates. Although similar data are not available in the sports medicine literature, these probably best reflect the current trend in our society. More miles is not always better. Certainly, beginners and marathon training types have the greatest number of injuries, thus programs should allow for gradual adaptation to training for beginners and limit the mileage for many running enthusiasts who become injured or who are prone to injury. The high injury rate associated with running and the data concerning the amount of benefit from training versus the number of injuries has led Cooper[78] to state that if one trains more than 15 miles per week it's for more than health.

Does it make any difference whether a participant divides the training program into two small workout sessions per day rather than one larger one? Other than the extra time it takes to change clothes and so forth, either method is satisfactory. For example, Fisher and Ebisu[79] trained 53 male college students three times per week for 10 weeks at 80 percent of their HRmax. Group I ran once a day, group II twice a day, and group III three times a day. The total mileage for all three groups was the same. The authors concluded that it made little difference in aerobic adaptation whether a participant trained one, two, or three times per day.

If an individual trains 3 days in a row compared with spreading the training sessions over the full week, will the same improvement occur? Other than the potential injury factor related to running on consecutive days, a person should expect the same results. This was found in a study in which one group ran every Monday, Tuesday, and Wednesday and was compared with a group who trained Monday, Wednesday, and Friday.[80] Both groups had similar improvements in aerobic capacity.

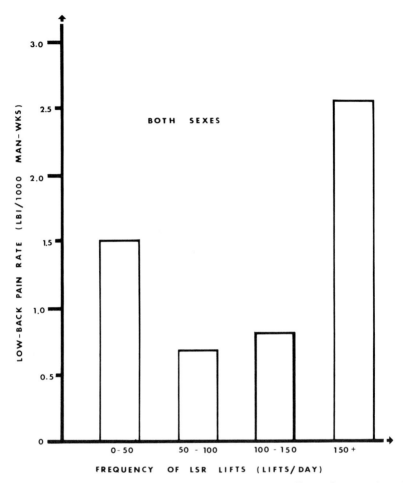

Figure 3–7. Mean low-back pain incidence rates with different frequencies of lifting. LSR refers to a lifting strength ratio. (From Chaffin, D. B., and Park, K. S.: A longitudinal study of low-back pain as associated with occupational weight lifting factors. **Am. Ind. Hyg. Assoc. J.** 34:513–515, 1973, with permission.)

DETRAINING AND REDUCED TRAINING

Closely related to frequency of training is the regularity with which one continues to participate and its subsequent effect on cardiorespiratory fitness. A significant reduction in aerobic capacity has been shown after one to two weeks of detraining.[81, 82] If training is not continued, the improvements gained in a program diminish rather rapidly.[81, 82] Cureton and Phillips,[83] using equal 8-week periods of training, nontraining, and retraining, found significant improvement, decrement, and improvement, respectively, in cardio-respiratory fitness.

Investigations in which subjects are put to bed for extended periods of time have shown decrements in aerobic capacity and related cardiovascular parameters.[84–86] Saltin and associates[85] confined five subjects to bed for 20 days, followed by a 60-day training period. Cardiovascular efficiency measures regressed during bed rest and improved steadily during training. Table 3–4 shows the results of bed rest on selected cardiovascular variables. Two of these subjects were initially trained, and the other three were untrained. It took the trained subjects significantly longer to reach their pre–bed rest fitness level once they began training again (40 days versus 14 days, respectively). It appears from more recent studies[86–88] that much of the so-called deconditioning that occurs with short-term bed-rest studies is related to postural fluid shifts and possibly other orthostatic factors. For example, peak $\dot{V}O_2$ was significantly reduced (16 percent) in subjects who were tested in the upright position after 10 days of bed rest but was only 6 percent (not statistically significant) when the subjects were tested in the supine position.[87] These studies have important implications toward the early treatment of cardiac patients as well as other hospitalized or convalescing patients. Early sitting and upright activity to re-establish or maintain normal upright hydrostatic and orthostatic mechanisms is important.

Participants in aerobic training programs who stop training have been shown to regress to pretraining levels after 10 weeks[89] to 8 or 9 months.[17, 90] A 50-percent reduction in improvement of aerobic capacity has been shown in just 4 to 12 weeks of detraining.[81, 89, 91] The time course for reduction in aerobic capacity was studied in seven habitually trained endurance runners and cyclists.[82] They were tested 12, 21, 56, and 84 days after stopping training. The largest reduction in $\dot{V}O_2$max occurred the first 12 to 21 days (-7 percent) and tended to stabilize after 56 days (-16 percent). Figure 3–8, from Coyle and associates,[82] showed that the

Table 3–4. Effects of Bed Rest and Subsequent Training on Cardiovascular Function of Young Men[85]

Variable	Units	Control	Bed Rest (20 days)	Training (60 days)
Maximal oxygen uptake	ml · kg^{-1} · min^{-1}	43.0	31.8	51.1
Maximal heart rate	beats/min	192.8	196.6	190.8
Maximal cardiac output	l/min	20.0	14.8	22.8
Maximal stroke volume	ml	104.0	74.2	119.8
Heart volume	ml	860.0	770	895

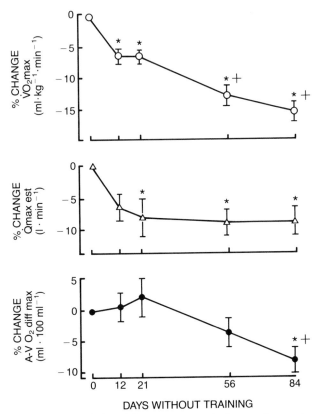

Figure 3–8. Effects of detraining on percent change in maximum oxygen uptake ($\dot{V}O_2$max), estimated cardiac output ($\dot{Q}$max), and calculated arteriovenous oxygen (A-V O_2) difference at $\dot{V}O_2$max. *Significantly lower than trained (day 0); $p < 0.05$. †Significantly lower than 21 days detraining; $p < 0.05$. (From Coyle, E. F., et al.: Time course of loss of adaptation after stopping prolonged intense endurance training. **J. Appl. Physiol.** 57:1857–1864, 1984.)

initial decline in $\dot{V}O_2$max was related to a reduction in cardiac output (mainly stroke volume) and later to reductions in A-V O_2 difference. They further stated that the muscle capillarization and oxidative enzyme activity remained above sedentary level and thus helped to explain why A-V O_2 difference and $\dot{V}O_2$max were higher than in untrained subjects after 84 days of detraining. These data and others[92] show that the loss of aerobic capacity is rapid but quite variable in rate among individuals after cessation of training. Factors such as level of fitness, age, and length of time in training add to this variability.

Once aerobic fitness has been attained, does a participant have to continue at the same training level to maintain this capacity? The answer to this question is not totally clear. As long as training intensity remains constant, it appears that some reduction in frequency of training over a period of 5 to 15 weeks will not greatly affect aerobic capacity.[81, 93, 94] Roskamm[81] trained two groups of soldiers 5 days a week for 4 weeks. The results showed that both groups improved significantly during this period (Fig. 3–9). A subsequent decrease in working capacity was found within 2 weeks after cessation of training for one of the two groups that refrained from training (group II). The group members who continued to train at least once every third day maintained their fitness for another 4 weeks (group I). After the eighth week, they stopped training, and cardiorespiratory fitness decreased significantly but not to the same level as that of group II, whose members had stopped training for a full 8 weeks.

Siegel and colleagues[95] trained nine sedentary middle-aged men for 12 minutes 3 days per week for 15 weeks and found an increase in $\dot{V}O_2$max of 19 percent. After completion of the program, five subjects continued to train once a week for another 14-week period. At this time, $\dot{V}O_2$max had decreased to 6 percent above the initial control level. The remaining four subjects who abstained from training fell below their original control values.

Brynteson and Sinning[93] trained 21 men (aged 20 to 38 years) for 30 minutes 5 days per week for 5 weeks at 80 percent of

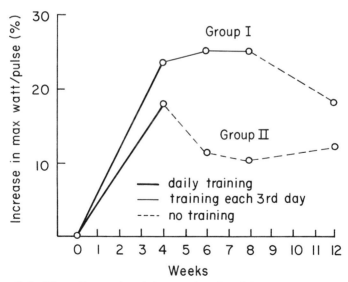

Figure 3–9. The effects of training, reduced training, and detraining on cardiorespiratory fitness. See text for explanation. (Originally published in Roskamm, H.: Optimum patterns of exercise for healthy adults. **Canad. Med. Assoc. J.** 96:895–899, 1967.)

maximum. They were then divided into four groups that trained one, two, three, or four times per week at the same intensity and duration for an additional 5 weeks. Only the groups that continued to train at least 3 days per week maintained their fitness.

An important series of studies concerning the effect of reduced training on aerobic capacity has been completed by Hickson and Rosenkoetter[94] (reduced frequency), Hickson and coworkers[96] (reduced duration), and Hickson and coworkers[97] (reduced intensity). All three studies trained 12 young college-aged men and women for 40 minutes 6 days per week for 10 weeks at nearly maximal intensities, i.e., training HR approached maximum by the end of each workout. After completion of 10 weeks of heavy training, the first experiment divided subjects into two groups that trained 2 or 4 days per week for an additional 15 weeks.[94] Intensity and duration remained the same as on the tenth week of training. The second[96] and third experiments[97] followed a design similar to that of the reduced frequency study, except one protocol reduced duration of training by one third and two thirds and one study reduced intensity by one third and two thirds for 15 weeks. In the reduced duration experiment, frequency and intensity of training were maintained at the level of the first 10 weeks of training, and in the reduced intensity study, frequency and duration of training were maintained. In all three studies, the first 10 weeks of training produced dramatic increases in $\dot{V}O_2$max: 20 percent (treadmill [Fig. 3–10]) and 25 percent (cycle ergometer). The results showed that when frequency and duration of training were reduced, $\dot{V}O_2$max essentially remained the same throughout the additional 15 weeks of reduced training. Only in the third experiment when intensity of training was reduced was there a significant reduction in $\dot{V}O_2$max. As shown in Figure 3–10, most of the reduction in $\dot{V}O_2$max occurred during the first 5 weeks of reduced intensity of training, with the two thirds–reduced intensity of training group showing the greatest loss. Because of the high intensity and rigorous nature of the latter investigations, their conclusions may not be completely generalized to the average population, who normally train at a significantly lower intensity. Nevertheless, these investigations provide additional important evidence that more exercise is required to increase $\dot{V}O_2$max than to maintain it. It also appears that if an exercise session is missed periodically or if training becomes reduced for up to 15 weeks, many important fitness variables will not be adversely affected as long as training intensity is maintained. Whether aerobic capacity can be maintained for longer periods is only speculative at this time.

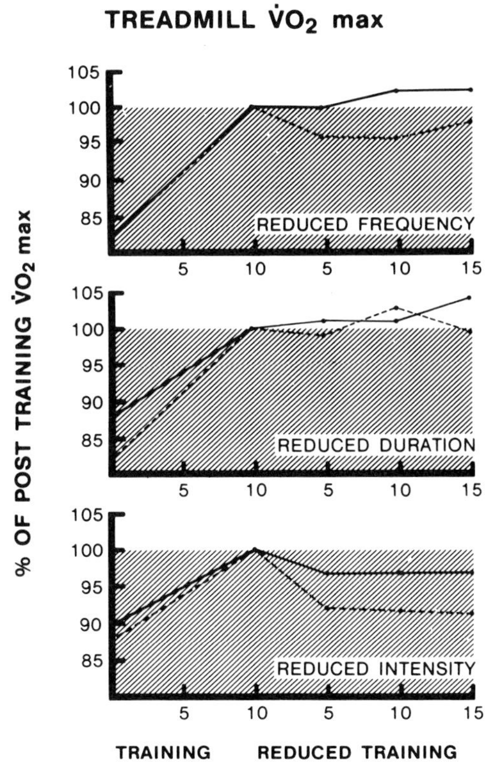

TREADMILL $\dot{V}O_2$ max

Figure 3–10. Effects of 10 weeks training and 15 weeks reduced training at one-third (solid lines) and two-thirds (broken lines) reductions in frequency, duration, and intensity on maximum oxygen uptake ($\dot{V}O_2$max). (Data from Hickson, R. C., et al.[94, 96, 97])

INTENSITY OF TRAINING

What is the optimal level of intensity to develop and maintain cardiorespiratory fitness? The levels most frequently mentioned are between 60 and 90 percent of the HRmax reserve.[27, 37, 98–100] The percentage of HRmax reserve is the percent difference between resting and maximal HR at which exercise is being performed. The methods for determining and calculating training HR are discussed in Chapter 7.

Two classic studies have been used to describe the minimal intensity threshold for improving cardiorespiratory fitness.[98, 99] Karvonen and associates[98] trained young men for 30 minutes 5 times per week on a motor-driven treadmill. They found no significant improvement in maximal working capacity for the group whose sustained HR did not reach 135 beats/min. Subjects whose sustained HRs were above 153 beats/min improved significantly. Hollmann and Venrath,[99] in a similar experiment conducted on a cycle ergometer, found that HR values of 130 beats/min or higher were needed to stimulate a training response. The group exercising at a rate lower than 130 beats/min increased only slightly in $\dot{V}O_2$max from 2.90 to 3.07 l/min, whereas the group that trained above this rate increased from 3.07 to 3.57 l/min. The data suggest that young men must exercise at a HR level equal to approximately 50 percent of their HRmax reserve. Åstrand and coworkers[101] state that persons should train at approximately 50 percent of their $\dot{V}O_2$max, which is in agreement with Karvonen and with Hollmann and Venrath. Figure 3–11 illustrates the relationship between $\dot{V}O_2$ expressed as a percentage of maximal HR in men of various ages in the United States and Sweden.[102] As a result of this relationship and ease of measurement, HR has been used as the standard means for quantifying and monitoring the intensity of physical training programs. Although these data are from men, the relationship is the same for women.

It must be remembered that the guideline of 60 percent of HRmax reserve to improve aerobic capacity was originally based on healthy young men. Shephard[60] and others[100, 103, 104] have since pointed out that this threshold value can fluctuate significantly, depending on level of fitness, i.e., persons with lower initial fitness have a lower threshold and persons with higher fitness a higher

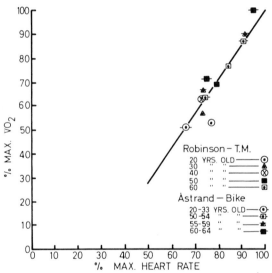

Figure 3–11. The relationship of submaximal oxygen uptake ($\dot{V}O_2$) expressed as percentage of maximum, and simultaneously measured heart rate as a percentage of maximum in men of various ages resident in the United States and Sweden. (From Taylor, H. L., et al.: Exercise tests: a summary of procedures and concepts of stress testing for cardiovascular diagnosis and function evaluation. In Blackburn, H. (ed.): **Measurement in Exercise Electrocardiography.** Courtesy of Charles C Thomas, Publisher, Springfield, Illinois, 1969, pp. 259–305.)

one. This point was well illustrated in a study by Gledhill and Eynon,[105] who trained college students for 20 minutes 5 days per week for 5 weeks. The subjects pedaled cycle ergometers at 120, 135, or 150 beats/min. Although the total group significantly improved their $\dot{V}O_2$max, when they were divided into low and high fitness levels, the group that initially had high fitness improved only at the higher training HR, whereas the low-fitness group improved at all three training intensities. Initial level of fitness and its effect on aerobic capacity are discussed again later in this chapter.

Kilbom[106] showed a positive relationship between intensity of training and improvement in $\dot{V}O_2$max. Sharkey and Holleman[107] found similar results when they walked young men on a treadmill 3 days per week at HR of 120, 150, and 180 beats/min. Faria[108] found no improvement in physical working capacity (PWC_{180}) with young men who bench-stepped at HR up to 120 to 130 beats/min.

Shephard[60] and Davies and Knibbs[59] designed experiments to look systematically at the training stimulus for improving aerobic capacity. Shephard trained men at 96, 75, or 39 percent of $\dot{V}O_2$max, and Davies and Knibbs trained their subjects at 80, 50, or 30 percent of $\dot{V}O_2$max. Both studies showed that improvements were in direct relation to intensity of training. In the Shephard study, improvements in $\dot{V}O_2$max ranged from 5 to 10 percent (depending on duration and frequency) for the 39-percent-intensity group to approximately 20 percent for the 96-percent-intensity group (Fig. 3–12). Davies and Knibbs found no improvement in $\dot{V}O_2$max for their 30-percent-intensity group.

If the total kilocalorie expenditure of the exercise regimen is approximately equal, does it matter whether one trains at a high or a moderate intensity? In general, as long as a person trains above the minimal training intensity threshold, programs that vary in intensity but have similar total kilocalorie expenditures appear to give similar improvements in aerobic capacity.[36, 69, 100, 106, 109, 110, 112–114A] There is only one study that does not support this concept of total kilocalorie expenditure.[114B] In this case, the high-intensity group improved $\dot{V}O_2$max by 17 percent and the low-intensity group by 8 percent when kilocalorie expenditure was equalized at approximately 350 kcal per exercise session. The fact that the low-intensity group started at a slightly higher $\dot{V}O_2$max than the high-intensity group and some of the subjects trained below 50 percent of $\dot{V}O_2$max may have influenced these results.[114B] To test the total kilocalorie expenditure hypothesis, Pollock and colleagues[112] trained four groups of men who were randomly assigned to a control (no training), continuous, interval, or combination of continuous

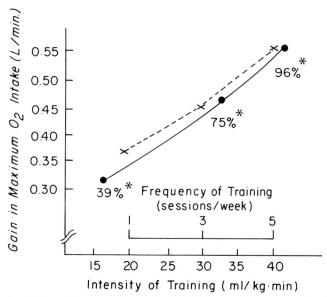

Figure 3–12. The influence of intensity (solid line) and frequency (broken line) of training on improvement of maximum oxygen uptake ($\dot{V}O_2$max). *Intensity of training expressed as a percentage of $\dot{V}O_2$max. (Data from Shephard, R. J.: Intensity, duration, and frequency of exercise as determinants of the response to a training regimen. **Int. Z. Angew. Physiol.** 26:272–278, 1968. Reproduced with permission.)

and interval training group. Training was for approximately 30 minutes, 3 days per week for 20 weeks. The interval training included repetitive nearly all-out bouts of 110- to 330-yard sprints with fast walking of equal distance interspersed. Total kilocalories among groups were equated on a regular basis. Figure 3–13 shows that improvement in aerobic capacity was similar for each of the three training groups.

In another study, Pollock and colleagues[69] trained middle-aged men at 80 or 90 percent of HRmax reserve for 20 weeks. Distance trained and total kilocalories expended per exercise session were similar between groups, but training HR averaged 15 beats/min lower for the 80-percent group (175 versus 160 beats/min). Figure 3–14 shows that the improvements in aerobic capacity were similar for both groups.

Many adults—particularly those more than 40 or 50 years of age, participants who are injury prone when jogging, and participants with heart disease—cannot or should not jog or run but can enjoy walking as an exercise program. How does walking compare as a training program? Again, it depends on the total kilocalories expended and on maintenance of the intensity level above the

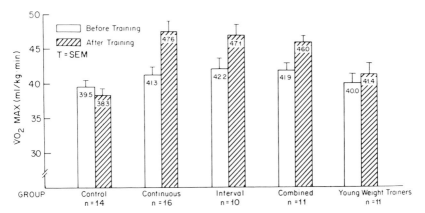

Figure 3–13. Effect of different intensities of running training on maximum oxygen uptake (VO₂max). Total kilocalories of energy expenditure were similar among running groups. (Data from Pollock, M. L., et al.: Physiological comparison of the effects of aerobic and anaerobic training. In Price, C. S., Pollock, M. L., Gettman, L. R., and Kent, D. A. [eds.]: **Physical Fitness Programs for Law Enforcement Officers: A Manual for Police Administrators.** Washington, D.C., U.S. Government Printing Office, No. 027-000-00671-0, 1978.)

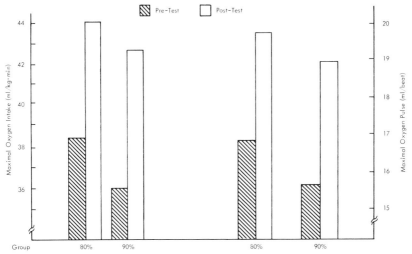

Figure 3–14. Effects of training two days per week at different intensities on maximal oxygen intake and oxygen pulse. (Data from Pollock, M. L., et al.: Effects of training two days per week at different intensities on middle-aged men. **Med. Sci. Sports** 4:192–197, 1972.)

minimal threshold. Pollock and colleagues[115] conducted a 20-week fast-walking study with men 40 to 57 years of age. The men walked for 40 minutes 4 days per week. The improvement found in this program (Fig. 3–15) was equal to that found in 30-minute, 3-day-per-week jogging programs for men of similar age.[10, 116, 117] The lower intensity of the walking program (65 to 75 percent of HRmax reserve) was offset by the increased duration and frequency of training.

The experiments described in the preceding paragraph have important implications for prescribing exercise. First, as long as kilocalorie expenditure is similar, a variety of intensities can elicit approximately the same training result. This gives participants latitude in developing their training program. Second, persons can train at a moderately lower intensity without significantly affecting their results, an important factor in long-term adherence to training regimens.[118]

High-intensity effort is often important for high-level competition, but because it is also related to increased musculoskeletal injuries,[118–120] and to cardiovascular symptoms and events,[121, 122] and has been found to be somewhat unattractive psychologically to noncompetitive middle-aged and older adults,[118, 123] it is not generally recommended for the average person. In the study comparing

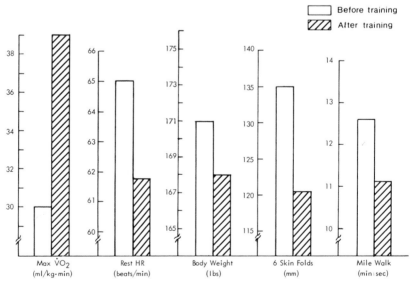

Figure 3–15. Effects of walking on the physical fitness of middle-aged men. (From Pollock, M. L., Wilmore, J. H., and Fox, S. M.: **Health and Fitness Through Physical Activity.** New York, copyright John Wiley and Sons, 1978, with permission.)

continuous, interval, and combination training, the interval training group had twice the number of dropouts as the continuous training group.[112] This was a result of both more injuries and a dislike for high-intensity effort. At the conclusion of the study, members of the combination group, who had experience in both programs, were queried about which regimen they preferred. Ninety percent of the group preferred continuous training rather than interval training, with 10 percent being neutral.

DURATION OF TRAINING

Improvement in aerobic capacity is directly related to duration of training.[10, 37, 100] Improvements in cardiovascular function have been found after 6 to 10 training sessions lasting only 5 to 10 minutes a day.[60] As a rule, the programs of shorter duration (10 to 15 minutes) of moderate intensity show a significantly lower training effect than do programs of 30 to 60 minutes duration.[27, 37, 100, 124–127] Figure 3–16 shows the results from a study conducted on men 20 to 35 years of age for a period of 20 weeks.[124] The intensity was standardized at 85 to 90 percent of HRmax reserve, and the men participated 3 days per week. Improvement in $\dot{V}O_2$max was 8.5, 16.1, and 16.8 percent for the 15-, 30-, and 45-minute groups, respectively.

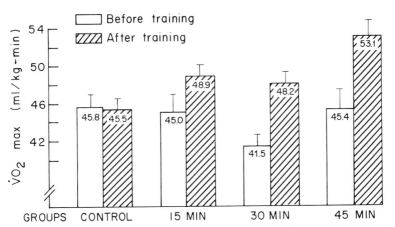

Figure 3–16. Effect of different training durations on maximum oxygen uptake ($\dot{V}O_2$max). (Data from Milesis, C. A., et al.: Effects of different durations of training on cardiorespiratory function, body composition and serum lipids. **Res. Q.** 47:716–725, 1976. From Pollock, M. L., Wilmore, J. H., and Fox, S. M.: **Health and Fitness Through Physical Activity.** New York, copyright John Wiley and Sons, 1978, with permission.)

In other experiments, Olree and coworkers[109] trained young men for 20, 40, or 60 minutes and found the longer duration to produce more significant improvements. Their training regimen included a 5-minute warm-up period, followed by a training period in which the resistance on the cycle ergometer was increased to produce a training HR of approximately 180 beats/min. Wilmore and associates[128] conducted a jogging program for middle-aged men three times per week for 10 weeks. Subjects trained either 12 or 24 minutes per exercise session. Both groups improved significantly in most cardiovascular variables, with the latter group showing an advantage in most values. Yeager and Brynteson[129] trained young women on a cycle ergometer for 10, 20, and 30 minutes 3 days per week for 6 weeks. The training HR averaged 144 beats/min. Their results were in agreement with the previously mentioned studies. In these experiments, attempts were made to keep the intensity and frequency of training equal among groups.

At this stage in the discussion, it is important to emphasize that duration and intensity are closely interrelated and that the total amount of work (energy cost) accomplished in a training program is an important criterion for fitness development. Sharkey[110] mentioned that previous studies were not designed to separate the effects of intensity from those of duration and that a cell sample size of only 1 or 2 is often limiting; thus, the interaction effects could not be determined. Therefore, he randomly assigned 36 college men to the cells of a 3×2 factorial design that included three intensities (training HR of 130, 150, and 170 beats/min) and two levels of work (7,500 or 15,000 kpm of total work). The 6-week training program was conducted on cycle ergometers 3 days per week. He concluded that intensity did not significantly influence the extent of training changes when the total amount of work was held constant. In addition, intensity and duration of training did not interact to produce significantly different training changes. These results are supported by the two previously described investigations by Pollock and associates[69, 112] (Figs. 3–13 and 3–14), Gaessner and Rich,[113] Burke and Franks,[114] Santiago and associates[114A] and Blair and associates.[130] Although more definitive investigations conducted at other levels of intensity and length of duration are necessary, the current studies appear to point to the importance of the total amount of work (energy cost) accomplished as the important criterion for cardiovascular improvement. That is, as long as training is performed above the minimum threshold of intensity, improvement in aerobic capacity will be similar for activities performed both at a lower intensity and longer duration and at a higher intensity and shorter duration if the total energy expenditure of the activities are equal. For many years, Cureton[36] has hypothesized this concept.

The American College of Sports Medicine guidelines suggest a minimum of 15 minutes per training session.[37] How does this relate to the above-mentioned research findings? In general, most training programs that meet the guideline standards show a 15 to 30 percent improvement in aerobic capacity. In addition, a 300 kcal expenditure per training session was recommended. The previously mentioned experiments support these guidelines. Thus, 15 to 20 minutes of very heavy, high-intensity activity (85 percent of HRmax reserve or higher), 20 to 30 minutes of heavy, high-intensity training (75 to 84 percent of HRmax reserve), or 40 to 50 minutes of moderate-intensity activity (50 to 74 percent HRmax reserve) will generally meet these standards. Because of the problems associated with and difficulty attaining and maintaining very high intensity exercise, the programs mentioned earlier, a 20- to 30-minute program is a more realistic minimal standard. This is why ACSM is changing its minimal duration standard from 15 to 20 minutes. In addition, because of the injury factor shown in Figure 3–6, beginning jogger-runners or aerobic dancers initially should keep their duration to within 30 minutes. As mentioned earlier, lesser combinations of duration and frequency result in significant improvements in $\dot{V}O_2$max but usually in the 5 to 10 percent range.[10, 37, 100]

MODE OF TRAINING

There are a multitude of training modes available. They range from individual to group activities requiring different levels of skill and varying degrees of competitiveness. The relative value of these activities in producing changes in cardiorespiratory fitness is in question. Previous parts of this review have shown that certain quantities and combinations of intensity, duration, and frequency are necessary to produce and maintain a training effect. Theoretically, in view of the results from the aforementioned training studies, it would appear that training effects would be independent of mode of activity if the various combinations of intensity, duration, and frequency are the same. Little information comparing the effects of various modes of training is available.

Olree and coworkers[109] compared the effects of running, walking (treadmill), and cycling (ergometer) training regimens on college men. Each group trained for 20 minutes 5 days per week for 10 weeks, at a HR of 150 to 160 beats/min. In general, they found running and cycling to be superior training modes when compared with walking. Pollock and associates,[111] in a similar experiment conducted with middle-aged men, found all three modes of training to be equally effective in producing a significant aerobic effect. In this study, the subjects trained for 30 minutes 3 days per week for 20 weeks, at 85 to 90 percent of HRmax reserve (approximately 175 beats/min) (Fig. 3–17). These studies agree except for the college-age walkers. This discrepancy is not clearly understood but may exist because the training intensity level was much less for the younger men and because the HR training data were not expressed as a percentage of maximum. Therefore, it is concluded that a variety of aerobic activities can be interchanged for improving and maintaining fitness, i.e., it is not necessarily what you do but how you do it that is important.

A variety of activities have been shown to elicit a significant improvement in aerobic capacity. These are generally known as moderate- to high-energy expenditure activities, e.g., running-jogging,[17, 64–67, 79, 80, 83, 85, 89, 91, 96–98, 100–148, 161] fast walking,[92, 107, 109, 111, 114A, 115, 127, 149, 150] cycling (bicycling),[68, 95, 109, 111, 113, 114, 130, 148, 150, 151, 161]

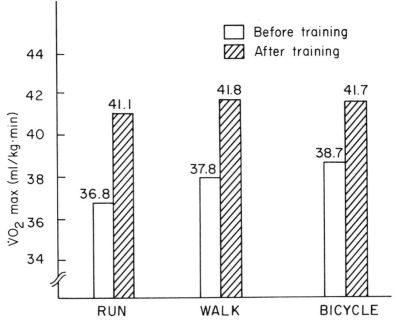

Figure 3–17. Effects of different modes of training on maximum oxygen uptake (VO$_2$max). (Data from Pollock, M. L., et al.: Effects of mode of training on cardiovascular function and body composition of middle-aged men. **Med. Sci. Sports** 7:139–145, 1975. From Pollock, M. L., Wilmore, J. H., and Fox, S. M.: **Health and Fitness Through Physical Activity.** New York, copyright John Wiley and Sons, 1978, with permission.)

swimming,[152-156A] cross-country skiing,[1, 157] aerobic dance,[158-160] tennis,[161] rope skipping,[145, 162, 163] soccer,[164] wheeling (wheelchair) or arm cranking,[165-174] and so on. In contrast, low-energy cost or highly intermittent activities (lots of rest breaks) show little or no effect. These activities include moderate calisthenics,[175, 176] golf,[177] and weight lifting.[178, 179]

Tables listing the energy expenditure (kcal/min and METs) of various activities are shown in Chapter 7.

Are weight lifting and circuit weight training suitable activities to improve cardiorespiratory fitness? In a review, Gettman and Pollock[180] showed that traditional weight lifting and training activities in which a participant lifted heavy weights with few repetitions and long rest periods resulted in no improvement in aerobic capacity. Circuit weight training that used moderately heavy weights and included many repetitions for each exercise (12 to 20 repetitions) with little rest between bouts of exercise showed only modest improvements in aerobic capacity. The average increase in $\dot{V}O_2$max of the seven studies reported was 5 percent.[181-187] Kimura and associates,[188] using fit and unfit young men, found no significant improvement in $\dot{V}O_2$max with the fit subjects and a 7-percent improvement with the unfit subjects. The subjects performed three circuits of eight exercises (45-second training and 15-second rest for each exercise) 3 days per week for 8 weeks, for approximately 24 minutes per session, at approximately 40 to 50 percent of one-repetition maximum. Gettman and associates[189] found a 12-percent improvement in $\dot{V}O_2$max with middle-aged men and women who performed 3 circuits of 10 stations, 3 days per week, at 40 percent of one-repetition maximum. More recently, the use of high-intensity circuit strength training showed increases of $\dot{V}O_2$max of 4.7 percent in middle-aged subjects[190] and 10.8 percent in young men.[191] Both of these studies used 12 Nautilus machines on their circuit and exercised their subjects to fatigue or failure using one set of eight to twelve repetitions. Two other studies using circuit weight training for exercise did not measure $\dot{V}O_2$max; one conducted on Navy personnel who also ran 3 days per week showed no more increase in work capacity on a stationary cycle than did a running-only group,[192] and one on cardiac patients showed improvement in treadmill walk time by 12 percent.[193] Caution should be taken when interpreting estimated $\dot{V}O_2$max data from treadmill time or cycle time with subjects doing strength training with the legs. Hickson, Rosenkoetter, and Brown[194] found a 12-percent increase in treadmill time and a 47-percent increase in cycle time after 10 weeks of leg strength training, with no concurrent increase in $\dot{V}O_2$max. Thus, improvements in $\dot{V}O_2$max with circuit weight training are generally significant (0 to 12 percent) but less than that found with the traditional aerobic training modes. Usually, the higher results (above 10 percent) were found with subjects who were less fit initially.

All of the circuit weight training studies mentioned above resulted in highly significant improvements in strength and favorable changes in body composition (in particular, increases in FFW). Strength changes are discussed in Chapter 5 and body composition in Chapter 4.

The results from weight lifting and circuit weight training studies show the effects of specificity of exercise training. It has been well documented that the muscles are trained and improved in the specific manner and rate that they are exercised.[1, 195–198] Thus, arm work favors changes in arm strength and endurance compared with the legs and vice versa.[199] For example, Harris and Holly[199A] assessed $\dot{V}O_2$max both by arm ergometry and treadmill performance before and after a 9-week circuit weight training program. They found a 21.2-percent increase in $\dot{V}O_2$max by arm ergometry and a 7.8-percent increase by treadmill. In addition, strength activities are primarily designed to improve strength and aerobic activities to improve cardiorespiratory fitness. Therefore, a well-rounded fitness program will include activities to enhance aerobic fitness, strength, and flexibility. Strength and flexibility programs should consist of a variety of exercises that train all the major muscle groups of the body.[27, 36]

Certain aspects of the results from circuit weight training may seem confusing at first glance. Circuit weight trainers tend to increase their HR within the acceptable training zone, and the activity uses large muscle groups and is rather continuous in nature. Why then the modest aerobic effect? Circuit weight training includes many arm exercises, and the energy expenditure for doing arm work compared with leg work is approximately 68 percent at the same HR level.[200] With arm training, $\dot{V}O_2$max for arm ergometry has been shown to increase from approximately 70 to 80 percent of $\dot{V}O_2$max of treadmill work.[166] Wilmore and colleagues,[201] using circuit weight training, trained men at 74 percent and women at 84 percent of their HRmax, but this corresponded only to 39 and 45 percent, respectively, of their $\dot{V}O_2$max. This was in agreement with Hurley and colleagues[190] and Hempel and Wells.[202] In addition, studies evaluating the energy cost of circuit weight training found it to correspond to that of a slow jog (11 to 12 minutes per mile).[201–204]

A study combining circuit weight training with a 30-second jog-run between each bout of exercise resulted in a 17 percent improvement in aerobic capacity.[189] Another study showed that once aerobic fitness had been attained by a jog-run program, a subsequent 8-week circuit weight training program was enough to maintain aerobic capacity.[185] This latter study supports the results mentioned earlier concerning reduced training, i.e., it takes less effort to maintain fitness than it does to attain it.

INITIAL LEVEL OF FITNESS

The level of fitness at which participants begin a program dictates their level of training and the rate of progression. These factors are discussed further in Chapter 7. The amount of improvement expected from a training program is directly related to the initial level of fitness, i.e., the lower the initial fitness level, the higher the expected change.[100, 106, 107, 205] Muller[206] first reported this observation after conducting a series of experiments dealing with improvement in strength. He concluded that the percentage of improvement was directly related to initial strength and its relative distance from a possible endpoint of improvement. This concept has also been true with training studies dealing with cardiorespiratory fitness parameters.[100, 106, 107, 205] Sharkey[106] noted that the magnitude of change was inversely related to the initial level of fitness ($r = -0.54$). He went on to say that the failure to account adequately for this factor in previous training studies may have resulted in erroneous conclusions or interpretations of results. To illustrate this point further, Saltin,[205] using the data of Rowell,[207] Ekblom and coworkers,[139] and Saltin and coworkers,[85] plotted the $\dot{V}O_2$max data of subjects at the start of physical conditioning against the percentage of improvement and found a moderately good relationship between the variables, excluding the data of older men (Fig. 3–18). The authors mentioned that the older men did not train as much as the younger men, which would account for some of their lack of improvement.

As mentioned earlier, the average improvement in $\dot{V}O_2$max with endurance training is between 15 and 30 percent.[10, 100] Other factors that tend to limit the amount of improvement include injury and poor health status, which can limit the amount of training that a participant can handle, and programs conducted over too short a time span. Particularly for middle-aged and older adults, adaptation to training takes weeks and months; thus short-term experiments usually show only small to moderate improvements. Kavanagh and associates[208] showed that some cardiac patients continued to improve their $\dot{V}O_2$max for up to 2 years. Young boys and young adults, who are generally more fit early in life, also may

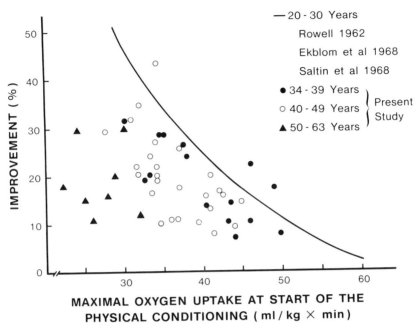

Figure 3–18. Improvement in maximum oxygen uptake ($\dot{V}O_2$max) in young individuals (line) and in middle-aged and older subjects in relation to initial level of $\dot{V}O_2$max. (From Saltin, B., et al.: Physical training in sedentary middle-aged men, II. **Scand. J. Clin. Lab. Invest.** 24:323–334, 1969, with permission from Blackwell Scientific Publications Limited.)

show more moderate improvements in aerobic capacity.[10] On the other hand, improvements may be inflated in individuals whose initial tests were stopped prematurely, i.e., true maximal tests were not initially performed,[83] or who lost large amounts of body weight during the course of the program. The latter is particularly true if $\dot{V}O_2$max is expressed in $ml \cdot kg^{-1} \cdot min^{-1}$. In addition, body weight is inversely related to treadmill performance time.[1, 209]

AGE AND TRAINABILITY

In general, aerobic capacity can be improved at all ages.[10, 27, 210] Saltin and colleagues[205] mention that even though this training effect occurs as readily in middle-aged and older men as in young men, the absolute change is less, i.e., there appears to be an aging effect. For example, Pollock and colleagues[211] trained a group of sedentary men who were 49 to 65 years of age three times per week for 20 weeks. The training included a walk-jog regimen with mainly jogging occurring during the latter weeks. Figure 3–19 shows an 18-percent improvement in $\dot{V}O_2$max. The relative values were what would be expected for younger persons, but the absolute values were lower.

The results of earlier studies by DeVries,[212] which showed only an 8-percent improvement in aerobic capacity, and by Benestad,[213] which showed no improvement, may be somewhat misleading. The latter program was of short duration, and the intensity and duration of training are considered minimal in relation to the criteria established by the ACSM.[37] DeVries' regimen was conducted over a much longer period, but the training intensity was minimal. Other more recent studies conducted with elderly subjects training at moderate intensities document an increase in $\dot{V}O_2$max of 10 to 15 percent.[214–216] The concern for protecting middle-aged and older subjects from overstress is important, and most investigators use much caution in their exercise prescription. As a result, sedentary groups need more time to adapt to training. This point was well illustrated in the investigation of Seals and coworkers[217] on 60- to 69-year-old participants. The first 6 months of training were conducted for 27 minutes, 4 days per week, at a low-moderate intensity (40 percent HRmax reserve). This walking training produced a 12% improvement in VO_2max. During the second 6 months of training, intensity was slowly increased from 75 to 85 percent of HRmax reserve. Depending on their orthopedic status, subjects went from fast walking to either jogging, stationary cycling, or graded treadmill walking. They averaged 3.6 days per week for 45 minutes. The higher-intensity program further increased their $\dot{V}O_2$max by 18 percent. Thus, these 63-year-old subjects increased their $\dot{V}O_2$max

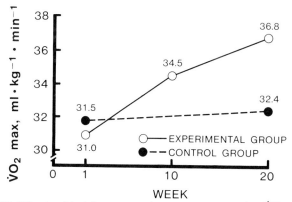

Figure 3–19. Effects of training on maximum oxygen uptake ($\dot{V}O_2$max) of men 49 to 65 years of age. (Data from Pollock, M. L., et al.: Physiologic responses of men 49 to 65 years of age to endurance training. **J. Am. Geriatr. Soc.** 24:97–104, 1976.)

from 25.2 to 32.9 ml • kg^{-1} • min^{-1} (30 percent). More recently, a 22-percent change in $\dot{V}O_2$max was found with 70- to 79-year-old participants.[218] Hagberg and associates[218] trained their subjects 3 days per week for 6 months. The first 3 months included moderate-intensity walking (60 to 70 percent of HRmax reserve) for 40 minutes, and during the second 3 months, training was slowly increased to 75 to 85 percent of HRmax reserve.

An important finding of this study with 70- to 79-year-olds relates to orthopedic injuries.[218A] When subjects went from a fast walking mode of training to interspersed bouts of slow jogging (approximately 50 to 100 yards), the leg injury rate increased dramatically; i.e., 8 of 14 subjects (57 percent) became significantly injured and could not continue jogging. All but one, who encountered a stress fracture in her tibia, were immediately placed on a stationary cycle or treadmill for grade walking for the remainder of the study. These subjects recovered from their injuries and were able to attain the 75 to 85 percent of HRmax level of intensity. The important implications of this study and the one of Seals and colleagues[217] show that healthy elderly subjects are capable of training at a high intensity but not if high-impact forces are associated with the training mode. Thus, it appears that as we age, not only are longer adaptation periods necessary, but modes of training that include high-impact forces, e.g., jogging and aerobic dance, may be contraindicated. The final major factor shown is that intensity of training in the elderly, as in younger participants, is an important factor in eliciting improvement in aerobic capacity.[219] Additional information on rate of adaptation to training is discussed in Chapter 7.

Can participants who continue to train their whole life or for periods of years maintain their aerobic capacity? Only a few longitudinal studies have been reported.[220–224] Earlier interpretation generally showed a rather linear reduction in $\dot{V}O_2$max with age for both athletic and sedentary groups. The slopes of the curves tended to remain parallel, so that the athlete remained at a higher capacity at every age. In a more recent review, Buskirk and Hodgson[225] found that the decline in $\dot{V}O_2$max with age did not appear linear and varied from 0.04 to 1.43 ml • kg^{-1} • min^{-1} per year.

In general, cross-sectional studies have shown less decline in $\dot{V}O_2$max per decade (4 to 5 percent) compared with longitudinal studies (8 to 10 percent).[225, 226] Dehn and Bruce[226] have stated that data from longitudinal studies are more accurate than data from cross-sectional ones because cross-sectional studies may represent a biased sample, generally including volunteer subjects who are probably more willing to perform maximal tests.

Buskirk and Hodgson[225] state that there appears to be a less significant drop per year for active individuals than for sedentary ones. They suggest that the decline in $\dot{V}O_2$max with age is probably curvilinear over the entire age range, with active persons declining more slowly if they maintain their exercise habit, and sedentary individuals declining more rapidly initially, followed by a slower rate of decline after their thirties. Buskirk and Hodgson[225] also suggest that women show a slower rate of decline in $\dot{V}O_2$max with age than do men. The data of Robinson and colleagues,[220] who evaluated champion distance runners from 1936 to 1942 and subsequently in 1971 (25 to 43 years of follow-up), showed different slopes, depending on whether the former champions continued to train. Their data suggest that elite runners who have a particularly high $\dot{V}O_2$max when young may have a greater decline in $\dot{V}O_2$max per decade if they become sedentary. In contrast, two who continued to train had significantly less drop-off in aerobic capacity than their sedentary counterparts. Because longitudinal data are scarce, most research has focused on the cross-sectional approach.

Cross-sectional data show trained athletes to be superior to their age-matched sedentary counterparts.[210, 227–232] Their superior $\dot{V}O_2$max is probably the result of both genetic endowment and physical training. The age decrement mentioned earlier also appears in the trained groups and becomes particularly evident after age 60 years. Can this decrement in $\dot{V}O_2$max be explained by age itself, or are training factors also apparent? Current evidence supports both notions. Young endurance runners train 100 to 200 miles per week (sometimes less if higher-intensity interval training is used), whereas middle-aged and older runners rarely accomplish this. In data collected from the 1971 National Master's Amateur Athletic Union (AAU) track and field meet and in subsequent laboratory evaluations conducted by Pollock, Miller, and Wilmore,[229] the average number of miles trained per week was 40, 40, 30, and 20 for the fourth, fifth, sixth, and seventh age decades, respectively (Fig. 3–20). Another interesting fact was that most of these men were former college athletes who had not trained all their lives. Most of the older athletes had been sedentary for many years and had been back in training for only 5 to 10 years. Grimby and Saltin's[227] data on middle-aged and older athletes who had trained all of their lives are comparable at the fourth decade but are lower for the fifth and sixth decades (Fig. 3–21). Other data of Pollock and coworkers[234] for men who had been training for more than 5.5 years are significantly higher than for men completing their first 6 months of training but are less than for the aforementioned athletic groups. Dill and associates'[224] and Costill and

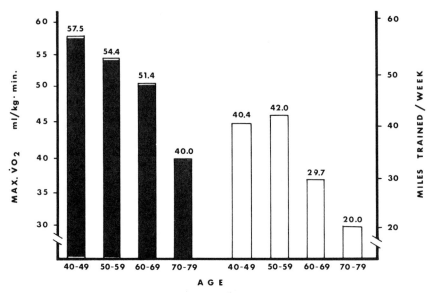

Figure 3–20. Maximum oxygen uptake ($\dot{V}O_2$max) and miles trained per week of American champion track athletes 40 to 75 years of age. (Data from Pollock, M. L., Miller, H. S., and Wilmore, J.: Physiological characteristics of champion American track athletes 40 to 75 years of age. **J. Gerontol.** 29:645–649, 1974. From Pollock, M. L., and Gushiken, T. T.: Aerobic capacity and the aged athlete. In Butts, N. K., Gushiken, T. T., and Zarins, B. [eds.]: **The Elite Athlete.** Champaign, IL, Human Kinetics Publishers, Inc., 1985, pp. 267–274. Reprinted with permission.)

Winrow's[235] data on competitive marathon runners agree. Thus, the conclusions from these longitudinal studies and others reviewed by Heath and associates[231] showed a 9-percent reduction per decade in $\dot{V}O_2$max with age, ranging from 20 to 70 years. The athletic groups showed the same percent decrease as their sedentary counterparts, and therefore their $\dot{V}O_2$max remained significantly higher at all ages.

In an attempt to rule out the training and mileage differences found in the studies comparing younger and older runners, Heath and colleagues[231] investigated a group of younger and older runners matched for mileage and training characteristics. Their data suggest less difference between groups by age than had been found by previous studies (approximately 5 percent per decade) (Fig. 3–21).

In contrast to these findings, Kasch and Wallace[223] found no reduction in aerobic capacity after a 10-year follow-up of middle-aged noncompetitive runners. The subjects were 45 years of age initially and continued to run approximately 15 miles per week. Maximal oxygen uptake (43.7 versus 44.4 ml $\cdot$ kg^{-1} $\cdot$ min^{-1}), resting

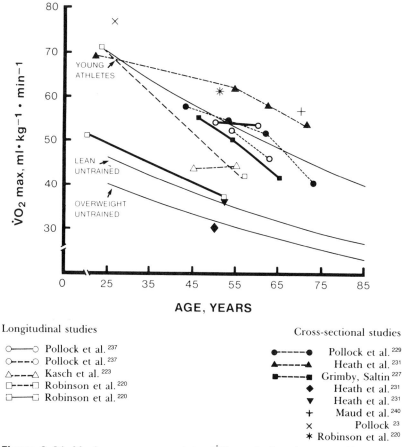

Longitudinal studies

O——O	Pollock et al. [237]
O----O	Pollock et al. [237]
△----△	Kasch et al. [223]
□----□	Robinson et al. [220]
□——□	Robinson et al. [220]

Cross-sectional studies

●----●	Pollock et al. [229]
▲----▲	Heath et al. [231]
■----■	Grimby, Saltin [227]
◆	Heath et al. [231]
▼	Heath et al. [231]
+	Maud et al. [240]
×	Pollock [23]
✻	Robinson et al. [220]

Figure 3–21. Maximum oxygen uptake ($\dot{V}O_2$max) of endurance athletes and nonathletes of various ages. See legend and text for group descriptions.

HR (63 versus 61 beats/min), and body weight (76.8 versus 76.0 kg) remained constant over the 10-year period. Only HRmax decreased significantly (178 versus 171 beats/min). Their 18-year follow-up continued a similar trend.[236] More recently, Pollock and colleagues[237] completed a 10-year follow-up study on champion master runners. Important questions include the following: (1) Is the aging curve linear over a wide age range? (2) If a person continues to train at the same level, will a reduction in aerobic capacity occur? The cross-sectional results from this group's 1971 data showed the expected decrease in $\dot{V}O_2$max up to approximately 65 years of age, with a more dramatic reduction occurring thereafter (see Fig. 3–20).[229, 233] As a result of the small sample studied who were older than the age of 70 years and the significant difference in the quantity and quality of training among the various age groups, conclusions were considered somewhat tenuous. Was the reduction in aerobic capacity a result of aging or the difference in training level? The follow-up data were collected on 24 men 50 to 82 years of age. All of the subjects had continued their training, but only 11 were training at approximately the same level and were still highly competitive. Training mileage remained unchanged for both groups, but the noncompetitors slowed their training pace by approximately 2 minutes per mile. Figure 3–21 shows the results in $\dot{V}O_2max$. The competitive group showed no significant change in $\dot{V}O_2max$ (54.2 versus 53.3 ml $\cdot$ kg^{-1} $\cdot$ min^{-1}), whereas the noncompetitive group decreased significantly (52.5 versus 45.9 ml $\cdot$ kg^{-1} $\cdot$ min^{-1}). The results of this study help to confirm the hypothesis that the reduction in aerobic capacity found with age is affected by maintenance of training. This hypothesis is in agreement with the results of Kasch, Wallace, and Van Camp,[223, 236] and of Åstrand.[238] Åstrand[238] describes a 33-year follow-up of former physical education students that were tested in 1949, 1970, and 1982. The data from 1970[239] showed a 20-percent reduction in $\dot{V}O_2max$ for both men and women. Those who continued or eventually resumed an active lifestyle had little decrement in $\dot{V}O_2max$[238] (personal communication, 1987). The data from Pollock and associates[237] also showed the aging curve for aerobic capacity to be curvilinear rather than linear, as reported by previous research.[225, 230, 231] The competitive group who continued to train at the same intensity level showed no reduction until after age 60 to 65 years (Fig. 3–22). After this age, a decrease was evident but not at the same rate as shown in the cross-sectional report. Although these longitudinal studies seem to answer important questions about how exercise may affect cardiorespiratory fitness, more data using larger numbers of subjects and longer follow-up periods are necessary before final conclusions can be drawn.

Although these studies of Kasch and Wallace,[223] Heath and associates,[231] and Pollock and associates[237] showed that the reduction in aerobic capacity with age is affected by training, there seemed to be no effect on maximum HRmax, i.e., HRmax declined with age, independent of training. Londeree and Moeschberger[242] in a review of data representing 23,000 independent subjects ranging from 5 to 81 years of age, found no difference in HRmax as related to sex or race. In contrast to the longitudinal data presented earlier, their data from cross-sectional studies showed active participants to have a lower HRmax at the younger ages and a higher value at the older ages. They felt that the lower HRmax shown in the cross-sectional studies was a result of less local muscle fatigue

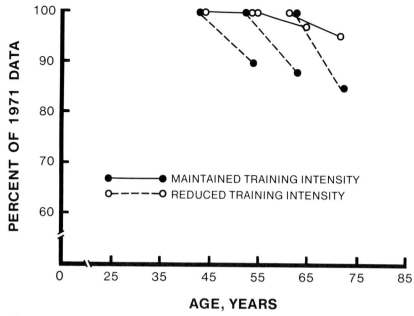

Figure 3–22. Reduction of maximum oxygen uptake after 10 years follow-up for master track athletes who maintained or reduced their training intensity. (Data from Pollock, M. L., et al.: Effect of age and training on aerobic capacity and body composition of master athletes. **J. Appl. Physiol.** 62:725–731, 1987.)

in the active versus the sedentary older subjects (Fig. 3–23). Although there appears to be an age-related reduction in the cardiovascular response to beta-adrenergic stimulation, the precise explanation of why HRmax declines with age is not clear.

If HRmax declines with age, how is $\dot{V}O_2$max maintained with age in habitually active individuals? The fact that oxygen pulse appears to remain the same in habitually active subjects suggests that cardiac output has been maintained by an accommodating increase in stroke volume or oxygen extraction.[231, 237, 243–245] Data of Rodeheffer and colleagues[244] from participants in the Baltimore longitudinal study, aged 25 to 79 years, found an age-related increase in end-diastolic volume and stroke volume, and an age-related decrease in HRmax. LaKatta and colleagues,[245] in a more recent review, mention that at higher workloads, end-diastolic and end-systolic volumes decrease and stroke volume plateaus in younger subjects. In contrast, in healthy older subjects, left ventricular volume and stroke volume continue to increase during exercise, thus compensating for the lower HR. Ehsani[243] agrees with Rodeheffer and colleagues[244] and LaKatta and colleagues[245]

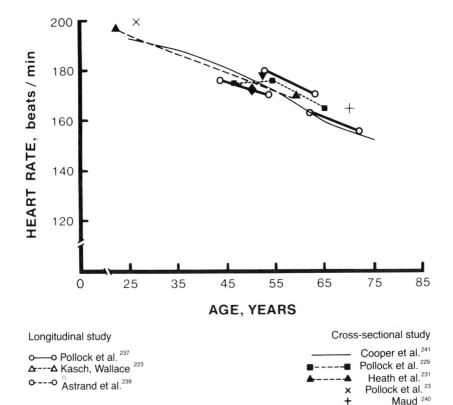

Figure 3–23. Maximum heart rate of groups of various ages. See illustration and text for group descriptions.

concerning ventricular function with age and adds that their data with master endurance athletes also showed a proportional increase in left ventricular wall thickness suggestive of volume overload hypertrophy. The magnitude of hypertrophy was similar to that found in young endurance athletes.

Is the aerobic capacity of children and youth affected the same as that of adults? The $\dot{V}O_2$max improvement with training in young boys is complicated somewhat by the maturation process, making interpretation more difficult.[246, 246A] This is clearly shown by Krahenbuhl, Skinner, and Kohrt[246A] in a review of the developmental aspects of $\dot{V}O_2$max in children. They showed that $\dot{V}O_2$max expressed in $l \cdot min^{-1}$ are similar for boys and girls from age 6 to 12 years of age. The regression lines are curvilinear (quadratic and cubic), with boys increasing through age 16 years and girls curving downward after age 14 years. Differences in FFW and exercise habits are the best explanations used to describe this phenomenon.[246A] The same values for $\dot{V}O_2$max expressed in ml • kg^{-1} • min^{-1} show that sedentary boys remain relatively constant from age 6 to 16 years (52.8 to 53.5 ml • kg^{-1} • min^{-1}), but sedentary girls decrease linearly from 52.0 to 40.5 ml • kg^{-1} • min^{-1} over the same time span.

The exercise training data of Ekblom,[247] Sherman,[248] Larsson and coworkers,[249] Lussier and Buskirk,[250] Elovainio and Sundberg,[251] and Rotstein and coworkers[252] show significant improvements with training, whereas those of Daniels and Oldridge[253] do not. Inspection of the results shows Daniels and Oldridge's initial values to be much higher than the others, thus again bringing up initial status of fitness and its relationship to possible improvement. The results of Elovainio and Sundberg[251] are not in agreement with those of Daniels and Oldridge[253]; in their 5-year follow-up elite runners show an increase in $\dot{V}O_2$max from 64.2 ml • kg^{-1} • min^{-1} at age 14 to 73.9 ml • kg^{-1} • min^{-1} at age 19. Their controls went from 58.7 to 61.0 ml • kg^{-1} • min^{-1} during the same time span. The age-related average $\dot{V}O_2$max values reported by Robinson,[34] Cumming,[254] and Krahenbuhl, Skinner, and Kohrt[246A] are in agreement with values found by Ekblom,[247] Sherman,[248] and Rotstein and associates,[252] whereas those of Larsson and associates[249] probably were related to the subjects' lower initial fitness. Thus, it appears that children and youth adapt to aerobic training about the same as adults.

Will training during youth give added benefits and advantages to aerobic performance capacity at maturity? Longitudinal studies conducted by Ekblom and associates,[139] Åstrand and associates,[155] Zauner and Benson,[255] and Elovainio and Sundberg[251] on young boys and girls showed higher than normal improvements in many physiological parameters with endurance training regimens, thus suggesting the probability of significant cardiopulmonary and anthropometric modifications occurring during the formative years. Although these results seem promising, further study is necessary before more definitive conclusions can be made.

Can aerobic training be harmful to younger children? Cureton and Barry[40] found that children adapt well to endurance training. In over 20 years of study with boys 7 to 14 years of age, no significant problems were noted. Although injuries in youth programs are mostly related to trauma from collision and contact sports, a number of overuse injuries have been reported.[246, 256] As far as endurance training is concerned, congenital defects, heat stress, and orthopedic problems related to overuse are reported most often. Whether a marathon type of training is detrimental for youngsters is not known. Possibly this type of activity creates more psychological problems, resulting from parental pressure and so on, than physical ones.

HEREDITY

The effects of training have been well documented, with clear differences being established between sedentary, moderately trained, and highly trained athletes.[1-3] Even with these differences, there are broad overlappings among these groups on most physiological variables. This fact, plus the aging process, makes various standards awkward and somewhat misleading. That is, much of our ability is endowed by heredity.[1, 257-261A] Åstrand[262] stated that the best way to become a champion athlete is to be selective in the manner in which you choose your parents. Therefore, the fact of having a high $\dot{V}O_2$max must be interpreted with caution. It is possible to have a high $\dot{V}O_2$max and be considered in poor condition and to have a low one and be considered fit. The former would be true with a highly trained endurance athlete who has become inactive. Klissouras[258] has suggested, somewhat speculatively, that genotype factors account for approximately 85 to 90 percent of biological variability in regard to aerobic capacity. More recent studies by Prud'homme and colleagues[260] and Hamel and colleagues[261] agree with Klissouras concerning the genetic predisposition to aerobic and anaerobic power and its trainability, but show that it may be more in the range of 60 to 80 percent genotype. In a review, Bouchard[261A] states that "age and sex of subjects as well as their prior training experience do not seem to contribute much to human variation in trainability. The major causes of human variation in the response to training are the current phenotype level, that is, the pretraining status of the trait considered, and a genetically determined capacity to adapt to exercise training, probably unique for each biological characteristic or family of characteristics." Even though the exact amount of influence heredity has is in question, it is still recommended that physiological results be interpreted with respect to both genetic makeup and environmental factors, as well as individual differences and variations.

TRAINING IN WOMEN

Treating the effects of aerobic training on women in a separate section should not be interpreted as a minimization of the subject's importance, but because of the more recent emergence of women in endurance training (for fitness and athletic purposes), a special section seems warranted. Only a few training investigations dealing with women have been designed to quantify training regimens as described earlier.[10, 28, 29, 37, 129] Several studies have evaluated working capacity and anthropometric measurements of young women[129, 159, 263–266, 276, 277] and middle-aged women.[106, 160, 267–271] Some investigations have evaluated highly trained women athletes.[1, 2, 21, 29, 30, 155, 272–275] Others[106, 129, 148, 151, 158–160, 182, 186, 263–271, 276, 277] have shown significant cardiovascular function and body composition changes with endurance training. The former data show significant differences between men and women, which become apparent after puberty.[1, 2, 246A] Most early studies show a 20- to 30-percent difference in $\dot{V}O_2$max (ml • kg^{-1} • min^{-1} of body weight) between men and women after maturity. A meta-analysis of studies comparing $\dot{V}O_2$max in men and women showed only a 12- to 15-percent difference when $\dot{V}O_2$max was expressed in terms of FFW.[278] These differences have been minimized in the last decade since women have begun training at the same level as men.[2, 30, 273, 274, 279] Tokmakidis and coworkers[275] found that $\dot{V}O_2$max differences between male and female Grecian athletes varied from sport to sport: 9 percent for basketball to 24 percent for distance runners. Recent data from studies conducted with American elite athletes show an approximate 10- to 13-percent difference when $\dot{V}O_2$max is expressed in ml • kg^{-1} • min^{-1} of body weight.[30, 273, 274] When $\dot{V}O_2$max is expressed in ml • kg^{-1} • min^{-1} of FFW, the difference is less than 5 percent.[30, 273] Pollock and coworkers[273] found an 11.9 percent difference in $\dot{V}O_2$max expressed in body weight between male and female speedskaters who were training for the 1984 Olympic games. When these values were expressed in terms of FFW, the difference was only 3.6 percent (nonsignificant statistically).

An interesting study by Cureton and Sparling[280] attempted to equalize sex differences in body composition of runners by adding an external weight to the trunk of male runners. When percent excess weight of the man was equal to the excess percent fat of the weight-matched woman, sex difference in treadmill time reduced 32 percent, and 12-minute run performance regressed by 30 percent. An average 38-percent reduction in the sex difference of oxygen required per unit of FFW to run at various submaximal speeds and a 65-percent reduction in the difference in $\dot{V}O_2$max per ml • kg^{-1} • min^{-1} of body weight were shown. The authors concluded that "since sex-specific, essential fat of women cannot be eliminated by diet or training, it provides part of a biological justification for separate distance running standards and expectations for men and women." Even though physiological and performance differences between men and women become less as women begin to train in a similar fashion as men, certain sex-specific differences related to relative hemoglobin content, heart size, muscle mass, and other anthropometric and body composition factors will continue to affect differences in absolute performance.

Most of the studies concerning training have been conducted on men. Although information on women is lacking, the available evidence indicates that women tend to adapt to endurance training in the same manner as men.[148, 263, 269, 271, 277]

TRAINING WITH CARDIAC PATIENTS

The effects of chronic endurance training on cardiac patients are shown in Table 3–1. Many of the adaptive changes are similar to those found in normal healthy subjects. Aerobic capacity and submaximal capacity improve in most patients,[281–299] including those with impaired left ventricular function.[300–305] While it is well established that healthy adults adapt to endurance training by improving both central and peripheral function mechanisms,[1–4, 199] many have suggested that cardiac patients improve solely or mainly through peripheral mechanisms.[1, 199, 288, 306–308]

In contrast to the previously mentioned view concerning the adaptive response of cardiac patients to endurance training, the more recent results of Ehsani and colleagues[281, 297–299, 309] have shown that high-intensity, high-volume endurance training elicits both a significant central and peripheral training effect with cardiac patients.

In an attempt to illustrate and clarify the contrasting views as to how cardiac patients adapt to endurance training, Pollock[310] compared the findings of two classic investigations. In this illustration, the results of Froelicher and associates[291, 294] were contrasted with those of Ehsani and associates.[281, 297–299, 309]

In order to determine whether endurance training had an effect on myocardial perfusion and function, Froelicher and associates[291] randomly assigned 146 male patients—who had had a myocardial infarction at least 4 months previously and who were considered stable—to an exercise training group (n = 72) or a control group (n = 74). The groups were 35 to 65 years of age ($\bar{x}$ = 53 years). The exercise group trained mainly by walking, but arm and leg ergometry and jogging were performed by some. Training was conducted three times per week for approximately 45 minutes for a year. The average intensity of training was 60 percent of HRmax reserve. The training was considered to be of moderate intensity and was representative of the training load used by many programs conducted in North America. The intensity of training was at the level that usually elicits a significant aerobic training response. As stated by Pollock,[310]

"The results of the program showed that the exercise group elicited the typical adaptations associated with such a program: reduced resting HR; reduced HR, systolic BP, and rate-pressure product (RPP) at a standard submaximal work load; increased maximal oxygen uptake ($\dot{V}O_2$max, 18 percent); and no change in maximum HR, systolic BP, and RPP. Less angina pectoris and S-T–segment depression were found during the standard submaximal work test; however, the RPP also was significantly lower as a result of training. At similar RPP values (pre- versus post-training tests), there was no change in symptoms or S-T–segment depression. In general, no improvement was found in physiological variables that could be related to improvement in central function, i.e., RPP at maximum, which correlates with myocardial blood supply, stroke volume, cardiac output, left ventricular ejection fraction (both at rest and during exercise), and thallium perfusion. A small but significant improvement in stroke volume and cardiac output was found in the trained patients who did not have angina. Also, thallium perfusion improved slightly in the exercise group who had angina. The improvement in thallium perfusion with the angina group is in agreement with animal studies that suggest ischemia stimulates collateral flow; thus, exercise may act as a facilitator of this response."

Pollock[310] further explains that

"Ehsani and associates,[281, 297, 299, 309] in a series of experiments dating from 1981 to the present have demonstrated consistent significant effects on central function in MI patients who participated in high-intensity training. The subjects for these investigations included 10 to 25 in the exercise groups and 10 to 14 in control groups. Although subjects were not randomized, they were initially of similar age (approximately 52 years), physical characteristics, fitness level ($\dot{V}O_2$max), and medical status. The controls could not participate in the formal program generally because they lived too far from the exercise center. The training of their patients was of similar intensity (50 to 70 percent of $\dot{V}O_2$max), duration, and frequency as described by Froelicher and associates[291] for the first 3 months. The next 9 months differed significantly through training of higher intensity (80 to 90 percent of $\dot{V}O_2$max), greater frequency (5 days per week), and increased duration (50 to 60 minutes, exclusive of warm-up and cool-down periods). An example of the rigorousness of the training showed the runners to average 18.1 ± 1.6 miles per week at a peak training intensity of 89.4 ± 1.3 percent of $\dot{V}O_2$max during the last 3 months of training.[299] With this higher volume and intensity of training, $\dot{V}O_2$max increased 35 to 40 percent. Their results clearly showed a significant improvement in markers of central function: increased stroke volume and maximal RPP, and increased left ventricular ejection fraction from rest to exercise only after the training period. The systolic BP–end-systolic volume relationship was shifted upward and to the left, with an increase in maximal systolic BP and a smaller end-systolic volume, suggesting an improved contractile state after training. Also, markers of ischemia showed improvement after training, i.e., reduced S-T–segment depression at maximal effort (higher RPP after training) and significantly less angina. No changes were found in the control group."

More recently, Martin and Ehsani[298] found a reversal of exertional hypotension with prolonged exercise training as described previously in myocardial infarction patients. Other physiological improvements found with patients after endurance exercise training include greater glucose tolerance and insulin sensitivity,[311] diminished catecholamine response to exercise,[312] inhibition of secondary platelet aggregation,[296] reduction in systolic and diastolic BP in hypertensive patients,[19] increase in high-density lipoprotein cholesterol and high-density lipoprotein cholesterol to total cholesterol ratio,[297, 299, 313, 314] and favorable changes in body composition.[297, 299]

The question as to how long benefits from endurance exercise training can be maintained in cardiac patients is not well documented. A recent 7-year follow-up study on myocardial infarction patients involved in high-intensity and high-volume training was reported by Rogers and colleagues.[299] Table 3–5 shows that the initial significant benefits in physiological function and other important variables found after a year of high-intensity and high-volume training were maintained for 7 years. The results included the maintenance of reduced S-T–segment changes and symptoms of angina pectoris.

"These new findings of Ehsani and colleagues are provocative but must be interpreted with caution. It appears that higher-intensity programs provide a greater potential benefit for the patient, i.e., increased aerobic capacity, which include adaptations of both central and peripheral factors, than the more traditional light- to moderate-intensity exercise regimens. But it is also known that high-intensity

Table 3–5. Effects of High-Intensity and High-Volume Endurance Training in Cardiac Patients: 7 Years Follow-up (n = 9)[299]

Variable	Time of Follow-up (years)		
	0	*1*	*7*
Intensity (% HRmax)	—	81*	84*
Miles/Week	—	18*	25*
$\dot{V}O_2$max (ml $\cdot$ kg^{-1} $\cdot$ min^{-1})	25	36*	37*
RPP (SBP $\times$ HR $\times$ 10^{-3})	23.5	26.8*	26.2*
Total Cholesterol (mg/dl)	218	208	210
High-Density Lipoprotein (mg/dl)	38	45*	53*

*$p \leq 0.05$ from initial test.

effort [and significant S-T–segment depression are] associated with greater risk of precipitation of a major cardiac event.[315–318] Hossack and Hartwig[316] found three significant factors that differentiated patients who required resuscitation from a major coronary event and those patients who did not during rehabilitation in the CAPRI program. Patients who had cardiac arrests had higher aerobic capacities, exercised more often above their recommended upper limit training HR, and had significant S-T–segment depression of more than 1 mm of flat or downsloping S-T–depression from the J-point in response to exercise than the comparison group. Shephard and colleagues[318] reported that five of the first seven deaths in the Ontario Exercise-Heart Collaborative Study were in patients who showed deep S-T–segment depression during exercise. Figure 8–1, from Hellerstein and Franklin,[317] diagrammatically shows the relationship between exercise intensity (percent $\dot{V}O_2$max), improvement in $\dot{V}O_2$max, and risk of cardiovascular events. The figure shows a greater improvement in $\dot{V}O_2$max with increased intensity of training, and a dramatic increase in cardiovascular events when training exceeded 85 percent of $\dot{V}O_2$max. It must be emphasized that Ehsani (personal communication [1988]) has had many patients training at a high intensity, 85 to 90 percent of $\dot{V}O_2$max, the past [8 to 10] years who had significant S-T–segment depression during exercise and were without incident."[310]

SUMMARY

The chronic effects of physical activity on cardiorespiratory functions were reviewed. Generally, $\dot{V}O_2$max, cardiac output, stroke volume, A-V O_2 difference, and working capacity improved with endurance training. At submaximal work loads, $\dot{V}O_2$ and cardiac output remain fairly constant, with HR and systolic BP decreasing and stroke volume increasing. Whether cardiac patients show both central and peripheral physiological adaptations to endurance training is not known. Central changes in cardiac patients may depend on increased intensity of training (85 percent HRmax reserve or higher) and normal left ventricular function.

Research findings show that improvement in cardiorespiratory endurance depends on the intensity, duration, and frequency of the training program. Intensity and duration of training were found to be interrelated, and total kilocalorie expenditure was the important factor. Although there appears to be a minimal threshold for improving cardiorespiratory fitness (50 to 60 percent of maximum), programs of 20 to 40 minutes of continuous activity, performed 3 to 5 days per week, generally produce significant improvement in cardiorespiratory fitness. Programs of lesser frequency, intensity, or duration will not normally elicit the 15- to 30-percent improvement in aerobic capacity found in the previously mentioned regimens but still may cause a significant improvement (usually 5 to 10 percent). Weight training results in increased muscular strength but little improvement in aerobic capacity. To help prevent musculoskeletal injuries and improve adherence to endurance training, moderate-intensity programs appear to be superior to high-intensity ones.

Although women have been shown to have a lower $\dot{V}O_2$max as compared with men, their adaptation to training is similar.

The aging curve for $\dot{V}O_2$max may not be the same for active and sedentary populations. Middle-aged and elderly men who continue to train in a consistent fashion show a less than 5-percent reduction in aerobic capacity per decade of follow-up.

References

1. Åstrand, P.O., and Rodahl, K.: **Textbook of Work Physiology,** 3rd Ed. New York, McGraw-Hill Book Co., 1986.
2. Wilmore, J.H., and Costill, D.L.: **Training for Sport and Activity: The Physiological Basis of the Conditioning Process,** 3rd Ed. Dubuque, IA, William C. Brown, 1988.
3. McArdle, W.D., Katch, F.I., and Katch, V.L.: **Exercise Physiology, Energy, Nutrition and Human Performance,** 2nd Ed. Philadelphia, Lea & Febiger, 1986.
4. Rowell, L.B.: **Human Circulation Regulation during Physical Stress.** New York, Oxford University Press, 1986.
5. Taylor, H.L., and Rowell, L.B.: Exercise and metabolism. In Johnson, W., and Buskirk, E.R. (eds.): **Science and Medicine of Exercise and Sport,.** 2nd Ed. New York, Harper and Row, 1974, pp. 84–111.
5A. Dempsey, J., Hanson, P., and Henderson, K.: Exercise-induced arterial hypoxemia in healthy persons at sea level. **J. Physiol. (Lond.)** 355:161–175, 1984.
5B. Williams, J., Powers, S., and Stuart, M.: Hemoglobin desaturation in highly trained athletes during heavy exercise. **Med. Sci. Sports Exerc.** 18:168–173, 1986.
6. Mitchell, J.H., Sproule, B.J., and Chapman, C.: The physiological meaning of the maximal oxygen intake test. **J. Clin. Invest.** 37:538–547, 1958.
7. Astrand, P.O.: Measurement of maximal aerobic capacity. **Can. Med. Assoc. J.** 96:732–735, 1967.
8. Taylor, H.L., Buskirk, E.R., and Henschel, A.: Maximal oxygen intake as an objective measure of cardiorespiratory performance. **J. Appl. Physiol.** 8:73–78, 1955.
9. Buskirk, E.R., and Taylor, H.L.: Maximal oxygen intake and its relation to body composition, with special reference to chronic physical activity and obesity. **J. Appl. Physiol.** 11:72–78, 1957.
10. Pollock, M.L.: The quantification of endurance training programs. In Wilmore, J.H. (ed.): **Exercise and Sport Sciences Reviews,** Vol. 1. New York, Academic Press, 1973, pp. 155–188.
11. Kitamura, K., Jorgenson, C.R., Gobel, F.L., Taylor, H.L., and Wang, Y.: Hemodynamic correlates of myocardial oxygen consumption during upright exercise. **J. Appl. Physiol.** 32:516–522, 1972.
12. Robinson, B.F.: Relationship of heart rate and systolic blood pressure to the onset of pain in angina pectoris. **Circulation** 35:1073–1083, 1967.

13. Tzankoff, S.P., Robinson, S., Pyke, F.S., and Brown, C.A.: Physiological adjustments to work in older men as affected by physical training. **J. Appl. Physiol.** 33:346–350, 1972.
14. Boyer, J., and Kasch, F.: Exercise therapy in hypertensive men. **JAMA** 211:1668–1671, 1970.
15. Choquette, G., and Ferguson, R.J.: Blood pressure reduction in borderline hypertensives following physical training. **Can. Med. Assoc. J.** 108:669–703, 1973.
16. Hagberg, J.M., Ehsani, A.A., Goldring, D., Hernandez, A., Sinacore, D.R., and Holloszy, J.O: Effect of weight training on blood pressure and hemodynamics in hypertensive adolescents. **J. Pediatr** 104:147–151, 1984.
16A. Duncan, J.J., Farr, J.E., Upton, J., Hagan, R.D., Oglesby, M.E., and Blair, S.N.: The effects of aerobic exercise on plasma catecholamines and blood pressure in patients with mild essential hypertension. **JAMA** 254:2609–2613, 1985.
17. Hagberg, J.M., Goldring, D., Ehsani, A.A., Heath, G.W., Hernandez, A., Schechtman, K., and Holloszy, J.O.: Effect of exercise training on blood pressure and hemodynamic features of hypertensive adolescents. **Am. J. Cardiol.** 52:763–768, 1983.
18. Bjorntorp, P.: Effects of physical training and blood pressure in hypertension. **Eur. Heart J.** 8(Suppl.):B71–B76, 1987.
19. Hagberg, J.M., and Seals, D.R.: Exercise and hypertension. **Acta Med. Scand.** (Suppl.)711:131–136, 1987.
20. Tipton, C.M., Overton, J.M., Pepin, E.B., Edwards, J.G., Wegner, J., and Youmans, E.M.: Influence of exercise training on resting blood pressures of Dahl rats. **J. Appl. Physiol.** 63:342–346, 1987.
21. Saltin, B., and Åstrand, P.O.: Maximal oxygen uptake in athletes. **J. Appl. Physiol.** 23:353–358, 1967.
22. Costill, D.L.: Physiology of marathon running. **JAMA** 221:1024–1029, 1972.
23. Pollock, M.L.: Submaximal and maximal working capacity of elite distance runners. **Ann. N.Y. Acad. Sci.** 301:310–322, 1977.
24. Weber, K.T., and Janicki, J.S.: **Cardiopulmonary Exercise Testing.** Philadelphia, W.B. Saunders Co., 1986.
25. Wasserman, K., Hansen, J.E., Sue, D.Y., and Whipp, B.J.: **Principles of Exercise Testing and Interpretation.** Philadelphia, Lea & Febiger, 1987.
26. Froelicher, V.F.: Exercise and the Heart: **Clinical Concepts,** 2nd Ed., Chicago, Year Book Medical Publishers, 1987.
27. Pollock, M.L., Wilmore, J.H., and Fox, S.M.: **Health and Fitness Through Physical Activity.** New York, John Wiley and Sons, 1978.
28. Drinkwater, B.L.: Physiological responses of women to exercise. In Wilmore, J.H. (ed.): **Exercise and Sport Sciences Reviews,** Vol. 1. New York, Academic Press, 1973, pp. 126–154.
29. Wilmore, J.H., and Brown, C.H.: Physiological profiles of women distance runners. **Med. Sci. Sports** 6:178–181, 1974.
30. Pate, R.R., Wilson, G.E., Cureton, K.J., and Miller, B.J.: Cardiorespiratory and metabolic responses to submaximal and maximal exercise in elite women distance runners. **Int. J. Sports Med.** (Suppl.) 2:91–95, 1987.
31. Cooper, K.H.: **The New Aerobics.** New York, J.B. Lippincott, 1970.
32. Buskirk, E.R., and Hodgson, J.L.: Age and aerobic power: the rate of change in men and women. **Fed. Proc.** 46:1824–1829, 1987.
33. Hurst, W.: **The Heart,** 6th Ed. New York, McGraw-Hill Book Co., 1986.
34. Robinson, S.: Experimental studies of physical fitness in relation to age. **Arbeitphysiol.** 10:251–323, 1938.
35. Asmussen, E., Fruensgaard, K., and Norgaard, S.: A follow-up longitudinal study of selected physiologic functions in former physical education students after forty years. **J. Am. Geriatr. Soc.** 23:442–450, 1975.
36. Cureton, T.K.: **The Physiological Effects of Exercise Programs upon Adults.** Springfield, IL, Charles C Thomas, 1969.

37. American College of Sports Medicine: Position statement on the recommended quantity and quality of exercise for developing and maintaining fitness in healthy adults. **Med. Sci. Sports** 10:vii–x, 1978.
38. Costill, D.L.: Inside Running: **Basics of Sports Physiology.** Indianapolis, Benchmark Press, 1986.
39. MacDougall, J.D., Wenger, H.A., and Green, H.J. (eds.): **Physiological Testing of the Elite Athlete.** Ottawa, Canada, The Canadian Association of Sports Sciences, 1982.
40. Cureton, T.K., and Barry A.J.: **Improving the Physical Fitness of Youth.** Monograph of the Society of Research for Child Development, Vol. 29, No.4, 1964.
41. Pollock, M.L., and Blair, S.N.: Action into analysis: exercise prescription. **J. Phys. Educ. Rec.** 52:30–35, 1981.
42. The Perrier Study: **Fitness in America.** New York, Perrier, Great Waters of France, 1979.
43. White, C.C., Powell, K.E., Hogelin, G.C., Gentry, E.M., and Foreman, M.R.: The behavioral risk factor surveys: IV. the descriptive epidemiology of exercise. **Am. J. Prev. Med.** In press.
44. Schoenborn, C.A.: Health habits of U.S. adults, 1985: the 'Alameda 7' revisited. **Public Health Rep.** 101:571–580, 1986.
45. Stephens, J.: Secular trends in adult physical activity: exercise boom or bust? **Res. Q. Exerc. Sport.** 58:94–105, 1987.
46. Casperson, C.J., Christenson, G.M., and Pollard, R.A.: Status of the 1990 physical fitness and exercise objectives—evidence from NHIS 1985. **Public Health Rep.** 101:587–592, 1986.
47. Department of Health and Human Services: **Promoting Health/Preventing Disease: Objectives for the Nation.** Washington, D.C., U.S. Goverment Printing Office, 1980.
48. Public Health Service and U.S. Department of Health and Human Services: **The 1990 Health Objectives for the Nation: A Mid Course Review.** Washington, D.C., U.S. Government Printing Office, 1986.
48A. Shephard, R.J.: Fitness boom or bust—a Canadian perspective. **Res. Q. Exerc. Sport** 59:265–269, 1988.
49. LaPorte, R.E., Adams, L.L., Savage, D.D., Brenes, G., Dearwater, S., and Cook, T.: The spectrum of physical activity, cardiovascular disease and health: an epidemiologic perspective. **Am. J. Epidemiol.** 120:507–517, 1984.
50. Haskell, W.L., Montoye, H.J., and Orenstein, D.: Physical activity and exercise to achieve health-related physical fitness components. **Public Health Rep.** 100:202–212, 1985.
51. Haskell, W.L.: Physical activity and health: need to define the required stimulus. **Am. J. Cardiol.** 55:4D–9D, 1985.
52. Wilmore, J.H.: Exercise prescription for widespread fitness. In Skinner, J.S., Corbin, C.B., Landers, D.M., Martin, P.E., and Wells, C.L. (eds.): **Future Directions in Exercise and Sport Research.** Champaign, IL, Human Kinetics Books, 1989.
53. Leon, A.S., Connett, J., Jacobs, D.R., and Rauramaa, R.: Leisure-time physical activity levels and risk of coronary heart disease and death; the multiple risk factor intervention trial. **JAMA** 258:2388–2395, 1987.
54. Smith, E.L., Reddan, W., and Smith, P.E.: Physical activity and calcium modalities for bone mineral increase in aged women. **Med. Sci. Sports Exerc.** 13:60–64, 1981.
55. Paffenbarger, R.S., Hyde, R.T., Wing, A.L., and Hsieh, C.: Physical activity and all-cause mortality, and longevity of college alumni. **N. Engl. J. Med.** 314:605–613, 1986.
56. Durnin, J.V.G.A., and Passmore, R.: **Energy, Work and Leisure.** London, Heinemann Educational Books, 1967.
57. Christensen, E.H.: Physiological evaluation of work in the Nykroppa iron works. In Floyd, W.F., and Welford, A.T. (eds): **Ergonomics Society Symposium on Fatigue.** London, Lewis, 1953, pp. 93–108.

58. Katch, F.I., and McArdle, W.D.: **Nutrition, Weight Control and Exercise,** 3rd Ed. Philadelphia, Lea & Febiger, 1988.

59. Davies, C.T.M., and Knibbs, A.V.: The training stimulus, the effects of intensity, duration and frequency of effort on maximum aerobic power output. **Int. Z. Angew. Physiol.** 29:299–305, 1971.

60. Shephard, R.J.: Intensity, duration, and frequency of exercise as determinants of the response to a training regimen. **Int. Z. Angew. Physiol.** 26:272–278, 1969.

61. Hill, J.S.: **The Effects of Frequency of Exercise on Cardiorespiratory Fitness of Adult Men.** M.S. Thesis. London, University of Western Ontario, 1969.

62. Jackson, J.H., Sharkey, B.J., and Johnson, P.L.: Cardiorespiratory adaptations to training at specified frequencies. **Res. Q.** 39:295–300, 1968.

63. Sidney, K.H., Eynon, R.B., and Cunningham, D.A.: Effect of frequency of exercise upon physical working performance and selected variables representative of cardiorespiratory fitness. In Taylor, A.W., and Howell, M.L. (Eds): **Training: Scientific Basis and Application.** Springfield, IL, Charles C Thomas, 1972, pp. 144–148.

64. Pollock, M.L., Cureton, T.K., and Greninger, L.: Effects of frequency of training on working capacity, cardiovascular function, and body composition of adult men. **Med. Sci. Sports** 1:70–74, 1969.

65. Pollock, M.L., Tiffany, J., Gettman, L., Janeway, R., and Lofland, H.: Effect of frequency of training on serum lipids, cardiovascular function, and body composition. In Franks, B.D. (ed.): **Exercise and Fitness.** Chicago, Athletic Institute, 1969, pp. 161–178.

66. Pollock, M.L., Miller, H.S., Linnerud, A.C., and Cooper, K.H.: Frequency of training as a determinant for improvement in cardiovascular function and body composition of middle-aged men. **Arch. Phys. Med. Rehabil.** 58:141–145, 1975.

66A. Bouchard, C., Boulay, M., Thibault, M.C., and Carrier, R.: Training of submaximal working capacity: frequency, intensity, duration, and their interactions. **J. Sports Med.** 20:29–40, 1980.

67. Gettman, L.R., Pollock, M.L., Durstine, J.L., Ward, A., Ayres, J., and Linnerud, A.C.: Physiological responses of men to 1, 3, and 5 day per week training programs. **Res. Q.** 47:638–646, 1976.

68. Fox, E.L., Bartels, R.L., Billings, C.E., O'Brien, R., Bason, R., and Mathews, D.K.: Frequency and duration of interval training programs and changes in aerobic power. **J. Appl. Physiol.** 38:481–484, 1975.

69. Pollock, M.L., Broida, J., Kendrick, Z., Miller, H.S., Janeway, R., and Linnerud, A.C.: Effects of training two days per week at different intensities on middle-aged men. **Med. Sci. Sports** 4:192–197, 1972.

70. Kilbom, A., Hartley, L., Saltin, B., Bjure, J., Grimby, G., and Åstrand, I.: Physical training in sedentary middle-aged and older men. **Scand. J. Clin. Lab. Invest.** 24:315–322, 1969.

71. Pollock, M.L., Gettman, L.R., Mileses, C.A., Bah, M.D., Durstine, J.L., and Johnson, R.B.: Effects of frequency and duration of training on attrition and incidence of injury. **Med. Sci. Sports** 9:31–36, 1977.

72. Pollock, M.L.: How much exercise is enough? **Phys. Sportsmed.** 6:50–64, 1978.

73. Blair, S.N., and Kohl, H.W.: Rates and risks for running and exercise injuries: studies in three populations. **Res. Q. Exerc. Sport** 58:221–228, 1987.

74. Richie, D.H., Kelso, S.F., and Bellucci, P.A.: Aerobic dance injuries: a retrospective study of instructors and participants. **Phys. Sportsmed.** 13:130–140, 1985.

75. Powell, K.E., Kohl, H.W., Casperson, C.J., and Blair, S.N.: An epidemiological perspective of the causes of running injuries. **Phys. Sportsmed.** 14:100–114, 1986.

76. Pollock, M.L.: Prescribing exercise for fitness and adherence. In Dishman, R.K.

(ed.): **Exercise Adherence: Its Impact on Public Health.** Champaign, IL., Human Kinetics Books, 1988, pp. 259–282.

77. Chaffin, B.D., and Park, K.S.: A longitudinal study of low-back pain as associated with occupational weight lifting factors. **Am. Ind. Hyg. Assoc. J.** 34:513–525, 1973.

78. Cooper, K.H.: **Running Without Fear.** New York, M. Evans and Company, 1985.

79. Fisher, A.G., and Ebisu, T.: Splitting the duration of exercise: effects on endurance and blood lipid levels. **Med. Sci. Sports Exerc.** (Abstr.) 12:90, 1980.

80. Moffatt, R.J., Stamford, B.A., and Neill, R.D.: Placement of tri-weekly training sessions: importance regarding enhancement of aerobic capacity. **Res. Q.** 48:583–591, 1977.

81. Roskamm, H.: Optimum patterns of exercise for healthy adults. **Can. Med. Assoc. J.** 96:895–899, 1967.

82. Coyle, E.F., Martin, W.H., Sinacore, D.R., Joyner, M.J., Hagberg, J.M., and Holloszy, J.O.: Time course of loss of adaptation after stopping prolonged intense endurance training. **J. Appl. Physiol.** 57:1857–1864, 1984.

83. Cureton, T.K., and Phillips, E.E.: Physical fitness changes in middle-aged men attributable to equal eight-week periods of training, non-training and retraining. **J. Sports Med. Phys. Fitness** 4:1–7, 1964.

84. Taylor, H.L., Henschel, A., Brozek, J., and Keys, A.: Effects of bed rest on cardiovascular function and work performance. **J. Appl. Physiol.** 2:233–239, 1949.

85. Saltin, B., Blomqvist, G., Mitchell, J., Johnson, R.L., Wildenthal, K., and Chapman, C.B.: Response to exercise after bed rest and after training. **Circulation** (Suppl.)37:1–78, 1968.

86. Convertino, V., Hung, J., Goldwater, D., and DeBusk, R.F.: Cardiovascular responses to exercise in middle-aged men after 10 days of bed rest. **Circulation** 65:134–140, 1982.

87. Hung, J., Goldwater, D., Convertino, V.A., McKillop, J.H., Goris, M.L., and DeBusk, R.F.: Mechanisms for decreased exercise capacity after bed rest in normal middle-aged men. **Am. J. Cardiol.** 51:344–348, 1983.

88. Gaffney, F.A., Nixon, J.V., Karlsson, E.S., Campbell, W., Dowdey, A.B.C., and Blomqvist, C.G.: Cardiovascular deconditioning produced by 20 hours of bed rest with head-down tilt ($-5°$) in middle-aged healthy men. **Am. J. Cardiol.** 56:634–638, 1985.

89. Fringer, M.N., and Stull, A.G.: Changes in cardiorespiratory parameters during periods of training and detraining in young female adults. **Med. Sci. Sports** 6:20–25, 1974.

90. Knuttgen, H.G., Nordesjo, L.O., Ollander, B., and Saltin, B.: Physical conditioning through interval training with young male adults. **Med. Sci. Sports** 5:220–226, 1973.

91. Kendrick, Z.B., Pollock, M.L., Hickman, T.N., and Miller, H.S.: Effects of training and detraining on cardiovascular efficiency. **Am. Corr. Ther. J.** 25:79–83, 1971.

92. Miyashita, M., Haga, S., and Mitzuta, T.: Training and detraining effects on aerobic power in middle-aged and older men. **J. Sports Med.** 18:131–137, 1978.

93. Brynteson, P., and Sinning, W.E.: The effects of training frequencies on the retension of cardiovascular fitness. **Med. Sci. Sports** 5:29–33, 1973.

94. Hickson, R.C., and Rosenkoetter, M.A.: Reduced training frequencies and maintenance of increased aerobic power. **Med. Sci. Sports Exerc.** 13:13–16, 1981.

95. Siegel, W., Blomqvist, G., and Mitchell, J.H.: Effects of quantitated physical training program on middle-aged sedentary males. **Circulation** 41:19–29, 1970.

96. Hickson, R.C., Kanakis, C., Davis, J.R., Moore, A.M., and Rich, S.: Reduced

training duration effects on aerobic power, endurance, and cardiac growth. **J. Appl. Physiol.** 53:225–229, 1982.

97. Hickson, R.C., Foster, C., Pollock, M.L., Galassi, T.M., and Rich, S.: Reduced training intensities and loss of aerobic power, endurance, and cardiac growth. **J. Appl. Physiol.** 58:492–499, 1985.

98. Karvonen, M., Kentala, K., and Musta, O.: The effects of training heart rate: a longitudinal study. **Ann. Med. Exp. Biol. Fenn.** 35:307–315, 1957.

99. Hollmann, W., and Venrath, H.: Experimentelle untersuchungen zur Bedeutung eines trainings unterhalb and oberhalb der Dauerbeltz strungsgranze. In Diem, C. (ed.): **Korbs, Festschrift.** Frankfurt/Wein, W.U.A., 1962.

100. Wenger, H.A., and Bell, G.J.: The interactions of intensity, frequency, and duration of exercise training in altering cardiorespiratory fitness. **Sports Med.** 3:346–356, 1986.

101. Astrand, I., Astrand, P.O., Christensen, E.A., and Hedman, R.: Intermittent muscular work. **Acta Physiol. Scand.** 48:448–453, 1960.

102. Taylor, H.L., Haskell, W., Fox, S.M., and Blackburn, H.: Exercise tests: a summary of procedures and concepts of stress testing for cardiovascular diagnosis and function evaluation. In Blackburn, H. (ed.): **Measurement in Exercise Electrocardiography.** Springfield, IL, Charles C Thomas, 1969, pp. 259–305.

103. Shephard, R.J.: Future research on the quantifying of endurance training. **J. Hum. Ergol.** 3:163–181, 1975.

104. Sidney, K.H., Shephard, R.J., and Harrison, H.: Endurance training and body composition of the elderly. **Am. J. Clin. Nutr.** 30:326–333, 1977.

105. Gledhill, N., and Eynon, R.B.: The intensity of training. In Taylor, A.W., and Howell, M.L. (eds.): **Training, Scientific Basis and Application.** Springfield, IL, Charles C Thomas, 1972, pp. 97–102.

106. Kilbom, A.: Physical training in women. **Scand. J. Clin. Lab. Invest.** (Suppl.) 119:1–34, 1971.

107. Sharkey, B.J., and Holleman, J.P.: Cardiorespiratory adaptations to training at specified intensities. **Res. Q.** 38:698–704, 1967.

108. Faria, I.E.: Cardiovascular response to exercise as influenced by training of various intensities. **Res. Q.** 41:44–50, 1970.

109. Olree, H.D., Corbin, B., Penrod, J., and Smith, C.: **Methods of Achieving and Maintaining Physical Fitness for Prolonged Space Flight.** Final Progress Report to NASA. Grant No. NGR-04-002-004, 1969.

110. Sharkey, B.J.: Intensity and duration of training and the development of cardiorespiratory endurance. **Med. Sci. Sports** 2:197–202, 1970.

111. Pollock, M.L., Dimmick, J., Miller, H.S. Jr., Kendrick, Z., and Linnerud, A.C.: Effects of mode of training on cardiovascular function and body composition of middle-aged men. **Med. Sci. Sports** 7:139–145, 1975.

112. Pollock, M.L., Gettman, L.R., Raven, P.B., Ayres, J., Bah, M., and Ward, A.: Physiological comparison of the effects of aerobic and anaerobic training. In Price, C.S., Pollock, M.L., Gettman, L.R., and Kent, D.A. (eds.): **Physical Fitness Programs for Law Enforcement Officers: A Manual for Police Administrators.** Washington, D.C., U.S. Government Printing Office, No. 027-000-00671-0, 1978.

113. Gaessner, G.A., and Rich, R.G.: Effects of high- and low-intensity exercise training on aerobic capacity and blood lipids. **Med. Sci. Sports Exerc.** 16:269–274, 1984.

114. Burke, E.J., and Franks, B.D.: Changes in $\dot{V}O_2$max resulting from bicycle training at different intensities holding total mechanical work constant. **Res. Q.** 46:31–37, 1975.

114A. Santiago, M.C., Alexander, J.F., Stull, G.A., Serfass, R.C., Hayday, A.M., and Leon, A.S.: Physiological responses of sedentary women to a 20-week conditioning program of walking or jogging. **Scand. J. Sports Sci.** 9:33–39, 1987.

114B. Gossard, D., Haskell, W.L., Taylor, C.B., Mueller, J.K., Rogers, F., Chandler,

M., Ahn, D.K., Miller, N.H., and DeBusk, R.F.: Effects of low- and high-intensity home-based exercise training on functional capacity in healthy middle-aged men. **Am. J. Cardiol.** 57:446–449, 1986.

115. Pollock, M.L., Miller, H., Janeway, R., Linnerud, A.C., Robertson, B., and Valentino, R.: Effects of walking on body composition and cardiovascular function of middle-aged men. **J. Appl. Physiol.** 30:126–130, 1971.

116. Hanson, J.S., Tabakin, B.S., Levy, A.M., and Nedde, W.: Long-term physical training and cardiovascular dynamics in middle-aged men. **Circulation** 38:783–799, 1968.

117. Hartley, L.H., Grimby, G., Kilbom, A., Nilsson, N.J., Åstrand, I., Bjure, J., Ekblom, B., and Saltin, B.: Physical training in sedentary middle-aged and older men. III. **Scand. J. Clin. Lab. Invest.** 24:335–344, 1969.

118. Pollock, M.L.: Prescribing exercise for fitness and adherence. In Dishman, R.K. (ed.): **Exercise Adherence: Its Impact on Public Health.** Champaign, IL, Human Kinetics Books, 1988, pp. 259–277.

119. Kilbom, A., Hartley, L., Saltin, B., Bjure, J., Grimby, G., and Åstrand, I.: Physical training in sedentary middle-aged and older men. I. **Scand. J. Clin. Lab. Invest.** 24:315–322, 1969.

120. Oja, P., Teraslinna, P., Partaner, T., and Karava, R.: Feasibility of an 18 months' physical training program for middle-aged men and its effect on physical fitness. **Am. J. Pub. Health** 64:459–465, 1975.

121. Froelicher, V.F.: Exercise testing and training: clinical applications. **J. Am. Coll. Cardiol.** 1:114–125, 1983.

122. Hossack, K.F., and Hartwig, R.: Cardiac arrest associated with supervised cardiac rehabilitation. **J. Cardiac Rehabil.** 2:402–408, 1982.

123. Price, C., Pollock, M.L., Gettman, L.R., and Kent, D.A.: **Physical Fitness Programs for Law Enforcement Officers: A Manual for Police Administrators.** Washington, D.C., U.S. Government Printing Office, No. 027-000-00671-0, 1978.

124. Milesis, C.A., Pollock, M.L., Bah, M.D., Ayres, J.J., Ward, A., and Linnerud, A.C.: Effects of different durations of training on cardiorespiratory function, body composition and serum lipids. **Res. Q.** 47:716–725, 1976.

125. Terjung, R.L., Baldwin, K.M., Cooksey, J., Samson, B., and Sutter, R.A.: Cardiovascular adaptation to twelve minutes of mild daily exercise in middle-aged sedentary men. **J. Am. Geriatr. Soc.** 21:164–168, 1973.

126. Hartung, G.H., Smolensky, M.H., Harrist, R.B., and Runge, R.: Effects of varied durations of training on improvement in cardiorespiratory endurance. **J. Hum. Ergol.** 6:61–68, 1977.

127. Liang, M.T., Alexander, J.F., Taylor, H.L., Serfrass, R.C., Leon, A.S., and Stull, G.A.: Aerobic training threshold, intensity, duration, and frequency of exercise. **Scand. J. Sports Sci.** 4:5–8, 1982.

128. Wilmore, J.H., Royce, J., Girandola, R.N., Katch, F.I., and Katch, V.L.: Physiological alterations resulting from a 10-week jogging program. **Med. Sci. Sports** 2:7–14, 1970.

129. Yeager, S.A., and Brynteson, P.: Effects of varying training periods on the development of cardiovascular efficiency of college women. **Res. Q.** 41:589–592, 1970.

130. Blair, S.N., Chandler, J.V., Ellisor, D.B., and Langley, J.: Improving physical fitness by exercise training programs. **South. Med. J.** 73:1594–1596, 1980.

131. Knehr, C.A., Dill, D.B., and Neufeld, W.: Training and its effect on man at rest and at work. **Am. J. Physiol.** 136:148–156, 1942.

132. Saltin, B., Hartley, L., Kilbom, A., and Åstrand, I.: Physical training in sedentary middle-aged and older men. II. **Scand. J. Clin. Lab. Invest.** 24:323–334, 1969.

133. Ismail, A.H., Corrigan, D., and McLeod, D.F.: Effect of an eight-month exercise program on selected physiological, biochemical, and audiological variables in adult men. **Br. J. Sports Med.** 7:230–240, 1973.

134. Mann, G.V., Garrett, H., Farhi, A., Murray, H., Billings, T.F., Shute, F., and Schwarten, S.E.: Exercise to prevent coronary heart disease. **Am. J. Med.** 46:12–27, 1969.

135. Naughton, J., and Nagle, F.: Peak oxygen intake during physical fitness program for middle-aged men. **JAMA** 191:899–901, 1965.

136. Ribisl, P.M.: Effects of training upon the maximal oxygen uptake of middle-aged men. **Int. Z. Angew. Physiol.** 26:272–278, 1969.

137. Oscai, L.B., Williams, T., and Hertig, B.: Effects of exercise on blood volume. **J. Appl. Physiol.** 24:622–624, 1968.

138. Skinner, J., Holloszy, J., and Cureton, T.: Effects of a program of endurance exercise on physical working capacity and anthropometric measurements of fifteen middle-aged men. **Am. J. Cardiol.** 14:747–752, 1964.

139. Ekblom, B., Åstrand, P.O., Saltin, B., Sternberg, J., and Wallstrom, B.: Effect of training on circulatory response to exercise. **J. Appl. Physiol.** 24:518–528, 1968.

140. Hickson, R.C., Bomze, H.A., and Holloszy, J.O.: Linear increase in aerobic power induced by a strenuous program of endurance exercise. **J. Appl. Physiol.** 42:372–376, 1977.

141. Pechar, G.S., McArdle, W.D., Katch, F.I., Magel, J.R., and Deluca, J.: Specificity of cardiorespiratory adaptation to bicycle and treadmill training. **J. Appl. Physiol.** 36:753–756, 1974.

142. Golding, L.: Effects of physical training upon total serum cholesterol levels. **Res. Q.** 32:499–505, 1961.

143. Kasch, F.W., Phillips, W.H., Carter, J.E.L., and Boyer, J.L.: Cardiovascular changes in middle-aged men during two years of training. **J. Appl. Physiol.** 314:53–57, 1972.

144. Wood, P.D., Haskell, W.L., Blair, S.N., Williams, P.T., Krauss, R.M., Lindgren, F.T., Albers, J.J., Ho, P.H., and Farquhar, J.W.: Increased exercise level and plasma lipoprotein concentrations: a one-year, randomized, controlled study in sedentary, middle-aged men. **Metabolism** 32:31–39, 1983.

145. Buyze, M.T., Foster, C., Pollock, M.L., Sennett, S.M., Hare, J., and Sol, N.: Comparative training responses to rope skipping and jogging. **Phys. Sportsmed.** 14:65–69, 1986.

146. Wood, P.D., Terry, R.B, and Haskell, W.L.: Metabolism of substrates: diet, lipoprotein metabolism, and exercise. **Fed. Proc.** 44:358–363, 1985.

147. Hartzell, A.A., Freund, B.J., Jilka, S.M., Joyner, M.J., Anderson, R.L., Ewy, G.A., and Wilmore, J.H.: The effect of beta-adrenergic blockade on ratings of perceived exertion during submaximal exercise before and following endurance training. **J. Cardiopul. Rehabil.** 6:444–456, 1986.

148. Pels, A.D., Pollock, M.L., McCole, S.D., Dohmeier, T.E., Lemberger, K.A., and Oehrlein, B.F.: Training adaptations of males and females to different exercise modes. In review.

149. Leon, A.S., Conrad, J., Hunninghake, D.B., and Serfass, R.: Effects of vigorous walking program on body composition, and carbohydrate and lipid metabolism of obese young men. **Am. J. Clin. Nutr.** 32:1776–1787, 1979.

150. Davis, J.A., Frank, M.H., Whipp, B.J., and Wasserman, K.: Anaerobic threshold alterations caused by endurance training in middle-aged men. **J. Appl. Physiol.** 46:1039–1046, 1979.

151. Atomi, Y., Ito, K., Iwasaski, H., and Miyashita, M.: Effects of intensity and frequency of training on aerobic work capacity of young females. **J. Sports Med.** 18:39, 1978.

152. Magle, J., Foglia, G.F., McArdle, W.D., Gutin, B., Pechar, G.S., and Katch, F.I.: Specificity of swim training on maximum oxygen uptake. **J. Appl. Physiol.** 38:151–155, 1975.

153. Stransky, A.W., Mickelson, R.J., Van Fleet, C., and Davis, R.: Effects of a swimming training regimen on hematological, cardiorespiratory and body composition changes in young females. **J. Sports Med.** 19:347–354, 1979.

154. Cureton, T.K.: Improvement in physical fitness associated with a course of U.S. Navy underwater trainees, with and without dietary supplements. **Res. Q.** 34:440–453, 1963.
155. Åstrand, P.O., Eriksson, B.O., Nylander, I., Engstrom, L., Karlberg, P., Saltin, B., and Thorn, C.: Girl swimmers with special reference to respiratory and circulatory adaptation and gynecological and psychiatric aspects. **Acta Paediatr.** (Suppl.) 147:1–75, 1963.
156. Holmer, I.: Physiology of swimming man. **Acta Physiol. Scand.** (Suppl.) 407:1–55, 1974.
156A. Martin, W.H., Montgomery, J., Snell, P.G., Corbett, J.R., Sokolov, J.J., Buckey, J.C., Maloney, D.A., and Blomqvist, C.G.: Cardiovascular adaptations to intense swim training in sedentary middle-aged men and women. **Circulation** 75:323–330, 1987.
157. Christensen, E.H., and Hogberg, P.: Physiology of skiing. **Arbeitsphysiol.** 14:292–303, 1950.
158. Daniels, S., Pollock, M.L., and Startsman, T.: Effects of dancing training on cardiovascular efficiency and body composition of young obese women. **Proceedings of the 37th Annual Convention of the Southern District American Association for Health, Physical Education, and Recreation,** 1970, pp. 99–101.
159. Vaccaro, P., and Clinton, M.: The effects of aerobic dance conditioning on the body composition and maximal oxygen uptake of college women. **J. Sports Med.** 21:291–294, 1981.
160. Rockefeller, K.A., and Burke, E.J.: Psycho-physiological analysis of an aerobic dance programme for women. **Br. J. Sports Med.** 13:77–80, 1979.
161. Wilmore, J.H., Davis, J.A., O'Brien, R.S., Vodak, P.A., Walder, G.R., and Amsterdam, E.A.: Physiological alterations consequent to 20-week conditioning programs of bicycling, tennis, and jogging. **Med. Sci. Sports Exerc.** 12:1–8, 1980.
162. Jones, D.M., Squires, C., and Rodahl, K.: Effect of rope skipping on physical work capacity. **Res. Q.** 33:236–238, 1962.
163. Baker, J.A.: Comparison of rope skipping and jogging as methods of improving cardiovascular efficiency of college men. **Res. Q.** 39:240–243, 1968.
164. Fardy, P.S.: Effects of soccer training and detraining upon selected cardiac and metabolic measures. **Res. Q.** 40:502–508, 1969.
165. Claussen, J.P., Trap-Jensen, T., and Lassen, N.A.: Effects of training on heart rate during arm and leg exercise. **Scand. J. Clin. Lab. Invest.** 26:295–301, 1970.
166. Pollock, M.L., Miller, H.S., Linnerud, A.C., Laughridge, E., Coleman, E., and Alexander, E.: Arm pedaling as an endurance training program regimen for the disabled. **Arch. Phys. Med. Rehabil.** 55:418–424, 1974.
167. Nilsson, S., Staff, P.H., and Pruett, E.D.R.: Physical work capacity and effect of training on subjects with long-standing paraplegia. **Scand. J. Rehabil. Med.** 7:51–56, 1975.
168. Stamford, B.A., Caddihee, R.W., Moffatt, R.J., and Rowland, R.: Task specific changes in maximal oxygen uptake resulting from arm versus leg training. **Ergonomics** 21:1–19, 1978.
169. Magel, J.R., McArdle, W.D., Toner, M., and Delio, D.J.: Metabolic and cardiovascular adjustment to arm training. **J. Appl. Physiol.** 45:75–79, 1978.
170. Gass, G.C., Watson, J., Camp, E.M., Court, H.J., McPherson, L.M., and Redhead, P.: The effects of physical training on high level spinal lesion patients. **Scand. J. Rehabil. Med.** 12:61–65, 1980.
171. Lewis, S., Thompson, P., Areskog, N.H., Vodak, P., Marconyak, M., DeBusk, R., Mellen, S., and Haskell, W.: Transfer effects of endurance training to exercise with untrained limbs. **Eur. J. Appl. Physiol.** 44:25–34, 1980.
172. Miles, P.S., Sawka, M.N., Wilde, S.W., Durbin, R.J., Gotshall, R.W., and Glaser, R.M.: Pulmonary function changes in wheelchair athletes subsequent to exercise training. **Ergonomics** 25:239–246, 1982.

173. DiCarlo, S.E., Supp, M.D., and Taylor, H.C.: Effect of arm ergometry training on physical work capacity of individuals with spinal cord injuries. **Phys. Ther.** 63:1104–1107, 1983.

174. Whiting, R.B., Dreisinger, T.E., Dalton, R.B., and Londeree, B.R.: Improved physical fitness and work capacity in quadriplegics by wheelchair exercise. **J. Cardiac Rehabil.** 3:251–255, 1983.

175. Campney, H.K., and Wehr, R.W.: Effects of calisthenics on selected components of physical fitness. **Res. Q.** 36:393–402, 1965.

176. Taddonio, D.A.: Effect of daily fifteen-minute periods of calisthenics upon the physical fitness of fifth grade boys and girls. **Res. Q.** 37:276–281, 1966.

177. Getchell, L.: **An Analysis of the Effects of a Season of Golf on Selected Cardiovascular, Metabolic, and Muscular Fitness Measures on Middleage Men.** Ph.D. Dissertation. Urbana, IL, University of Illinois, 1965.

178. Nagle, F., and Irwin, L.: Effects of two systems of weight training on circulorespiratory endurance and related physiological factors. **Res. Q.** 31:607–615, 1960.

179. Fahey, T.D., and Brown, C.H.: The effects of an anabolic steroid on the strength, body composition, and endurance of college males when accompanied by a weight training program. **Med. Sci. Sports** 5:272–276, 1973.

180. Gettman, L.R., and Pollock, M.L.: Circuit weight training: a critical review of its physiological benefits. **Phys. Sportsmed.** 9:44–60, 1981.

181. Allen, T.E., Byrd, R.J., and Smith, D.P.: Hemodynamic consequences of circuit weight training. **Res. Q.** 47:299–306, 1976.

182. Wilmore, J.H., Parr, R.B., Girandola, R.N., Ward, P., Vodak, P.A., Barstow, T.J., Pipes, T.V., Romero, G.T., and Leslie, P.: Physiological alterations consequent to circuit weight training. **Med. Sci. Sports** 10:79–84, 1978.

183. Gettman, L.R., Ayres, J.J., Pollock, M.L., and Jackson, A.: The effect of circuit weight training on strength, cardiorespiratory function, and body composition of adult men. **Med. Sci. Sports** 10:171–176, 1978.

184. Gettman, L.R., and Ayres, J.J.: Aerobic changes through 10 weeks of slow and fast speed isokinetic training (abstract). **Med. Sci. Sports** 10:47, 1978.

185. Gettman, L.R., Ayres, J.J., Pollock, M.L., Durstine, J.L., and Grahtham, W.: Physiological effects on adult men of circuit strength training and jogging. **Arch. Phys. Med. Rehabil.** 60:115–120, 1979.

186. Garfield, D.S., Ward, P., Cobb, R., Disch, J., and Southwick, D.: **The Syracuse circuit weight training study report.** Houston, Dynamics Health Equipment, 1979.

187. Gettman, L.R., Culter, L.A., and Stratman, T.: Physiologic changes after 20 weeks of isotonic vs. isokinetic circuit training. **J. Sports Med. Phys. Fitness** 20:265–274, 1980.

188. Kimura, Y., Itow, H., and Yamazakie, S.: The effects of circuit weight training on $\dot{V}O_2$max and body composition of trained and untrained college men. **J. Physiol. Soc. Jpn.** 43:593–596, 1981.

189. Gettman, L.R., Ward, P., and Hagan, R.D.: A comparison of combined running and weight training with circuit weight training. **Med. Sci. Sports Exerc.** 14:229–234, 1982.

190. Hurley, B.F., Seals, D.R., Ehsani, A.A., Cartier, L.J., Dalsky, G.P., Hagberg, J.M., and Holloszy, J.O.: Effects of high-intensity strength training on cardiovascular function. **Med. Sci. Sports Exerc.** 16:483–488, 1984.

191. Messier, J.P., and Dill, M.: Alterations in strength and maximal oxygen uptake consequent to Nautilus circuit weight training. **Res. Q. Exerc. Sport** 56:345–351, 1985.

192. Marcinik, E.J., Hodgdon, J.A., Mittleman, K., and O'Brien, J.J.: Aerobic/calisthenics and aerobic/circuit weight training programs for Navy men: a comparative study. **Med. Sci. Sports Exerc.** 17:482–487, 1985.

193. Kelemen, M.H., Stewart, K.J., Gillian, R.E., Ewart, C.K., Valenti, S.A., Manley, J.D., and Kelemen, M.D.: Circuit weight training in cardiac patients. **J. Am. Coll. Cardiol.** 7:38–42, 1986.

194. Hickson, R.C., Rosenkoetter, M.A., and Brown, M.M.: Strength training effects on aerobic power and short-term endurance. **Med. Sci. Sports Exerc.** 12:336–339, 1980.
195. Hubbard, A.W.: Homokinetics: muscular function in human movement. In Johnson, W.R., and Buskirk, E.R. (eds): **Science and Medicine of Exercise and Sport,** 2nd Ed. New York, Harper and Row, 1974, pp. 523.
196. Brouha, L.: Training. In Johnson, W.R., and Buskirk, E.R. (eds): **Science and Medicine of Exercise and Sport,** 2nd Ed. New York, Harper and Row, 1980, pp. 276–286.
197. Saltin, B., Nazar, K., Costill, D.L., Stein, E., Jansson, E., Essen, B., and Gollnick, P.D.: The nature of the training response: peripheral and central adaptations to one legged exercise. **Acta Physiol. Scand.** 96:289–297, 1976.
198. Graves, J.E., Pollock, M.L., Jones, A.E., Colvin, A.B., and Leggett, S.H.: Specificity of limited range of motion variable resistance training. **Med. Sci. Sports Exerc.** 21:84–89, 1989.
199. Clausen, J.P.: Circulatory adjustments to dynamic exercise and effect of physical training in normal subjects and in patients with coronary disease. **Progr. Cardiovasc. Dis.** 18:459–493, 1976.
199A. Harris, K.A., and Holly, R.G.: Physiological response to circuit weight training in borderline hypertensive subjects. **Med. Sci. Sports Exerc.** 19:246–252, 1987.
200. Åstrand, P.O., and Saltin, B.: Maximal oxygen uptake and heart rate in various types of muscular activity. **J. Appl. Physiol.** 16:977–981, 1961.
201. Wilmore, J.H., Parr, R.B., Ward, P., Vodak, P., Barstow, T.J., Pipes, T.V., Grimditch, G., and Leslie, P.: Energy cost of circuit weight training. **Med. Sci. Sports** 10:75–78, 1978.
202. Hempel, L.S., and Wells, C.L.: Cardiorespiratory cost of the Nautilus express circuit. **Phys. Sportsmed.** 13:82–97, 1985.
203. Strathman, T., Gettman, L., and Culter, L.: The oxygen cost of an isotonic circuit strength program (abstract). **American Alliance for Health, Physical Education, and Recreation Research Papers,** 1979, p. 70.
204. Gettman, L.R.: The aerobic cost of isokinetic slow- and fast-speed circuit training programs (abstract). **American Alliance for Health, Physical education, and Recreation Research Papers,** 1979, p. 31.
205. Saltin, B., Hartley, L., Kilbom, A., and Astrand, I.: Physical training in sedentary middle-aged men, II. **Scand. J. Clin. Lab. Invest.** 24:323–334, 1969.
206. Muller, E., and Rohmert, W.: Die Geschwindigkeit der Muskelkraft-Zunahme bei isometrischem Training. **Arbeitsphysiol.** 19:403–419, 1963.
207. Rowell, L.B.: **Factors Affecting the Prediction of the Maximal Oxygen Intake from Measurements Made during Submaximal Work.** Ph.D. Dissertation. Minneapolis, University of Minnesota, 1962.
208. Kavanagh, T., Shephard, R.J., Doney, H., and Pandit, V.: Intensive exercise in coronary rehabilitation. **Med. Sci. Sports** 5:34–39, 1973.
209. Cooper, K.H., Pollock, M.L., Martin, R., and White, S.R.: Levels of physical fitness versus selected coronary risk factors—a cross sectional study. **JAMA** 236:166–169, 1976.
210. Skinner, J.: The cardiovascular system with aging and exercise. In Brunner, D., and Jokl, E. (eds): **Physical Activity and Aging.** Baltimore, University Park Press, 1970, pp. 100–108.
211. Pollock, M.L., Dawson, G.A., Miller, H.S. Jr., Ward, A., Cooper, D., Headly, W., Linnerud, A.C., and Nomeir, M.M.: Physiologic responses of men 49 to 65 years of age to endurance training. **J. Am. Geriatr. Soc.** 24:97–104, 1976.
212. DeVries, H.A.: Physiological effects of an exercise training regimen upon men aged 52 to 88. **J. Gerontol.** 24:325–336, 1970.
213. Benestad, A.M.: Trainability of old men. **Acta Med. Scand.** 178:321–327, 1965.

214. Suominen, H., Heikkinen, E., and Tarkatti, T.: Effect of eight weeks physical training on muscle and connective tissue of the m. vastus lateralis in 69-year-old men and women. **J. Gerontol.** 32:33–37, 1977.
215. Badenhop, D.T., Cleary, P.A., Schaal, S.F., Fox, E.L., and Bartels, R.L.: Physiological adjustments to higher- or lower-intensity exercise in elders. **Med. Sci. Sports Exerc.** 15:496–502, 1983.
216. Thomas, S.G., Cunningham, D.A., Rechnitzer, P.A., Donner, A.P., and Howard, J.H.: Determinants of the training response in elderly men. **Med. Sci. Sports Exerc.** 17:667–672, 1985.
217. Seals, D.R., Hagberg, J.M., Hurley, B.F., Ehsani, A.A., and Holloszy, J.O.: Endurance training in older men and women, I. cardiovascular responses to exercise. **J. Appl. Physiol.** 57:1024–1029, 1984.
218. Hagberg, J.M., Graves, J.E., Limacher, M., Woods, D.R., Leggett, S.H., Cononie, C., Gruber, J.J., and Pollock, M.L.: Cardiovascular responses of 70-79 year old men and women to exercise training. **J. Appl. Physiol.** 66:2589–2594, 1989.
218A. Pollock, M.L., Graves, J., Leggett, S., Braith, R., and Hagberg, J.M.: Injuries and adherence to aerobic and strength training exercise programs for the elderly. **Med. Sci. Sports Exerc.** 21:S59 (Abstract), 1989.
219. Hagberg, J.M.: Effect of training on the decline of $\dot{V}O_2$max with aging. **Fed. Proc.** 46:1830–1833, 1987.
220. Robinson, S., Dill, D.B., Robinson, R.D., Tzankoff, S.P., and Wagner, J.A.: Physiological aging of champion runners. **J. Appl. Physiol.** 41:46–51, 1976.
221. Robinson, S., Dill, D.B., Ross, J.C., Robinson, R.D., Wagner, J.A., and Tzankoff, S.P.: Training and physiological aging in man. **Fed. Proc.** 32:1628–1634, 1973.
222. Asmussen, E., Fruensgaard, K., and Norgaard, S.: A follow-up longitudinal study of selected physiologic functions in former physical education students after forty years. **J. Am. Geriatr. Soc.** 23:442–450, 1975.
223. Kasch, F., and Wallace, J.P.: Physiological variables during 10 years of endurance exercise. **Med. Sci. Sports** 8:58, 1967.
224. Dill, D.B., Robinson, S., and Ross, J.C.: A longitudinal study of 16 champion runners. **J. Sports Med. Phys. Fitness** 7:127, 1967.
225. Buskirk, E.R., and Hodgson, J.L.: Age and aerobic power: the rate of change in men and women. **Fed. Proc.** 46:1824–1829, 1987.
226. Dehn, M.M., and Bruce, R.A.: Longitudinal variations in maximal oxygen intake with age and activity. **J. Appl. Physiol.** 33:805–807, 1972.
227. Grimby, G., and Saltin, B.: Physiological analysis of physically well-trained middle-aged and old athletes. **Acta Med. Scand.** 179:513–526, 1966.
228. Pollock, M.L., Miller, H.S., Linnerud, A.C., Royster, C.L., Smith, W.E., and Sonner, W.H.: Physiological findings in well-trained middle-aged American men. **Br. Assoc. Sport Med. J.** 7:222–229, 1973.
229. Pollock, M.L., Miller, H.S., and Wilmore, J.: Physiological characteristics of champion American track athletes 40 to 75 years of age. **J. Gerontol.** 29:645–649, 1974.
230. Hodgson, J.L., and Buskirk, E.R.: Physical fitness and age, with emphasis on cardiovascular function in the elderly. **J. Am. Geriatr. Soc.** 25:385–392, 1977.
231. Heath, G.W., Hagberg, J.M., Ehsani, A.A., and Holloszy, J.O.: A physiological comparison of young and older endurance athletes. **J. Appl. Physiol.** 51:634–640, 1981.
232. Drinkwater, B.L., Horvath, S.M., and Wells, C.L.: Aerobic power of females, ages 10 to 68. **J. Gerontol.** 30:385–394, 1975.
233. Pollock, M.L., and Gushiken, T.T.: Aerobic capacity in the aged athlete. In Butts, N.K., Gushiken, T.T., and Zarins, B. (eds.): **The Elite Athlete.** New York, Spectrum Publications, 1985, pp. 267–274.
234. Pollock, M.L., Miller, H.S., and Ribisl, P.M.: Effect of fitness on aging. **Phys. Sportsmed.** 6:45–48, 1978.

235. Costill, D.L., and Winrow, E.: Maximal oxygen intake among marathon runners. **Arch. Phys. Med. Rehabil.** 51:317–320, 1970.
236. Kasch, F.W., Wallace, J.P., and Van Camp, S.P.: Effects of 18 years of endurance exercise on physical work capacity of older men. **J. Cardiopul. Rehabil.** 5:308–312, 1985.
237. Pollock, M.L., Foster, C., Knapp, D., Rod, J.S., and Schmidt, D.H.: Effect of age and training on aerobic capacity and body composition of master athletes. **J. Appl. Physiol.** 62:725–731, 1987.
238. Åstrand, P.O.: Exercise physiology of the mature athlete. In Sutton, J.R., and Brock, R.M. (eds.): **Sports Medicine for the Mature Athlete.** Indianapolis, Benchmark Press, 1986, pp. 3–16.
239. Åstrand, I., Åstrand, P.O., Hallback, I., and Kilbom, A.: Reduction in maximal oxygen uptake with age. **J. Appl. Physiol.** 35:649–654, 1973.
240. Maud, P.J., Pollock, M.L., Foster, C., Anholm, J., Guten, G., Al-Nouri, M., Hellman, C., and Schmidt, D.H.: Fifty years of training and competition in the marathon: Wally Hayward aged 70—a physiological profile. **S. Afr. Med. J.** 59:153–157, 1981.
241. Cooper, K.H., Purdy, J.G., White, S.R., Pollock, M.L., and Linnerud, A.C.: Age-fitness adjusted maximal heart rates. In Brunner, D., and Jokl, E. (eds.): **Medicine and Sport, Vol. 10, The Role of Exercise in Internal Medicine.** Basel, S. Karger, 1977, pp. 78–88.
242. Londeree, B.R., and Moeschberger, M.L.: Effect of age and other factors on maximal heart rate. **Res. Q. Exerc. Sport** 53:297–304, 1982.
243. Ehsani, A.A.: Cardiovascular adaptations to exercise training in the elderly. **Fed. Proc.** 46:1840–1843, 1987.
244. Rodeheffer, R.J., Gerstenblith, G., Becker, L.C., Fleg, J.L., Weisfeldt, M.L., and LaKatta, E.G.: Exercise cardiac output is maintained with advancing age in healthy human subjects: cardiac dilatation and increased stroke volume compensate for a diminished heart rate. **Circulation** 69:203–213, 1984.
245. LaKatta, E.G., Mitchell, J.H., Pomerance, A., and Rowe, G.G.: Human aging: changes in structure and function. **J. Am. Coll. Cardiol.** 10:42A–47A, 1987.
246. Bar-Or, O.: **Pediatric Sports Medicine for the Practitioner: From Physiological Principles to Clinical Applications.** New York, Springer-Verlag, 1983.
246A. Krahenbuhl, G.S., Skinner, J.S., and Kohrt, W.M.: Developmental aspects of maximal aerobic power in children. In Terjung, R.L. (ed.): **Exercise and Sport Sciences Reviews.** New York, MacMillan, 1985, pp. 503–538.
247. Ekbolm, B.: Effect of physical training in adolescent boys. J. Appl. Physiol. 27:350–355, 1969.
248. Sherman, M.: **Maximal Oxygen Intake Changes of Experimentally Exercised Junior High School Boys.** Ph.D. Dissertation. Urbana, IL, University of Illinois, 1967.
249. Larsson, Y., Persson, B., Sterky, G., and Theren, C.: Functional adaptations to rigorous training and exercise in diabetic and non-diabetic adolescents. **J. Appl. Physiol.** 19:629–635, 1964.
250. Lussier, L., and Buskirk, E.R.: Effects of an endurance training regimen on assessment of work capacity in prepubertal children. **Ann. N.Y. Acad. Sci.** 301:734–747, 1977.
251. Elovainio, R., and Sundberg, S.: A five-year follow-up study on cardiorespiratory function in adolescent elite endurance runners. **Acta Paediatr. Scand.** 72:1–6, 1983.
252. Rotstein, A., Dotan, R., Bar-Or, O., and Tenenbaum, G.: Effect of training on anaerobic threshold, maximal aerobic power and anaerobic performance of preadolescent boys. **Int. J. Sports Med.** 7:281–286, 1986.
253. Daniels, J., and Oldridge, N.: Changes in oxygen consumption of young boys during growth and running training. **Med. Sci. Sports** 3:161–165, 1971.
254. Cumming, G.R.: Current levels of fitness. **Can. Med. Assoc. J.** 96:868–977, 1967.

255. Zauner, C.W., and Benson, N.Y.: Physiological alterations in young swimmers during three years of intensive training. **J. Sports Med.** 21:179–185, 1981.

256. Kozar, B., and Lord, R.M.: Overuse injury in young athletes: reasons for concern. **Phys. Sportsmed.** 11:116–122, 1983.

257. Gedda, L.: Sports and genetics: a Study on twins (351 pairs). In Larson, L.A. (ed.): **Health and Fitness in the Modern World.** Chicago, Athletic Institute, 1961, pp. 43–64.

258. Klissouras, V.: Heritability of adaptive variation. **J. Appl. Physiol.** 31:338–344, 1971.

259. Klissouras, V., Pirnay, F., and Petit, J.: Adaptation to maximal effort: genetics and age. **J. Appl. Physiol.** 35:288–293, 1973.

260. Prud'homme, D., Bouchard, C., Leblanc, C., Lambry, F., and Fontaine, E.: Sensitivity of maximal aerobic power to training is genotype dependent. **Med. Sci. Sports Exerc.** 16:489–493, 1984.

261. Hamel, P., Simoneau, J.A., Lortie, G., Boulay, M.R., and Bouchard, C.: Heredity and muscle adaptation to endurance training. **Med. Sci. Sports Exerc.** 18:690–696, 1986.

261A. Bouchard, C.: Gene-environment interaction in human adaptability. In Malina, R.B., and Eckert, H.M. (eds.): **The Academy Papers.** Champaign, IL, Human Kinetics Publishers, 1988, pp. 56–66.

262. Åstrand, P.O.: Do we need physical conditioning? **J. Phys. Educ.** Mar.–Apr.: 129–135, 1972.

263. Kearney, J.J., Stull, G.A., Ewing, J.L., and Strein, J.W.: Cardiorespiratory responses of sedentary college women as a function of training intensity. **J. Appl. Physiol.** 41:822–825, 1976.

264. Smith, D.P., and Stransky, F.W.: The effects of jogging on body composition and cardiovascular response to submaximal work in young women. **J. Sports Med.** 15:26–32, 1975.

265. Marigold, E.A.: The effect of training at predetermined heart rate levels for sedentary college women. **Med. Sci. Sports** 6:14–19, 1974.

266. Mayhew, J.L., and Gross, P.M.: Body composition changes in young women with high resistance weight training. **Res. Q.** 45:433–439, 1974.

267. Flint, M.M., Drinkwater, B.L., and Horvath, S.M.: Effects of training on women's response to submaximal exercise. **Med. Sci. Sports** 6:89–94, 1974.

268. Cunningham, D.A., and Hill, J.S.: Effect of training on cardiovascular response to exercise in women. **J. Appl. Physiol.** 39:891–895, 1975.

269. Getchell, L.H., and Moore, J.C.: Physical training: comparative responses of middle-aged adults. **Arch. Phys. Med. Rehabil.** 56:250–254, 1975.

270. Franklin, B., Buskirk, E., Hodgson, J., Gahagan, H., Kollias, J., and Mendez, J.: Effects of physical conditioning on cardiorespiratory function, body composition and serum lipids in relatively normal weight and obese middle-aged women. **Int. J. Obesity** 3:97–109, 1979.

271. Hanson, J.S., and Nedde, W.H.: Long-term physical training effect in sedentary females. **J. Appl. Physiol.** 37:112–116, 1974.

272. Daniels, J., Krahenbuhl, G., Foster, C., Gilbert, J., and Daniels, S.: Aerobic responses of female distance runners to submaximal and maximal exercise. **Ann. N.Y. Acad. Sci.** 301:726–733, 1977.

273. Pollock, M.L., Pels, A.E., Foster, C., and Holum, D.: Comparison of male and female Olympic speedskating candidates. In Landers, D.M. (ed.): **Sport and Elite Performers.** Champaign, IL, Human Kinetics Publishers, 1986, pp. 143–152.

274. Daniels, J., Scardina, N., and Foley, P.: Elite and subelite female middle- and long-distance runners. In Landers, D.M. (ed.): **Sport and Elite Performers.** Champaign, IL, Human Kinetics Publishers, 1986, pp. 57–72.

275. Tokmakidis, S.P., Tsopanakis, A., Tsarouchas, E., and Klissouris, V.: Physiological profile of elite athletes to maximal effort. In Landers, D.M. (ed.): **Sport**

and Elite Performers. Champaign, IL, Human Kinetics Publishers, 1986, pp. 177–184.

276. Smith, D.P., and Stransky, F.W.: The effect of training and detraining on the body composition and cardiovascular response of young women to exercise. **J. Sports Med.** 16:112–120, 1976.

277. Burke, E.J.: Physiological effects of similar training programs in males and females. **Res. Q.** 48:510–517, 1977.

278. Sparling, P.B.: A meta-analysis of studies comparing maximal oxygen uptake in men and women. **Res. Q. Exerc. Sport** 51:542–552, 1980.

279. Wilmore, J.: Inferiority of female athletes: myth or reality. **J. Sports Med.** 3:1–6, 1975.

280. Cureton, K.J., and Sparling, P.B.: Distance running performance and metabolic responses to running in men and women with excess weight experimentally equated. **Med. Sci. Sports Exerc.** 12:288–294, 1980.

281. Ehsani, A.A., Heath, G.H., Hagberg, J.M., Sobel, B.E., and Holloszy, J.O.: Effects of 12 months of intense exercise training on ischemic ST-segment depression in patients with coronary artery disease. **Circulation** 64:1116–1124, 1981.

282. Hellerstein, H.K.: Exercise therapy in coronary disease. **Bull N.Y. Acad. Med.** 44:1028–1047, 1968.

283. Kavanagh, T., and Shephard, R.J.: Conditioning of postcoronary patients: comparison of continuous and interval training. **Arch. Phys. Med. Rehabil.** 56:72–76, 1975.

284. Naughton, J., Bruhn, J.G., and Lategola, M.T.: Effects of physical training on physiologic and behavioral characteristics of cardiac patients. **Arch. Phys. Med. Rehabil.** 49:131–137, 1968.

285. Ferguson, R.J., Petitclerc, R., Choquette, G., Chamiotis, L., Gauthier, P., Huot, R., Allard, C., Jankowski, L., and Campeau, L.: Effect of physical training on treadmill exercise capacity, collateral circulation, and progression of disease. **Am. J. Cardiol.** 34:764–769, 1974.

286. Detry, J.M., and Bruce, R.A.: Effects of physical training on exertional ST-segment depression in coronary heart disease. **Circulation** 44:390–396, 1971.

287. Clausen, J.P., and Trap-Jensen, J.: Effects of training on distribution of cardiac output in patients with coronary artery disease. **Circulation** 42:611–624, 1970.

288. Kasch, F.W., and Boyer, J.L.: Changes in maximum work capacity resulting from six months training in patients with ischemic heart disease. **Med. Sci. Sports** 1:156–159, 1969.

289. Bjernulf, A., Boberg, J., and Froberg, S.: Physical training after myocardial infarction: metabolic effects during short and prolonged exercise before and after physical training in male patients after myocardial infarction. **Scand. J. Clin. Lab. Invest.** 33:173–185, 1974.

290. Letac, B., Cribier, A., and Desplanches, J.F.: A study of left ventricular function in coronary patients before and after physical training. **Circulation** 56:375–378, 1977.

291. Froelicher, V., Jensen, D., Genter, F., Sullivan, M., McKirnan, M.D., Witzum, K., Scharf, J., Strong, M.L., and Ashburn, W.: A randomized trial of exercise training in patients with coronary heart disease. **JAMA** 252:1291–1297, 1984.

292. Foster, C., Pollock, M.L., Anholm, J.D., Squires, R.W., Ward, A., Dymond, D.S., Rod, J.L., Saichek, R.P., and Schmidt, D.H.: Work capacity and left ventricular function during rehabilitation after myocardial revascularization surgery. **Circulation** 69:748–755, 1984.

293. Miller, N.H., Haskell, W.L., Berra, K., and DeBusk, R.F.: Home versus group exercise training for increasing functional capacity after myocardial infarction. **Circulation** 70:645–649, 1984.

294. Froelicher, V., Jensen, D., and Sullivan, M.: A randomized trial of the effects

of exercise training after coronary artery bypass surgery. **Arch. Intern. Med.** 145:689–692, 1985.

295. Laslett, L.J., Paumer, L., and Amsterdam, E.A.: Increase in myocardial oxygen consumption indexes by exercise training at onset of ischemia in patients with coronary artery disease. **Circulation** 71:958–962, 1985.

296. Rauramaa, R., Salonen, J.T., Sappanen, K., Salonen, R., Venalainen, J.M., Ihanainen, M., and Rissanen, V.: Inhibition of platelet aggregability by moderate-intensity physical exercise: a randomized clinical trial in overweight men. **Circulation** 74:939–944, 1986.

297. Ehsani, A.A., Biello, D.R., Schultz, J., Sobel, B.E., and Holloszy, J.O.: Improvement of left ventricular contractile function by exercise training in patients with coronary artery disease. **Circulation** 74:350–358, 1986.

298. Martin, W.H., and Ehsani, A.A.: Reversal of exertional hypotension by prolonged exercise training in selected patients with ischemic heart disease. **Circulation** 76:548–555, 1987.

299. Rodgers, M.A., Yamamoto, C., Hagberg, J.M., Holloszy, J.O., and Ehsani, A.A.: The effect of 7 years of intense exercise training on patients with coronary artery disease. **J. Am. Coll. Cardiol.** 10:321–326, 1987.

300. Lee, A.P., Ice, R., Blessey, R., and Sanmarco, M.E.: Long-term effects of physical training on coronary patients with impaired ventricular function. **Circulation** 60:1519–1526, 1979.

301. Conn, E.H., Williams, R.S., and Wallace, A.G.: Exercise responses before and after physical conditioning in patients with severely depressed left ventricular function. **Am. J. Cardiol.** 49:296–300, 1982.

302. Smith, L.K., Layton, K., Newmark, J.L., and Dietrich, E.B.: An intensive cardiovascular rehabilitation program for patients with disabling angina and diffuse coronary artery disease. **J. Cardiopul. Rehabil.** 7:425–429, 1987.

303. Musch, T.I., Moore, R.L., Leathers, D.J., Bruno, A., and Zelis, R.: Endurance training in rats with chronic heart failure induced by myocardial infarction. **Circulation** 74:431–441, 1986.

304. Kellermann, J.J.: The role of exercise therapy in patients with impaired ventricular function and chronic heart failure. **J. Cardiovas. Pharmacol.** 10(Suppl.):S172–S177, 1987.

305. Sullivan, M.J., Higgenbotham, M.B., and Cobb, F.R.: Exercise training in patients with severe left ventricular dysfunction: hemodynamic and metabolic effects. **Circulation** 78:506–515, 1988.

306. Haskell, W.L.: Mechanisms by which physical activity may enhance the clinical status of cardiac patients. In Pollock, M.L., and Schmidt, D.H. (eds.): **Heart Disease and Rehabilitation,** 2nd Ed. New York, John Wiley and Sons, 1986, pp. 303–324.

307. Froelicher, V.F.: Exercise testing and training: clinical applications. **J. Am. Coll. Cardiol.** 1:114–125, 1983.

308. Hagberg, J.M.: Central and peripheral adaptations to training in patients with coronary artery disease. In Saltin, B. (ed.): **Biochemistry of Exercise, VI.** Champaign, IL, Human Kinetics Publishers, 1986, pp. 267–277.

309. Hagberg, J.M., Ehsani, A.A., and Holloszy, J.O.: Effect of 12 months of intense exercise training on stroke volume in patients with coronary artery disease. **Circulation** 67:1194–1199, 1983.

310. Pollock, M.L.: Benefits of exercise: effect on mortality and physiological function. In Kappagoda, C.T., and Greenwood, P.V. (eds.): **Long-Term Management of Patients after Myocardial Infarction.** Boston, Martinus Nijhoff Publishing, 1988, pp. 189–205.

311. Holloszy, J.O., Schultz, J., Kusnierkiewiez, J., Hagberg, J.M., and Ehsani, A.A.: Effects of exercise on glucose tolerance and insulin resistance. **Acta Med. Scand.** (Suppl.) 711:55–65, 1987.

312. Cousineau, D., Ferguson, R., deChamplain, J., Gauthier, P., Cote, P., and Bourassa, M.: Catecholamines in coronary sinus during exercise in man before and after training. **J. Appl. Physiol.** 43:801–806, 1977.

313. Hartung, G.H., Squires, W.G., and Gotto, A.M.: Effect of exercise training on plasma high-density lipoprotein cholesterol in coronary patients. **Am. Heart J.** 101:181–184, 1981.
314. Cowan, G.O.: Influence of exercise on high-density lipoproteins. **Am. J. Cardiol.** 52:13B–15B, 1983.
315. Haskell, W.L.: Cardiovascular complications during training of cardiac patients. **Circulation** 57:920–924, 1974.
316. Hossack, K.F., and Hartwig, R.: Cardiac arrest associated with supervised cardiac rehabilitation. **J. Cardiac Rehabil.** 2:402–408, 1982.
317. Hellerstein, H.K., and Franklin, B.A.: Exercise testing and prescription. In Wenger, N.K., and Hellerstein, H.K. (eds.): **Rehabilitation of the Coronary Patient,** 2nd Ed. New York, John Wiley and Sons, 1984, pp. 197–284.
318. Shephard, R.J.: Cardiac rehabilitation in prospect. In Pollock, M.L., and Schmidt, D.H. (eds.): **Heart Disease and Rehabilitation,** 2nd Ed. New York, John Wiley and Sons, 1986, pp. 713–740.

4

BODY COMPOSITION ALTERATIONS WITH EXERCISE

INTRODUCTION

What role does exercise play in the prevention, control, and treatment of obesity? For many years, it has been a common belief that exercise has little or no value in programs of weight reduction and control. Many examples are given demonstrating the tremendous number of hours of vigorous exercise necessary to obtain even small losses in body weight. It is a fact that compared with starvation or semi-starvation diets, exercise is not an efficient means of losing body fat. To complete a 26.2-mile marathon requires an energy expenditure of approximately 100 kcal per mile, or 2,620 kcal for the entire race. With 3,500 kcal representing the energy equivalent of a single pound of adipose tissue, this race could be completed using less than a pound of fat, provided fat was the primary energy source. In reality, carbohydrate is the predominant fuel source for such an activity, so the total fat loss would be only 0.25 pounds or less. However, evidence shows that physical inactivity may be a major cause of obesity in the United States and may even be a more significant factor than overeating.[1] In addition, many studies to be reviewed in this chapter have shown that substantial changes in body composition do result from an exercise program, even when diet remains unchanged.

When weight is lost by diet alone, a substantial amount of the total weight loss comes from the lean tissue, primarily as a result of water and protein loss. This was discussed in Chapter 2. Most of the recent fad diets have emphasized low carbohydrate intake, which results in a depletion of the body's carbohydrate stores. With the loss of 1 g of carbohydrate from the body stores, there is a concomitant loss of approximately 3 g of water. With a total storage capacity of 400 to 500 g of carbohydrate, there is the potential for a water loss of 1.2 to 1.5 kg with total depletion of the carbohydrate stores.[2] The ketosis resulting from these typical diets also promotes additional water loss (refer to Chapter 2). Thus, up to 1.5 to 2.5 kg (3 to 5 pounds) of weight loss per week can come from water loss associated with carbohydrate depletion and ketosis. Although the large decreases in scale weight resulting from this water loss are very rewarding on a day-to-day basis, the individual will eventually discontinue a particular diet when a target or goal weight is achieved. Typically, this individual will then revert to previous eating habits, and water storage will accompany the replenishment of the depleted carbohydrate stores. This initial water storage can approximate up to 2.0 to 2.5 kg (4 to 5 pounds) in the first 24 to 48 hours and is usually a devastating experience for the faithful dieter.

When exercise is used for weight loss or weight control purposes, there is often a gain in fat-free weight because of an increase in muscle mass, i.e., exercise-induced hypertrophy.[3] In addition, there is a loss of body fat, the magnitude of which depends on many variables to be discussed later in this chapter. Typically, body weight changes little, if at all, during the first 6 to 8 weeks of an exercise program, since gains in fat-free weight are compensating for losses in body fat.[3] This frequently leads to frustration on the part of the individual attempting to lose weight, whose scale reads "no change" after weeks of hard work. It is important to alert those in exercise programs to this basic fact. Scale weight is not a good index of those changes in body composition that are taking place as a result of the exercise program. The tightness or looseness of clothing is probably a better index of the body composition changes.

When using exercise as a means of weight reduction and control, the total energy cost of the physical activity program is the most important consideration in program design. Activities that are continuous in nature and have a moderate to high rate of caloric expenditure are recommended, e.g., walking, jogging, running, cycling, swimming, dancing, and vigorous sports or games. By increasing caloric expenditure by 300 to 500 kcal per exercise session through a properly prescribed physical activity program, it is possible to lose a pound of fat in 7 to 12 exercise sessions, provided food intake remains constant. For most people, this would mean a moderate jog for 30 minutes per day or a brisk walk for 45 to 60 minutes. If a modest diet was also followed, weight and fat reduction would occur at an even faster rate. Reducing food intake by one buttered slice of bread or one glass of dry white wine per day (approximately 100 kcal), combined with a 30-minute per day jogging program 3 days per week, would result in a fat weight loss of approximately 0.4 to 0.5 pounds per week, or 20 to 25 pounds in a year.

The remainder of this chapter investigates the role of exercise in weight control. First, the role of exercise in appetite regulation is discussed. Second, studies that have investigated alterations in body composition with physical training are reviewed. Finally, the body composition of athletic populations is presented.

EXERCISE IN APPETITE REGULATION

A common myth that has been perpetuated for decades suggests that exercise is ineffective in weight loss programs owing to the stimulating effect of the exercise on one's appetite, i.e., the exercise leads to a greater intake of kilocalories, negating the caloric expenditure of the exercise itself. Does exercise stimulate the appetite? The following review is divided into those studies conducted on animals and those conducted on humans, for the data are not totally consistent. For additional information on this topic, the reader is referred to the excellent review articles of Oscai,[4] Thompson and associates,[5] Pace and associates,[6] and Titchenal.[7]

Animal Studies

Oscai,[4] in his review of the research literature through 1972, concluded that exercise does tend to suppress the appetite in male animals, and the appetite suppression effect appears to be related to the intensity of the exercise. With long-duration, low-intensity exercise, animals that exercised had appetites similar to those of control animals that had not exercised. With high-intensity, short-term exercise, there was a distinct difference between the two groups, with the exercised groups consuming substantially fewer calories. Katch and colleagues[8] investigated the effects of exercise intensity on subsequent food consumption and body weight changes in two groups of male rats. One group exercised at a considerably higher intensity, but the total caloric expenditure during exercise was equated between the two groups. The high-intensity group demonstrated a reduction in food consumption and a reduction in body weight gain that exceeded that of the low-intensity group. However, both groups had depressed food consumption and rate of body weight gain compared with nonexercised control animals. Richard and colleagues[9] reported similar findings in two groups of male rats exercising at two different environmental temperatures,

24°C and 4°C, when their food intakes were compared with those
of sedentary control rats living under identical environmental
conditions. Both exercise groups consumed approximately 10 percent fewer calories per day compared with their sedentary controls.

Mayer and coworkers[10] investigated the role of exercise and
food intake on body weight in normal rats and genetically obese
mice. The results of this study are presented in Figure 4–1. Animals
were exercised for each of the specified durations for a minimum of
14 days or until a steady state of weight had been achieved. The
results indicated that exercise durations of 20, 40, and 60 minutes
were not accompanied by increases in food intake above the
amounts consumed by the group that was totally inactive. In fact,
a small decrease in food intake was observed at each of these
exercise durations. At durations of 2 hours or more, there was a
linear increase in food intake through 6 hours, at which point the
animals reached the stage of exhaustion. Body weight was reduced
below the control level, i.e., the level of the physically inactive
group, at each duration of exercise, with the weight stabilizing at
durations of 1 to 6 hours per day. A more recent study by Bulbulian
and associates,[11] repeating the Mayer and associates[10] protocol on

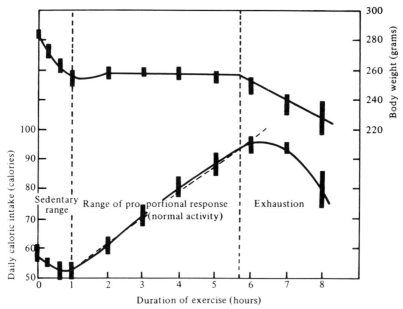

Figure 4–1. Food intake and body weight as functions of duration of exercise
in normal adult rats. (From Mayer, J., et al.: Exercise, food intake and body
weight in normal rats and genetically obese adult mice. **Am. J. Physiol.**
177:544–548, 1954.)

Swiss albino mice, demonstrated similar trends, but not to the same extent.

Studies using female animals have produced results that are not totally consistent with those for males as cited previously. In the reviews of Oscai[4] and Titchenal,[7] several studies were cited that reported increased appetites in female animals exercised for long durations as compared with sedentary controls. Oscai and colleagues[12] investigated the responses of both male and female rats to the same swimming program. The female rats that swam and were permitted unrestricted access to food took in an average of 75 kcal per day compared with 61 kcal per day for the sedentary female rats. In contrast, exercise had no effect on the voluntary intake of food in the male animals. Mazzeo and Horvath[13] found similar results in female rats, but the response was age related. Rats that started training at 6 months of age ate 28 percent more than their sedentary, age-matched controls; those who started training at 15 months of age ate 18 percent more than their sedentary, age-matched controls; and those who started training at 27 months of age ate the same as their sedentary, age-matched controls. Applegate and coworkers[14] found no change in 24-hour food intakes in either exercising male or female rats as compared with sedentary controls. The physiological basis for this sex-related paradox has not been elucidated. This phenomenon has not been observed in humans.[7]

What physiological mechanisms underlie the appetite suppression response to high-intensity exercise in animals? Oscai concluded that the appetite suppression induced by exercise is possibly mediated through increased levels of catecholamines associated with the stress of exercise.[4] It is well recognized that catecholamine levels increase in direct response to exercise intensity, i.e., the higher the intensity, the greater the levels of the circulating catecholamines.[2] Thus, high-intensity exercise leading to marked increases in catecholamine levels would result in a greater suppression of appetite than would low-intensity exercise, during which catecholamine levels would only be moderately elevated. Brobeck,[15] however, postulates that increased core temperature results in appetite suppression, which could also explain, at least in part, the appetite suppression effect of exercise. In addition, the increase in core temperature with exercise varies with the medium (swimming in water versus running through air) and the environmental conditions (heat, humidity, wind, and radiation). These factors must be considered when comparing studies conducted under different experimental conditions. Wirth and associates[16] have reported both a decreased insulin secretion and increased plasma clearance in trained as compared with untrained rats, resulting in lowered plasma insulin concentrations. Elevations in plasma insulin concentration are known to increase appetite markedly.

Human Studies

With humans, does exercise increase or decrease the appetite, or does the appetite remain unchanged? Similarly, if the appetite is increased in response to exercise, is this increase in caloric intake equal to, greater than, or less than that which was expended directly as a result of that exercise? These are very difficult questions to answer owing to the inherent problems associated with accurately measuring both energy intake and energy expenditure. An increase or decrease in caloric intake of 100 kcal per day above or below maintenance level would result in a 10-pound weight gain or loss, respectively, over the period of a year. To assess caloric intake to within ± 100 kcal per day is extremely difficult, perhaps impossible, even when subjects are monitored directly and their food intake is measured very accurately with a balance scale.[17] Assessment of energy expenditure is even more difficult. Although direct calorimetry is a reasonably accurate method of measuring caloric expenditure, it is highly impractical, and more indirect techniques have been utilized. Activity diaries, mechanical and electronic activity monitors, and heart rate monitors all provide relative indices of activity, but the conversion of these indices to actual caloric expenditures is not precise.[17] Although the animal model for investigating the relationship between exercise and appetite suffers from the very basic fact that "man is not a rat"[17] i.e., the applicability of data derived from studies on rats to humans is not well established, the human model suffers from its lack of control and precision. Thus, in reviewing the following data, these potential limitations must be recognized.

Mayer and colleagues[18] observed the relationship between caloric intake, body weight, and physical work in a group of 213 mill workers in West Bengal, India. The workers covered a wide range of on-job physical activity levels, from sedentary to very hard work. It was found that caloric intake increased with activity only within a certain zone, i.e., normal activity. With sedentary employees, the actual food intake was higher than that of the employees in the normal activity zone. For those employees in the medium to very heavy work zones, the caloric intake increased in proportion to the energy expenditure demands of the job. From this study and from his study on the food intake patterns of exercising rats, Mayer has concluded that when activity is reduced to below a minimal level, a corresponding decrease in food intake does not result, and obesity develops.[19] This has led to the theory that a certain minimal level of physical activity is necessary before the body can precisely regulate food intake to balance energy expenditure. An appropriate analogy might be the television set, in which a program can be selected by the use of both a channel selector and a fine tuner. The channel selector brings the viewer into the appropriate region, and the fine tuner allows for a precise regulation of the picture (M.J. Joyner, personal communication). It is possible that a certain level of physical activity is necessary before the body can exactly control food intake to match energy expenditure. Thus, a sedentary lifestyle may reduce the ability of the fine tuning device to control food intake precisely, resulting in a positive energy balance. This may amount to only a 10- to 100-kcal error, or the equivalent of a potato chip to a slice of buttered bread, but this would produce a net yearly weight gain of one to ten pounds. Mayer and colleagues[10] have referred to the sedentary "nonresponsive" zone, in which a decrease in activity is *not* accompanied by a reduction in appetite and food intake. Mayer and Bullen[20] state that this has been known empirically by farmers for centuries and explains the practice of penning up or cooping up cattle, hogs, and geese for fattening.

Other studies have attempted to investigate experimentally the role of increased physical activity on appetite and food intake. Dempsey[21] studied a small group of obese and nonobese young men undergoing a program of vigorous physical exercise. Initially, overweight subjects experienced significant losses of body weight and subcutaneous and total body fat and increases in fat-free body weight and muscular mass. Daily caloric intake was unchanged over the 18-week program, when compared with a 3-week pretraining phase in which the subjects were relatively sedentary. These results could be interpreted in two ways. It would be logical to conclude that exercise had no effect on appetite; in fact, the trend was for a 100- to 200-kcal increase in food intake, although this was not statistically significant. However, it must be remembered that the subjects were increasing their energy expenditures through an hour per day of vigorous exercise. Although the caloric equivalent of this exercise was not provided, walking 4 miles in 60 minutes (15 minutes per mile) or jogging 6 miles in 60 minutes (10 minutes per mile) would result in an average caloric expenditure of 400 to 600 kcal per day in addition to the normal caloric expenditure for 24 hours. Thus, the fact that the appetite did not increase implies a 300- to 500-kcal deficit in intake over expenditure (allowing a resting metabolic rate of 100 kcal per hour), provided the individual was in energy balance at the beginning of the study. The point to be made is that energy intake should not be expected to remain the same with increased caloric expenditure if caloric balance is to be maintained. It is therefore possible to interpret this study as showing a *relative* decrease in appetite even though caloric intake did not change, since intake did not increase proportionally to expenditure.

Holloszy and associates[22] observed the effects of a 6-month program of endurance exercise on the serum lipids of middle-aged men. Skinner and associates[23] reported on the work capacity and anthropometric measurement changes in this same group of men. In these two reports of this single study, the men who were placed on a 6-month exercise program of endurance calisthenics and distance running (2 to 4 miles per day) on the average of 3.3 times per week had no change in either body weight or average daily caloric intake, although there were changes in body composition, i.e., decreased body fat and increased lean weight. These results are in agreement with the study of Dempsey cited previously and could be interpreted to indicate that there was a net loss in appetite, since caloric intake did not increase with increasing caloric expenditure.

Jankowski and Foss[24] measured the postexercise changes in the 24-hour energy intake of 14 sedentary men after either a 440-yard or a one-mile run on a treadmill. They found that the performance of these running tasks had no measurable effect on the 24-hour energy intake. This study can be criticized on the basis of the short period of the exercise bout, in which the energy expenditure would be 100 kcal or less, and on the basis that it was an acute bout of exercise. Although the controls used in this study were excellent, the study would have been much more valuable if the observations would have been extended over a period of several weeks and the duration and intensity of the exercise bouts would have been more substantive.

Johnson and colleagues[25] studied 32 college women who participated in a 10-week cycle ergometer endurance training program 30 minutes per day, 5 days per week. Although body weight remained unchanged, four skinfold thicknesses were reduced substantially, and the relative body fat estimated from skinfolds decreased from an initial value of 24.9 percent to 22.8 percent. Mean caloric intake decreased from 1,751 kcal per day to 1,584 kcal per day from the beginning to the end of the exercise program.

Woo and colleagues[26, 27] observed the effect of formalized exercise training on spontaneous caloric intake. In the first of two studies,[26] six obese women (167 percent of ideal weight) went through three 19-day treatment periods: sedentary control, mild daily activity of treadmill walking to increase daily expenditure to 110 percent of control values, and moderate daily activity of treadmill walking to increase daily expenditure to 125 percent of control values. The energy intake over the course of the three treatment periods did not change; thus, the difference between caloric intake and expenditure was +11 kcal per day for the sedentary period, −114 kcal per day for the mild activity, and −369 kcal per day for the moderate activity. This is illustrated in Figure 4–2.

In their second study, Woo and colleagues[27] observed three obese women (187 percent of ideal weight) for a period of 57 days. Activity levels were adjusted to 125 percent of control values. Daily energy expenditure was maintained through treadmill walking at 2,882 kcal per day, while intake was constant at 1,903 kcal per day. Intake did not change over the course of the study even though the subjects were provided food in extra quantity. Both of these studies have demonstrated an uncoupling, or an independence, of intake and expenditure.[28]

McGowan and coworkers[29] studied the effects of both increasing and decreasing normal energy expenditure over periods of one week on the self-reported caloric intake of seven male joggers. Periods of

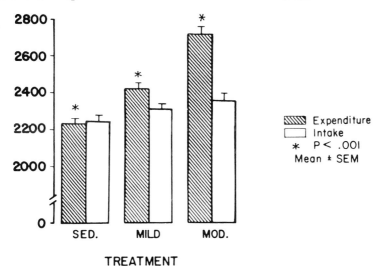

Figure 4–2. Alterations in energy intake and expenditure in obese women undergoing 19-day treatment periods of no exercise, mild exercise (110% of normal energy expenditure), and moderate exercise (125% of normal energy expenditure). (From Woo, R.: The effect of increasing physical activity on voluntary food intake and energy balance. **Int. J. Obesity** 9 [Suppl. 2]:155–160, 1985.)

no exercise, regular exercise (3.5 miles per day), and double exercise (7.0 miles per day) resulted in no significant changes in caloric intake, i.e., 2,529, 2,535, and 2,695 kcal per day under the three conditions, respectively.

If exercise does act to suppress the appetite or to maintain food intake at a constant level while energy expenditure is increasing, how can this be explained physiologically? In the previous section on animal studies, Oscai[4] concluded that appetite suppression could be mediated through increases in plasma catecholamine levels. The possible influence of elevations in core temperature was also mentioned. Belbeck and Critz[30] have investigated the possibility of increased levels of a urinary anorexigenic substance with exercise as a contributing cause to appetite suppression. Stevenson and associates[31] first demonstrated the existence of this substance in 1964. Belbeck and Critz[30] found that 60 to 90 minutes after exhaustive treadmill exercise in seven healthy young men, there was a 21 percent increase in the plasma concentration of this anorexigenic substance. The injection of this substance in amounts sufficient to cause a 50-percent increase in its plasma concentration in rats had previously been shown to decrease food intake for 24 to 48 hours. They concluded that this substance may be responsible for the decreased appetite and food intake after exercise in humans. Unfortunately, no further studies have been conducted to determine more precisely the specific physiological mechanisms involved in appetite suppression with vigorous physical exercise. The reduction in insulin levels noted in the previous section[16] may play an important role.

BODY COMPOSITION ALTERATIONS WITH PHYSICAL TRAINING

To investigate those alterations in body composition that occur consequent to physical training, both animal and human models have been used. Although the animal model is much easier to control, the validity of drawing conclusions for humans from animal studies is still being debated. Thus, there is a need for human research as well, recognizing the inherent limitations in exerting tight controls. The following review of the literature is divided into two sections: animal studies and human studies. The animal studies are reviewed briefly, with a much more comprehensive review of the human investigations. The reader is referred to several extensive review articles for a more comprehensive overview of this area.[4–6]

Animal Studies

Oscai,[4] in a general review of the role of exercise in weight control published in 1973, provided a comprehensive summary of the animal studies that had been conducted through 1972. He concluded that male animals subjected to programs of regularly performed treadmill running or swimming gain weight more slowly and have lower final body weights than comparable freely eating sedentary controls. The slower rate of weight gain was due to an increased caloric expenditure associated with the exercise and, in some cases, to a significant reduction in food intake. Female rats, in contrast, gain weight at approximately the same rate as sedentary, freely eating controls. This is due to an increase in food intake that apparently balances the increase in caloric expenditure associated with exercise.

Analysis of the body composition changes in these animals after physical training reveals that the male animals are much lighter, have considerably lower fat weights, and have lower fat-free weights as compared with the sedentary, freely eating controls. The female exercisers have similar body weights, greatly reduced total body fat weights, and increased fat-free weights.[4]

To better understand the physiological mechanisms involved, several investigators have attempted to determine actual cellular changes consequent to physical training. Oscai and Holloszy[32] studied five groups of rats matched for weight under the following conditions: a baseline group sacrificed at the beginning of the study; a freely eating, swimming group; a freely eating, sedentary group; and two paired-weight groups who were calorie restricted to match the weight loss of the exercise group, with the protein intake of the one paired-weight group matched to that of the exercise group. With an initial mean weight of 706 g for all five groups, the exercising group lost 182 g over 18 weeks as a result of both an increase in caloric expenditure and a decrease in appetite. The sedentary, food-restricted animals lost an average of 182 g, and the sedentary, freely eating animals gained 118 g. The composition of the weight lost by the exercising animals was 78 percent fat, 5 percent protein, 1 percent minerals, and 16 percent water, compared with 62 percent fat, 11 percent protein, 1 percent minerals, and 26 percent water for the sedentary, food-restricted animals. Thus, exercise provided greater increases in fat loss and reduced the loss of the lean tissue.

Oscai and coworkers[33] divided young rats, 8 days of age, into one of three groups: swim-trained for 14 to 16 weeks; sedentary, paired-weight, with caloric intake regulated to match the weight gain of the exercising group; and sedentary, freely eating. At the conclusion of the study, the sedentary, freely eating rats weighed 418 g, compared with 260 g for the exercising rats and 266 g for the sedentary, paired-weight rats, with fat weights of 102 g (24.4 percent fat), 26 g (10.0 percent fat), and 45 g (16.9 percent fat), respectively. The average caloric intake after weaning was 60 kcal per day for the sedentary, freely eating rats, 59 kcal per day for the exercising, freely eating rats, and 34 kcal per day for the sedentary, paired-weight rats. Compared with the sedentary, freely eating control animals, the exercising and sedentary paired-weight animals had significantly lighter epididymal fat pads with fewer and smaller adipocytes. Compared with the food-restricted animals, the exercising animals had fewer and smaller adipocytes. The researchers concluded that exercise in addition to food restriction early in life is effective in reducing the rate of adipocyte proliferation consequent to growth.

Oscai and coworkers[34] investigated the influence of both exercise and food restriction on adipose tissue cellularity in rats, starting at 5 days of age. The rats were divided into the following six groups: two groups of rats exercised by swimming 6 days per week, 360 minutes a day for 23 weeks; two groups of rats that were sedentary but whose caloric intake was restricted to match the body weights of the exercised groups; and two groups of freely eating, sedentary rats. One group from each condition was sacrificed at the end of the 23-week exercise program, and the other group from each condition was studied through 62 weeks of age. During the final 34 weeks of the study, all three remaining groups were maintained sedentary without the opportunity to exercise and were allowed to eat freely. The body weight changes in these animals are illustrated in Figure 4–3. The average daily food intakes for the first 28 weeks were 19, 11, and 20 g for the exercising; sedentary, paired-weight; and sedentary, freely eating groups, respectively, and were 20, 19, and 20 g, respectively, from week 28 to week 62. The exercised animals, even after 34 weeks of a sedentary existence, had epididymal fat pads that were lighter and contained less fat than either of the sedentary groups. The lower fat content in the exercised group was the result of fewer adipocytes, as the cell diameters were similar among the three groups. The authors concluded that exercise in early life is effective in significantly reducing the rate of adipocyte proliferation, resulting in significantly lower body fat later in life.

Taylor and associates[35] observed the effects of fat pad removal

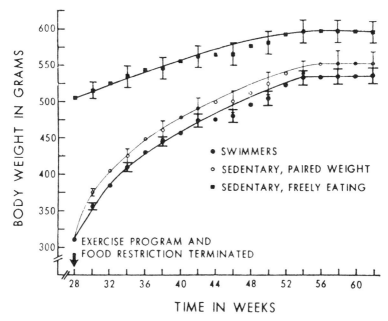

Figure 4–3. Influence of exercise and food restriction during the first 28 weeks of life on subsequent gains in body weight using male Wistar strain rats. (From Oscai, L. B., et al.: Exercise or food restriction: effect on adipose tissue cellularity. **Am. J. Physiol.** 227:901–904, 1974.)

in 54 exercised and control male Wistar rats. The animals were divided into three feeding pattern groups: freely eating, pair-fed, and paired-weight. The exercise program consisted of running on a motor-driven treadmill for a period of 16 weeks, an hour a day, 5 days per week. Animals had either one or both fat pads removed before starting the exercise program. Fat pad regeneration was noted in all animals. When one fat pad was removed, the regeneration was not as great per pad as after bilateral lipidectomy. Exercise further inhibited fat pad regeneration when both pads were removed. This inhibition was the result of a smaller cell diameter and a lower cell number in the fat pads of the exercised rats.

Studies conducted on adult animals demonstrate a slightly different response to exercise training. Deb and Martin[36] investigated the effects of exercise and of food restriction on Zucker obese and lean rats. Zucker obese rats pair-fed to match their lean littermates gained more body fat on the same caloric intake, indicating greater efficiency of diet utilization. Exercise significantly reduced the fat pad weights and the body fat content of the obese rats. However, exercise had no effect on adipocyte number. Askew and colleagues[37] reported similar results, i.e., decreases in body weight, epididymal fat pad weight, and adipocyte size, with no change in adipocyte number, in a group of mature rats trained on a motor-driven treadmill for a period of 13 weeks. Taylor[38] also reported decreased fat cell diameter and lipid content, but no change in fat cell number after running or swimming programs in mature rats of 4 months' duration. In the study by Applegate and colleagues,[14] described in a previous section of this chapter, exercising male rats weighed less and had a lower relative body fat content as compared with their sedentary controls, and female rats weighed the same but had lower relative body fat values as compared with their sedentary controls, after a 22-day period of treadmill running.

From the preceding studies, a fairly consistent pattern is apparent. In young, growing animals, physical training slows the rate of increase in body weight, total fat weight, and fat cell number. At maturity, the exercised animal has a lower body weight, lower total fat weight, and fewer adipocytes. The reduced number of adipocytes is the result of a decreased rate of proliferation, not a decrease in existing fat cell number. This latter point is an important one, for there appears to be no way, other than surgical removal, to decrease the number of adipocytes. When exercise is started later in life, after the attainment of maturity, there is a subsequent reduction or decreased rate of increase in total body weight, in total fat weight, and in adipocyte cell size, with no change in cell number.

One additional factor, which is of considerable importance, concerns the alterations in lean tissue with weight loss. When weight is lost solely through caloric restriction, considerable losses in lean tissue of 35 to 45 percent of the total weight loss are common.[4] With exercise or a combination of caloric restriction and exercise, there is a sparing of lean tissue and substantially greater losses in body fat.[32] Oscai[4] attributes the above alterations to the lipid-mobilizing effect of exercise, an effect that he feels is mediated, in part, by increased activity of the sympathetic nervous system. He states that the fat-mobilizing effect, which persists for a considerable time after the cessation of exercise, could play a role in the conservation of lean tissue by making available to the muscle and organ cells more of the energy stored as fat. Richard and Trayhurn have demonstrated that exercise training reduces the rate of fatty acid synthesis in the major lipogenic tissues.[39] It is clear that exercise training plays an important role in controlling the adipose tissue mass in animals both early in life and after attaining full maturity.

Normal Human Populations

A number of studies have investigated body composition alterations with physical training. It would not be practical, nor serve any useful purpose, to review each of these studies. Thus, the following review includes only those studies that have made a unique contribution to this body of knowledge. There also appears to be a trend emerging from the existing literature that should be acknowledged. The response to physical training programs appears to be a function of the degree of obesity exhibited by the subjects at the start of the study. This is an inverse relationship, with those who are only moderately obese receiving the greatest benefits.

Parizkova and Poupa[40] conducted a longitudinal study of seven female gymnasts on the Czechoslovakian National Team and an additional group of female gymnasts attending a sports school for 3 to 4 years. Their observations were carried out over a period of several years. They found that there was a direct correlation between the intensity of training and alterations in body composition. With intense training, body density increased, reflecting a loss in relative body fat, and skinfold thicknesses decreased. During periods of rest or reduced activity, these changes were reversed. Interestingly, the caloric intake was highest during intense training when body fat levels were low and energy expenditure high, and was lowest during rest periods when body fat levels were elevated. Parizkova's[41] study of 11 female gymnasts over a period of 5 years confirms these findings (Fig. 4–4).

Wells and coworkers[42] found that after 4 weeks of intensive physical training, adolescent girls showed an increase in specific gravity of 1.053 to 1.058, a decrease in the sum of 10 skinfolds from 102 to 85 mm, and a slight increase in body weight of 1.0 kg. These data are approximations, as they were estimated from the original data that were presented in figure format. These changes reflect an increase in fat-free tissue and a decrease in the total body fat content.

Parizkova[43] studied a group of 143 boys from the age of 11 through 18 years. The group was divided into three subgroups on the basis of their habitual levels of activity. Relative fat-free mass increased linearly with age, and relative body fat decreased linearly with age, with the more active groups exhibiting the more favorable body compositions. At each age, the most active groups had lower absolute body fat and higher absolute fat-free mass.

Numerous studies have been conducted on the adult population. In one of the first studies to observe body composition changes with physical training, Thompson and coworkers[44] evaluated body

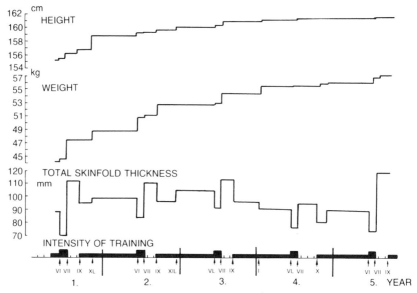

Figure 4–4. Changes in height, weight, and skinfold thickness in girl gymnasts during periods of various intensity of training. (From Parizkova, J.: Body composition and exercise during growth and development. In Rarick, G. L. [ed.]: **Physical Activity, Human Growth and Development.** New York, Academic Press, 1973, p. 109, with permission.)

weights and skinfold thicknesses on basketball and hockey players before and after a season of play in their respective sports. Although weight remained relatively stable, there were rather major decreases in subcutaneous skinfold fat measurements. In a similar study of football players, Thompson[45] reported no change in body weight, substantial decreases in skinfold thicknesses, and significant increases in estimated body density, indicating an overall decrease in total body fat and an increase in fat-free weight resulting from a season of training.

Skinner and associates[23] used densitometry to determine longitudinal changes in body composition with training in a group of men who exercised a minimum of three times per week, approximately 40 minutes per session for a period of 6 months. Specific gravity increased from 1.058 to 1.063, and the sum of six skinfolds decreased from 107.7 to 99.3 mm. Oscai and Williams[46] studied five middle-aged men who ran three times per week, a minimum of 30 minutes per session for a total of 16 weeks. Compared with a group of five sedentary controls, the experimental group lost 4.5 kg of body weight, 3.6 kg of body fat, and 0.9 kg of fat-free weight, as estimated from changes in skinfold thickness. Carter and Phillips[47] observed 13 subjects, 7 experimentals and 6 controls, for a 3-year period, with body composition evaluations occurring every 6 months. The experimental subjects participated in one-hour sessions of calisthenics and jogging 3 days per week, with jogging mileage progressing from 1.5 to 7.5 miles per week. The experimental group made significant decreases in body weight, percentage of fat, skinfolds, girths, and the somatotype component of mesomorphy while significantly increasing specific gravity, as estimated from underwater weighing. The majority of the change in each of these variables occurred during the first year of the program.

Pollock and colleagues[48] randomly assigned 19 middle-aged men to an exercise regimen of either 2 days per week or 4 days per week, with an additional 8 subjects serving as sedentary controls. The experimental subjects performed approximately 30 minutes of jog-run training per day for either 2 or 4 days per week, for a total of 20 weeks. The group training 2 days per week had no significant changes in body composition, whereas the group that trained 4 days per week decreased total body weight (79.7 to 76.8 kg), the sum of six skinfold thicknesses (131.4 to 107.8 mm), and relative body fat estimated from skinfold thicknesses (19.6 to 18.6 percent). Katch and colleagues[49] studied 10 members of the women's tennis team and 5 members of the women's swimming team at the University of California, Santa Barbara, before and after a season of competition. They found no significant alterations in body composition over 16 weeks of sports training.

Wilmore and coworkers[50] investigated body composition alterations in 55 men between the ages of 17 and 59 years after a 3-day per week, 10-week program of jogging. Small but significant decreases were found in total body weight, relative body fat, and four of seven skinfold measurements, and a significant increase was found in body density. Boileau and coworkers[51] studied 23 college men who participated in a walking and running exercise program 60 minutes per day, 5 days per week for 9 weeks. From the initial evaluations, 8 subjects were classified as obese (29 to 46 percent fat) and the remaining 15 as normal (10 to 21 percent fat). Total weight decreased by 3.2 kg in the obese and 1.0 kg in the normal groups, whereas fat-free, or lean, weight increased by 2.7 and 1.4 kg, respectively. Relative fat decreased by 3.9 percent in the obese and 3.0 percent in the normal groups. In this study, as well as in the study by Wilmore and coworkers,[50] the actual fat loss was more than could be accounted for by the energy equivalent of the actual exercise performed.

Pollock and associates[52] investigated the effects of a 20-week walking program (40 minutes per day, 4 days per week) on the body composition of middle-aged men. Reductions were found in total body weight (-1.3 kg) and in relative body fat (-1.1 percent). In a subsequent study, Pollock and associates[53] determined the physiological responses to training 2 days per week at different intensities, 45 minutes per day for 20 weeks. The group training at 90 percent of maximal heart rate demonstrated small but significant decreases in the sum of seven skinfold measurements and in relative fat estimated from skinfolds. The group training at 80 percent of maximal heart rate exhibited no change in body composition. In a third study by Pollock and associates,[54] the effects of mode of training on cardiovascular function and body composition were determined. Sedentary middle-aged men were assigned to one of four groups: running, walking, cycling, or control. All training groups exercised for 30 minutes per day, 3 days per week for 20 weeks at 85 to 90 percent of maximal heart rate. The experimental groups had significant decreases in body weight, skinfold fat, and relative body fat estimated from skinfolds. The studies of Pollock and associates are summarized in Figures 4–5 to 4–7.

Kollias and colleagues[55] conducted a 15-week weight reduction study, with 19 women assigned to a volitional dieting, a volitional exercise, or a combined dieting and exercising group. Body weight decreased by 5.3, 5.7, and 3.4 kg, and relative body fat decreased

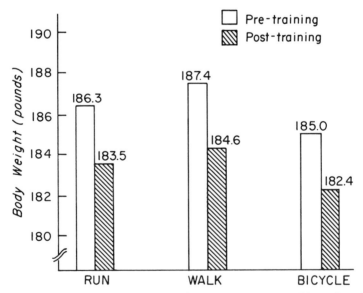

Figure 4–5. Alterations in body weight consequent to a 20-week training program of running, walking, or bicycling. (Data from Pollock, M. L., et al.: Effects of mode of training on cardiovascular functions and body composition of adult men. **Med. Sci. Sports** 7:139–145, 1975.)

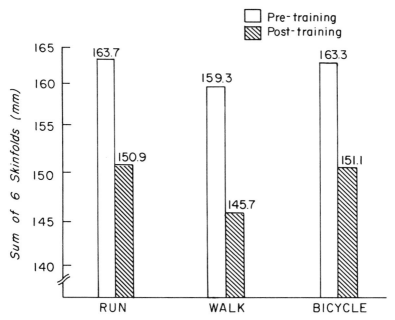

Figure 4–6. Alterations in skinfold fat consequent to a 20-week training program of running, walking, or bicycling. (Data from Pollock, M. L., et al.: Effects of mode of training on cardiovascular functions and body composition of adult men. **Med. Sci. Sports** 7:139–145, 1975.)

by 2.2, 2.5, and 1.7 percent in the diet, exercise, and combined groups, respectively. Girandola and Katch[56] studied the effects of 9 weeks of physical training on the aerobic capacity and body composition of college men. The exercise program consisted of calisthenics, running, and weight lifting, 2 days per week, in a circuit training format. Relative body fat decreased by 1.0 percent, but total and fat-free weights remained unchanged.

Getchell and Moore[57] studied the adaptations of middle-aged men and women to a 10-week physical training program consisting of 30 minutes of walking and jogging 3 to 4 days per week. Both groups lost a negligible amount of body weight, − 0.7 and − 0.8 kg for men and women, respectively. However, the sum of six skinfold measurements decreased substantially, from a mean value of 144.6 to 115.4 mm in women and from 148.8 to 110.6 mm in men. These changes suggest that there were losses of total body fat and gains in fat-free weight. Girandola[58] investigated the effects of high- and low-intensity exercise training on body composition changes in college women. Twenty women participated in a 10-week program three times per week, which consisted of riding a cycle ergometer at either 420 or 840 kpm/min for varying intervals of time. Body

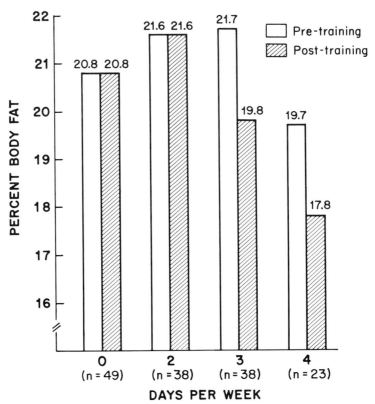

Figure 4–7. Effects of frequency of cardiorespiratory endurance training on percentage of body fat. (Data from Pollock, M. L., et al.: Frequency of training as a determinant for improvement in cardiovascular function and body composition of middle-aged men. **Arch. Phys. Med. Rehab.** 56:141–145, 1975.)

weight did not change over the course of the study; however, there was an increase in body density and a decrease in relative body fat in the low-intensity group (420 kpm/min). The high-intensity group exhibited no significant changes in body composition.

Wilmore and coworkers[59] observed changes in body composition after 20 weeks of bicycle, tennis, or jogging training. The subjects exercised for 30 minutes per day, 3 days per week at a prescribed training heart rate. The only alteration noted in body composition was an increase in the lean weight of members of the bicycle group. Although those in the jogging and bicycling group demonstrated rather major decreases in total body weight and relative and absolute body fat, these decreases were not statistically significant owing to similar unexplained changes in the control group.

Most of the studies cited thus far have involved an aerobic type of exercise. There have been several studies that have evaluated the effects of weight training, in either a standard or a circuit format, on alterations in body composition. Fahey and Brown[60] investigated changes in strength, body composition, and endurance of college men performing a weight-training program 3 times per week for 9 weeks under placebo or steroid treatment. Body weight and fat-free weight increased in both groups, whereas relative body fat decreased. Misner and associates[61] assigned 24 adult men to a weight-training, jogging, or control group, with the groups exercising 30 minutes per day, 3 days per week for 8 weeks. After the training period, the weight-training group gained body weight (1.0 kg) and fat-free, or lean, body weight (3.1 kg) while losing absolute (−2.3 kg) and relative (−2.9 percent) body fat. The jogging group lost body weight (−0.8 kg) and absolute (−2.3 kg) and relative (−2.5 percent) body fat.

Wilmore[62] conducted a 10-week weight-training program, 2 days per week for 40 minutes per day, involving 47 women and 26 men. Neither group changed total body weight, but both groups decreased absolute body fat by 1.2 and 0.9 kg and relative body fat by 1.9 and 1.3 percent and increased fat-free weight by 1.1 and 1.2 kg in the women and men, respectively. Mayhew and Gross[63] conducted a similar study on 17 college women and reported nearly identical results. Brown and Wilmore[64] observed body composition changes in seven nationally ranked track and field throwing event athletes, 16 to 23 years of age, after 6 months of maximal resistance training for 3 days a week, 60 to 90 minutes per day. Body weight decreased slightly, as did relative and absolute body fat, and fat-free weight increased.

Circuit weight training has also been shown to alter body composition. Wilmore and coworkers[65] circuit weight trained men and women subjects 3 days per week, approximately 30 minutes per day for a period of 10 weeks. Although increases were found in fat-free weight of 1.7 and 1.3 kg for men and women, respectively, there were no significant changes in body weight, and only the women exhibited a significant decrease in relative body fat (−1.8 percent). Gettman and Pollock[66] summarized the circuit weight-training literature in 1981 and found either small or no changes in body weight, increases in fat-free weight, and decreases in relative body fat.

In a series of studies, O'Hara and associates[67–70] have observed rather remarkable losses in fat mass and gains in lean mass after exercise in the cold. In one study,[67] 55 soldiers were observed over a vigorous 10-day sledding patrol in the Canadian arctic and subarctic. The authors claimed a fat loss of 3.9 kg and a gain in fat-free weight of 3.9 kg in this relatively short exposure. In the second study,[68] 10 men spent one week in a cold climatic facility, performing simulated arctic military exercises. The subjects lost an average of 2.6 kg of body weight and sustained a reduction in mean skinfold thickness of 2.6 mm. Body fat decreased by 2.35 kg, and fat-free weight decreased by 0.25 kg. In the third study,[69] six obese men, 25 to 46 years of age, exercised vigorously in a cold chamber for 3.5 hours on 10 consecutive days. Fat-free weight increased slightly, fat weight decreased by 3.1 kg,, and body weight decreased by a mean of 3.2 kg. In their fourth study, O'Hara and associates[70] reported similar results for a group of 15 middle-aged, moderately obese men who exercised 2.5 hours per day for 2 weeks. Cold exposure and exercise led to reductions in skinfold thicknesses and body fat and to an increase in fat-free weight. The researchers thought the observed fat loss in the cold can be explained by new protein synthesis, ketosis, and a small energy deficit.

In 1985, Timmons and colleagues[71] studied substrate utilization during cold temperature exercise in seven men who performed 60 minutes of continuous cycle ergometer exercise at $-10°C$ and $+22°C$. The cumulative total energy expenditure for 60 minutes of exercise in the cold was 13 percent higher than that of the control condition, and the cumulative fat expenditure was 35 percent higher. These studies certainly indicate a new area of research that could have major implications for the treatment of obesity. Murray and colleagues[72] observed the effects of cold stress and exercise on fat loss in somewhat obese, relatively fit, young women. They found that 5-day trials of 200-minute bouts of exercise in the cold resulted in a fat loss of only 0.5 kg, well below that found in men in the previous studies.

To summarize this section, rather substantial alterations occur in body composition consequent to exercise training. Although body weight usually decreases over long periods of time, i.e., 3 months or longer, it is not unusual for body weight to change very little during the initial few months of training. This lack of substantial change in the early phases of an exercise program is primarily the result of alterations in body composition, i.e., losses in body fat accompanied by similar gains in fat-free weight. As the exercise program is extended beyond 3 months, lean weight changes very little, and decreases in body weight now start to reflect actual changes in body fat. The exercise program should be of an aerobic nature, although substantial alterations in body composition can occur with either traditional or circuit strength training. Pollock and coworkers[73] have established that frequency of training is important relative to body composition alterations; regimens of 3 and 4 days per week provide significant changes, whereas only small or no changes have been found with regimens of 2 days per week. There may, in fact, be a threshold for the minimal number of kilocalories expended per exercise session or per week, in addition to a minimal duration and intensity, in order to achieve significant alterations in lean and fat weight (see Fig. 4–7).

OBESE AND LEAN POPULATIONS

The next part of this chapter is reserved for a review of those studies that have been conducted on obese or extremely lean populations. These studies were separated from the others, as there does appear to be a somewhat different response to physical training in these two subgroups.

Parizkova and coworkers[74] studied 18 obese boys and 15 obese girls with a mean age of 12.7 years, before and after 7 weeks of reducing treatment in a summer camp where they performed considerable physical activity and received a diet of 1,700 kcal per day. The girls lost 12.8 percent of their initial body weight compared with 11.1 percent loss for the boys. The absolute fat-free mass did not change; however, there were major increases in relative fat-free mass and decreases in relative body fat. Sprynarova and Parizkova[75] observed seven obese boys before and after a 7-week regimen of dietary restriction and regular exercise. All subjects experienced marked increases in body density and relative fat-free weight and decreases in total body weight (mean loss of 6.6 kg, or 14.5 pounds) and in relative body fat.

Christakis and associates[76] studied the effect of a combined nutrition education and physical fitness program on the course of obesity in 55 randomly selected obese freshmen high school students. A control group of 35 obese boys was used for comparison. After an 18-month period of observation, the experimental group gained an average of 5.8 pounds, and the control group gained 13.5 pounds. With respect to percentage of overweight, there was a major shift toward normal weight in the experimental group as compared with the control group.

Epstein and associates[77] observed the effect of diet and controlled exercise on weight loss in obese girls who were randomly assigned to one of two groups: diet or diet plus exercise. During the first 6 weeks of treatment, the children in the combination group exercised in a formal exercise program three times per week, walking or running 3 miles in addition to 10 minutes of stationary aerobic activity and warm-up games. For the remainder of the year, the children were under the supervision of their parents for the exercise program. The diet-only group decreased their percent overweight from the beginning of the program through the second month. The diet-plus-exercise group demonstrated similar reductions in their percent overweight for the first two months and continued to decrease their percent overweight through 6 months. At the end of one year there were no differences between the two groups.

Moody and colleagues[78] measured body composition changes in 40 normal and obese high school girls after participation in a 15- or 29-week physical activity program of walking, jogging, and running 4 days per week, covering up to 3 to 3.5 miles per day. Total weight decreased by 1.15 kg; fat weight decreased by 2.66 kg; and relative body fat decreased by 3.1 percent in the obese group after 29 weeks of activity. Moody and colleagues[79] placed 11 overweight college women on a physical activity program for 8 weeks, expending approximately 500 kcal per day. Total body weight decreased by an average of 2.4 kg, and the mean skinfold thickness of the ten sites decreased by an average of 7.5 mm. Relative body fat, estimated from skinfolds, decreased from 38.6 to 28.5 percent; fat weight decreased by 5.3 kg; and fat-free weight increased by 2.9 kg. Kollias and colleagues[80] reported similar results for a group of eight obese college students after 9 weeks of physical conditioning for 5 days per week. Weight decreased by 3.2 kg, and relative body fat decreased from 38.5 to 34.6 percent.

Gwinup[81] placed 11 obese women on a progressively increasing program of walking each day for a year or longer, with no dietary restriction imposed. No weight loss occurred until walking exceeded 30 minutes per day. Generally, the weight loss paralleled the length of time spent walking. Weight loss varied from 10 to 38 pounds, with an average of 22 pounds. The rate of weight loss seldom exceeded 0.5 pounds per week. There was also a striking decrease in skinfold thickness, which could have indicated an even larger fat loss and a possible increase in fat-free weight. Lewis and coworkers[82] evaluated the effects of physical activity on weight reduction in obese middle-aged women. They observed 22 obese women, 30 to 52 years of age, through a 17-week exercise program consisting of 2.5 miles of walking-jogging and one hour of calisthenics per week. Caloric restriction was also allowed on an individual basis and was felt to account for approximately 60 percent of the total mean energy deficit. Relative body fat decreased by 5 percent; absolute body fat decreased by 5.4 kg; and total body weight decreased by 4.2 kg.

Leon and colleagues[83] studied the effects of a vigorous walking program on the body composition of six sedentary obese men, 19 to

31 years of age. After 16 weeks of vigorous walking for 90 minutes a day, 5 days per week, on a treadmill at up to 3.2 mph on a 10 percent grade, i.e., approximately 1,100 kcal per session, fat-free weight increased 0.2 kg, fat weight decreased 5.9 kg, and body fat decreased from 23.3 to 17.4 percent. Monitored food intake initially increased and then progressively decreased below pretraining levels. Ballor and colleagues[84] observed the effects of resistance training only, diet only, and resistance training plus diet as compared with not dieting and not exercising (control group) on changes in body composition in 40 obese women. The two groups that dieted had significantly greater losses in total body weight and fat weight as compared with the resistance training only and control groups. However, the two groups that exercised had significant gains in fat-free body mass, whereas the diet-only group lost fat-free mass.

Gwinup[85] randomly assigned a group of 45 obese women to one of three exercise modalities—swimming, stationary cycling, or walking—building from 5 to 10 minutes up to 60 minutes per day over a period of 6 months. Weight losses were not significant until the duration of exercise reached 30 minutes per day. At the end of the 6 months of training, the walkers and cyclists had lost approximately 10 and 12 percent of their initial weight, respectively, whereas the swimmers experienced no weight change over the course of the study (Fig. 4–8). There was no obvious explanation for these results, although there is some evidence that indicates that swimming in cold water does act as an appetite stimulant.

Franklin and coworkers[86] and MacKeen and coworkers[87] studied 36 sedentary women who participated in a 12-week physical conditioning program consisting of jogging 15 to 25 minutes per day for 4 days a week. Of the total group, 23 were classified as obese and 13 as normal. Although caloric intake remained unaltered throughout the training program, the obese subjects lost body weight and fat weight, whereas fat-free weight was not significantly altered. Fifteen of the obese subjects were re-evaluated 18 months after termination of the training program and were found to have returned to their pretraining values.

Krotkiewski and coworkers[88] observed the effects of long-term physical training on adipose tissue cellularity and body composition in patients with either hypertrophic or hyperplastic obesity. The patients were trained as hard as possible for 45 minutes per session, 3 times per week for a period of 6 months. Hypertrophic patients reduced body fat 6 kg after 3 months, which was the result of a decreased fat cell weight, as fat cell number was unchanged. In hyperplastic patients, there was no change in body fat. Thus, the form of obesity does appear to have an influence on the subsequent

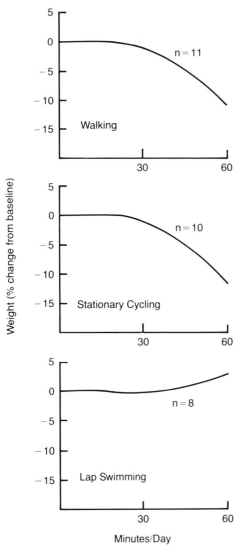

Figure 4–8. Changes in body weight with 6 months of walking, stationary cycling, or swimming in obese women. (Adapted from Gwinup, G.: Weight loss without dietary restriction: efficacy of different forms of aerobic exercise. **Am. J. Sports Med.** 15:275–279, 1987.)

results from physical training programs. In a second study, Krotkiewski and coworkers[89] trained 27 women with varying degrees of obesity, for a period of 6 months. Again, body fat changes were positively correlated with the number of fat cells in adipose tissue. Obese women with fewer fat cells decreased in weight during training, whereas women with severe obesity and an increased number of fat cells even gained weight. A third study by Krotkiewski and coworkers[90] reported essentially the same results. Warwick and Garrow[91] have found similar results with three obese women studied for periods of 12 to 13 weeks. Adding 2 hours per day of cycle ergometer exercise did not change the rate of weight loss in these women, who were on an 800-kcal reducing diet. Judging from their weights, these women were most probably obese as a result of hypercellularity.

Few studies have been conducted on the body composition changes of the extremely lean or underweight individual. Dempsey[21] reported substantial gains in total weight, fat weight, and lean weight after an 18-week exercise program in one of his subjects who had initial relative body fat of only 3 percent. Wilmore[92] placed seven women, classified as being chronically underweight, on a 15-week exercise program consisting of walking-jogging for 30 minutes a day, 5 days per week. Body weight and fat-free weight increased slightly, and absolute and relative fat decreased slightly.

DIET IN COMBINATION WITH EXERCISE

In this chapter, an attempt has been made to review selected studies that have investigated alterations in body composition with physical training. In all but one of the studies reviewed, diet was not manipulated as an experimental variable. In some studies, diet was monitored simply to observe spontaneous changes with training, but in most studies, diet was assumed to remain constant. Zuti and Golding[93] designed a study to investigate changes in body composition with diet, exercise, and a combination of diet and exercise. A caloric deficit of 500 kcal per day was maintained by each of three groups of adult women during a 16-week period of weight loss. The diet group simply reduced their daily caloric intake by 500 kcal. The exercise group increased their energy expenditure by 500 kcal per day, exercising 5 days per week. The combination group reduced their caloric intake by 250 kcal per day and increased their caloric expenditure by 250 kcal per day. The results of this study are illustrated in Figure 4–9. Although all three groups lost the same amount of weight over 16 weeks, there was a substantial difference in the alterations in body composition. The exercise group and the exercise and diet group both increased their fat-free weights, whereas the diet group lost fat-free weight. In addition, the two exercise groups both lost substantially more body fat. These findings have particular relevance for those individuals who are on a weight-reducing regimen with dietary intervention. Exercise does appear to protect the lean tissue, particularly when moderate dietary restriction is imposed upon the individual.

A more recent study by Pavlou and associates[94] supports the

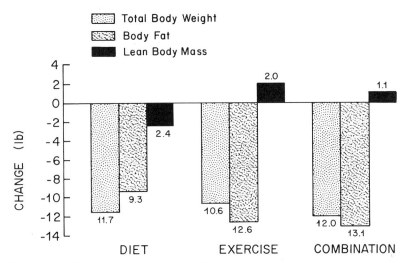

Figure 4–9. Changes in body weight, body fat, and lean body weight for diet, exercise, and combination groups. (From Zuti W. B., and Golding, L. A.: Comparing diet and exercise as weight reduction tools. **Phys. Sportsmed.** 4:49–53, 1976.)

data of Zuti and associates and is illustrated in Figure 4–10. Seventy-two mildly obese male subjects were assigned to one of several treatment programs, which included either exercise or nonexercise in combination with different dietary treatments. Although the exercise and nonexercise groups lost similar amounts of weight, the exercise group lost significantly more fat weight and did not lose a significant amount of fat-free weight. The nonexercising group lost a significant amount of fat-free weight.

McMurray and colleagues[95] observed 7-day periods of 1,000

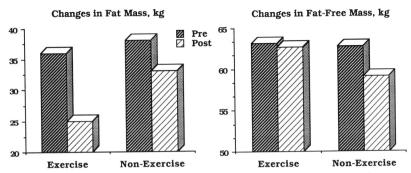

Figure 4–10. Alterations in fat mass and fat-free body mass in mildly obese individuals with or without exercise training. (Adapted from Pavlou, K. N., et al.: Effects of dieting and exercise on lean body mass, oxygen uptake, and strength. **Med. Sci. Sport Exerc.** 17:466–471, 1985.)

kcal per day deficits induced by diet or exercise in six endurance-trained men, each subject undergoing both protocols. Total weight loss during the exercise week was 0.76 kg compared with a loss of 2.16 kg during the dietary restriction week. Although body composition measures were not obtained, the authors did measure cumulative nitrogen loss over both treatment periods, and the loss during the dietary period (-24.5 g) was significantly greater than the loss over the exercise period (-11.1 g). This did not include estimates of sweat loss of nitrogen. This study is difficult to interpret without estimates of change in body composition. It is quite likely that at least part of the greater weight loss during the dietary restriction period was due to both protein loss and the obligatory loss of water that accompanies protein loss. The use of only one-week interventions is also somewhat problematic with respect to interpretation of this data.

Hagan and coworkers[96] compared the effects of exercise, caloric restriction, or both for 12 weeks on body composition changes in 48 men and 48 women who were overweight (120 to 140 percent of ideal weight). The subjects were randomly assigned to one of four groups: diet, exercise, diet plus exercise, and sedentary control. The dietary regimen consisted of 1,200 kcal per day, whereas the exercise consisted of 5 days per week, 30 minutes per day, of walking-running. The weight changes over the 12-week program for the four groups are illustrated in Figure 4–11. The greatest changes in body weight occurred in the diet-plus-exercise group for both men and women, with weight remaining relatively stable in the exercise group. Relative body fat decreased from 26.2 to 20.3 percent and from 34.4 to 29.2 percent in the diet-plus-exercise group, and from 25.5 to 21.0 percent and from 34.5 to 29.9 percent in the diet group, for men and women, respectively. Relative body fat did not change in either the control or the exercise-only group. No attempt was made to balance the caloric deficit across the three experimental groups. The dietary regimen of 1,200 kcal per day represented approximately a 1,000 kcal per day deficit for men and a 500 kcal per day deficit for women, whereas those exercising were expending only 700 to 900 kcal per week for men and 500 to 600 kcal per week for women. This would be considered to be a very minimal exercise dose, i.e., less than 200 kcal per day. It was also interesting to note that there was not a preservation of fat-free tissue in the dietary group that exercised as compared with the dietary group that did not exercise.

One last point needs to be made regarding the composition of weight loss in obese subjects whether from diet, exercise, or a combination of both. It is now well established that gains in fat-

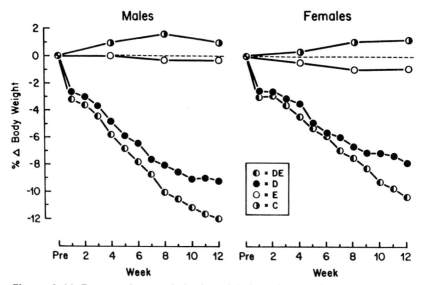

Figure 4–11. Percent changes in body weight in males and females according to treatment effects of diet and exercise (DE), diet (D), exercise (E), and control (C). (From Hagan, R. D., et al.: The effects of aerobic conditioning and/or caloric restriction in overweight men and women. **Med. Sci. Sport Exerc.** 18:87–94, 1985.)

free tissue occur in addition to gains in fat in studies of overfeeding in humans.[97] Obese subjects gain considerable amounts of fat-free tissue as they become obese, at least in part to support their new, increased body weight. Thus, losses of fat-free tissue should be expected with weight loss in obese subjects. As total weight decreases, there is no longer the need for the excess lean tissue to support the lower body weight in normal daily activity.

SPOT REDUCTION AND SPECIAL EXERCISE DEVICES

Many individuals undertake an exercise program in an attempt to reduce fat in certain areas of the body, a practice that has been referred to as spot reduction. Many, including athletes, believe that by exercising a specific area, the fat in that area will be selectively utilized, thus reducing the locally stored fat. A study by Olson and Edelstein, published in 1968,[98] in fact did demonstrate selective loss of fat at the triceps skinfold site with three sets of seven repetitions of maximal one-arm curls either on a daily or alternate day protocol. The other arm, acting as the control, did not experience similar changes in triceps skinfold fat. Roby[99] in a study of almost identical design, using one-arm elbow extension exercises, found no differences in triceps skinfold fat between the exercised and control arm. More recent studies have shown the concept of spot reduction to be a myth, and they have revealed that exercise, even when localized, draws from all of the fat stores of the body, not just from the local deposits.

A study by Gwinup and associates[100] demonstrated that the dominant arm of professional tennis players had greater muscular development than the nondominant arm because of the differences in activity levels of the two arms. However, no differences were found between the arms in localized fat stores, as assessed by multiple skinfold determinations.

Katch and associates[101] observed the effects of a 27-day sit-up training program on adipose cell size and adiposity. Fat biopsies were obtained from the abdominal, subscapular, and gluteal regions both before and after this extensive training regimen (5,004 sit-ups total). Weight, total body fat, skinfold fat thickness, and girths remained unaltered, and there was no evidence from the fat biopsy data to indicate a selective or preferential use of fat from the abdominal region compared with the subscapular and gluteal regions.

With the popularity of exercise increasing, many gimmicks, gadgets, and fads have flooded the retail market. Although some of these are legitimate and effective, many are of no practical value for either exercise or weight loss. Three such devices were recently evaluated to determine the legitimacy of the claims that were being made as to their efficacy in changing the morphology and composition of the body: the Mark II bust developer, the Astro-Trimmer exercise belt, and the Slim-Skins vacuum pants. Although rather remarkable claims were made in newspaper and magazine advertisements for each of these devices, they failed to produce any changes whatsoever when evaluated in tightly controlled scientific studies.[102, 103]

BODY COMPOSITION OF ATHLETIC POPULATIONS

Advances in sports physiology have led to an interest in the development of physiological profiles to describe the qualities and characteristics of elite athletes in their various sports. These profiles have considerable application in developing a better understanding of the sport and in providing data on elite athletes, with which data from aspiring athletes can be compared. With respect to understanding the sport better, the profile of the elite athlete provides insights into those areas of training that should be emphasized and those areas that would need little, if any, attention.

With respect to body composition, those profiles reflect both the levels of training that are necessary for the sport and the genetic endowments of the athlete who finds success in that sport. Height, weight, and relative body fat for athletes in various sports are presented in Table 4–1. From this table, it is apparent that the female athlete is typically fatter than her male counterpart and that athletes who are involved in endurance activities or who must control their weight to meet a certain competitive weight classification have very low relative body fat. It is generally thought that a low relative body fat is desirable for successful competition in almost any sport. There is a negative correlation between percentage of body fat and performance in those activities in which the body mass must be moved through space either vertically, as in jumping, or horizontally, as in running.

Figure 4–12 illustrates the relative body fat values for a number of national and international class track and field female athletes. This figure illustrates several very important points. First, although not obvious from the figure, the better runners generally had low relative body fat values, usually below 12 percent body fat. However, one of the best runners, who held most of the American middle-distance records, had over 17 percent body fat. She was training very intensely, with a great volume of both high-intensity training and long-distance running. It is unlikely that this athlete could have reduced her relative body fat to levels below 12 percent without having a negative influence on her subsequent performance. It is possible that each individual has a certain minimal body fat level, and reductions below this level are met with considerable resistance to fat loss and may result in loss of fat-free tissue. This points to the importance of treating each athlete as an individual and not as a member of a group in which all athletes in the same sport, or even within an event, have to achieve the same level of body fat. It is appropriate to establish guidelines for a sport, but consideration must be given to the exceptions.

SUMMARY

It has been the purpose of this chapter to ascertain those alterations in body composition that occur consequent to physical training. From the literature on both humans and animals, exercise does appear to have an influence on appetite, with either a reduction in food intake after intensive exercise or an increase in caloric

Table 4–1. Body Composition Values in Male and Female Athletes

Athletic Group or Sport	Sex	Age (yr)	Height (cm)	Weight (kg)	Relative Fat (%)	Reference
Baseball	male	20.8	182.7	83.3	14.2	Novak
	male	—	—	—	11.8	Forsyth
	male	26.0	185.4	87.5	16.2	Gurry
	male	27.3	185.8	86.4	12.6	Coleman
	male	27.4	183.1	88.0	12.6	Wilmore
Pitchers	male	26.7	188.1	89.8	14.7	Coleman
Infielders	male	27.4	183.1	83.2	12.0	Coleman
Outfielders	male	28.3	185.9	85.6	9.9	Coleman
Basketball	female	19.1	169.1	62.6	20.8	Sinning
	female	19.4	173.0	68.3	20.8	Vaccaro
	female	19.4	167.0	63.9	26.9	Conger
Centers	male	27.7	214.0	109.2	7.1	Parr
Forwards	male	25.3	200.6	96.9	9.0	Parr
Guards	male	25.2	188.0	83.6	10.6	Parr
Bicycling	male	—	180.3	67.1	8.8	Burke
	female	—	167.7	61.3	15.4	Burke
Canoeing/Paddlers	male	23.7	182.0	79.6	12.4	Rusko
	male	20.1	179.9	76.3	10.4	Vaccaro
Dancing, Ballet	female	15.0	161.1	48.4	16.4	Clarkson
General	female	21.2	162.7	51.2	20.5	Novak
Fencers	male	20.4	174.9	68.0	12.2	Vander
Football	male	19.3	186.8	93.1	13.7	Smith
	male	20.3	184.9	96.4	13.8	Novak
	male	—	—	—	13.9	Forsyth
Defensive	male	17–23	178.3	77.3	11.5	Wickkiser
Backs	male	24.5	182.5	84.8	9.6	Wilmore
Offensive	male	17–23	179.7	79.8	12.4	Wickkiser
Backs	male	24.7	183.8	90.7	9.4	Wilmore
Linebackers	male	17–23	180.1	87.2	13.4	Wickkiser
	male	24.2	188.6	102.2	14.0	Wilmore
Offensive	male	17–23	186.0	99.2	19.1	Wickkiser
Linemen	male	24.7	193.0	112.6	15.6	Wilmore
Defensive	male	17–23	186.6	97.8	18.5	Wickkiser
Linemen	male	25.7	192.4	117.1	18.2	Wilmore
Quarterbacks, Kickers	male	24.1	185.0	90.1	14.4	Wilmore
Golf	female	33.3	168.9	61.8	24.0	Crews
Gymnastics	male	20.3	178.5	69.2	4.6	Novak
	female	14.0	—	—	17.0	Parizkova
	female	15.2	161.1	50.4	13.1	Moffatt
	female	19.4	163.0	57.9	23.8	Conger
	female	20.0	158.5	51.5	15.5	Sinning
	female	23.0	—	—	11.0	Parizkova
	female	23.0	—	—	9.6	Parizkova
Ice Hockey	male	22.5	179.0	77.3	13.0	Rusko
	male	26.3	180.3	86.7	15.1	Wilmore
Jockeying	male	30.9	158.2	50.3	14.1	Wilmore
Orienteering	male	31.2	—	72.2	16.3	Knowlton
	female	29.0	—	58.1	18.7	Knowlton
Pentathalon	female	21.5	175.4	65.4	11.0	Krahenbuhl
Racketball	male	25.0	181.7	80.3	8.1	Pipes
Lightweight	male	21.0	186.0	71.0	8.5	Hagerman
	female	23.0	173.0	68.0	14.0	Hagerman
Rowing	male	25.6	192.0	93.0	6.5	Secher
Rugby	male	28.1	181.6	86.3	9.1	Maud

Table continued on following page

Table 4–1. Body Composition Values in Male and
Female Athletes *Continued*

Athletic Group or Sport	Sex	Age (yr)	Height (cm)	Weight (kg)	Relative Fat (%)	Reference
Skiing	male	25.9	176.6	74.8	7.4	Sprynarova
Alpine	male	16.5	173.1	65.5	11.0	Song
	male	21.0	178.0	78.0	9.9	Veicsteinas
	male	21.2	176.0	70.1	14.1	Rusko
	male	21.8	177.8	75.5	10.2	Haymes
	female	19.5	165.1	58.8	20.6	Haymes
Cross-country	male	21.2	176.0	66.6	12.5	Niinimaa
	male	22.7	176.2	73.2	7.9	Haymes
	male	25.6	174.0	69.3	10.2	Rusko
	female	20.2	163.4	55.9	15.7	Haymes
	female	24.3	163.0	59.1	21.8	Rusko
Nordic	male	21.7	181.7	70.4	8.9	Haymes
Combination	male	22.9	176.0	70.4	11.2	Rusko
Skijumping	male	22.2	174.0	69.9	14.3	Rusko
Soccer	male	26.0	176.0	75.5	9.6	Raven
US Junior	male	17.5	178.3	72.3	9.4	Kirkendahl
US Olympic	male	20.6	179.3	72.5	9.1	Kirkendahl
US Collegiate	male	20.0	175.3	72.4	10.9	Kirkendahl
US National	male	22.5	178.6	76.2	9.9	Kirkendahl
MISL	male	26.9	177.3	74.5	10.5	Kirkendahl
Skating, Speed	male	21.0	181.0	76.5	11.4	Rusko
	male	—	181.0	73.6	9.0	Vanlugen
Figure	male	21.3	166.9	59.6	9.1	Niinimaa
	female	16.5	158.8	48.6	12.5	Niinimaa
Swimming	male	15.1	166.8	59.1	10.8	Vaccaro
	male	20.6	182.9	78.9	5.0	Novak
	male	21.8	182.3	79.1	8.5	Sprynarova
	female	19.4	168.0	63.8	26.3	Conger
Sprint	female	—	165.1	57.1	14.6	Wilmore
Middle Distance	female	—	166.6	66.8	24.1	Wilmore
Distance	female	—	166.3	60.9	17.1	Wilmore
Synchronized Swimming	female	20.1	166.2	55.8	24.0	Roby
Tennis	male	—	—	—	15.2	Forsyth
	male	42.0	179.6	77.1	16.3	Vodak
	female	39.0	163.3	55.7	20.3	Vodak
Track and Field	male	21.3	180.6	71.6	3.7	Novak
	male	—	—	—	8.8	Forsyth
Running	male	22.5	177.4	64.5	6.3	Sprynarova
Distance	male	26.1	175.7	64.2	7.5	Costill
	male	26.2	177.0	66.2	8.4	Rusko
	male	26.2	177.1	63.1	4.7	Pollock
	male	40–49	180.7	71.6	11.2	Pollock
	male	47.2	176.5	70.7	13.2	Lewis
	male	55.3	174.5	63.4	18.0	Barnard
	male	50–59	174.7	67.2	10.9	Pollock
	male	60–69	175.7	67.1	11.3	Pollock
	male	70–75	175.6	66.8	13.6	Pollock
	female	19.9	161.3	52.9	19.2	Malina
	female	32.4	169.4	57.2	15.2	Wilmore
	female	37.8	165.1	54.1	15.5	Upton
	female	43.8	161.5	53.8	18.3	Vaccaro
Middle Distance	male	20.1	178.1	71.9	6.9	Wilmore
	male	24.6	179.0	72.3	12.4	Rusko
Sprint	female	20.1	164.9	56.7	19.3	Malina
	male	20.1	178.2	72.8	5.4	Wilmore
	male	46.5	177.0	74.1	16.5	Barnard
Cross-country	female	15.6	164.2	51.1	15.3	Butts
	female	15.6	163.3	50.9	15.4	Butts

Table 4–1. Body Composition Values in Male and Female Athletes *Continued*

Athletic Group or Sport	Sex	Age (yr)	Height (cm)	Weight (kg)	Relative Fat (%)	Reference
Race Walking	male	26.7	178.7	68.5	7.8	Franklin
Discus	male	26.4	190.8	110.5	16.3	Wilmore
	male	28.3	186.1	104.7	16.4	Fahey
	female	21.1	168.1	71.0	25.0	Malina
Jumping and Hurdling	female	20.3	165.9	59.0	20.7	Malina
Shot put	male	22.0	191.6	126.2	19.6	Behnke
	male	27.0	188.2	112.5	16.5	Fahey
	female	21.5	167.6	78.1	28.0	Malina
Triathalon	male	—	—	—	7.1	Holly
	female	—	—	—	12.6	Holly
Volleyball	male	26.1	192.7	85.5	12.0	Puhl
	female	19.4	166.0	59.8	25.3	Conger
	female	19.9	172.2	64.1	21.3	Kovaleski
	female	21.6	178.3	70.5	17.9	Puhl
Weight Lifting	male	24.9	166.4	77.2	9.8	Sprynarova
Power	male	25.5	173.6	89.4	19.9	Hakkinen
	male	26.3	176.1	92.0	15.6	Fahey
Olympic	male	25.3	177.1	88.2	12.2	Fahey
Body Builders	male	25.6	176.9	87.6	13.4	Hakkinen
	male	27.6	178.8	88.1	8.3	Pipes
	male	29.0	172.4	83.1	8.4	Fahey
	female	27.0	160.8	53.8	13.2	Freedson
Wrestling	male	11.3	141.2	34.2	12.7	Sady
	male	15–18	172.3	66.3	6.9	Katch
	male	19.6	174.6	74.8	8.8	Sinning
	male	20.6	174.8	67.3	4.0	Stine
	male	22.0	—	—	5.0	Parizkova
	male	23.0	—	79.3	14.3	Taylor
	male	24.0	173.3	77.5	12.7	Hakkinen
	male	26.0	177.8	81.8	9.8	Fahey
	male	27.0	176.0	75.7	10.7	Gale

(From Wilmore, J. H., and Costill, D. L.: **Training for Sport and Activity: The Physiological Basis of the Conditioning Process,** 3rd Ed. Copyright 1988, Wm. C. Brown Publishers, Dubuque, Iowa. All rights reserved. Reprinted by permission. See this publication for specific references.)

intake that is less than that expected on the basis of the caloric expenditure. With respect to body composition alterations with exercise, there do appear to be slight decreases in total body weight, increases in fat-free weight, and decreases in fat weight.[4, 5, 6, 104] The magnitude of these changes will vary directly with the intensity and duration of the activity, the total daily caloric expenditure, and the type of activity, e.g., aerobic versus strength training. Current research is focusing on the effects of exercise training on those factors that affect energy balance and thermogenesis. Initial data are pointing to potential alterations in resting metabolic rate and in the thermic effect of food, or dietary-induced thermogenesis, as possible mechanisms to explain the beneficial effects of exercise in weight control.[105, 106] In conclusion, exercise appears to be a major factor in both the prevention and the treatment of obesity.

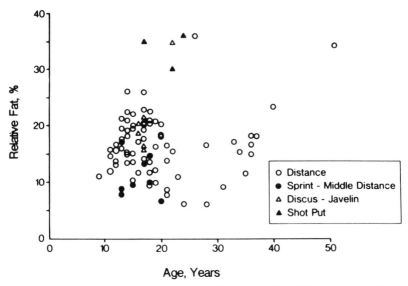

Age, Years

Figure 4–12. Relative body fat values for female track and field athletes. (From Wilmore, J. H., Brown, C. H., and Davis, J. A.: Body physique and composition of the female distance runner. **Ann. N.Y. Acad. Sci.** 301:764–776, 1977, with permission.)

References

1. Mayer, J.: **Overweight: Causes, Cost, and Control.** Englewood Cliffs, NJ, Prentice-Hall, 1968.
2. McArdle, W.D., Katch, F.I., and Katch, V.L.: **Exercise Physiology: Energy, Nutrition, and Human Performance,** 2nd Ed. Philadelphia, Lea & Febiger, 1986.
3. Behnke, A.R., and Wilmore, J.H.: **Evaluation and Regulation of Body Build and Composition.** Englewood Cliffs, NJ, Prentice-Hall, 1974.
4. Oscai, L.B.: The role of exercise in weight control. **Exerc. Sport Sci. Rev.** 1:103–123, 1973.
5. Thompson, J.K., Jarvie, G.J., Lahey, B.B., and Cureton, K.J.: Exercise and obesity: etiology, physiology, and intervention. **Psychol. Bull.** 91:55–79, 1982.
6. Pace, P.J., Webster, J., and Garrow, J.S.: Exercise and obesity. **Sports Med.** 3:89–113, 1986.
7. Titchenal, C.A.: Exercise and food intake: what is the relationship? **Sports Med.** 6:135–145, 1988.
8. Katch, V.L., Martin, R., and Martin, J.: Effects of exercise intensity on food consumption in the male rat. **Am. J. Clin. Nutr.** 32:1401–1407, 1979.
9. Richard, D., Arnold, J., and LeBlanc, J.: Energy balance in exercise-trained rats acclimated at two environmental temperatures. **J. Appl. Physiol.** 60:1054–1059, 1986.
10. Mayer, J., Marshall, N.B., Vitale, J.J., Christensen, J.H., Mashayekhi, M.B., and Stare, F.J.: Exercise, food intake and body weight in normal rats and genetically obese adult mice. **Am. J. Physiol.** 177:544–548, 1954.
11. Bulbulian, R., Grunewald, K.K., and Haack, R.R.: Effect of exercise duration on feed intake and body composition of Swiss albino mice. **J. Appl. Physiol.** 58:500–505, 1985.
12. Oscai, L.B., Mole, P.A., and Holloszy, J.O.: Effects of exercise on cardiac weight

and mitochondria in male and female rats. **Am. J. Physiol.** 220:1944–1948, 1971.

13. Mazzeo, R.S., and Horvath, S.M.: Effects of training on weight, food intake, and body composition of aging rats. **Am. J. Clin. Nutr.** 44:732–738, 1986.

14. Applegate, E.A., Upton, D.E., and Stern, J.S.: Food intake, body composition and blood lipids following treadmill exercise in male and female rats. **Physiol. Behav.** 28:917–920, 1982.

15. Brobeck, J.R.: Food intake as a mechanism of temperature regulation. **Yale J. Biol. Med.** 20:545, 1948.

16. Wirth, A., Holm, G., Nilsson, B., Smith, U., and Bjorntorp, P.: Insulin kinetics and insulin binding to adipocytes in physically trained and food-restricted rats. **Am. J. Physiol.** 238:E108–E115, 1980.

17. Garrow, J.S.: **Energy Balance and Obesity in Man,** 2nd Ed. New York, Elsevier/North Holland Biomedical Press, 1978.

18. Mayer, J., Roy, P., and Mitra, K.P.: Relation between caloric intake, body weight, and physical work: studies in an industrial male population in West Bengal. **Am. J. Clin. Nutr.** 4:169–175, 1956.

19. Mayer, J.: Inactivity and etiological factors in obesity and heart disease. In Blix, G. (ed.): **Nutrition and Physical Activity.** Symposium of the Swedish Nutrition Foundation V. Uppsala, Almqvist and Wiksells, 1967.

20. Mayer, J., and Bullen, B.A.: Nutrition, weight control, and exercise. In Johnson, W.R., and Buskirk, E.R. (eds.): **Science and Medicine of Exercise and Sport,** 2nd Ed. New York, Harper and Row, 1974.

21. Dempsey, J.A.: Anthropometrical observations on obese and nonobese young men undergoing a program of vigorous physical exercise. **Res. Q.** 35:275–287, 1964.

22. Holloszy, J.O., Skinner, J.S., Toro, G., and Cureton, T.K.: Effects of a 6 month program of endurance exercise on the serum lipids of middle-aged men. **Am. J. Cardiol.** 14:753–760, 1964.

23. Skinner, J.S., Holloszy, J.O., and Cureton, T.K.: Effects of a program of endurance exercises on physical work capacity and anthropometric measurements of 15 middle-aged men. **Am. J. Cardiol.** 14:747–752, 1964.

24. Jankowski, L.W., and Foss, M.L.: The energy intake of sedentary men after moderate exercise. **Med. Sci. Sports** 4:11–13, 1972.

25. Johnson, R.E., Mastropaolo, J.A., and Wharton, M.A.: Exercise, dietary intake, and body composition. **J. Am. Diet. Assoc.** 61:399–403, 1972.

26. Woo, R., Garrow, J.S., and Pi-Sunyer, F.X.: Effect of exercise on spontaneous calorie intake in obesity. **Am. J. Clin. Nutr.** 36:470–477, 1982.

27. Woo, R., Garrow, J.S., and Pi-Sunyer, F.X.: Voluntary food intake during prolonged exercise in obese women. **Am. J. Clin. Nutr.** 36:478–484, 1982.

28. Woo, R.: The effect of increasing physical activity on voluntary food intake and energy balance. **Int. J. Obesity** 9 (Suppl. 2):155–160, 1985.

29. McGowan, C.R., Epstein, L.H., Kupfer, D.J., and Bulik, C.M.: The effect of exercise on non-restricted caloric intake in male joggers. **Appetite** 7:97–105, 1986.

30. Belbeck, L.W., and Critz, J.B.: Effect of exercise on the plasma concentration of anorexigenic substance in man. **Proc. Soc. Exp. Biol. Med.** 142:19–21, 1973.

31. Stevenson, J.A.F., Fox, B.M., and Szlavko, A.J.: A fat mobilizing and anorectic substance in the urine of fasting rats. **Proc. Soc. Exp. Biol. Med.** 115:424, 1964.

32. Oscai, L.B., and Holloszy, J.O.: Effects of weight changes produced by exercise, food restriction, or overeating on body composition. **J. Clin. Invest.** 48:2124–2128, 1969.

33. Oscai, L.B., Spirakis, C.N., Wolff, C.A., and Beck, R.J.: Effects of exercise and of food restriction on adipose tissue cellularity. **J. Lipid Res.** 13:588–592, 1972.

34. Oscai, L.B., Babirak, S.P., Dubach, F.B., McGarr, J.A., and Spirakis, C.N.:

Exercise or food restriction: effect on adipose tissue cellularity. **Am. J. Physiol.** 227:901–904, 1974.

35. Taylor, A.W., Garrod, J., McNulty, M.E., and Secord, D.C.: Regenerating epididymal fat pad cell size and number after exercise training and three different feeding patterns. **Growth** 37:345–354, 1973.
36. Deb, S., and Martin, R.J.: Effects of exercise and of food restriction on the development of spontaneous obesity in rats. **J. Nutr.** 105:543–549, 1975.
37. Askew, E.W., Barakat, H., Kuhl, G.L., and Dohm, G.L.: Response of lipogenesis and fatty acid synthetase to physical training and exhaustive exercise in rats. **Lipids** 10:491–496, 1975.
38. Taylor, A.W.: The effects of different feeding regimens and endurance exercise programs on carbohydrate and lipid metabolism. **Can. J. Appl. Sport Sci.** 4:126–130, 1979.
39. Richard, D., and Trayhurn, P.: Effect of exercise training on the rates of fatty acid synthesis in mice. **Can. J. Physiol. Pharmacol.** 62:695–699, 1984.
40. Parizkova, J., and Poupa, O.: Some metabolic consequences of adaptation to muscular work. **Br. J. Nutr.** 17:341–345, 1963.
41. Parizkova, J.: Impact of age, diet, and exercise on man's body composition. **N.Y. Acad. Sci.** 110:661–674, 1963.
42. Wells, J.B., Parizkova, J., and Jokl, E.: Exercise, excess fat and body weight. **Assoc. Phys. Med. Ment. Rehabil.** 16:35–40, 58, 1962.
43. Parizkova, J.: Somatic development and body composition changes in adolescent boys differing in physical activity and fitness: a longitudinal study. **Anthropologie** 10:3–36, 1972.
44. Thompson, C.W., Buskirk, E.R., and Goldman, R.F.: Changes in body fat, estimated from skinfold measurements of college football players during a season. **Res. Q.** 27:418–430, 1956.
45. Thompson, C.W.: Changes in body fat, estimated from skinfold measurements of varsity college football players during a season. **Res. Q.** 30:87–93, 1959.
46. Oscai, L.B., and Williams, B.T.: Effect of exercise on overweight middle-aged males. **J. Am. Geriatr. Soc.** 16:794–797, 1968.
47. Carter, J.E.L., and Phillips, W.H.: Structural changes in exercising middle-aged males during a 2-year period. **J. Appl. Physiol.** 27:787–794, 1969.
48. Pollock, M.L., Cureton, T.K., and Greninger, L.: Effects of frequency of training on working capacity, cardiovascular function, and body composition of adult men. **Med. Sci. Sports** 1:70–74, 1969.
49. Katch, F.I., Michael, E.D., and Jones, E.M.: Effects of physical training on the body composition and diet of females. **Res. Q.** 40:99–104, 1969.
50. Wilmore, J.H., Royce, J., Girandola, R.N., Katch, F.I., and Katch, V.L.: Body composition changes with a 10-week program of jogging. **Med. Sci. Sports** 2:113–117, 1970.
51. Boileau, R.A., Buskirk, E.R., Horstman, D.H., Mendez, J., and Nicholas, W.C.: Body composition changes in obese and lean men during physical conditioning. **Med. Sci. Sports** 3:183–189, 1971.
52. Pollock, M.L., Miller, H.S., Janeway, R., Linnerud, A.C., Robertson, B., and Valentino, R.: Effects of walking on body composition and cardiovascular function of middle-aged men. **J. Appl. Physiol.** 30:126–130, 1971.
53. Pollock, M.L., Broida, J., Kendrick, Z., Miller, H.S., Janeway, R., and Linnerud, A.C.: Effects of training two days per week at different intensities on middle-aged men. **Med. Sci. Sports** 4:192–197, 1972.
54. Pollock, M.L., Miller, H.S., Jr., Kendrick, Z., and Linnerud, A.C.: Effects of mode of training on cardiovascular functions and body composition of adult men. **Med. Sci. Sports** 7:139–145, 1975.
55. Kollias, J., Skinner, J.S., Bartlett, H.L., Bergsteinova, B.S., and Buskirk, E.R.: Cardiorespiratory responses of young overweight women to ergometry following modest weight reduction. **Arch. Environ. Health** 27:61–64, 1973.
56. Girandola, R.N., and Katch, V.: Effects of nine weeks of physical training on aerobic capacity and body composition in college men. **Arch. Phys. Med. Rehabil.** 54:521–524, 1973.

57. Getchell, L.H., and Moore, J.C.: Physical training: comparative responses of middle-aged adults. **Arch. Phys. Med. Rehabil.** 56:250–254, 1975.

58. Girandola, R.N.: Body composition changes in women: effects of high and low exercise intensity. **Arch. Phys. Med. Rehabil.** 57:297–300, 1976.

59. Wilmore, J.H., Davis, J.A., O'Brian, R.S., Vodak, P.A., Walter, G.R., and Amsterdam, E.A.: Physiological alterations consequent to 20-week conditioning programs of bicycling, tennis, and jogging. **Med. Sci. Sports Exerc.** 12:1–8, 1980.

60. Fahey, T.D., and Brown, C.H.: The effects of anabolic steroid on the strength, body composition, and endurance of college males when accompanied by a weight training program. **Med. Sci. Sports** 5:272–276, 1973.

61. Misner, J.S., Boileau, R.A., Massey, B.H., and Mayhew, J.L.: Alterations in the body composition of adult men during selected physical training programs. **Am. J. Geriatr. Soc.** 22:33–38, 1974.

62. Wilmore, J.H.: Alterations in strength, body composition and anthropometric measurements consequent to a 10-week weight training program. **Med. Sci. Sports** 6:133–138, 1974.

63. Mayhew, J.L., and Gross, P.M.: Body composition changes in young women with high resistance weight training. **Res. Q.** 45:433–440, 1974.

64. Brown, C.H, and Wilmore, J.H.: The effects of maximal resistance training on the strength and body composition of women athletes. **Med. Sci. Sports** 6:174–177, 1974.

65. Wilmore, J.H., Parr, R.B., Girandola, R.N., Ward, P., Vodak, P.A., Barstow, T.J., Pipes, T.V., Romero, G.T., and Leslie, P.: Physiological alterations consequent to circuit weight training. **Med. Sci. Sports** 10:79–84, 1978.

66. Gettman, L.R., and Pollock, M.L.: Circuit weight training: a critical review of its physiological benefits. **Phys. Sportsmed.** 9:44–60, 1981.

67. O'Hara, W.J., Allen, C., and Shephard, R.J.: Loss of body fat during an arctic winter expedition. **Can. J. Physiol. Pharmacol.** 55:1235–1241, 1977.

68. O'Hara, W.J., Allen, C., and Shephard, R.J.: Loss of body weight and fat during exercise in a cold chamber. **Eur. J. Appl. Physiol.** 37:205–218, 1977.

69. O'Hara, W.J., Allen, C., and Shephard, R.J.: Treatment of obesity by exercise in the cold. **Can. Med. Assoc. J.** 117:773–779, 1977.

70. O'Hara, W.J., Allen, C., Shephard, R.J., and Allen, G.: Fat loss in the cold—a controlled study. **J. Appl. Physiol.** 46:872–877, 1979.

71. Timmons, B.A., Araujo, J., and Thomas, T.R.: Fat utilization enhanced by exercise in a cold environment. **Med. Sci. Sports Exerc.** 17:673–678, 1985.

72. Murray, S.J., Shephard, R.J., Greaves, S., Allen, C., and Radomski, M.: Effects of cold stress and exercise on fat loss in females. **Eur. J. Appl. Physiol.** 55:610–618, 1986.

73. Pollock, M.L., Miller, H.S., Jr., Linnerud, A.C., and Cooper, K.H.: Frequency of training as a determinant for improvement in cardiovascular function and body composition of middle-aged men. **Arch. Phys. Med. Rehabil.** 56:141–145, 1975.

74. Parizkova, J., Vaneckova, M., and Vamberova, M.: A study of changes in some functional indicators following reductions of excessive fat in obese children. **Physiol. Bohemoslov.** 11:351–357, 1962.

75. Sprynarova, S., and Parizkova, J.: Changes in aerobic capacity and body composition in obese boys after reduction. **J. Appl. Physiol.** 20:934–937, 1965.

76. Christakis, G., Sajecki, S., Hillman, R.W., Miller, E., Blumenthal, S., and Archer, M.: Effect of a combined nutrition education and physical fitness program on the weight status of obese high school boys. **Fed. Proc.** 25:15–19, 1966.

77. Epstein, L.H., Wing, R.R., Penner, B.C., and Kress, M.J.: Effect of diet and controlled exercise on weight loss in obese children. **J. Pediatr.** 107:358–361, 1985.

78. Moody, D.L., Wilmore, J.H., Girandola, R.N., and Royce, J.P.: The effects of a jogging program on the body composition of normal and obese high school girls. **Med. Sci. Sports** 4:210–213, 1972.

79. Moody, D.L., Kollias, J., and Buskirk, E.R.: The effect of a moderate exercise program on body weight and skinfold thickness in overweight college women. **Med. Sci. Sports** 1:75–80, 1969.
80. Kollias, J., Boileau, R.A., Barlett, H.L., and Buskirk, E.R.: Pulmonary function and physical conditioning in lean and obese subjects. **Arch. Environ. Health** 25:146–150, 1972.
81. Gwinup, G.: Effect of exercise alone on the weight of obese women. **Arch. Int. Med.** 135:676–680, 1975.
82. Lewis, S., Haskell, W.L., Wood, P.D., Manoogian, N., Bailey, J.E., and Pereira, M.: Effects of physical activity on weight reduction in obese middle-aged women. **Am. J. Clin. Nutr.** 29:151–156, 1976.
83. Leon, A.S., Conrad, J., Hunninghake, D.B., and Serfass, R.: Effects of a vigorous walking program on body composition, and carbohydrate and lipid metabolism of obese young men. **Am. J. Clin. Nutr.** 33:1776–1787, 1979.
84. Ballor, D.L., Katch, V.L., Becque, M.D., and Marks, C.R.: Resistance training during caloric restriction enhances lean body weight maintenance. **Am. J. Clin. Nutr.** 47:19–25, 1988.
85. Gwinup, G.: Weight loss without dietary restriction: efficacy of different forms of aerobic exercise. **Am. J. Sports Med.** 15:275–279, 1987.
86. Franklin, B.A., MacKeen, P.C., and Buskirk, E.R.: Body composition effects of a 12-week physical conditioning program for normal and obese middle-aged women, and status at 18-month follow-up. **Int. J. Obesity** 2:394, 1978.
87. MacKeen, P.C., Franklin, B.A., Nicholas, W.C., and Buskirk, E.R.: Body composition, physical work capacity and physical activity habits at 18-month follow-up of middle-aged women participating in an exercise intervention program. **Int. J. Obesity** 7:61–71, 1983.
88. Krotkiewski, M., Sjostrom, L., and Sullivan, L.: Effects of long-term physical training on adipose tissue cellularity and body composition in hypertrophic and hyperplastic obesity. **Int. J. Obesity** 2:395, 1978.
89. Krotkiewski, M., Mandroukas, K., Sjostrom, L., Wetterqvist, H., and Bjorntorp, P.: Effects of long-term training on body fat, metabolism, and blood pressure in obesity. **Metabolism** 28:650–658, 1979.
90. Krotkiewski, M., Bjorntorp, P., Holm, G., Marks, V., Morgan, L., Smith, U., and Feurle, G.E.: Effects of physical training on insulin, connecting peptide (C-peptide), gastric inhibitory polypeptide (GIP) and pancreatic polypeptide (PP) levels in obese subjects. **Int. J. Obesity** 8:193–199, 1984.
91. Warwick, P.M., and Garrow, J.S.: The effect of addition of exercise to a regime of dietary restriction on weight loss, nitrogen balance, resting metabolic rate and spontaneous physical activity in three obese women in a metabolic ward. **Int. J. Obesity** 5:25–32, 1981.
92. Wilmore, J.H.: Exercise-induced alterations in weight of underweight women. **Arch. Phys. Med. Rehabil.** 54:115–119, 1973.
93. Zuti, W.B., and Golding, L.A.: Comparing diet and exercise as weight reduction tools. **Phys. Sportsmed.** 4:49–53, 1976.
94. Pavlou, K.N., Steffee, W.P., Lerman, R.H., and Burrows, B.A.: Effects of dieting and exercise on lean body mass, oxygen uptake, and strength. **Med. Sci. Sport Exerc.** 17:466–471, 1985.
95. McMurray, R.G., Ben-Ezra, V., Forsythe, W.A., and Smith, A.T.: Responses of endurance-trained subjects to caloric deficits induced by diet or exercise. **Med. Sci. Sport Exerc.** 17:574–579, 1985.
96. Hagan, R.D., Upton, S.J., Wong, L., and Whittam, J.: The effects of aerobic conditioning and/or caloric restriction in overweight men and women. **Med. Sci. Sport Exerc.** 18:87–94, 1986.
97. Forbes, G.B.: Body composition as affected by physical activity and nutrition. **Fed. Proc.** 44:343–347, 1985.
98. Olson, A.L., and Edelstein, E.: Spot reduction of subcutaneous adipose tissue. **Res. Q.** 39:647–652, 1968.
99. Roby, F.B.: Effect of exercise on regional subcutaneous fat accumulations. **Res. Q.** 33:273–278, 1962.

100. Gwinup, G., Chelvam, R., and Steinberg, T.: Thickness of subcutaneous fat and activity of underlying muscles. **Ann. Int. Med.** 74:408–411, 1971.
101. Katch, F.I., Clarkson, P.M., Kroll, W., McBride, T., and Wilcox, A.: Effects of sit-up exercise training on adipose cell size and adiposity. **Res. Q. Exerc. Sport** 55:242–247, 1984.
102. Wilmore, J.H., Atwater, A.E., Maxwell, B.D., Wilmore, D.L., Constable, S.H., and Buono, M.J.: Alterations in breast morphology consequent to a 21-day bust developer program. **Med. Sci. Sport Exerc.** 17:106–112, 1985.
103. Wilmore, J.H., Atwater, A.E., Maxwell, B.D., Wilmore, D.L., Constable, S.H. and Buono, M.J.: Alterations in body size and composition consequent to Astro-Trimmer and Slim-Skins training programs. **Res. Q. Exerc. Sport** 56:90–92, 1985.
104. Hagan, R.D.: Benefits of aerobic conditioning and diet for overweight adults. **Sports Med.** 5:144–155, 1988.
105. Woo, R., Daniels-Kush, R., and Horton, E.S.: Regulation of energy balance. **Ann. Rev. Nutr.** 5:411–433, 1985.
106. Horton, E.S.: Metabolic aspects of exercise and weight reduction. **Med. Sci. Sport Exerc.** 18:10–18, 1985.

MUSCULOSKELETAL FUNCTION

INTRODUCTION

Sound musculoskeletal function is essential to optimal health and physiological function. Although it is true that very few people die from a lack of strength or poor flexibility, a number of otherwise healthy people suffer from chronic lower back problems and decreases in muscle mass. As the body loses fat-free tissue, there is a concomitant reduction in its basal and resting metabolic rate. Frequently, food intake is not reduced in proportion to the decrease in metabolic rate, and increases in fat stores result. Finally, without proper stimulation, bones lose strength through loss of the bone matrix and minerals. Osteoporosis and hip and vertebral fractures often are the result of this degenerative process.

Back pain is a major malady of modern society. In 1974, insurance companies reported more claims for back disability than for any other cause.[1] Kraus and Raab have demonstrated that over 80 percent of low back pain is due to muscular deficiency.[2] Further, in a 2- to 8-year follow-up study of 233 low back pain patients on a muscle strengthening and flexibility program, 82 percent reported good, 15.5 percent reported fair, and only 2.5 percent reported poor responses to the exercise regimen.[2] It is now clearly recognized that inadequate muscular strength and flexibility can lead to serious musculoskeletal disorders that result in considerable pain and discomfort, losses in income, increased disability, and premature retirement.

Losses of fat-free tissue with aging have been associated with physical inactivity. Existing longitudinal data using both whole-body potassium-40 (^{40}K) and densitometry indicate rates of loss ranging from 0.13 to 0.36 kg per year, with the higher rates of loss occurring later in life, when individuals are less active.[3] This decline in fat-free body mass has been associated with decreases in basal metabolic rate (BMR) with aging.[3] From cross-sectional studies, Quenouille and associates[4] have concluded that the BMR declines at a rate of 3 percent per decade from the age of 3 to over 80 years. Keys and associates[5] conducted both a cross-sectional and a longitudinal study of changes in BMR with aging. Comparing men 21.9 years of age with men 49.8 years of age indicated a 4.5 to 5.0 percent decrease in BMR per decade. Of the original group of younger men, 63 were evaluated a second time 19.4 years later. There was an average decrease in BMR of 3.2 percent per decade. A reduction in BMR with age without a concomitant reduction in energy intake will lead to increases in body fat stores. This is one of several mechanisms postulated for the increases in body fat identified with aging, which was referred to in Chapter 2. Thus, maintaining one's fat-free body weight through a carefully designed exercise program should help in the prevention of obesity.

Bone also undergoes deterioration with aging, which is again related to reduced physical activity. Bed rest and immobilization are accompanied by calcium deficits. Birge and Whedon,[6] summarizing the research literature through 1967, concluded that disuse atrophy of bone has been observed to be clinically associated with varying degrees of immobilization, resulting largely from bone resorption. Vogel and Whittle,[7] in reviewing the changes in bone mineral content in the Skylab astronauts, concluded that mineral losses do occur from the bones of the lower extremities during missions of up to 84 days and that these mineral losses generally follow the loss patterns observed in the bed rest situation. Although the astronauts are mobile in space, they are working in a gravity-free environment, and weight-bearing bones are not placed under the same degree of stress that they experience in a normal 1 G environment. Thus, with reduced use, bone loses both structure and function, which will eventually lead to osteoporosis.[8]

Aloia and colleagues[9] and Smith and colleagues[10] have demonstrated that exercise can prevent involutional bone loss in women with an average age of 52.3 and 81.0 years, respectively. In fact, exercise resulted in increases in bone mineral content[10] and in total body calcium,[9] whereas the nonexercising control groups demonstrated losses in both. Darby and colleagues[11] reported increases in calcium deposition in mature female rats after only four months of exercise training. Chow and colleagues[12] observed the effects of both an aerobic exercise program and an aerobic plus strength exercise program on bone mass in postmenopausal women 50 to 62 years of age. Both exercise groups increased bone mass, whereas the control, nonexercising group lost bone mass over the course of the year. Dalsky and colleagues[13] observed both the effects of training and detraining on the bone mineral content of postmenopausal women 55 to 70 years of age. Walking, jogging, and stair climbing led to increases of 5.2 percent after 13 months and 6.1 percent after 22 months, whereas there was no change in the control group and losses back to 1.1 percent above baseline with 13 months of reduced training.

Several cross-sectional studies have also supported the hypothesis that physical activity plays a major role in maintaining bone health. Aloia and coworkers[14] and Kanders and coworkers[15] reported significant correlations between physical activity and lumbar spine bone mineral density in samples of premenopausal women. Pocock and coworkers[16] found that physical fitness (predicted maximal oxygen uptake) was significantly correlated with both femoral neck and lumbar spine bone mineral density in postmenopausal subjects. Kriska and coworkers[17] evaluated physical activity patterns over the life span of 223 postmenopausal women and found a significant relationship of activity status with cortical bone density and area of the radius.

Smith and Raab[18] and Martin and Houston,[19] in review articles, have concluded that both middle-aged and elderly women increase bone mass or reduce the rate of bone loss in response to physical activity intervention programs. The reader is referred to these excellent reviews for more details on proposed mechanisms.

It is apparent that regular exercise is important for optimal musculoskeletal function. The remainder of this chapter includes a discussion of the physiology of strength and flexibility and procedures for the development of strength and flexibility.

PHYSIOLOGY OF STRENGTH AND FLEXIBILITY

Definitions

Before discussing the physiology of strength and flexibility, it is important to define several key words that are used frequently in the literature. Strength refers to the ability of the muscle or muscle group to apply force.[20] Typically, strength is defined relative to maximal force-producing capabilities. The individual who can maximally curl a barbell weighing 150 pounds is twice as strong as the individual who can curl only 75 pounds. The scientist takes a purer approach, defining strength precisely as the maximal force one can generate in a single isometric (static) contraction of unrestricted duration.[21] With the advent of isokinetic dynamometers, it is now possible to obtain a strength curve, i.e., the maximal force of contraction possible at each point in the full range of motion (Fig. 5–1). In fact, these can be obtained at different speeds of

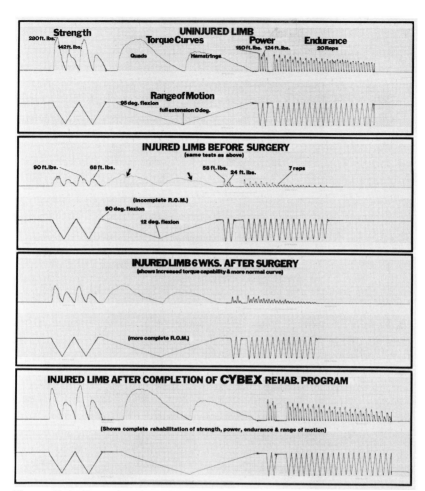

Figure 5–1. Example of an isokinetic strength curve taken from a Cybex isokinetic dynamometer.

contraction, providing additional information on the muscle fiber characteristics of the contracting muscles.[22, 23] A study by Graves and associates,[24] however, suggests that multiple isometric tests at various points in the full range of motion may provide more accurate estimates of pure strength.

When sophisticated laboratory equipment is unavailable for assessing strength, having the individual lift as much as he or she can just one time provides a simple but accurate estimate of strength. This is referred to as the one-repetition maximum (1-RM). In many fitness programs, the 1-RM is assessed for both the bench press and the leg press, providing estimates of both upper and lower body strength. In addition, an estimate of abdominal strength is also usually obtained. Factor analytic studies have shown that strength typically clusters in three areas: upper body, trunk, and lower body.[25, 26] Thus, obtaining only a single strength measure would not be representative of the total body, whereas assessments at each of these three sites would collectively provide an accurate estimate of total body strength.

Power is a term that refers to the maximal strength-producing capacity of the individual expressed relative to time,[20] i.e., (force × distance)/time. An individual who can bench press 200 pounds a distance of 2 feet in 0.5 seconds would have a power output of 800 foot-pounds per second. For training athletes, power is most likely the most important component, but it is often ignored. The basketball player leaping for a rebound, the football player lunging across the line to block the opponent, and the tennis player serving to the opponent are all relying on power for peak performance.

Muscular endurance refers to the ability of the muscle or muscle group to sustain contractions of a given force over time.[20] A simple measure of muscular endurance involves determining the number of repetitions a person can complete while lifting a fixed percentage of his or her 1-RM. If two individuals have identical 1-RM for the bench press of 200 pounds, the individual who performs more repetitions at 75 percent of that 1-RM, i.e., 150 pounds, would have the greater muscular endurance. More accurate estimates of endurance can be performed in the laboratory with specific dynamometers and strain gauges that are attached to recording devices. Endurance is related to the fiber-type characteristics of the individual.[22, 23]

Flexibility refers to the looseness or suppleness of the body or specific joints and involves the interrelationships between bones, muscles, fascia, tendons, ligaments, adipose tissue, and the joint capsule itself.[27] Limited flexibility is usually the result of muscles and tendons that are too tight, restricting the range of motion; however, excessive fatness is also a contributing factor. Flexibility is not easy to measure, even in a laboratory setting. Several tests, such as the sit and reach test, have been devised, but they provide only estimates, not absolute measures of flexibility. Hoeger[28] has proposed a simple battery of flexibility tests that appear to be relevant for inclusion in a fitness test battery. Chapter 6 provides more information concerning the testing for strength, muscular endurance, and flexibility.

Mechanisms of Strength Gains

When one gains strength through a planned program of strength training exercises, what physiological alterations occur to allow these gains? For many years, it was assumed that gains or losses in strength simply reflected changes in the size of the muscle or muscle groups: as the muscles increased in size, or underwent hypertrophy, there was an increase in strength, and as the muscles decreased in size, or underwent atrophy, there was a decrease in strength. It is now recognized that changes in strength are not so simply explained. Wilmore[29] demonstrated substantial gains in strength in college-aged women after a 10-week strength training program, with little or no change in muscle girth. In fact, some women were able to double their strength for certain weight training exercises but experienced no perceptible hypertrophy.

It is important to recognize that in the intact human, it is impossible to separate the muscle from its motor nerve. More specifically, a single motor nerve innervates a few to several thousand individual muscle fibers that compose the motor unit. When a motor nerve is activated by a simple reflex or by the higher brain centers, all of the muscle fibers innervated by that motor unit contract. The grading of a muscle's force production capabilities is accomplished by any one or a combination of the following: an increase in the number of motor units activated, the rate of activation, and an increased synchronization of motor unit firing. Thus, strength and gains in strength must be discussed relative to neuromuscular integration, i.e., the muscle's ability to produce tension and the nervous system's ability to activate the muscle. Sale[30, 31] has summarized the importance of the motor unit in this respect, as human motor units vary considerably in twitch force, contractile speed, axonal conduction velocity, fatigue resistance, recruitment thresholds, firing rates, and firing patterns. Enoka[32] has conducted an extensive review of the research literature on the role of the nervous system in the development of strength. He presents a convincing argument that neural mechanisms make significant contributions to the gains in strength with short-term training.

Examples of the neural component in the expression of strength are available from human experiences as well as from controlled laboratory studies. Periodically, newspapers provide detailed accounts of superhuman feats of strength, as illustrated by the small, middle-aged woman who lifts the automobile that has slipped off of its jack, freeing her son who was trapped beneath.[20] In one of the first laboratory experiments to investigate this phenomenon, Ikai and Steinhaus[33] measured the strength of the right forearm flexors during normal testing conditions and after hypnosis, a gunshot, a loud shout, alcohol ingestion, an injection of epinephrine, and ingestion of an amphetamine. Compared with control conditions, strength was affected $+26.5$ percent to -31.0 percent by the various interventions. This study pointed to the importance of specific inhibitory mechanisms employed by the body to protect the integrity of the muscles, tendons, ligaments, joints, and other tissues that might be subject to tear or injury consequent to the generation of high peak forces. Overcoming these inhibitory mechanisms appears to be an important adaptation in allowing the body to express greater levels of strength.

Moritani and deVries[34] proposed a model to differentiate the mechanisms for gains in strength into the components of "neural factors" and hypertrophy. If the gains in strength are attributed solely to neural factors, such as learning to disinhibit, then increases in maximal integrated electromyographic activation without any change in force per fiber or motor units innervated would be expected. If strength gains are attributable solely to muscular hypertrophy, increases in force production capabilities without increases in maximal integrated electromyographic activation would be expected. With this model, they demonstrated in seven young men and eight women that neural factors accounted for the larger proportion of the initial strength gains, with hypertrophy becoming the dominant factor after the first 3 to 5 weeks (Fig. 5–2). Coyle and colleagues[35] identified a neural component explaining at least a portion of the gains in strength they observed after a program of maximal two-legged knee extensions performed at one of three different velocities.

Milner-Brown and colleagues[36] found strength increases after training to be associated with significantly greater levels of synchronization of the various motor units. Komi and colleagues[37] also suggest improved synchronization of motor units to explain increases in strength. Finally, Gerchman and colleagues[38] have identified enlargement of the nucleolus in motor neurons with training, providing morphological evidence of motor neuron involvement in training adaptations. The reader is referred to the excellent review by Enoka[32] for elaboration in this area.

Thus, strength is the result of complex neuromuscular integrations. Strength is more than just a simple linear function of muscle size. Although size is possibly the most important determinant of strength, neurological and psychological factors must also be considered.

Muscle Hypertrophy and Atrophy

To understand how a muscle can undergo both hypertrophy with training and atrophy with disuse or immobilization, it is first

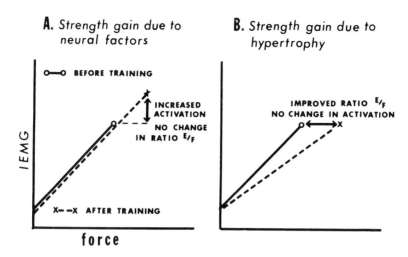

A. Strength gain due to
neural factors

B. Strength gain due to
hypertrophy

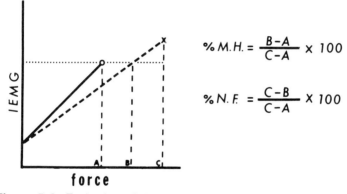

C. Evaluation of % contributions of neural
factors (N.F.) vs hypertrophy (M.H.)

$$\% \, M.H. = \frac{B-A}{C-A} \times 100$$

$$\% \, N.F. = \frac{C-B}{C-A} \times 100$$

Figure 5–2. Evaluation of the percent contributions of neural factors and hypertrophy to gains in strength through strength training exercise. (From Moritani, T., and deVries, H.A.: Potential for gross muscle hypertrophy in older men. **J. Gerontol.** 35:672–682, 1980.)

necessary to review the basic morphology of muscle. For many years, muscle was assumed to be composed of two major types of fibers, red and white. Red fibers were considered to be oxidative, or endurance, fibers, owing to their high concentration of myoglobin. White fibers were considered to be glycolytic fibers with high force-producing capabilities but with low endurance capacity. More recently, with the use of the muscle biopsy procedure (Fig. 5–3) pioneered by Bergstrom in 1962,[39] muscle fibers have been classified into three basic types: (1) slow, or type I, (2) fast-oxidative-glyco-lytic, or type IIa, and (3) fast glycolytic, or type IIb (Fig. 5–4). A

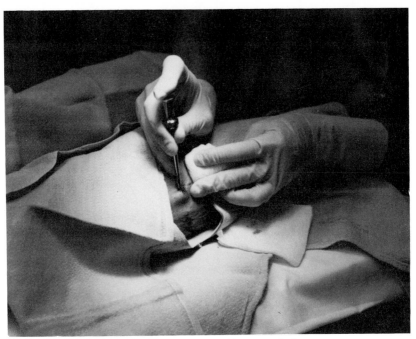

Figure 5–3. The muscle biopsy technique.

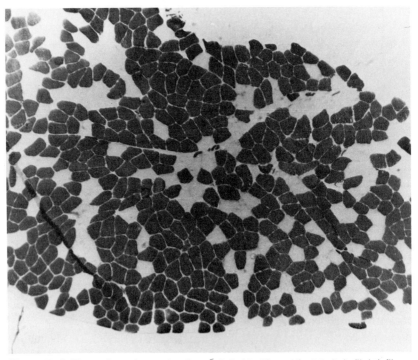

Figure 5–4. Illustration of muscle slow-twitch (dark) and fast-twitch (light) fiber types.

210

1986 review article by Gollnick and Hodgson[40] has pointed to the complexities involved in fiber typing and classifying muscle fibers. Classification nomenclature appears to be in a constant state of flux.

Endurance athletes typically have a preponderance of type-I fibers, whereas sprint-type athletes have a preponderance of type-II fibers.[20] In addition, it appears that fiber type is largely genetically determined and that the relative proportions of the type-I and type-II fibers do not change under normal conditions of training.[41, 42] The genetic influence is illustrated in Figure 5–5. Research with animals has shown that fiber type conversion is possible under conditions of cross-innervation, in which a fast-twitch motor unit is innervated by a slow-twitch motor neuron and vice versa. Further, chronic stimulation of fast-twitch motor units with low-frequency nerve stimulation transforms fast-twitch into slow-twitch motor units within a matter of weeks.[43] Several more recent studies

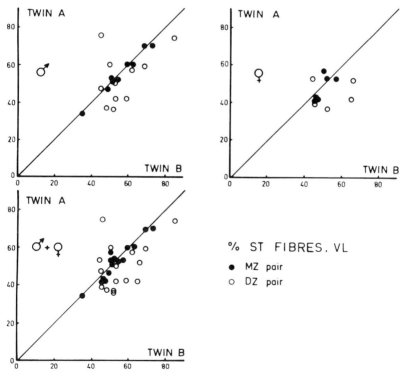

Figure 5–5. The heritability of fiber type in the vastus lateralis: percentage of type I, or slow-twitch, fibers comparing Twin A with Twin B. (From Komi, P.V., et al.: Skeletal muscle fibres and muscle enzyme activities in monozygous and dizygous twins of both sexes. **Acta Physiol. Scand.** 100:385–392, 1977.)

in both rats[44] and humans[45, 46] (Coyle, unpublished observations), have suggested a shift in fiber type as a result of long-term, high-intensity training.

Muscle hypertrophy represents a normal response to exercise training and is characterized by an increase in the size of the individual muscle fibers. This response could also involve an increase in the number of muscle fibers, the latter phenomenon being referred to as hyperplasia.[47, 48] Goldberg and coworkers[47] concluded that hypertrophy is the result of both an increased protein synthesis and a decreased protein degradation, alterations that could reflect either or both individual fiber hypertrophy and hyperplasia.

Morpurgo (see reference 49), in 1897, trained dogs on the treadmill after removal of the sartorius muscle to induce a compensatory hypertrophy. He found muscle hypertrophy to be solely the result of increases in fiber size, with no increase in fiber number. In 1970, Goldspink[48] reported similar results and concluded that individual fiber enlargement was the result of myofibril proliferation. In the late 1960's and early 1970's, researchers began to report muscle fiber hyperplasia under certain exercise training conditions, and these increases in fiber number were attributed to longitudinal fiber splitting.[49]

Gonyea,[50] in a series of studies in which cats were trained to lift weights with their right forelimb, reported a 20.5 percent increase in muscle fiber number after training, with a maximal increase in fiber diameter of only about 11 percent. This hyperplasia was attributed to muscle fiber splitting. Gollnick and associates[51] produced muscular hypertrophy in groups of rats by both surgical ablation of a synergist and the combination of synergist ablation and formal exercise training. Counting each fiber of the hypertrophied muscles, they were unable to identify any evidence of hyperplasia and concluded that hypertrophy was the result of enlarged fiber size, not hyperplasia. Similar results were found by Gollnick and coworkers[52] and Timson and coworkers[53] when the total fiber population was counted individually. Gollnick, Timson, and their associates[51-53] felt that Gonyea's histological sectioning method produced artifacts leading to an incorrect conclusion of fiber hyperplasia.

This led Gonyea and his colleagues[54] to repeat their strength training study with cats, this time using actual fiber counts to determine the existence of hyperplasia. They found a 9 percent increase in actual fiber number after training, confirming the original findings of hyperplasia reported by Gonyea.[50] The difference in the results between the studies of Gonyea and those of Gollnick and Timson and their colleagues is quite possibly due to both methodological differences and, most likely, to differences in the training protocol. Gonyea used a purer form of strength training, i.e., high-resistance, low-repetition training, whereas Gollnick and Timson used more endurance types of activity, i.e., low-resistance, high-repetition training. The reader is referred to an excellent, extensive review of the hypertrophy versus hyperplasia issue by Taylor and Wilkinson for additional information and the potential applications in humans.[55]

Atrophy, or the reduction in the size of a muscle or a muscle group, represents a normal response to disuse or immobilization. When aging is accompanied by an increasingly sedentary lifestyle and when a limb is immobilized in a cast consequent to a broken bone or surgery, muscle atrophy is almost always the result. Goldberg and associates[47] make the important observation that whereas hypertrophy of a muscle can help the organism improve physical performance, acquire new skills, or compensate for disease or injury to other body parts, atrophy of inactive muscle ensures that the organism does not have to maintain structures that are metabolically expensive but physiologically unnecessary.

Larsson[56] has reported that the proportion and the cross-sectional area of type-II muscle fibers decrease with aging, with no change in type-I fibers. This decrease in the type-II fibers correlates with decreases in strength observed with aging. Grimby and associates[57] reported a different aging pattern in their subjects. They did not find a decrease in type-II fiber numbers, or the percentage of the total represented by type-II fibers, but they did confirm the decrease in type-II fiber area with aging. Thus, it does appear that aging has a specific effect on the type-II fiber, with decreased fiber area being associated with decreased physical activity. Grimby and Saltin,[58] in their review of the literature in this area, have concluded that the main cause of the reduction in muscle mass with aging is a loss of muscle fibers.

Once the muscle undergoes atrophy with aging, it is difficult to regain that muscle mass with strength training. Moritani and deVries[59] found that increases in strength with strength training, in 67- to 72-year-old men, were predominantly the result of neural factors, as described earlier in this chapter, with muscle hypertrophy accounting for less than 30 percent of the strength gains. However, Panton and colleagues[60] found significant increases in biceps girth with resistance training in men and women 70 to 79 years of age. Grimby and Saltin[58] concluded from their review that both type-I and type-II fibers can continue to increase in fiber area with strength training in men in their 60's and 70's.

Muscle atrophy has also been studied during periods of immobilization. Haggmark and Eriksson[61] studied 16 patients who had been placed in either standard cylinder casts or in a mobile cast brace after anterior cruciate ligament reconstructive surgery of the knee. Patients with the standard cast showed a significant atrophy of type-I muscle fibers in the vastus lateralis, whereas those patients in the mobile brace demonstrated no significant changes in cross-sectional area of either type-I or type-II fibers. Evidently, the mobile brace, while maintaining the integrity of the surgical repair, still allowed sufficient stimulus of the involved muscles to prevent muscle atrophy. Grimby and colleagues[62] reported somewhat lower fiber areas, particularly in type-II fibers, when comparing the operated leg with the nonoperated leg in 30 subjects who had undergone surgery for knee ligament injuries. Sargeant and colleagues[63] studied seven patients who had suffered unilateral leg fractures after removal of their immobilizing plaster casts. After a mean casting period of 131 days, leg volume was reduced by 12 percent in the injured leg, and this was accompanied by a reduction of 42 percent in the cross-sectional area of the muscle fibers sampled from the vastus lateralis of the injured leg. Both type-I and type-II fibers were equally affected. MacDougall and colleagues[64] found decreases in fiber area of the triceps brachii of 33 percent to the fast-twitch and 25 percent to the slow-twitch fibers after 5 to 6 weeks of immobilization in elbow casts, coincident with a 41 percent decrease in elbow extension strength.

Muscle atrophy has been shown to occur very rapidly. The studies of Booth and coworkers[65, 66] have demonstrated that during the first 6 hours of hindlimb immobilization in rats, a significant decline of 37 percent occurs in the fractional rate of protein synthesis. In addition, the position in which the limb is immobilized is extremely important. Atrophy exhibited a half-time response, i.e., the time to reach one half of the final decrease, of 4 to 6 days when the muscle was casted in a shortened position. When the muscle was fixed in a stretched position, i.e., greater than resting length, the onset of atrophy was delayed. In fact, in some cases, muscles hypertrophied when fixed in the stretched position. Wilmore and coworkers[67] casted a human subject for a period of 17 days and reported a net protein breakdown of 40 and 59 percent on days 10 and 17 of casting, respectively. Graves and coworkers[68] have observed the effects of reduced training on gains in strength from a regular training program. They found that muscular strength can be maintained for up to 12 weeks with reduced training frequency (see Fig. 7–6).

Strength Training in Women

Women are generally considered to be the weaker sex. Is this stereotype justified? In a review article of nine separate studies, Laubach[69] compared basic strength abilities of men and women. He reported the following: (1) upper extremity strength measurements in women range from 35 to 79 percent of men's, averaging 55.8 percent, (2) lower extremity strength measurements in women range from 57 to 86 percent of men's, averaging 71.9 percent, and (3) trunk strength measurements for women range from 37 to 70 percent of men's, averaging 63.8 percent. Wilmore[29] compared the absolute strength of college-aged men and women for both the upper and the lower body, finding the women to have only 36.9 percent of the bench press strength and 73.4 percent of the leg press strength of men. When strength was expressed relative to body weight, the women had only 46.2 percent of the bench press strength but 92.4 percent of the leg press strength of men. When expressed relative to fat-free body weight, removing the influence of body fat, women had only 53.4 percent of the bench press strength but 106.0 percent of the leg press strength of men. In other words, relative to the fat-free body weight, women were as strong as men when equated for fat-free weight, but only with respect to leg strength. Hosler and Morrow[70] reported similar findings in young women and men for leg and arm isokinetic strength. They found that once body composition and size were controlled, gender accounted for only 2 percent of the variance in leg strength and 1 percent in arm strength. Thus, it would appear that the quality of the muscle is similar for men and women, but the larger size of the man will always be a distinct advantage relative to absolute strength.

There is also evidence that women respond in a manner similar to men when placed in a strength training program. Brown and Wilmore[71] trained seven female throwing-event athletes for a period of 6 months using a heavy resistance strength training program. After 6 months, bench press strength increased by 15 to 44 percent and half-squat strength increased by 16 to 53 percent. In a study of nonathletic young women, Wilmore[29] observed a 29.5 percent increase in leg press strength and a 28.6 percent increase in bench press strength after a 10-week strength training program. A comparison group of men exhibited increases of 26.0 percent and 16.5 percent, respectively. In both of these studies, strength gains in women were accompanied by little or no change in muscle girth, indicating that hypertrophy was not a necessary concomitant to gains in strength. This may not be true with higher-intensity programs. Mayhew and Gross[72] reported similar results for a group of college women who strength trained for a period of 9 weeks. Thus, it appears that women can gain benefits from strength training similar to those of men and that these benefits do not necessitate major increases in muscle bulk.

Strength Training in Men

Several reviews have summarized the magnitude of improvement with strength training in men.[73, 74] Obviously, as discussed in Chapter 7, improvements in strength will depend largely on the frequency, duration, and intensity of the training program. In the review of Kraemer and associates,[74] increases in bench press strength from studies conducted on men can range between 8 and 44 percent, whereas improvements in leg press strength can vary between 7 and 71 percent. Pollock and associates[75] have reported increases of over 100 percent in lumbar extension strength. It should be noted that percent improvements are a direct function of the initial starting level as well as the true gains in strength.[74] In studies in which men and women have been compared, the relative increases in strength are similar, although the men generally have greater absolute increases.[73] Further, men typically have significantly greater muscle hypertrophy with resistance training.[73]

Muscle Soreness

Muscle soreness may be present during the latter stages of exercise, during immediate recovery, between 12 and 48 hours after a strenuous bout of exercise, or at each of these times. The pain that is felt during and immediately after exercise is probably due to the accumulation of the end products of exercise and to tissue edema caused by the high hydrostatic pressure that forces fluid to shift from the blood plasma into the tissue.[20] This pain and soreness is usually of short duration, disappearing within an hour after cessation of exercise.[76]

The muscle soreness that is felt a day or two after a heavy bout of exercise has been explained by several recent theories, but there is not total agreement about which of these most adequately explains the soreness phenomenon. DeVries[77] developed the spasm theory to explain muscle soreness. According to this theory, exercise brings about localized muscle ischemia, the ischemia causes pain, the pain generates increased reflex motor activity, and greater motor activity creates even greater local muscle tension, which results in even greater degrees of ischemia. His research supports this theory, and he has also found that static stretching procedures help to prevent soreness, as well as to relieve soreness when it is present.

More recently, Abraham[78, 79] has provided data supporting Hough's torn-tissue hypothesis, which was originally formulated in 1902.[80] Abraham found muscle soreness to correlate with the appearance of myoglobin in the urine, with myoglobin being a marker of muscle fiber trauma. Since myoglobin in the urine is associated with all strenuous work, independent of muscle soreness, he also looked at hydroxyproline excretion, indicative of connective tissue breakdown. He found a significant correlation between the day of maximal hydroxyproline excretion and the day when the subjects experienced their greatest soreness.

There are several interesting characteristics of muscle soreness that may eventually be important considerations when attempting to identify potential contributing mechanisms. First, muscle soreness is usually a transient phenomenon. The individual typically experiences extreme muscle soreness only during the first few weeks of a new exercise program. After this initial training period, there is relatively little soreness, even with substantially higher levels of exercise, provided the form of exercise is the same. Second, muscle soreness appears to be associated with only the eccentric phase of muscle contraction, i.e., the lengthening of a muscle, as when a weight is gradually lowered back to its starting position after the completion of a lift.[20] With eccentric contraction, the force of gravity brings the weight down, and the muscles execute a controlled lengthening to reduce the speed of this downward movement. Talag[81] investigated the relationship of muscle soreness to eccentric, concentric, and isometric contractions and found that the group that trained solely with eccentric contractions experienced extreme muscle soreness, whereas the isometric and concentric contraction groups experienced little muscle soreness. Assmussen[82] and Komi and associates[83, 84] suggest that eccentric work overloads and overstretches the muscle's elastic components and that this insult results in muscle soreness.

Armstrong[85] has reviewed the possible mechanisms responsible for this muscle soreness, which he refers to as delayed onset muscular soreness (DOMS); DOMS is associated with elevations in plasma enzymes, myoglobinemia, and abnormal muscle histology and ultrastructure. He has proposed a model of DOMS that states (1) high tensions in the contractile/elastic system of muscle result in structural damage; (2) this cell membrane damage leads to a disruption of calcium ion homeostasis in the injured fibers, resulting in necrosis that peaks about 48 hours after exercise; and (3) the products of macrophage activity and the intracellular contents accumulate in the interstitium, which, in turn, stimulate the free nerve endings of the group-IV sensory neurons in the muscle. This process appears to be accentuated in eccentric exercise in which large forces are distributed over relatively small cross-sectional areas of the muscle.

More recent studies have confirmed that muscle soreness results predominantly from eccentric activity.[86-88] Further, McCully and Faulkner[89] have demonstrated that the extent of muscle damage is inversely related to the peak force developed.

Flexibility

Flexibility is limited in some joints by either the bony structure or the bulk of the surrounding muscle, or both. These mechanical factors cannot be greatly modified. However, for most joints, the limitation of movement through the range of movement is imposed by the soft tissues, including (1) the muscle and its fascial sheaths; (2) the connective tissue, with tendons, ligaments, and joint capsules; and (3) the skin.[27] John and Wright,[90] studying wrist flexion and extension in the cat, found the muscles, the joint capsule, and the tendons to be the most important factors limiting free movement about the joint.

DeVries[27] has cited a number of factors other than those listed previously that influence the flexibility of joints. First, the more active the individual, generally the more flexible he or she is. It appears that this activity must be performed through the full range of motion of each specific joint in order to gain benefits. Most long-distance runners who do little or no stretching before or after their workouts have limited or poor flexibility. The mechanics of the running movement are such that the runner does not utilize the full range of movement while running. Thus, even those who are very active must evaluate the nature of their activity to determine if that activity is promoting or reducing general body flexibility.

Second, there appears to be a gender difference in flexibility, with girls and women being much more flexible than boys and men. Third, flexibility is age related, with flexibility decreasing to the age of 10 to 12 years and then increasing into adulthood. With aging, flexibility begins a progressive decline. Fourth, flexibility is greatly influenced by temperature. Local warming of a joint increases the flexibility of that joint, whereas local cooling brings about the opposite effect. Finally, there is the possibility that overstretching may result in joint laxity, which may increase the risk of injury.

STRENGTH AND FLEXIBILITY TRAINING PROCEDURES

Strength, power, muscular endurance, and flexibility can be altered through specific muscle and flexibility training programs. Although the intent of this chapter is to provide a basic overview of the physiological foundations of strength and flexibility, it is also important to understand basic procedural concepts in order to prescribe strength and flexibility training programs most effectively. The remainder of this chapter gives a brief overview of training procedures specific to strength and flexibility programs. Much more detail is provided in Chapters 7 and 8.

Strength Training Procedures

Strength training procedures can be classified according to whether the contraction is static or dynamic and whether the contraction is concentric, i.e., shortening, or eccentric, i.e., lengthening. In a static, or isometric, contraction, the muscle contracts, but there is no visible movement about the joint. With dynamic contraction, there is movement about the joint, and this movement can take one of several forms. With isotonic contraction, there is movement of a specific weight through the full range of motion, as illustrated by the two-arm curl, in which the barbell is lifted from a position with the elbows fully extended to a position of complete flexion (Fig. 5–6). When curling a weight of 105 pounds, there is a constant resistance of 105 pounds that must be overcome by the application of a force in excess of 105 pounds. Owing to the mechanics of the elbow joint, however, the force of 105 pounds represents different fractions of the maximal potential at each angle in the range of motion. Strength is the result of the contractile force and the mechanics of movement about a joint. Thus, the 105 pounds in the biceps curl may represent maximal strength at the angles of 60 degrees and 180 degrees, but only 75 percent of maximal strength at 100 degrees, when the contractile force and joint mechanics are optimal. In isotonic movements, therefore, the muscle is not contracting at its capacity or at a constant percentage of its capacity throughout the entire range of motion.

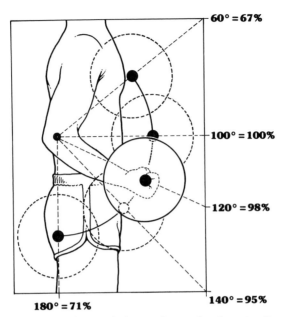

60° = 67%

100° = 100%

120° = 98%

140° = 95%

180° = 71%

Figure 5–6. Variation in force relative to the angle of contraction, with 100% representing the angle at which force is optimal. (From Wilmore, J.H., and Costill, D.L.: **Training for Sport and Activity: The Physiological Basis of the Conditioning Process,** 3rd Ed. Dubuque, IA, William C. Brown Publishers, 1988.)

Isokinetic contraction is a form of dynamic contraction in which the speed of limb movement is constant. Typically, the muscle applies force against a resistance that is moving at a constant speed. Figure 5–7 illustrates a Cybex II isokinetic testing device. The lever arm, against which the individual is applying force, moves at a fixed rate of movement. The rate of movement can be adjusted to any speed ranging from an isometric contraction at 0 degrees per second to a relatively fast speed of 300 degrees per second. Theoretically, if properly motivated, the individual can apply maximal force throughout the entire range of motion. This would be an apparent advantage over isotonic procedures, in which the muscle is taxed to its capacity only in the weakest portion of its range of motion.

Accommodating resistance training is a form of training in which the resistance is varied in a systematic manner in an attempt to match the force-producing capabilities of the muscle or muscle group. Although similar to the loading achievable with isokinetic training, there is no attempt to control the speed of movement. Variable resistance training is another form of dynamic contraction

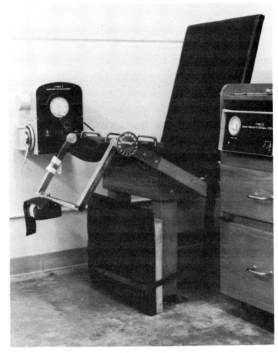

Figure 5–7. The Cybex II isokinetic muscle testing device.

in which the resistance is altered throughout the range of motion. This is illustrated by the Nautilus machine in Figure 5–8.

Isometric training procedures are based on the theory that strength can be efficiently gained by training the muscle or muscle group against a fixed, immovable resistance. Although isometric training has been practiced for many years, it was popularized in the mid-1950's by the research of Hettinger and Muller[91] in Germany. Their initial studies indicated that strength gains of 5 percent of the original strength value could be obtained each week as a result of only one 6-second contraction per day at only 67 percent of maximal effort. Little additional improvement resulted with maximal effort or with repeated contractions totaling 45 seconds. Subsequent research from these investigators indicated that maximal contractions provided better results.[92] Clarke,[93] in reviewing the research literature through 1972, concluded that the best results from isometric training appear to be obtained by using maximal contractions held for a period of 6 seconds, repeated five to ten times per day. In a more recent review, Atha[21] concluded that isometric contractions, to have their greatest effect, should

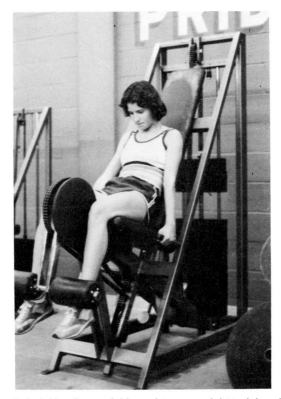

Figure 5–8. A Nautilus variable resistance weight training device.

probably be performed at nearly maximal effort, should last long enough for all fibers in a muscle group to be fully recruited, and should be repeated several times daily.

Isotonic strength training typically involves the use of weights in the form of dumbbells, barbells, pulleys, and machines that use stacked weights. Two important principles govern isotonic strength training and, in fact, all forms of dynamic strength training. The principle of overload refers to the well-known fact that to gain strength through muscle training procedures, it is necessary to load the muscle beyond the point at which it is normally loaded. Closely related, the principle of progressive resistance exercise refers to the fact that as the muscle becomes stronger, it must work against a progressively greater resistance in order to continue to achieve gains in strength. To illustrate, the male weightlifter who can perform only ten repetitions of a bench press using 150 pounds of weight will, as he weight trains and gets stronger, be able to increase his repetitions for the same weight, e.g., 14 or 15 repetitions. By adding 5 pounds of weight to the bar for a total of 155 pounds, he will reduce the maximal number of repetitions he can perform to eight to ten. As he continues to train, his maximal number of repetitions for this new weight will continue to increase until it is time to add an additional 5 pounds of weight. Thus, there is a progressive increase in the amount of resistance, or weight, lifted.[20]

With isotonic procedures, what is the most effective procedure for training? DeLorme,[94] and later DeLorme and Watkins,[95] are credited with the initial efforts to systematize isotonic training procedures. They emphasized the use of heavy resistance and a low number of repetitions to develop muscular strength, as opposed to light resistance and a high number of repetitions to develop muscular endurance. Originally working with 100 repetitions divided into seven to ten sets, they modified this to three sets of ten repetitions each. In 1951, Zinovieff[96] proposed the Oxford technique, in which 100 repetitions were performed over ten sets, with the resistance decreasing with each progressive set as the individual fatigued.

Subsequent research has attempted to identify the best possible combination of sets, repetitions, and resistance to maximize strength gains. Clarke,[97] in the January 1974 issue of the *Physical Fitness Research Digest*, summarized the research literature through 1973, and Atha[21] conducted a review that was published in 1982. From these two reviews, it appears that weight training should be performed at five to seven repetitions per set, with three sets of each exercise executed per training session, to maximize gains in muscle strength. The weight used for each set should be sufficient to tax the muscle maximally to fatigue by the last repetition of the set. Training frequency should be three times per week, although this can be increased to five times per week if the muscles have been preconditioned. It should be noted that these guidelines have been established for maximizing strength gains, where strength training is the primary training mode. For a more balanced "total fitness" training program, refer to Chapter 7.

Isokinetic training procedures are relatively new in concept and in practice. This concept, which was introduced by Perrine in 1968,[98] is rather unique in that it does allow maximal force production throughout the full range of movement, provided the subject is properly motivated. Most isokinetic training devices also provide variation in the speed of the movement, allowing the subject to train at different velocities. Traditional weight training is performed at very slow velocities, whereas most human movement, particularly with respect to sport, is performed at relatively fast velocities. For the training of athletes for sport, this raises the following question: would athletes be better off to train at faster velocities that more closely approximate the speeds at which they perform? Preliminary research suggests that fast speed training may, in fact, have important benefits,[35] although additional research is needed. Isokinetic training would seem to have at least two potential advantages over static or other dynamic forms of training: opportunity for maximal force production throughout the full range of motion at the slower speeds of contraction, and variable speed training.

Actual training procedures for isokinetic training are similar to those listed earlier for isotonic training. Typically, three sets are performed for each exercise, with five to seven repetitions at maximal force production. There may be some advantage to mixing slow and fast speed training, but this has yet to be confirmed by experimental research. As mentioned previously, accommodating resistance training is considered to be similar to isokinetic training in that the resistance can be matched to the force-producing capabilities of the muscles at all points in the range of motion. However, with several of the commercial devices, although the resistance accommodates to the force-producing capabilities of the muscle, the movements are not truly isokinetic, since the speed of movement is not absolutely constant. The Hydra-Gym and the Cam II strength training devices are examples of accommodating resistance devices, using hydraulics and air, respectively, to provide the accommodating resistance.

Variable resistance devices typically use several different means to alter the mechanical advantage of the lever arm, thus altering the resistance to the subject through the range of motion, even though the weight on the weight stack remains constant. The variable resistance cam used by Nautilus was illustrated in Figure 5–8. This is an ingenious device that attempts to alter the resistance of the weight stack to match the force-producing capabilities of the muscles throughout the full range of motion. The Universal Gym Centurion reduces the length of the lever arm as the subject progresses through the range of motion, decreasing the mechanical advantage and increasing the resistance.

Two additional training procedures that do not fit within the definitions of the training procedures noted previously are eccentric training and plyometric training. Eccentric training has received much interest, since a muscle can be loaded with considerably more weight eccentrically than concentrically. The research literature indicates that eccentric training is effective for increasing strength, but no more effective than concentric training.[21] Plyometric training was described by Wilt in 1975,[99] but is considered to be an extension of the work of Verkhoshanski in 1966.[100] Verkhoshanski advocated a rebound jump after dropping from a fixed height. The muscle is loaded so suddenly that it is forced to yield and stretch before developing sufficient tension to arrest the motion of the load and to reverse the direction of movement. Atha has described plyometric loading as a rhythmical hybrid of eccentric plus concentric activity, loading the elastic as well as the contractile components of the muscle.[21] Although the theory of plyometrics appears sound, there has not been sufficient research conducted to demonstrate its effectiveness relative to other training procedures. It has been used successfully in the training of athletes, but there is certainly an increased potential for injury because of the high impact forces.

Which of the previously named training procedures provides the greatest gains in strength? Much early work compared isometric with isotonic training procedures and found that both procedures led to substantial increases in strength, with the isotonic procedures providing slightly greater gains in strength and substantially greater gains in muscular endurance and in muscular hypertrophy.[101] Few studies have compared isokinetic with isotonic and isometric training procedures. Atha[21] concludes that at the present time, isokinetic procedures have not been demonstrated to have superiority over other training procedures, but this may be due to an inadequate number of well-designed and controlled investigations. With respect to variable and accommodating resistance devices, despite the claims of the manufacturers, no experimental evidence exists to demonstrate the superiority of one system over another.

Specificity of Strength Training Procedures

Over the years, the scientific community has become much more aware of the specificity of different training procedures. It is obvious that strength training will do very little to improve one's time in the marathon or that distance running will have little effect on improving the strength of the competitive weight lifter. Strength training improves strength and distance running improves cardiorespiratory endurance capacity. This does not mean that the distance runner should not lift weights or that the weight lifter should not run, but simply that training is very specific in what it accomplishes.

With respect to strength training, there are currently two conflicting theories regarding training to improve sports performance. One theory states that the training should simulate the sport movement as closely as possible relative to anatomical movement pattern, velocity, contraction type, and contraction force.[102] The opposing theory holds that it is necessary to train only the appropriate muscle groups, i.e., there is no need to have movement-specific exercises.[102] Sale and MacDougall,[102] in a review of research in this area, conclude that the scientific evidence to date strongly favors specificity in training.

The pattern of movement is highly specific and has been shown to be very important relative to increases in strength with training. Thorstensson and colleagues[103] demonstrated this very clearly in a study in which they trained their subjects by having them perform barbell squats. The subjects were tested before and after training by performing 1-RM barbell squats and by performing an isometric leg press, both using the same muscle groups in approximately the same position. Strength gains after 8 weeks of training approached 75 percent for the barbell squat test but averaged less than 30 percent for the isometric leg press.

Velocity of training is also highly specific, as illustrated by Coyle and colleagues.[35] Training subjects at either a fast speed of 300 degrees per second or a relatively slow speed of 60 degrees per second, or a combination of fast and slow speeds, for maximal two-legged isokinetic knee extensions three times per week for 6 weeks, they found the improvements in strength, i.e., peak torque, to be highly specific to the speed of training. The group that trained at the high speed improved most when tested at high speeds; the group that trained at the slow speed demonstrated improvement only at the slow speed; and the combination group demonstrated intermediate changes.

Specificity is also a factor with respect to the angle within the range of motion at which training takes place. Graves and colleagues[104] studied limited range of motion dynamic resistance training on the full range of motion strength development. Using knee extension training, Group A trained from 120 to 60 degrees, Group B trained from 60 to 0 degrees, and Group AB trained through the full range of motion. Strength gains for the limited-range-of-motion–trained groups (Groups A and B) were greater within the trained range than outside the training range. This is illustrated in Figure 5–9. Thus, it is important to emphasize full range of motion training, including exercises for all major muscle groups.

Since specificity is a factor in strength development, is it also a factor when training to develop muscle power? Since most athletic events depend on power, should training be structured to emphasize

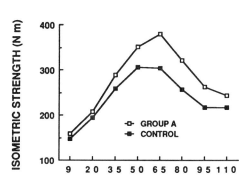

Figure 5–9. Specificity of strength training with respect to the range of motion of training within the total range of motion. Relative changes (%) in isometric strength after 10 weeks of variable resistance training. Group A trained from 120° to 60° of knee flexion, Group B trained from 60° to 0° of knee flexion, and Group AB trained from 120° to 0° knee flexion. The control group did not train. (From Graves, J.E., et al: Specificity of limited range of motion variable resistance training. **Med. Sci. Sports Exerc.** 21:84–89, 1989.)

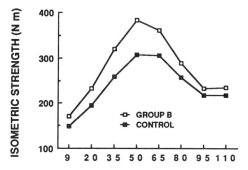

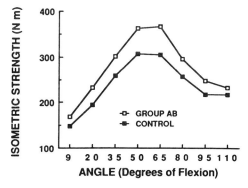

power movements? Although these questions have not yet been answered, the evidence previously presented relative to the specificity of training for strength suggests that there is probably a high degree of specificity associated with training to maximize gains in power. Assuming that specificity does exist, how would one train to maximize power development? McLario[105] investigated the relative contribution of force and velocity to the development of peak power output in the bench press. Peak power was achieved when force production was at approximately 50 percent of the 1-RM for the bench press. This would suggest that at least part of an individual's training should be performed at these low relative force outputs, emphasizing both speed and explosiveness of movement when executing the lift.

Circuit Weight Training

Circuit training is an innovative type of conditioning program that was developed by Morgan and Adamson in 1953 at the University of Leeds in London.[106] Circuit training can be designed to develop strength, power, muscular endurance, speed, agility, flexibility, and cardiovascular endurance. With circuit training, the individual proceeds through a series of selected exercises or activities that are performed in sequence or in a circuit. There are usually six to ten stations in a circuit, which can be located inside gymnasiums, exercise rooms, or hallways, or outside on courts, fields, or rooftops. The individual performs a specific exercise at each station and then proceeds to the next station. The idea is to progress through the circuit as rapidly as possible, attempting to improve either by decreasing the total time to complete the circuit or by increasing the amount of work accomplished at each station, or both.

Allen and associates[107] investigated the possibility of placing traditional weight training into a circuit training format. Traditional weight training is usually performed in a slow, methodical manner, with very short work periods and very long rest intervals. With circuit weight training, individuals work at approximately 40 to 60 percent of their 1-RM for periods of approximately 30 seconds, with 15-second rest intervals interspersed between work periods, although both the length of these intervals and the work-to-rest ratio can be altered. They start at the first station, completing as many repetitions as possible in 30 seconds, take a 15-second rest, during which they move to the next station, and then begin their second 30-second work period. This continues until they complete the six to twelve stations in the circuit, and then they start their second set. The work and rest intervals can be varied to match the needs of the individual or group.

Gettman and Pollock[108] have published an excellent review of all research that has been conducted on circuit weight training from the original study of Allen and associates[107] through 1980. Circuit weight training provides modest increases in maximal oxygen uptake (see Chapter 3); major increases in strength, muscular endurance, and flexibility; and substantial alterations in body composition, i.e., increases in fat-free body weight and decreases in body fat. More recent studies have shown similar results in patient populations.[109-111]

Flexibility Training Procedures

Flexibility training is not difficult, requires little time and effort, and can be accomplished during either or both the warm-up and cool-down phases of the daily workout. Most advocates are now promoting true flexibility training at the end of the workout when the body is warm and pliable. In the performance of stretching exercises, the movement can be either static or dynamic. Dynamic stretching involves slow to rapid or ballistic movements, e.g., bobbing or jerking, whereas static stretching involves a slow positioning of the body followed by a static stretch. As an example, with the hip flexion movement, the ballistic approach would have the individual, from the sitting position on the floor, bending forward at the waist attempting to touch his or her toes with the fingers and hands extended forward using five or six rapid, jerking or bouncing motions. In the static stretch, the individual grabs his or her ankles with the hands and slowly stretches forward, attempting to place the head on the knees. Research has shown both methods to be effective. However, it is believed that there is less danger of injury and soreness with static stretching. If a muscle contracts quickly or in a jerky motion, it will stretch the antagonist muscles, causing them to contract, thus limiting the range of dynamic motion. A firm static stretch involves the inverse myotatic reflex, which results in an inhibition of the antagonist group of muscles, allowing them to relax and enhancing the range of motion.[27]

During the late 1970's and early 1980's a new form of stretching received considerable attention. Proprioceptive neuromuscular facilitation (PNF) is a technique first used by physical therapists for treating patients with various types of neuromuscular paralysis. This technique requires the use of a partner and uses one or more of several different procedures, i.e., contract-relax, hold-relax, and slow-reversal-hold.

With the hold-relax procedure, a partner pushes or pulls the individual in the direction of the desired stretch while the individual applies active resistance, i.e., contraction, against the partner's efforts. This results in a static or isometric contraction that is to be held for a period of 4 to 5 seconds. After this period of static contraction, the muscles that have been contracting are relaxed and the partner continues to apply force in the direction of the desired stretch. This process can be repeated several times during the same stretch.

In the contract-relax procedure, the individual performs a concentric contraction, slowly overcoming the resistance of the partner, moving in a direction opposite to that of the stretch. As in the hold-relax procedure, the individual then totally relaxes those muscles that were contracting, and the partner continues to apply force, gradually increasing the degree of stretch. In the slow-reversal-hold procedure, the partner applies pressure in the direction of the stretch. Once the limb reaches that point where the individual feels slight discomfort in the muscle, he or she begins to contract the antagonistic muscles against his or her partner's resistance. Following a 10-second contraction, the antagonists are relaxed and the agonists are contracted for a period of 10 seconds, allowing the partner to increase the range of motion in the desired direction.

Moore and Hutton[112] have compared the improvement in hip flexion resulting from static, contract-relax, and contract-relax with agonist contraction (similar to slow-reversal-hold) techniques in young female gymnasts. They found that the contract-relax with agonist contraction produced the largest gains in hip flexion, although the differences were not that great. Etnyre and Lee,[113] in reviewing the literature on PNF through 1987, concluded that there is no clear advantage to any one stretching technique over any other. Ballistic, static, and PNF techniques all appear to improve flexibility to a similar extent.

When flexibility is increased with stretching, the muscles, tendons, and ligaments appear to be the site of any change. The mechanism of change appears to be a simple stretching of the involved connective tissue, primarily the ligamentous joint capsule, the tendons, and the connective tissue framework and sheathing within and around the muscle.[114]

SUMMARY

Attention must be given to maintaining optimal functioning of the musculoskeletal system. Prevention of poor posture, lower back complaints, fat-free tissue loss, and osteoporosis depends on the incorporation of a comprehensive strength and flexibility training program into the daily workout. This chapter has presented the physiological foundations for both strength and flexibility and has attempted to review the most current thoughts relative to training procedures. A number of excellent reviews are available for the reader who would like additional information.[21, 30–32, 55, 73, 74, 85, 88, 93, 108, 115–119] Specific strength and flexibility exercises are presented in Chapters 7 and 8.

References

1. Massachusetts Mutual Insurance Company: **Disability Income Protection Approved Claims, 1974.** World Supplement, June 1975.
2. Kraus, H., and Raab, W.: **Hypokinetic Disease.** Springfield, IL, Charles C Thomas, 1961.
3. Forbes, G.B.: The adult decline in lean body mass. **Hum. Biol.** 48:161–173, 1976.
4. Quenouille, M.H., Boyn, A.W., Fisher, W.B., and Leitch, I.: Statistical studies of recorded energy expenditure in man. Part 1. Basal metabolism related to sex, stature, age, climate and race. **Commonw. Agr. Bur. Tech. Comm.** No. 17. Bucks, England, Farnham Royal, 1951.
5. Keys, A., Taylor, H.L., and Grande, F.: Basal metabolism and age of adult man. **Metabolism** 22:579–587, 1973.
6. Birge, S.J., Jr., and Whedon, G.D.: Bone. In McCally, M. (ed.): **Hypodynamics and Hypogravics.** New York, Academic Press, 1968.
7. Vogel, J.M., and Whittle, M.W.: **The Proceedings of the Skylab Life Sciences Symposium. NASA Technical Memorandum JSC-09275.** Washington, D.C., 1974.
8. Bortz, W.M.: Disuse and aging. **JAMA** 248:1203–1208, 1982.
9. Aloia, J.F., Cohn, S.H., Ostuni, J.A., Cane, R., and Ellis, K.: Prevention of involutional bone loss by exercise. **Ann. Intern. Med.** 89:356–358, 1978.
10. Smith, E.L., Reddan, W., and Smith, P.E.: Physical activity and calcium modalities for bone mineral increase in aged women. **Med. Sci. Sports Exerc.** 13:60–64, 1981.
11. Darby, L.A., Pohlman, R.L., and Lechner, A.J.: Increased bone calcium following endurance exercise in the mature female rat. **Lab. Anim. Sci.** 35:382–386, 1985.
12. Chow, R., Harrison, J.E., and Notarius, C.: Effect of two randomised exercise programmes on bone mass of healthy postmenopausal women. **Br. Med. J.** 295:1441–1444, 1987.
13. Dalsky, G.P., Stocke, K.S., Ehsani, A.A., Slatopolsky, E., Lee, W.C., and Birge, S.J.: Weight-bearing exercise training and lumbar bone mineral content in postmenopausal women. **Ann. Intern. Med.** 108:824–828, 1988.
14. Aloia, J.F., Vaswani, A.N., Yeh, J.K., and Cohn, S.H.: Premenopausal bone mass is related to physical activity. **Arch. Phys. Med.** 148:121–123, 1988.
15. Kanders, B., Dempster, D.W., and Lindsay, R.: Interaction of calcium nutrition and physical activity on bone mass in young women. **J. Bone Miner. Res.** 3:145–149, 1988.
16. Pocock, N.A., Eisman, J.A., Yeates, M.G., Sambrook, P.N., and Eberl, S.: Physical fitness is a major determinant of femoral neck and lumbar spine bone mineral density. **J. Clin. Invest.** 78:618–621, 1986.
17. Kriska, A.M., Sandler, R.B., Cauley, J.A., LaPorte, R.E., Hom, D.L., and

Pambianco, G.: The assessment of historical physical activity and its relation to adult bone parameters. **Am. J. Epidemiol.** 127:1053–1063, 1988.

18. Smith, E.L., and Raab, D.M.: Osteoporosis and physical activity. **Acta Med. Scand.** (Suppl.) 711:149–156, 1986.

19. Martin, A.D., and Houston, C.S.: Osteoporosis, calcium and physical activity. **Can. Med. Assoc. J.** 136:587–593, 1987.

20. Wilmore, J.H., and Costill, D.L.: **Training for Sport and Activity: The Physiological Basis of the Conditioning Process,** 3rd Ed. Dubuque, IA, William C. Brown, 1988.

21. Atha, J.: Strengthening muscle. **Exerc. Sport Sci. Rev.** 9:1–73, 1982.

22. Thorstensson, A., Larsson, L., Tesch, P., and Karlsson, J.: Muscle strength and fiber composition in athletes and sedentary men. **Med. Sci. Sports** 9:26–30, 1977.

23. Gregor, R.J., Edgerton, V.R., Perrine, J.J., Campion, D.S., and DeBus, C.: Torque-velocity relationships and muscle fiber composition in elite female athletes. **J. Appl. Physiol.** 47:388–392, 1979.

24. Graves, J.E., Pollock, M.L., Carpenter, D.M., Leggett, S.H., Jones, A., Mac-Millan, M., and Fulton, M.: Quantitative assessment of full range-of-motion isometric lumbar extension strength. **Spine** in press, 1990.

25. Clarke, H.H.: Toward a better understanding of muscular strength **Phys. Fitness Res. Digest** 3:1–20, 1973.

26. Jackson, A., Watkins, M., and Patton, R.W.: A factor analysis of twelve selected maximal isotonic strength performances on the Universal Gym. **Med. Sci. Sports Exerc.** 12:274–277, 1980.

27. deVries, H.A.: **Physiology of Exercise for Physical Education and Athletics,** 4th Ed. Dubuque, IA, William C. Brown, 1986.

28. Hoeger, W.W.K.: **Lifetime Physical Fitness and Wellness: A Personalized Program.** Englewood, CO, Morton Publishing Co., 1986, pp. 45–52.

29. Wilmore, J.H.: Alterations in strength, body composition and anthropometric measurements consequent to a 10-week weight training program. **Med. Sci. Sports** 6:133–138, 1974.

30. Sale, D.G.: Influence of exercise and training on motor unit activation. **Exerc. Sport Sci. Rev.** 15:95–151, 1987.

31. Sale, D.G.: Neural adaptation to resistance training. **Med. Sci. Sports Exerc.** 20:S135–S145, 1988.

32. Enoka, R.M.: Muscle strength and its development: new perspectives. **Sports Med.** 6:146–168, 1988.

33. Ikai, M., and Steinhaus, A.H.: Some factors modifying the expression of human strength. **J. Appl. Physiol.** 16:157–163, 1961.

34. Moritani, T., and deVries, H.A.: Neural factors versus hypertrophy in the time course of muscle strength gain. **Am. J. Phys. Med.** 58:115–130, 1979.

35. Coyle, E.F., Feiring, D.C., Rotkis, T.C., Cote, R.W., III, Roby, F.B., Lee, W., and Wilmore, J.H.: Specificity of power improvements through slow and fast isokinetic training. **J. Appl. Physiol.** 51:1437–1442, 1981.

36. Milner-Brown, H.S., Stein, R.B., and Lee, R.G.: Synchronization of human motor units: possible roles of exercise and supraspinal reflexes. **Electroencephalogr. Clin. Neurophysiol.** 38:245–254, 1975.

37. Komi, P.V., Viitasalo, J.T., Rauramaa, R., and Vihko, V.: Effect of isometric strength training on mechanical, electrical and metabolic aspects of muscle function. **Eur. J. Appl. Physiol.** 40:45–55, 1978.

38. Gerchman, L., Edgerton, V.R., and Carrow, R.: Effects of physical training on the histochemistry and morphology of the ventral motor neurons. **Exp. Neurol.** 49:790–801, 1975.

39. Bergstrom, J.: Muscle electrolytes in man. **Scand. J. Clin. Lab. Invest.** 68:11–13, 1962.

40. Gollnick, P.D., and Hodgson, D.R.: The identification of fiber types in skeletal muscle: a continual dilemma. **Exerc. Sport Sci. Rev.** 14:81–104, 1986.

41. Komi, P.V., and Karlsson, J.: Physical performance, skeletal muscle enzyme activities, and fibre types in monozygous and dizygous twins of both sexes. **Acta Physiol. Scand.** (Suppl.) 462, 1972.

42. Komi, P.V., Viitasalo, J.H.T., Havu, M., Thorstensson, A., Sjodin, B., and Karlsson, J.: Skeletal muscle fibres and muscle enzyme activities in monozygous and dizygous twins of both sexes. **Acta Physiol. Scand.** 100:385–392, 1977.

43. Pette, D.: Activity-induced fast to slow transitions in mammalian muscle. **Med. Sci. Sports Exerc.** 16:517–528, 1984.

44. Green, H.J., Klug, G.A., Reichmann, H., Seedorf, U., Wiehrer, W., and Pette, D.: Exercise-induced fibre type transitions with regard to myosin, parvalbumin, and sarcoplasmic reticulum in muscles of the rat. **Pflugers Arch.** 400:432–438, 1984.

45. Simoneau, J.A., Lortie, G., Boulay, M.R., Marcotte, M., Thibault, M.C., and Bouchard, C.: Human skeletal muscle fiber type alteration with high-intensity intermittent training. **Eur. J. Appl. Physiol.** 54:250–253, 1985.

46. Tesch, P.A., and Karlsson, J.: Muscle fiber types and size in trained and untrained muscles of elite athletes. **J. Appl. Physiol.** 59:1716–1720, 1985.

47. Goldberg, A.L., Etlinger, J.D., Goldspink, D.F., and Jablecki, C.: Mechanisms of work-induced hypertrophy of skeletal muscle. **Med. Sci. Sports** 7:248–261, 1975.

48. Goldspink, G.: The proliferation of myofibrils during muscle fibre growth. **J. Cell. Sci.** 6:593–604, 1970.

49. Edgerton, V.R.: Exercise and the growth and development of muscle tissue. In Rarick, G.L. (ed.): **Physical Activity, Human Growth and Development.** New York, Academic Press, 1973.

50. Gonyea, W.J.: Role of exercise in inducing increases in skeletal muscle fibre number. **J. Appl. Physiol.** 48:421–426, 1980.

51. Gollnick, P.D., Timson, B.F., Moore, R.L., and Riedy, M.: Muscular enlargement and number of fibers in skeletal muscles of rats. **J. Appl. Physiol.** 5:936–943, 1981.

52. Gollnick, P.D., Parsons, D., Riedy, M., and Moore, R.L.: Fiber number and size in overloaded chicken anterior latissimus dorsi muscle. **J. Appl. Physiol.** 54:1292–1297, 1983.

53. Timson, B.F., Bowlin, B.K., Dudenhoeffer, G.A., and George, J.B.: Fiber number, area, and composition of mouse soleus muscle following enlargement. **J. Appl. Physiol.** 58:619–624, 1985.

54. Gonyea, W.J., Sale, D.G., Gonyea, F.B., and Mikesky, A.: Exercise induced increases in muscle fiber number. **Eur. J. Appl. Physiol.** 55:137–141, 1986.

55. Taylor, N.A.S., and Wilkinson, J.G.: Exercise-induced skeletal muscle growth: hypertrophy or hyperplasia? **Sports Med.** 3:190–200, 1986.

56. Larsson, L.: Morphological and functional characteristics of the aging skeletal muscle in man: a cross-sectional study. **Acta Physiol. Scand.** (Suppl.) 457:1–36, 1978.

57. Grimby, G., Danneskiold-Samsoe, B., Hvid, K., and Saltin, B.: Morphology and enzymatic capacity in arm and leg muscles in 78–81 year old men and women. **Acta Physiol. Scand.** 115:125–134, 1982.

58. Grimby, G., and Saltin, B.: The ageing muscle. **Clin. Physiol.** 3:209–218, 1983.

59. Moritani, T., and deVries, H.A.: Potential for gross muscle hypertrophy in older men. **J. Gerontol.** 35:672–682, 1980.

60. Panton, L.B., Graves, J.E., Pollock, M.L., Hagberg, J.M., and Leggett, S.H.: Effect of aerobic and variable resistance exercise training on strength and body composition of men and women 70–79 yrs of age. Unpublished abstract, 1988.

61. Haggmark, T., and Eriksson, E.: Cylinder or mobile cast brace after knee ligament surgery. **Am. J. Sports Med.** 7:48–56, 1979.

62. Grimby, G., Gustafsson, E., Peterson, L., and Renstrom, P.: Quadriceps function and training after knee ligament surgery. **Med. Sci. Sports Exerc.** 12:70–75, 1980.

63. Sargeant, A.J., Davies, C.T.M., Edwards, R.H.T., Maunder, C., and Young, A.: Functional and structural changes after disuse of human muscle. **Clin. Sci. Mol. Med.** 52:337–342, 1977.

64. MacDougall, J.D., Elder, G.C.B., Sale, D.G., Moroz, J.R., and Sutton, J.R.: Effects of strength training and immobilization on human muscle fibers. **Eur. J. Appl. Physiol.** 43:25–34, 1980.
65. Booth, F.W.: Time course of muscular atrophy during immobilization of hindlimbs in rats. **J. Appl. Physiol.** 43:656–661, 1977.
66. Booth, F.W., and Seider, M.J.: Early change in skeletal muscle protein synthesis after limb immobilization of rats. **J. Appl. Physiol.** 47:974–977, 1979.
67. Wilmore, J.H., Tischler, M.E., Percy, E.C., Rotkis, T.C., Roby, F.B., Stanforth, P.R., Constable, S.H., Buono, M.J., Maxwell, B.D., and Sather, T.M.: Alterations in cardiovascular, metabolic and muscle function consequent to 17 days of single-leg casting (abstr.). **Int. J. Sports Med.** 4:142, 1983.
68. Graves, J.E., Pollock, M.L., Leggett, S.H., Braith, R.W., Carpenter, D.M., and Bishop, L.E.: Effect of reduced training frequency on muscular strength. **Int. J. Sports Med.** In press, 1989.
69. Laubach, L.L.: Comparative muscular strength of men and women: a review of the literature. **Aviat. Space Environ. Med.** 47:534–542, 1976.
70. Hosler, W.W., and Morrow, J.R.: Arm and leg strength compared between young women and men after allowing for differences in body size and composition. **Ergonomics** 25:309–313, 1982.
71. Brown, C.H., and Wilmore, J.H.: The effects of maximal resistance training on the strength and body composition of women athletes. **Med. Sci. Sports** 6:174–177, 1974.
72. Mayhew, J.L., and Gross, P.M.: Body composition changes in young women with high resistance weight training. **Res. Q.** 45:433–440, 1974.
73. Fleck, S.J., and Kraemer, W.J.: **Designing Resistance Training Programs.** Champaign, IL, Human Kinetics Books, 1987.
74. Kraemer, W.J., Deschenes, M.R., and Fleck, S.J.: Physiological adaptations to resistance exercise: implications for athletic conditioning. **Sports Med.** 6:246–256, 1988.
75. Pollock, M.L., Leggett, S.H., Graves, J.E., Jones, A., Fulton, M., and Cirulli, J.: Effect of resistance training on lumbar extension strength. **Am. J. Sports Med.** in press, 1990.
76. Fox, E.L., and Mathews, D.K.: **The Physiological Basis of Physical Education and Athletics**, 3rd Ed. Philadelphia, W.B. Saunders College Publishing, 1981.
77. deVries, H.A.: Quantitative electromyographic investigation of the spasm theory of muscle pain. **Am. J. Phys. Med.** 45:119–134, 1966.
78. Abraham, W.M.: Factors in delayed muscle soreness. **Med. Sci. Sports** 9:11–20, 1977.
79. Abraham, W.M.: Exercise-induced muscle soreness. **Phys. Sportsmed.** 7:57–60, 1979.
80. Hough, T.: Ergographic studies in muscular soreness. **Am. J. Physiol.** 7:76–92, 1902.
81. Talag, T.S.: Residual muscular soreness as influenced by concentric, eccentric and static contractions. **Res. Q.** 44:458–469, 1973.
82. Assmussen, E.: Observations on experimental muscle soreness. **Acta Rheumatol. Scand.** 1:19–116, 1956.
83. Komi, P.V., and Buskirk, E.R.: The effect of eccentric and concentric muscle activity on tension and electrical activity of human muscle. **Ergonomics** 15:417–434, 1972.
84. Komi, P.V., and Rusko, H.: Quantitative evaluation of mechanical and electrical changes during fatigue loading of eccentric and concentric work. **Scand. J. Rehabil. Med.** (Suppl.) 3:121–126, 1974.
85. Armstrong, R.B.: Mechanisms of exercise-induced delayed-onset muscular soreness: a brief review. **Med. Sci. Sports Exerc.** 6:529–538, 1984.
86. Evans, W.J., Meredith, C.N., Cannon, J.G., Dinarello, C.A., Frontera, W.R., Hughes, V.A., Jones, B.H., and Knuttgen, H.G.: Metabolic changes following

eccentric exercise in trained and untrained men. **J. Appl. Physiol.** 61:1864–1868, 1986.

87. Friden, J., Sfakianos, P.N., and Hargens, A.R.: Muscle soreness and intramuscular fluid pressure: comparison between eccentric and concentric load. **J. Appl. Physiol.** 61:2175–2179, 1986.

88. Evans, W.J.: Exercise-induced skeletal muscle damage. **Phys. Sportsmed.** 15:89–100, 1987.

89. McCully, K.K., and Faulkner, J.A.: Characteristics of lengthening contractions associated with injury to skeletal muscle fibers. **J. Appl. Physiol.** 61:293–299, 1986.

90. Johns, R.J., and Wright, V.: Relative importance of various tissues in joint stiffness. **J. Appl. Physiol.** 17:824–828, 1962.

91. Hettinger, T., and Muller, E.A.: Muskelleistung und muskel training. **Arbeitsphysiol.** 15:111–126, 1953.

92. Hettinger, T.: **Physiology of Strength.** Springfield, IL: Charles C. Thomas, 1961.

93. Clarke, D.H.: Adaptations in strength and muscular endurance resulting from exercise. **Exerc. Sport Sci. Rev.** 1:73–102, 1973.

94. DeLorme, T.L.: Restoration of muscle power by heavy resistance exercise. **J. Bone Joint Surg.** 27:645–667, 1945.

95. DeLorme, T.L., and Watkins, A.L.: Technics of progressive resistance exercise. **Arch. Phys. Med.** 29:263–273, 1948.

96. Zinovieff, A.N.: Heavy resistance exercises: the Oxford technique. **Br. J. Phys. Med.** 14:129–132, 1951.

97. Clarke, H.H.: Development of muscular strength and endurance. **Phys. Fitness Res. Digest** Series 4, No. 1, January 1974.

98. Perrine, J.J.: Isokinetic exercise and the mechanical energy potentials of muscle. **J. Health Phys. Educ. Rec.** 39:40–44, 1968.

99. Wilt, F.: Plyometrics: what it is—how it works. **Athlet. J.** 55:89–90, 1975.

100. Verkhoshanski, Y.: Perspectives in the improvement of speed-strength preparation of jumpers. **Track and Field** 9:11–12, 1966.

101. Clarke, H.H.: Strength development and motor-sports improvement. **Phys. Fitness Res. Digest** Series 4, No. 4, October 1974.

102. Sale, D., and MacDougall, D.: Specificity in strength training: a review for the coach and athlete. **Science Periodical on Research and Technology in Sport.** Ottawa, The Coaching Association of Canada, March 1981.

103. Thorstensson, A., Karlsson, J., Viitasalo, J.T., Luhtanen, P., and Komi, P.V.: Effect of strength training on EMG of human skeletal muscle. **Acta Physiol. Scand.** 94:313–318, 1975.

104. Graves, J.E., Pollock, M.L., Jones, A.E., Colvin, A.B., and Leggett, S.H.: Specificity of limited range of motion variable resistance training. **Med. Sci. Sports Exerc.** 21:84–89, 1989.

105. McLario, D.J.: **The Contribution of Force and Velocity in the Development of Peak Power Output.** M.S. Thesis. Tucson, University of Arizona, 1981.

106. Morgan, R.E., and Adamson, G.T.: **Circuit Weight Training.** London, G. Bell and Sons, 1961.

107. Allen, T.E., Byrd, R.J., and Smith, D.P.: Hemodynamic consequences of circuit weight training. **Res. Q.** 47:299–306, 1976.

108. Gettman, L.R., and Pollock, M.L.: Circuit weight training: a critical review of its physiological benefits. **Phys. Sportsmed.** 9:44–60, 1981.

109. Kelemen, M.H., Stewart, K.J., Gillilan, R.E., Ewart, C.K., Valenti, S.A., Manley, J.D., and Kelemen, M.D.: Circuit weight training in cardiac patients. **J. Am. Coll. Cardiol.** 7:38–42, 1986.

110. Stewart, K.J., Mason, M., and Kelemen, M.H.: Three-year participation in circuit weight training improves muscular strength and self-efficacy in cardiac patients. **J. Cardiopulmonary Rehabil.** 8:292–296, 1988.

111. Harris, K.A., and Holly, R.G.: Physiological response to circuit weight training

in borderline hypertensive subjects. **Med. Sci. Sports Exerc.** 19:246–252, 1987.

112. Moore, M.A., and Hutton, R.S.: Electromyographic investigation of muscle stretching techniques. **Med. Sci. Sports Exerc.** 12:322–329, 1980.

113. Etnyre, B.R., and Lee, E.J.: Comments on proprioceptive neuromuscular facilitation stretching techniques. **Res. Q. Exerc. Sport** 58:184–188, 1987.

114. Sapega, A.A., Quendenfeld, T.C., Moyer, R.A., and Butler, R.A.: Biophysical factors in range-of-motion exercise. **Phys. Sportsmed.** 9:57–65, 1981.

115. Vogel, J.A.: Introduction to the symposium: physiological responses and adaptations to resistance exercise. **Med. Sci. Sports Exerc.** 20:S131, 1988.

116. Fleck, S.J., and Kraemer, W.J.: Resistance training: basic principles (part 1 of 4). **Phys. Sportsmed.** 16:160–171, 1988.

117. Fleck, S.J., and Kraemer, W.J.: Resistance training: physiological responses and adaptations (part 2 of 4). **Phys. Sportsmed.** 16:108–124, 1988.

118. Fleck, S.J., and Kraemer, W.J.: Resistance training: physiological responses and adaptations (part 3 of 4). **Phys. Sportsmed.** 16:63–76, 1988.

119. Kraemer, W.J., and Fleck, S.J.: Resistance training: exercise prescription (part 4 of 4). **Phys. Sportsmed.** 16:69–81, 1988.

PRESCRIPTION FOR PROGRAMS OF PREVENTION AND REHABILITATION

It was not too many years ago that people electing to start an exercise program would go to their local YW/YMCA or health/fitness club and be placed in a general class with 20 to 30 other people who had similar goals. Each participant would receive the same exercise program without consideration of the fact that people differ greatly in their health status, abilities, capacities, and interests. The era of a single group program to fit people of all ages and capacities has come and gone. The exercise sciences have progressed to the point where individualized exercise programs can be prescribed and tailored to the likes, needs, capacity, and health status of the individual participant.

When prescribing exercise, it is important to know the family history and medical status of the participant, in addition to his or her fitness status. Once this has been determined, it is then possible to prescribe an exercise program on the basis of the type or mode of activity to be used; the frequency, duration, and intensity of participation; and the specific goals of the participant. At the same time, the participant can be educated in areas including the following: consumer tips when purchasing shoes and clothing; how best to avoid injury, particularly overuse injuries; how to prepare for exercising under unique environmental conditions; how to adapt exercise programs for the middle-aged and elderly participant; and how to stay motivated to continue the prescribed exercise program.

The final four chapters of this book address the areas of medical screening and evaluation, the prescription of exercise for healthy and diseased populations, and special considerations when prescribing exercise. These chapters provide the scientific foundation for medical screening, physiological assessment, exercise prescription, and general theory on the safe and efficacious use of exercise in disease prevention and rehabilitation.

6

MEDICAL SCREENING AND EVALUATION PROCEDURES

PRELIMINARY CONSIDERATIONS

This chapter focuses on the medical screening and evaluation procedures necessary for participants to enter an exercise program safely. These procedures should be helpful in giving participants advice about their health and behavior as related to physical fitness and risk for the development of coronary artery disease (CAD), an exercise prescription, and monitoring the progress of their health maintenance and exercise program. Information and test procedures usually include a medical history, CAD risk factor analysis, and physical fitness assessment. The physical fitness assessment includes test items in the following areas: cardiorespiratory (functional capacity), body composition, muscular strength and endurance, and flexibility. The diagnosis and medical treatment of CAD is discussed in detail in other texts;[1, 2] thus, this chapter emphasizes the use of tests as they relate to participants entering a health maintenance and rehabilitation exercise program.

Preliminary information should include such items as a physical examination or consultation with the family physician, or both; completion of a medical history questionnaire and its discussion; explanation and signing of an informed consent form; and, if possible, a symptom-limited graded exercise test (SL-GXT). The SL-GXT is used to determine functional capacity and to monitor the electrocardiogram (ECG) and blood pressure (BP) as well as other signs of exercise intolerance.

Medical History Questionnaire

The medical history form should include a record of personal and family history of CAD and the associated risk factors, present medication and treatment, eating habits and diet analysis, smoking history, and current physical activity pattern. In addition, any other pertinent medical problems and physical disabilities should be listed. Thus, the information obtained in the preliminary evaluation should help to identify in advance the person who might be classified at high risk for CAD and thus benefit from testing and program participation. Data from Bruce and associates[3] show the importance of a medical history in differentiating high- and low-risk patients. As is discussed later in this chapter, knowledge of risk for CAD has importance in the diagnostic and prognostic interpretation of the exercise test. See Appendix A, Figure A–1, for an example of a medical history questionnaire. For mass screening to determine who needs a more extensive medical follow-up before entering an exercise program, a less complex, briefer medical history, and physical readiness questionnaire, the physical activity readiness questionnaire (PAR-Q, see Appendix A, Figure A–2) has been used successfully and adopted by the Canadian government.[4-6]

Informed Consent

The informed consent form should provide the participant with an adequate explanation and understanding of the tests and program and the potential risk and discomforts that may be involved. In this way, an individual should know exactly what is involved before testing and participating in an exercise program.[7, 8] All testing information should be held in strict confidence and not be released to anyone without permission. In addition, participants should not be coerced or inadequately advised with the objective of obtaining a better performance on a test or increasing adherence to a program. Such procedures are unethical, violate human rights, and are against policy established by the federal government and most professional organizations.[7-10] If the consent form is being used for research purposes, a statement concerning withdrawal without prejudice of future care is appropriate. See Appendix A, Figures A–3 and A–4, for examples of informed consent forms for exercise testing and exercise training. In addition, refer to publications provided by the American College of Sports Medicine (ACSM),[10] the American Heart Association,[11] and others.[12-16] The informed consent form shown in Appendix A, Figure A–3, is used when the main purpose of the GXT is diagnostic, and the form in Figure A–4 is used for the purpose of entering an exercise program. An example of a form used for an outpatient cardiac rehabilitation program is shown in Appendix B, Figure B–7. In general, the informed consent form should contain certain basic components but must be individualized for each laboratory or program. For example, the Canadian Association of Sport Sciences[13] has developed a special consent form for testing athletes, and the YMCA of America[16] has developed special forms for fitness testing and exercise participation.

Herbert and Herbert[8] have listed ten common potential areas for liability that may be associated with an exercise program:

1. Failure to monitor an exercise test properly and/or to stop an exercise test in the application of competent professional judgement

2. Failure to evaluate the participant's physical capabilities or impairments competently, factors that would proscribe or limit certain types of exercise

3. Failure to prescribe a safe exercise intensity in terms of cardiovascular, metabolic, and musculoskeletal demands

4. Failure to instruct participants adequately as to safe performance of the recommended physical activities or as to the proper use of exercise equipment

5. Failure to supervise properly the participant's exercise during program sessions or to advise individuals regarding any restrictions or modifications that should be imposed in performing conditioning activities during unsupervised periods

6. Failure to assign specific participants to an exercise setting with a level of physiologic monitoring, supervision, and emergency medical support commensurate with their health status

7. Failure to perform or render performance in a negligent manner in a variety of other situations[7]

8. Rendition of advice to a participant that is later construed to represent diagnosis of a medical condition or is deemed tantamount to medical prescription to relieve a disease condition and that subsequently and/or proximately causes injury and/or deterioration of health and/or death

9. Failure to refer a participant to a physician or other appropriately licensed professional in response to the appearance of signs or symptoms suggestive of health problems requiring medical or other professional attention

10. Failure to maintain proper and confidential records documenting the informed consent process, the adequacy of participant instructions with regard to performance of program activities, and the adequacy of their physical responses to physical activity regimens.[7]

Most of the allegations against professionals are in the realm of negligence or malpractice. How many of the previous factors, e.g., items 5 and 6, affect cardiac rehabilitation programs in which patients are given home programs or are recommended to participate in unsupervised exercise, soon after myocardial infarction (MI) or coronary artery bypass graft (CABG) surgery, is not known. The authors presume that as long as physicians and health professionals are following standard accepted procedures for GXT and exercise prescriptions, litigation will be minimal.

Medical Evaluation and Supervision

Is it important to have a physical examination and undergo tests before starting an exercise program? Ideally, the answer is yes, although there should be some flexibility in the requirements, depending upon the participant's age, health status, family history, and current fitness level. It is desirable for participants to have a complete physical examination, including a 12-lead resting and exercise ECG before their physical fitness evaluation. As mentioned earlier, the more information known about a participant before testing and training, the safer and more accurate is the exercise prescription. In reality, the ideal situation is not always practical or medically indicated. The risk for a major coronary event for young, low-risk persons is extremely low, and the predictive value of an SL-GXT for the diagnosis of CAD in a young asymptomatic population is limited.[10] See the section later in this chapter on the safety of the GXT and see Chapter 8 for more details on the risk of major coronary events in cardiac and noncardiac patients involved in exercise training programs. The impracticality and considerable cost to the medical system or individual for doing mass medical testing (GXT) have been discussed by Shephard.[17] Thus, it does not appear to be realistic to recommend comprehensive medical evaluations for the total population. Mass nonmedical fitness evaluations have been successfully used by the YMCA of America and in Canada for years.[13, 16–18]

If a GXT is for a diagnostic purpose or is performed on persons with known CAD or who are at high risk for such disease, direct medical supervision is necessary. Nondiagnostic tests on apparently healthy individuals can be safely administered without direct physician supervision. Examples of nondiagnostic tests are the physical fitness test used and administered by the YMCA[16] or an SL-GXT given to athletes in a university setting for the purpose of determining their maximal oxygen uptake ($\dot{V}O_2$max). For years, thousands of assessments of cardiorespiratory fitness for the purpose of entering an exercise program have been safely administered by allied health (nonphysician) personnel.

What is meant by low- and high-risk individuals? The term "at risk" is usually associated with a person's risk for having CAD. A low-risk person might be asymptomatic (no chest discomfort, shortness of breath, and so on), with no previous history of CAD and no known primary risk factors for CAD (see Chapter 1 for CAD risk factors). Therefore, for persons who are symptomatic for CAD or who have known significant risk factors for CAD, a medical examination, including a resting and exercise ECG, is strongly recommended.

Is age alone a criterion for having a medical examination and diagnostic GXT before entering an exercise program? There is no set answer to this question. When the guidelines for exercise testing and exercise prescription were first developed by the ACSM (1976) there was a wide variety of opinion: some recommended that everyone (young and old) should have a GXT, and some favored a minimal age of 45 to 50 years. Most felt that a GXT was important or necessary for men between 30 and 45 years of age. The original agreed-upon recommendation was age 35. Now the recommendation is age 45 for healthy individuals.[10] A publication by the National Heart, Lung, and Blood Institute recommends that asymptomatic, low risk individuals over 60 years of age should see their doctor before starting an exercise program.[19] The recent popular application of the old theory developed by Bayes[20, 21] suggests that the new recommendation by the ACSM is about right. The ability of a GXT to predict future events in an asymptomatic population is not significant until after age 40 for men and 50 for women.[20, 21] In summary, in the absence of symptoms and primary risk factors for CAD, age in itself does not seem to be a strong indicator for requiring a physical examination or diagnostic GXT before age 40 to 45 for men and 50 to 55 for women. This summary statement is related to persons starting an exercise program. The need for a physical examination may be recommended sooner, e.g., individuals at risk for cancer or postmenopausal women concerned about osteoporosis.

Risk Factor Analysis

Several risk factor profile charts are available for use. The problem with most charts is their lack of validity; that is, they have been developed on the basis that risk factors for CAD are important predictors but include arbitrarily determined cut-off points (high and low) and weighting factors (relative strength of predictor). The general cardiovascular risk profile developed from the Framingham Study[22, 23] is one of the few validated profiles. It uses age, sex, serum cholesterol level, cigarette smoking, systolic BP, glucose intolerance, and left ventricular hypertrophy by ECG criteria for calculating risk. From these data, a Coronary Risk Handbook was published by the American Heart Association.[24]

Does this mean that nonvalidated risk factor profile charts should not be used? No, not necessarily. As mentioned in Chapter 1, many significant risk factors have been identified, and an increased number of risk factors dramatically increases the risk for premature manifestations of CAD.[23] As teaching tools for identifying risk factors and planning for their modification, many of these profiles can be useful. Problems lie in their application to the prediction of future events.

How accurately can future events be predicted from coronary risk profiles? The Framingham Study cardiovascular risk profile was developed from 5,209 men and women who had clinical evaluations every 2 years and continuous surveillance for morbidity and mortality.[22] The 10 percent of persons (ninetieth percentile) identified as at the highest risk accounted for 20 percent of the 8-year incidence of CAD and 33 percent of the 8-year incidence of atherothrombotic brain infarction, hypertensive heart disease, and intermittent claudication. These data show that the profile is significant in predicting high and low risk persons but is less than perfect. Thus, it is suggested that risk factor analyses (profiles) be used with caution and their predictability not be overstated.

Table 6–1 is a risk factor profile chart recommended for use with participants entering a health maintenance and exercise program. In addition, see Appendix A, Tables A–1 to A–12, for age- and sex-adjusted norms for many of these variables. For variables listed in Table 6–1, the relative risk scale has not been validated but is estimated from published data. Additional years of inquiry will be necessary before more definite results can be presented. As mentioned earlier, the chart should be used only for educational and descriptive purposes. In interpreting the risk factor profile for others, one should tell people that being at high risk in more than one factor greatly increases their chance of developing CAD. For example, the chances of developing CAD jumps from onefold to nearly fourfold when a person proceeds from having one to three primary risk factors.[22–24]

For the purpose of rating potential risk, whether a patient has primary or secondary risk factors is important. As mentioned in Chapter 1, cigarette smoking, hypercholesterolemia, and hypertension are the three primary risk factors for the development of CAD. Having one primary risk factor places a person at moderate risk,

Table 6–1. Risk of Developing Heart Disease

Risk Factor	Very Low	Low	Moderate	High	Very High
Relative Level of Risk					
Blood Pressure (mmHg)					
Systolic	< 110	120	130–140	150–160	> 170
Diastolic	< 70	76	82–88	94–100	> 106
Cigarettes (per day)	Never or none in 1 yr	5	10–20	30–40	> 50
Cholesterol (mg/dl)	< 180	< 200	220–240	260–280	> 300
Cholesterol ÷ HDL (mg/dl)	< 3.0	< 4.0	< 4.5	> 5.2	> 7.0
Triglycerides (mg/dl)	< 50	< 100	130	200	> 300
Glucose (mg/dl)	< 80	90	100–110	120–130	> 140
Body Fat (%)					
Men	12	16	25	30	> 35
Women	16	20	30	35	> 40
Body Mass Index*	< 25	25–30	30–40	> 40	
Stress-Tension	Never	Almost never	Occasional	Frequent	Nearly constant
Physical Activity (min/ wk)					
Above 6 kcal/min (5 METs)† or Above 60% HRmax	240	180–120	100	80–60	< 30
Reserve	120	90	30	0	0
ECG Abnormality (S-T–depression [mV])‡	0	0	0.05	0.10	0.20
Family History of Premature Heart Attack (blood relative)§	0	0	1	2	3+
Age	< 30	40	50	60	> 70

HDL = high-density lipoprotein; HRmax = maximal heart rate.

*Body Mass Index = weight (kg)/height^2 (m). Risk information from Bray, G. A.: Obesity and the heart. **Mod. Concepts Cardiovasc. Dis.** 56:67–71, 1987.

†A MET is equal to the oxygen cost at rest. One MET is generally equal to 3.5 ml • kg^{-1} • min^{-1} of oxygen uptake or 1.2 kcal/min.

‡Other ECG abnormalities are also potentially dangerous and are not listed here.

§Premature heart attack refers to persons younger than 60 years of age.

(Adapted with permission from Pollock, M. L., Wilmore, J. H., and Fox, S. M.: **Health and Fitness Through Physical Activity.** New York, John Wiley and Sons, 1978.)

and two to three factors mean high risk. Having one or two secondary factors puts one in a low to moderate risk category, and having three to four factors or more puts one in the moderate- and high-risk categories, respectively.

Percentile norms and an estimated health risk by age (15 to 69 years) and gender are also available for the waist-to-hip ratio.[6] These tables show that a ratio above 1.0 for men and 0.80 for women puts one at a higher health risk.

Although most people with risk factors can be safely evaluated and started on an exercise program, under certain conditions it might be recommended that individuals not exercise. Conditions contraindicating exercise include congestive heart failure, acute MI, acute infectious diseases, severe valvular heart disease, dangerous dysrhythmias, severe angina pectoris with and without effort, and active myocarditis. Chapter 8 lists absolute and relative contraindications to exercise that can also be used for GXT. It also names other medical conditions that are considered of a less serious nature but still require special precautions during exercise testing and training.

PHYSICAL FITNESS EVALUATION

Thus far, we have discussed the desirability of having certain preliminary information and a medical examination before entering an exercise program. The ACSM has recommended a minimal physical examination and set of laboratory tests as part of the medical evaluation.[10] In addition to medical screening, a thorough physical fitness evaluation is also recommended. Although there is some duplication in classifying tests, the main difference between medical screening tests and physical fitness tests are as follows: (1) medical tests classify a person's status relative to health and disease and can provide an estimation of risk of developing disease, and (2) physical fitness evaluations classify a person relative to his or her status of fitness. The results from both the medical and the fitness tests are used as a basis for an exercise prescription and as a baseline for future comparison. Like the medical examination, there can be some flexibility in the fitness testing program, depending upon individual health status, age, current fitness, and activity level, as well as the presence of CAD and other risks. Table 6–2 lists the major categories of fitness and the test items that will be discussed. Although the physical fitness evaluation can be thought of in broader terms, we feel that these categories and test items are sufficient for the basic needs of the adult population entering an exercise program.

Table 6–2. Recommended Testing Program for Adults

Fitness Category	Plan A*	Plan B†	Plan C‡
Cardiorespiratory	Heart rate, blood pressure, ECG	Same as Plan A	Heart rate, blood pressure
Rest	Symptom-limited GXT with heart rate, blood pressure, and ECG monitoring and actual assessment of aerobic capacity	Symptom-limited GXT with heart rate, blood pressure, and ECG monitoring (aerobic capacity estimated)	Submaximal test without ECG and blood pressure monitoring, and maximal field-type tests (aerobic capacity estimated)
Exercise			
Body Composition	Percent fat by underwater weighing or equivalent (should include determination of residual volume), anthropometry (skinfold and girth measures, height, and weight)	Percent fat by skinfold and/or girth measures, height, and weight	Same as Plan B
	Determine ideal/goal weight	Same as Plan A	Same as Plan A
Blood Measures	Serum cholesterol, triglycerides, glucose, high-density lipoprotein (HDL-C)	Serum cholesterol, triglycerides, and glucose	Serum cholesterol
Strength§	One-repetition maximal bench press or multiple repetitions with fixed weight	Same as Plan A	Same as Plan A
Muscular endurance§	All-out push-ups, bent-leg sit-ups for 1 minute	Same as Plan A	Same as Plan A
Flexibility	Sit and reach	Same as Plan A	Same as Plan A

*Most preferred plan of testing physical fitness and risk factors for coronary heart disease.

†Next most preferred plan of testing.

‡Least preferred plan of testing, and cardiorespiratory tests not used for diagnostic purposes.

§May not be appropriate for hypertensive and high-risk individuals.

(Adapted with permission from Pollock, M. L., Wilmore, J. H., and Fox, S. M.: **Health and Fitness Through Physical Activity.** New York, John Wiley and Sons, 1978.)

With the knowledge that the needs of patients and nonpatients often differ and that the amount of equipment and of technical and medical expertise varies with laboratories, three plans for testing are suggested. The test items listed in Table 6–2 become less complex and expensive from Plan A to Plan C. In some cases, the level of accuracy and diagnostic capability of the tests are also less between plans. For example, exercise tests listed under Plan C, cardiorespiratory, should not be used as diagnostic tests. The maximal field type of test, which includes a one- to two-mile run, is not recommended for patients with CAD or at high risk for CAD or for those without recent jogging-running experience. A newly developed one-mile walking test is available and recommended for persons over 40 years of age and who are unaccustomed to vigorous exercise.[25] Medical advisors and program directors, as well as the participants, should take the cost, risk, and feasibility aspects of testing into consideration before setting up a test battery. Except for the blood sample measures, each aspect of testing listed in Table 6–2 is discussed in the following sections.

Special Consideration in the Selection of Tests and Personnel

Often the type of test battery administered to participants depends on four major factors: time, expense, qualifications of personnel, and the population to be tested. If large numbers of individuals have to be tested in a short time, the test items may be limited to a less sophisticated test battery. If high-risk patients are involved, the SL-GXT with ECG and BP monitoring should be used.

With low-risk sedentary persons younger than 45 years of age a physician may not be required to be present for the test, whereas with high-risk individuals, a physician should be present during exercise testing.[10] Although field tests for determination of cardiorespiratory fitness, e.g., a one- to two-mile run, should not be attempted in these same groups, they are acceptable for use with young persons or middle-aged individuals who have been carefully screened and have had recent experience in jogging or running. The American Heart Association's Committee on Exercise[26] states that:

> **Emergency equipment and qualified personnel should be available for exercise testing of all patients. Patients with known or suspected heart disease or dysfunction should not be tested without a qualified physician at the site or in the immediate area (within 30 seconds) in order to provide life saving emergency care.**

They also feel that for nondiagnostic tests and, in particular, tests on younger individuals and persons without known CAD and risk factors for CAD, direct physician presence is not considered necessary provided the health care personnel directing the tests are trained to the satisfaction of the responsible physician in cardiopulmonary resuscitation and emergency cardiac care.

The expense often dictates the kind of equipment that will be available for testing. If funds are limited, the most important pieces of equipment for GXT would be an ergometer, ECG recorder, and BP apparatus. For diagnostic testing, the availability of emergency supplies and equipment (crash cart, defibrillator) is mandatory. Most new ECG GXT systems have a built-in or an attachable oscilloscope with a cardiotachometer. The oscilloscope allows the tester to observe the ECG at all times, and the cardiotachometer provides an instant visual readout of heart rate (HR). Multiple-channel recorders have become the standard for diagnostic ECG evaluation, with many having special computers with averaging, storing, and arrhythmia-detection capabilities.

As mentioned in earlier chapters, $\dot{V}O_2max$ is considered one of the best measures of cardiorespiratory fitness. If so, why has not anything been mentioned about the purchase of equipment to be used for this procedure? In general, $\dot{V}O_2max$ can be estimated accurately from performance time on a treadmill, cycle ergometer, or field tests (running, walking, or stair climbing); thus actual measurement may not be necessary (Table 6–3, Figure 6–1).[6, 10, 26–31] Although this is true, methodological problems have been shown potentially to cause gross errors in estimation.[30–33] More details concerning the issue of predicting $\dot{V}O_2max$ rather than its actual measurement are be discussed in more detail later in this chapter. Other equipment, e.g., skinfold fat calipers, hydrostatic weighing tanks, and so on, is discussed later.

Having the right personnel available for various phases of a physical fitness program is important. Although the physician and the program director have overall control of the program, they must have qualified exercise leaders (specialists, fitness instructors) and laboratory technicians to help them conduct the program. Exercise leaders should have a background in functional anatomy, exercise physiology, behavioral psychology and group dynamics, emergency procedures, and exercise prescription. The laboratory technician should have expertise in the mechanics of individual test procedures, screening a participant before exercise testing, administration of tests, emergency procedures, and data analysis. Programs for training personnel for such positions are becoming readily available in many universities.[34] A certification program

Table 6–3. Estimation of Maximal Oxygen Uptake and METs* for Various Protocols and Fitness Classifications for Exercise Prescription for Different Levels of Cardiorespiratory Fitness

Fitness Classification	Maximum O₂ Uptake ml/kg⁻¹/min⁻¹	METs	Treadmill Protocols					Åstrand (mph)	1.5-Mile Run (min:sec)
			Bruce†	Ellestad†	Balke†‡ (3.3 mph)	Balke†§ (3.0 mph)	Naughton†‖		
1	7	2	—	—	—	—	2:07	—	—
	10.5	3	—	—	1:00	3:00	4:17	—	—
	14	4	2:30	2:00	2:00	4:00	6:28	—	—
2	17.5	5	4:00	3:00	3:00	7:30	8:38	—	—
	21.0	6	6:00	4:45	6:00	10:30	10:49	—	—
	24.5	7	7:20	5:00	8:00	13:30	12:59	—	—
3	28.0	8	8:20	5:45	9:45	17:00	15:10	5.00	18:45
	31.5	9	9:15	6:40	12:00	19:30	17:20	5.25	16:30
	35.0	10	10:10	7:30	14:30	22:00	19:30	5.50	15:00
4	38.5	11	11:00	8:20	17:00	24:00	21:40	5.75	13:00
	42.0	12	12:00	9:10	19:00	27:00	23:51	6.25	12:00
5	45.5	13	12:45	10:15	21:30	30:00	26:01	6.50	11:00
	49.0	14	13:40	11:15	24:15	33:00	28:12	7.00	10:00
6	52.5	15	14:30	—	26:15	36:00	30:22	7.50	9:30
	56.0	16	15:15	—	27:45	—	32:33	8.00	9:00
7	59.5	17	16:10	—	29:00	—	—	8.50	8:15
	63.0	18	17:00	—	30:00	—	—	9.00	7:45
	66.5	19	18:00	—	31:15	—	—	9.25	7:15
8	70.0	20	19:20	—	32:00	—	—	9.75	6:52
	73.5	21	21:00	—	33:45	—	—	10.50	6:30
	77.0	22	22:30	—	35:45	—	—	11.00	6:10

*MET refers to metabolic equivalent above the resting metabolic level. Value at rest is approximately 3.5 ml · kg⁻¹ · min⁻¹.

†Data expressed in minutes and seconds of test protocol (duration) completed.

‡Balke protocol, 3.3 mph, at 1% grade increase in work level per minute (Fig. 6–2).

§Balke protocol, 3.0 mph, at 2.5% grade increase in work level every 3 minutes.

‖Naughton protocol, modified to use 2-minute rather than 3-minute stages.

(Adapted with permission from Pollock, M. L., Wilmore, J. H., and Fox, S. M.: **Health and Fitness Through Physical Activity.** New York, John Wiley and Sons, 1978.)

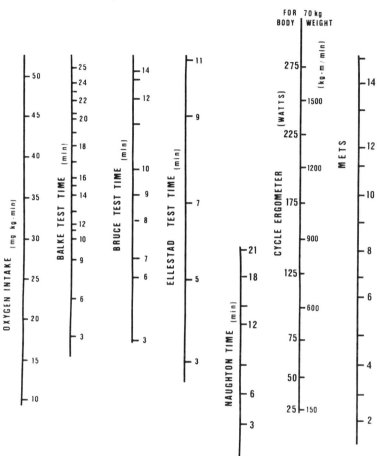

Figure 6–1. Exercise intensity equivalents can be estimated by drawing a horizontal line from the time on a given treadmill or cycle ergometer protocol to oxygen uptake (on the left) or MET level (on the right). (Modified from Pollock, M. L., et al.: A comparative analysis of four protocols for maximal treadmill stress testing. **Am. Heart J.** 92:39–46, 1976. Published with permission from ACSM: **Guidelines for Exercise Testing and Exercise Prescription,** 3rd Ed. Philadelphia, Lea & Febiger, 1986.)

for exercise program directors, health fitness directors, exercise specialists, health fitness instructors, and exercise test technologists is now available through the auspices of the ACSM.[10] The ACSM describes the competencies required for each level or category of certification:

> **The exercise test technologist must demonstrate competence in exercise testing of various individuals in states of illness and health; the health fitness instructor must demonstrate competence in exercise testing, designing and executing an exercise program, leading exercise, and organizing and operating fitness facilities for healthy individuals or those with controlled diseases; the exercise specialist, in addition to the competencies expected of the exercise test technologist and health fitness instructor, must demonstrate competency in implementing exercise prescriptions and leading exercise for individuals with known cardiovascular, pulmonary, or metabolic disease; the health fitness director, in addition to the competencies expected of a health fitness instructor, must demonstrate competence in preventive program administration, supervising staff, and program evaluation. The exercise program director, in addition to the competencies expected of the exercise test technologist, health fitness instructor, exercise specialist, and health fitness director, must demonstrate competence in administering preventive and rehabilitative programs, designing and implementing exercise programs, educating staff and community, and designing and conducting research.[10]**

For more details on these certification programs and their respective testing dates and sites write

ACSM, Director of Certification
P.O. Box 1440
401 W. Michigan Street
Indianapolis, IN 46206–1440, USA
(317) 637–9200

Procedure

In general, if the medical history form is filled out at home before the testing session, the testing procedure can be completed in approximately 2 to 3 hours. If possible, a 15- to 30-minute orientation to the laboratory and various procedures may be helpful before the test day. The orientation may relieve apprehensions associated with testing and improve performance on the GXT.[31, 33, 35–37] The orientation should include an explanation of all tests, familiarization with laboratory facilities, and, if possible, practice in treadmill walking (or the use of other ergometers) and the use of head gear (mouthpiece) and other equipment used in determining aerobic capacity.

Precise instructions should be given to the participant before he or she reports to the laboratory. These instructions should include date and time of test; shoe and clothing requirements; and information concerning eating, drinking of alcohol or stimulants (coffee and so forth), taking medications, and prior exercise. If testing is in the morning, avoidance of fluids (except water), smoking, and breakfast is appropriate. Most laboratories require a minimum of 2 to 3 hours of abstention from eating, drinking, and smoking before reporting for testing.[10, 35–37] If serum lipid levels are to be determined, refraining from alcohol consumption and vigorous exercise for 24 hours and having, at minimum, a 12-hour fast is recommended (a 12-hour fast is not necessary for a simple cholesterol screening).[38, 39] Vigorous exercise within 24 hours may also affect serum glucose.[39] Diabetics should be allowed to keep their dietary habits and injections of insulin as regular as possible. Extremes in hydration or dehydration should be avoided, since they can affect endurance performance, body weight, and results from hydrostatic weighing (body composition).[40, 41] The 24-hour history questionnaire shown in Appendix A, Figure A–5, may be helpful for use in standardizing and keeping a record of the participant's condition when reporting to the laboratory.

For standardization purposes, the organization of the testing session is important. The testing session should begin with quiet (resting) tests. Under Plan A, Table 6–2, this includes resting HR, BP, ECG, and blood drawing. Depending on the standardized length of time used for relaxation before determining HR and BP and the time taken for drawing a blood sample, the quiet tests should take approximately 20 to 30 minutes. Before quiet testing, usually a 5 to 15 minute rest period is recommended.

Body composition measures should be administered next. If both anthropometric and underwater weighing measures are taken, allow 30 to 45 minutes for testing. Anthropometric measures take approximately 5 minutes. Body composition measures are followed by the determination of strength, muscular endurance, and flexibility (30 minutes) and then by the GXT (45 minutes). Depending on the population being tested, the GXT may be scheduled on a separate day.

Once the testing has been completed, time should be scheduled to go over test results and give recommendations.

INITIAL EVALUATION

The medical and fitness evaluations are used as a basis for exercise prescription. The results of the initial tests are also used as a baseline for future comparisons. With respect to the latter, tests are excellent motivators for the participants in that they provide objective evidence about their initial status (health and fitness), as well as the progress and benefits attained from a regular exercise program. In contrast, if one is irregular in attendance or not devoting sufficient time and effort to training, testing may give added motivation to improve adherence or change the exercise prescription.

For the first evaluation, many persons are apprehensive and thus may not do as well on some test items. Apprehension will adversely affect most of the resting and submaximal cardiorespiratory tests but has little effect on maximal values. Resting and submaximal HR, BP, and metabolic measures are elevated under these conditions.[33] Many tests are sensitive to time of day and to the effects of eating or smoking before testing.[33, 42] These factors adversely affect resting and submaximal cardiorespiratory tests. Individuals usually improve their performance on a GXT with some practice. If a tester cannot use ideal conditions (fasting, time of day) for testing, then the conditions in which the tests are administered should be noted and standardized for future comparisons.

Heart rate and BP are particularly susceptible to time of day, smoking, apprehension, coffee and other stimulants, food, anxiety, temperature, and similar influences. Therefore, it is particularly important to standardize conditions for resting and submaximal HR tests. Maximal HR, $\dot{V}O_2$max, performance, and other related variables are usually not significantly affected by time of day, moderate amounts of food or drink, apprehension, or anxiety. Most cardiorespiratory tests should allow a minimum of 2 to 3 hours of controlled conditions before testing. For more details on the standardization and interpretation of submaximal and maximal tests, refer to the work of Taylor and colleagues.[33]

FOLLOW-UP EVALUATIONS

How often should follow-up examinations be administered? Unless something unusual is found in one's initial tests or unless a participant is considered at high risk or has had a change in health status, a regular medical examination may not be necessary. There is varied opinion on this subject. Many recommend a physical examination every 2 to 3 years for persons older than 40 years of age and yearly after 50 years of age. Under usual circumstances, a physical fitness test battery should be administered after approximately 3 to 6 months and again after a year of training. Yearly fitness evaluations are recommended after the first year.

Although fitness takes many months to attain, a check at 3 to 6 months is important for evaluating the participant's progress.

With this information, the participant's exercise prescription can be verified and modified as necessary. Not only does the progress check give the physician and program director vital information about how the participant is responding to the program but it also acts as a motivational tool to the participant. Most dropouts occur during the first 10 weeks of training, and many times interest wanes about 10 to 15 weeks after beginning training; therefore, a motivational lift can help at this stage.[43, 44]

RESTING EVALUATION

The resting, or quiet test, will vary between Plans A, B, and C but could include the determination of resting HR, BP, and serum lipid and glucose levels, as well as a standard 12-lead ECG. Standards for HR, BP, and serum cholesterol, triglyceride, and glucose levels, subdivided by age and sex, are shown in Appendix A, Tables A–1 to A–12. A comfortable armchair should be used for determining sitting HR and BP, and a stretcher bed or padded table should be used for the resting ECG. Blood drawing should occur after the HR and BP check, for minor discomfort may produce an "alarm reaction." Also, time of the resting period, subject position (sitting or supine), exercise or alcohol consumption the previous day, fasting or no fasting, and so forth can add to the variability of lipid and glucose measures.[38]

For persons who have a family history of heart disease, are over 40 years of age, or are at a high risk for CAD, a preliminary cardiovascular examination is important. The medical history is reviewed, and the physician listens for specific heart and blood vessel abnormalities (auscultation). This is considered an important part of the physical examination, since many dangerous valve or vessel dysfunctions are found in this way. If the physical fitness evaluation is for nondiagnostic purposes, this part of the examination is usually omitted (nonphysician evaluations).

The HR is usually counted for 15 to 30 seconds, then multiplied appropriately to obtain beats per minute. To help ensure accuracy and stabilization of BP, two to three readings are necessary.[47] For best results in taking blood pressure, do the following (see references 45 to 50):

1. **Take the measurement in a quiet room with a temperature approximately 70 to 74°F (21 to 23°C).**

2. **Have both men and women dressed in a T-shirt or sleeveless blouse (this makes it easier to adjust the pressure cuff properly).**

3. **Have the person sit in a comfortable chair with the arm at midchest level.**

4. **Take the BP from both the left and the right arms (because of arterial obstructions, sometimes the pressure in one arm is different from in the other). In subsequent evaluations, the arm found to have the higher pressure initially should be used.**

5. **Use the proper-sized cuff (a large cuff on a small arm will cause the readings to be lower and vice versa). The three most frequently used cuff sizes are child (13 to 20 cm), adult (17 to 26 cm), and large adult (32 to 42 cm). The measurement shown in parentheses refers to the arm circumference at midpoint. Refer to the American Heart Association Standards booklet for more details on cuff size.**[45]

6. **Take the measure fairly rapidly, and leave the pressure cuff deflated for approximately 30 seconds to a minute between determinations (this allows normal circulation to return to the arm).**

The white coat phenomenon is present in a significant number of patients, that is an apparent artificially high resting BP resulting from the anxiety associated with a physician taking the BP.[50] Thus, before a patient can clearly be classified as hypertense, taking multiple readings on different days with a trained technician is recommended.[45, 47, 49, 50]

The width of the inflatable bladder should be 40 percent of the circumference of the arm on which it is used; the length should be 80 percent of the circumference. The bladder should be applied directly over the compressible artery, approximately 2.5 cm above the antecubital space. With the stethoscope in place, the pressure cuff should be inflated rapidly to approximately 30 mmHg above the point at which the pulse disappears and then deflated at a rate of 2 to 4 mmHg per second. Usually just the systolic and fifth phase diastolic pressures are recorded at rest. During exercise and recovery from exercise, the fifth phase diastolic BP is often heard all the way to zero; thus both fourth and fifth phase should be noted. Sphygmomanometers should be calibrated at least once a year. More detailed information concerning the methods of taking BP and calibration of sphygmomanometers is found in American Heart Association Standards booklets.[45, 46]

The BP ranges shown at the top of page 257 have been recommended by the Joint National Committee on Detection, Evaluation, and Treatment of High Blood Pressure for the classification of BP in adults 18 years of age and older.

Persons with a resting systolic BP more than 180 mmHg or a diastolic BP higher than 100 mmHg may need to be referred to a physician before further testing or training.[48] In these extreme cases, it would be wiser to have persons achieve a reduction in BP (by drugs or dietary control program or both) before letting them begin a training program. If someone is hypertensive, the initial

BP Range (mmHg)	Category
Diastolic	
< 85	Normal blood pressure
85–89	High normal blood pressure
90–104	Mild hypertension
105–114	Moderate hypertension
≥ 115	Severe hypertension
Systolic, When Diastolic Blood Pressure Is < 90	
< 140	Normal blood pressure
140–159	Borderline isolated systolic hypertension
≥ 160	Isolated systolic hypertension

program should be of a low to moderate intensity. The hypertensive person should also avoid heavy static holds or lifting or pushing exercises. These types of exercises have a dramatic effect on elevating the BP.[51–53]

The blood serum measures listed in Table 6–2 are standard procedures and can be determined rather easily and economically by most medical laboratories. The determination of high-density lipoprotein-cholesterol (HDL-C) is the most expensive of the lipid profile analyses. To complete the risk factor profile shown in Table 6–1, the determination of serum cholesterol, triglyceride, HDL-C, and glucose levels is necessary. In general, if the serum cholesterol level is above 300 mg/dl or below 150 mg/dl, the measurement of HDL-C becomes less important. At these levels, the low-density lipoprotein cholesterol fraction of serum cholesterol measure would already be considered clinically high or low, respectively. Standards for serum lipid levels and treatment for hyperlipidemia have been published by the American Heart Association and National Cholesterol Education Program.[54, 55] The national goal is to lower the serum cholesterol of Americans below 200 mg/dl.

Cardiorespiratory Fitness

Maximal oxygen uptake is measured in the laboratory setting and can be directly assessed as part of a diagnostic GXT. Consolazio, Johnson, and Pecora[56] give a detailed description of the principles and methodology involved in the measurement of $\dot{V}O_2$max. More recently, reliable semiautomated and automated systems to measure aerobic capacity have become commercially available.[57, 58] Although the automated systems make it comparatively easy to measure $\dot{V}O_2$max directly, the equipment and supplies needed for its measurement, as well as the added technical assistance required during testing and analysis, add to the expense of the GXT procedure. In addition, regular technical assistance is required to keep equipment calibrated and in good working condition. When research is involved and when evaluating pulmonary patients, the actual measurement of $\dot{V}O_2$max is advisable.[59]

The estimation of $\dot{V}O_2$max can be made with relative accuracy from HR response at submaximal work loads and from performance time or distance on a standardized test protocol. Thus, because of time, expense, and the ease of estimating $\dot{V}O_2$max indirectly, the direct measurement of $\dot{V}O_2$max may not be practical for use in the general clinical setting.

Test retest reliability of the $\dot{V}O_2$max directly measured is r = 0.95 and higher with a standard error of 1 ml $\cdot$ kg^{-1} $\cdot$ min^{-1} (0.3 MET).[31, 32] There is no question that by not actually measuring $\dot{V}O_2$max, large potential errors in its estimation are possible. Methodology problems—e.g., holding onto the handrails during treadmill walking—can cause overestimation of the $\dot{V}O_2$max by as much as 30 percent (1 to 3 METs).[60–63] Average standard errors of estimate range from 2 to 5 percent (r = 0.8 to 0.95, $\pm$ 3 ml $\cdot$ kg^{-1} $\cdot$ min^{-1} or $\pm$ 0.9 METs) for tests listed under Plan B (Table 6–2) and from 5 to 10 percent (r = 0.7 to 0.9, $\pm$ 5 to 6 ml $\cdot$ kg^{-1} $\cdot$ min^{-1} or $\pm$ 1.8 METs) under Plan C.[13, 16, 25, 28, 29, 31, 64–66] The section on test interpretation further discusses errors of estimation and suggestions that generally help decrease them.

In reference to the testing plans suggested in Table 6–2, the protocols shown under Plans A and B are identical, except that $\dot{V}O_2$max is directly measured under Plan A and is estimated from performance under Plan B. Tests under Plan C are not diagnostic tests, but rather are tests to measure functional capacity. Most of the tests listed under Plan C are submaximal tests and use HR and work load to predict $\dot{V}O_2$max.[6, 16, 31] The one- to two-mile run (12-minute run-walk) tests require a maximal effort and are generally used for mass testing in the schools, for police, and in the military.[31, 67–69] More recently, the one-mile walk test has been recommended for use with the sedentary adult population.[25]

When deciding whether to use direct or indirect measurements of $\dot{V}O_2$max, the purpose of the test should be considered as well as the impact the error may have on test interpretation. In general, $\dot{V}O_2$max is used mainly for identifying status of cardiorespiratory fitness and showing serial results; thus, a consistent (under- or over-prediction) 5 to 10 percent error may not be crucial. When procedures are carefully standardized, errors have been shown to be consistent on repeated tests.[31, 70] Thus, results from serial testing, comparing one test with the next, should not be greatly affected.

As is discussed later in this chapter, knowledge of functional capacity can have certain diagnostic implications and is important for designing the initial exercise prescription. Even so, the actual exercise prescription is usually based on HR, on signs and symptoms, or both.

Going to a physician's office or other establishments (universities, YMCAs) to obtain a sophisticated GXT is impractical for many persons. Even so, the diagnostic test should be mandatory for high-risk persons and strongly recommended for sedentary persons who are more than 45 years of age and who are going to participate in moderate- to high-intensity activities. Once the status is determined and the participant begins his or her program, less sophisticated tests can often be used for future evaluations. If one has any difficulty deciding what to do, a physician should be consulted and, if available in the community, an expert in evaluation and fitness. Along with medical centers and clinics, many local YMCAs, Jewish Community Centers, health clubs/wellness centers, and colleges and universities have experts in adult fitness who can give the participant good advice.

TESTING PROTOCOLS

Maximal oxygen uptake is generally estimated from standardized tests administered on a treadmill, cycle ergometer, or steps.[6, 10, 30, 31, 35–37, 71–76] A national survey of 1,400 exercise testing facilities showed that the treadmill was the most used mode of testing (71 percent), followed by the cycle ergometer (17 percent), and steps (12 percent).[77] The cycle ergometer continues to be the testing device of choice in Scandinavia and Europe.[71] Although a more recent survey is not available at this time, the authors feel that the treadmill has become even more popular in North America in the 1980's. Recently, a motorized stair-climbing device has been developed and has shown to be an acceptable mode of conducting a GXT for moderately to highly fit populations.[79]

Of the treadmill protocols, the Bruce (65.5 percent),[29] Balke (9.7 percent),[73] Naughton (6 percent),[78] and Ellestad (3.1 percent)[36] protocols were the most widely used.

Treadmill. As mentioned above, several protocols can be used for diagnostic purposes and for the determination of $\dot{V}O_2$max. Figure 6–2 describes the most commonly used treadmill protocols. The modified Åstrand protocol includes a 5-minute warm-up walk (3.5 mph, 2.5-percent grade for nonathletes and 5-minute jog-run for fit adults or athletes) followed by a continuous, multistage run to exhaustion.[65, 71] The speed of the run is adjusted to exhaust each participant in 7 to 10 minutes; this time period is considered

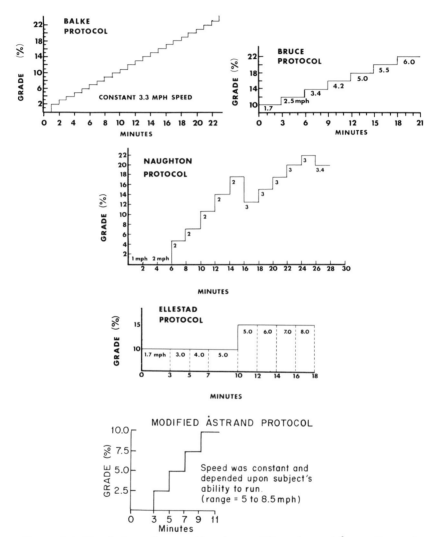

Figure 6–2. The Balke,[74] Bruce,[29] Naughton,[78] Ellestad,[36] and Åstrand[65] treadmill protocols are the most commonly used. Ellestad has modified his testing protocol. The treadmill speed of 5 mph is maintained from minutes 10 to 12 and is increased to 6 mph from minutes 12 to 14, and so on. (Reprinted with permission from Pollock, M. L., Wilmore, J. H., and Fox, S. M.: **Health and Fitness Through Physical Activity.** New York, copyright John Wiley and Sons, 1978; Pollock, M. L., Schmidt, D. H., and Jackson, A. S.: Measurement of cardiorespiratory fitness and body composition in the clinical setting. **Compr. Ther.** 6:12–27, 1980. Published with permission of the Laux Company, Inc., Harvard, MA.)

adequate for maximal physiological adjustments to occur.[71] The proper starting speed for the modified Åstrand test can be estimated from an initial screening test or from knowledge of the participant's current status of fitness. Usually, sedentary middle-aged participants who are starting an exercise program will run at 5 to 6 mph, moderately trained persons at 7 to 8 mph, and elite runners at 10 to 11 mph.[65, 80–82] The other protocols have a built-in warm-up and begin as illustrated in Figure 6–2.

Figure 6–3 illustrates different rates of increase in $\dot{V}O_2$max (METs) with the various protocols but similar maximal values.[65] Few differences among tests are noted with other maximal values, e.g., BP, rate-pressure product (RPP), respiratory exchange ratio (RER), pulmonary ventilation ($\dot{V}_E$), and rating of perceived exertion (RPE). At a submaximal level, the rate of increase differs among tests when results are compared by time of the test (Fig. 6–3). When work loads are standardized among tests (equal MET values), testing protocols vary little at submaximal levels (Fig. 6–4).[66] Some controversy exists concerning testing protocols, in that the Bruce protocol, which has a more abrupt increase in work load between stages of the test, may be more sensitive to picking up ischemic ECG responses than the protocols that have slower incremental increases (Naughton).[83] These findings have not been replicated or

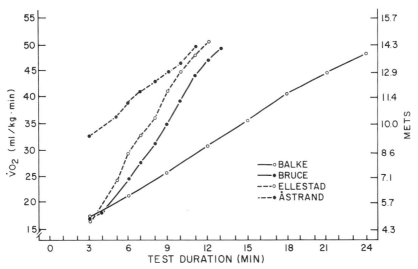

Figure 6–3. Rate of increase in oxygen uptake in four graded exercise test protocols on 51 men, aged 35 to 55 years. Data for women show similar results.[66] (Reprinted with permission from Pollock, M. L., et al.: A comparative analysis of four protocols for maximal treadmill stress testing. **Am. Heart J.** 92:39–46, 1976.)

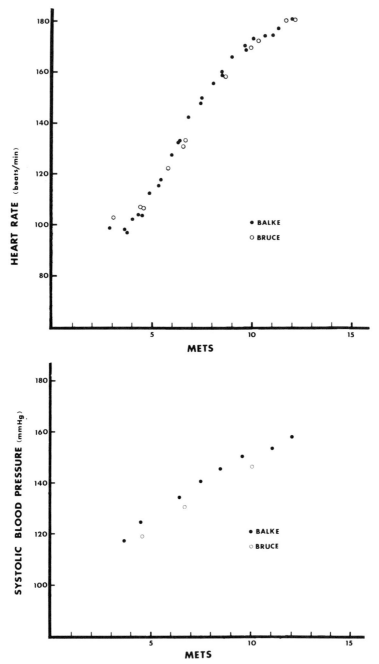

Figure 6-4. Rate of increase in heart rate (upper figure) and systolic blood pressure (lower figure) by MET increments on the Bruce and Balke graded exercise test protocols. (Reprinted with permission from Pollock, M. L., et al.: Comparative analysis of physiologic responses to three different maximal graded exercise test protocols in healthy women. **Am. Heart J.** 103:363–373, 1982.)

validated on a large sample; thus, at this time it is suggested that a variety of protocols can be used, and similar results should be expected.

How can a laboratory make a logical decision about what protocol to use for GXT? Special factors—e.g., population (patient, athlete, young, or old) and available time—should be considered. In general, a continuous, multistage test that starts at a low MET level (2 to 3 METs), has one- to three-minute stages, and increases the work load by no more than 1 to 3 METs per stage is recommended.[10, 11] The test should allow time for a warm-up and general cardiovascular-respiratory adaptation period and enough time and stages to allow for an incremental HR, BP, ECG, and RPE response curve. A test with a minimal time of 6 minutes and no longer than 15 minutes is recommended. A period longer than 15 minutes is generally not necessary to attain the needed physiological and clinical information and may add more discomfort to the patient (because of the mouthpiece, and other factors) and cause subjects to stop prematurely owing to boredom (lack of motivation), plasma volume shifts, and other conditions. Certainly, laboratories that evaluate a diverse population and use a common protocol should not be criticized. For research and other long-term comparative purposes, there are advantages in using the same protocol.

Experience with poorly fit, obese, elderly, and cardiac patients and, in particular, with patients who are relatively close to their cardiac event (one to twelve weeks after MI or surgery), has shown that an incremental work load of approximately 1 MET per stage that starts at approximately 2 METs is advisable. Under this condition, the standard Bruce, Balke, and Ellestad protocols start at too high a MET level. The Naughton protocol is particularly well suited for this situation. Bruce has designed a lower level 12-minute test for use with patients of low fitness.[84] The test includes four 3-minute stages: stage I, 1.2 mph, 0-percent grade; stage II, 1.2 mph, 3-percent grade; stage III, 1.2 mph, 6-percent grade; and stage IV, 1.7 mph, 6-percent grade. In addition, some have modified the original Bruce test by adding two 3-minute stages to the existing test protocol: step I, 1.7 mph, 0-percent grade; and step II, 1.7 mph, 5-percent grade.[85] The Balke protocol has been modified by adding a preliminary 2- to 3-minute stage at 2 mph, 0-percent grade.

Schauer and Hanson[86] have revived interest in the branching treadmill protocol that was described earlier by Adams, McHenry, and Bernauer.[87] Conceptually it has merit in that the subject walks at a comfortable speed between 2.0 and 3.5 mph. Once the speed is determined (speed increased by 0.25 mph increments), the workload is increased 1 MET every 2 minutes by adjusting the grade. This protocol is versatile and allows the tester to advance subjects at a walking pace that is compatible with their age, gait, and fitness.

From the criteria listed previously, it is obvious that the modified Åstrand protocol is not suitable for diagnostic testing. This protocol was designed to evaluate $\dot{V}O_2$max in normal, healthy individuals and is particularly well suited for use with runners.

In summary, there are many excellent treadmill protocols, and the one used is often dictated by the population being evaluated and by personal preference. The Bruce and Ellestad tests have been shown to be the most flexible tests used with a diverse population (men-women, nonathlete-athlete, young–middle-aged).

Although these tests are very popular (particularly the Bruce test), they are not without criticism. For example, the Bruce test is often criticized because of its abrupt increase in work load between stages and because stage IV for men (4.2 mph, 16-percent grade) and stage III for women (3.4 mph, 14-percent grade) are awkward in speed, thus it is difficult to decide whether to walk or run. One of the major advantages of using the Bruce test is its wide application and, thus, its yield of an abundance of comparative data.

The main criticism of the Balke test is its duration. The same would be true of the Naughton test if it were used with healthy and fit individuals. Because of their shorter stride length, a modified Balke (3.0 mph) protocol may be preferable for use with women.[66] The Naughton test has been most suitable for predischarge testing of cardiac patients and other patients and elderly persons who have low functional capacities (less than 6 METs). Most have modified the original Naughton protocol to incorporate 2-minute rather than 3-minute stages.

Cycle Ergometer, Arm Ergometer, and Step Test. Although the mode of testing is different with cycle and arm ergometers and with step test protocols, the general guidelines for GXT mentioned for treadmill testing are similar. Cycle ergometers are less expensive than treadmills. The advent of electronically controlled cycle ergometers has narrowed the price differential with treadmills. Whether the treadmill or cycle ergometer is used, frequent calibration for speed, grade, and resistance (kpm/min or watts) is necessary.[88] The manufacturer's instruction manual and the recommendations established by the American Heart Association[89] provide information and guidelines on the calibration of ergometric equipment. More specific instructions on the calibration of cycle ergometers, treadmills and sphygmomanometers are discussed by Howley.[90] The purchase of equipment that cannot be readily calibrated is not recommended.

Cycle Ergometry. The cycle ergometer test for determination of $\dot{V}O_2$max is usually performed on a mechanically or electronically braked cycle ergometer that is calibrated at 100 to 150 kpm/min (17- to 25-watt) increments. Most multistage protocols have 1- to 3-minute stages, with initial resistance for leg testing being set at 100 or 150 to 300 kpm/min. Power output increases by 100 to 150 kpm/min increments per stage. Middle-aged, less fit, cardiac patients generally begin at 100 or 150 to 300 kpm/min and increase their power output by 100 to 150 kpm/min per stage. Younger, more fit persons usually begin at 300 to 600 kpm/min (50 to 100 watts) and increase their power output by 150 to 300 kpm/min (25- to 50-watt) increments.

Cycle ergometers that do not internally adjust the power output to compensate for change in pedaling rate have to be pedaled at a constant rate, i.e., revolutions per minute (rpm). Some tests recommend a pedal rate of 50 rpm,[16, 91] but at the same power output, efficiency varies little between 50 and 80 rpm.[71] Competitive cyclists generally pedal at a minimum of 90 rpm and often up to 120 rpm.[92] Most of the commercially built cycle ergometers are not designed to test elite cyclists.

Recently, a resistance device in which your own bicycle is attached has been developed (Schwinn, Velodyne, Chicago, IL). It offers cyclists the advantage of using their own bicycle and pedaling at faster rates. Calibration may be difficult with these new devices, but they are adaptable for training and maximal testing.

In cycle ergometers that do not internally adjust resistance to compensate for a change in pedal speed, the use of a metronome assists the participant in keeping the proper pedal speed. Metronomes should be checked for calibration. In addition, calibration of all mechanical types of cycle ergometers is important. The friction type is the easiest to calibrate. With this kind of cycle ergometer, the friction belt expands as heat is generated by the flywheel, thus periodic tightening of the belt corrects for change in power output.[16, 90]

Another important point to remember when using a cycle ergometer is to make sure the height of the seat is properly adjusted. The seat should be adjusted so that there is a slight bend in the knee joint when the ball of the foot is on the pedal with the pedal in its lowest position.[92]

In comparison with the treadmill, there are some advantages in using the cycle ergometer. It is generally more portable. In addition, it is quieter and may involve less upper body movement, and thus, BP may be easier to assess. This is particularly true at the higher work levels. When taking BP of patients on a cycle ergometer, have them relax their grip and arm on the side being measured. Finally, in some cases, ECG recordings may show less skeletal muscle interference with cycle ergometry.

The major disadvantage of cycle ergometer testing in comparison with treadmill testing is that most Americans are unaccustomed to cycle riding; hence, their maximal values (HR and $\dot{V}O_2max$) are often underestimated. The lower values found on cycling can range from 5 to 25 percent, depending upon the participant's conditioning and leg strength.[83, 93–96] Since a lower measurement of functional capacity has obvious limitations in evaluation and exercise prescription, most testers prefer to use the treadmill. Persons trained on bicycles or cycle ergometers can often elicit equally high maximal physiological values on the cycle ergometer and the treadmill.[95, 96]

Arm Ergometry. Arm ergometry can be substituted when traditional leg testing is not possible owing to disability. Commercial arm ergometers are available, and cycle ergometers can be modified for use with the arms.[97–101] Either arm cranking or push-pull (Air-dyne) types of devices are appropriate for GXT.[98, 100, 102–104]

Some disadvantages of arm ergometry when compared with leg testing (treadmill and cycle) are as follows: a smaller muscle mass is used, thus $\dot{V}O_2max$ is lower by 20 to 30 percent;[97–100] HRmax is lower; BP may be difficult to assess; ECG quality can be affected; and it may not be recommended initially for patients with recent MI or heart surgery.[105] Arm training increases the arm $\dot{V}O_2max$ relative to the leg $\dot{V}O_2max$ by 5 to 10 percent.[99] Probably as a result of a greater use of muscle mass (arms and back muscles), the Air-dyne apparatus (arms only) appears to elicit a higher $\dot{V}O_2max$ than does arm cranking.[102] Although $\dot{V}O_2max$ and $\dot{V}_Emax$ do not differ with wheelchair ergometry as compared with arm cranking, power output and HRmax are significantly reduced with wheelchair ergometry.[106] The data now available on the value of arm ergometry in evaluating arrhythmias and ischemic responses to exercise are sufficient to support its use.[103, 104, 106, 107]

The same protocol recommended for leg ergometry can be used with arm ergometry, except that the initial power output and the incremental increases in power output between stages are lower for arm ergometry.[100] For patients who are considered of low fitness, the initial power output may be set at zero, and for moderately fit individuals, it may be set at 75 to 150 kpm/min (12 to 25 watts). Incremental increases in power output between stages of 75 and 100 kpm/min are generally recommended.

Since $\dot{V}O_2max$ and HRmax are significantly lower for arm work than for leg work, estimation of maximal values of leg work from arm work and its use for prescribing exercise for leg work are not recommended. With arm training, $\dot{V}O_2$max and HRmax significantly increase.[99] In prescribing exercise for arm training, the arm ergometer results should be used, and the same method of calculating training HR should be used as recommended for leg exercise (see Chapter 7). When the percentage of HRmax reserve is calculated from arm ergometry and compared with treadmill results, the same RPE score is often found, i.e., approximately 13 at 70 percent of HRmax reserve and 15 to 16 at 85 percent.[102]

Data are now available for GXT of paraplegic and quadriplegic subjects on various testing devices. Although paraplegics elicit slightly reduced to similar values for $\dot{V}O_2$max (ml $\cdot$ kg^{-1} $\cdot$ min^{-1}) and HRmax as compared with able-bodied subjects doing arm ergometry, quadriplegics show significantly lower values.[99, 109] Wheelchair ergometers have also been developed and compared with other types of arm ergometers.[110, 111] These data show similar findings among wheelchair, Monark arm cranking, Cybex upper body exercise, and Schwinn Air-dyne Ergometers. Thus a variety of equipment may be used to evaluate these patient populations. In general, the recommended GXT protocols for use with disabled groups are similar to those that are recommended for able-bodied subjects. The greater the disability, the lower the initial power output setting.[109] Wheeling protocols are often administered with the wheelchair placed on the treadmill.[112] Protocols use 2- to 3-minute stages, with speed usually beginning at 2 mph. Speed is increased by 0.5 mph, grade by 2 percent, or both, at each stage. Dreisinger and Londeree[113] give more detailed information on wheelchair exercise.

Stair/Bench Stepping. When neither a treadmill nor a cycle ergometer is available, a graded step test can be used as an alternative. The graded step test designed by Nagle, Balke, and Naughton[73] is recommended by the American Heart Association.[11] An adjustable platform permits the height to be varied from 2 to 50 cm while the patient continues to exercise. The platform height is initially set at 3 cm. At the end of the second minute, the platform is raised 2 cm; it is raised 4 cm each minute thereafter. The rhythm of stepping is regulated by a metronome at 30 steps/min. The stepping procedure is completed in four counts: at counts one and two, the patient steps up to an erect standing position with both feet on the platform; at counts three and four, he or she returns to the starting position standing in front of the platform. To help avoid local muscle fatigue, the lead leg may be changed periodically. The test is terminated when the patient is unable to maintain the required rhythm.

The Stairmaster step-treadmill is a revolutionary new device and can be used as an alternative ergometer for the GXT.[79] The

Stairmaster device is composed of revolving steps that are 21 cm high. The steps are propelled by the subject's weight as she or he climbs beginning at 30 steps/min. Stepping speed (work-load) can be adjusted mechanically to over 100 steps/min. Using 3-minute stages and stepping in place at 15 steps/min (2.8 METs) followed by stepping on the Stairmaster at 30 (4.6 METs), 50 (7.0 METs), 75 (10.0 METs), and 100 (13.0 METs) steps/min produced similar energy requirements as the Bruce treadmill protocol stages ½, 1, 2, 3, and 4.[79] Although this protocol and testing device are acceptable under most conditions recommended for GXT, the fact that the Stairmaster cannot be regulated by less than 30 steps/min is limiting. The MET level would be too high initially for screening patients with recent MI or CABG surgery or who are low fit.

Submaximal Tests and Field Tests to Determine Functional Capacity. The submaximal exercise testing protocols recommended here are found under Plan C (Table 6–2). The tests do not monitor ECG and BP and are not used for diagnostic purposes. The tests under Plan C are generally used for physical fitness testing of apparently healthy, low-risk youth and adults. They are primarily used by agencies that do mass testing, e.g., schools or the military, or that do not have extensive equipment or personnel with advanced training in test administration and interpretation, e.g., YMCAs, Jewish Community Centers, and health clubs. They also can be used as a follow-up test for persons who have had a diagnostic test and are considered at low risk and free from heart disease.

Submaximal tests to estimate VO_2max are based on the premise that there is a linear relationship between increased HR and VO_2 at submaximal levels. During this time, stroke volume has plateaued, and the major increase found in cardiac output is by an increase in HR. A fit person's HR is lower at any given work-load or power output, and thus the slope of his or her curve is lower (Fig. 6–5A). To estimate VO_2max, the steady state submaximal HR is projected to an estimated HRmax, with VO_2max being projected by a line drawn down to the horizontal axis. A multistage model would be the same as the single-stage model except that there would be 2 or 3 HR values to project to HRmax (Fig. 6–5B). To get the best prediction of VO_2max steady-state HR between 115 to 150 beats/min has been recommended for both single and multistage tests.[16, 71] More recently, Baumgartner and Jackson[31] have recommended an HR between 130 and 150 beats/min for the multistage model. In general, the higher the steady-state HR elicited during a test, the better the estimation of VO_2max.

Submaximal Treadmill Tests. Two protocols have been developed to estimate VO_2max from submaximal treadmill exercise.

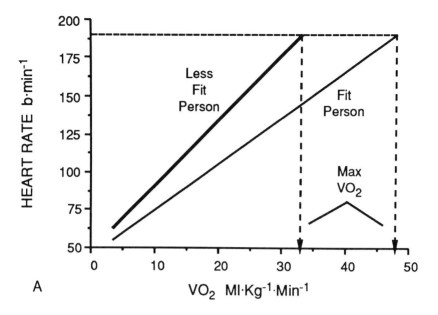

A

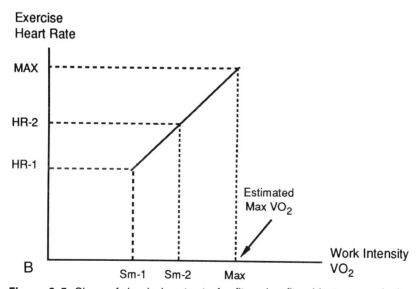

B

Figure 6–5. Slope of rise in heart rate for fit and unfit subjects on a single-stage exercise test *(A)*. Heart rate is projected to an estimated HRmax of 190 beats/min. Maximum oxygen uptake (V̇O₂max) is estimated by projecting a line down to the abscissa. A multi-stage test result is shown in *B*. (Reprinted with permission from Baumgartner, J. A., and Jackson, A. S.: **Measurement for Evaluation in Physical Education and Exercise Science,** 3rd Ed. Dubuque, IA, Wm. C. Brown Publishers, 1987. Copyright 1987, Wm. C. Brown Publishers, Dubuque, IA. All rights reserved.)

A single-stage model[114] was developed from the Bruce protocol[29] and a two-stage model[115] from a modification of the Balke protocol (Table 6–4).[74] The advantage of the modified Balke protocol is that it goes up more gradually from stage to stage, and thus a higher steady-state HR may be attained. The objective is to reach a steady-state HR between 115 and 155 beats/min. Usually the fourth stage of the Bruce protocol is not recommended because the speed of the treadmill is 4.2 mph, and most subjects will jog and a few will walk.

The following steps should be taken to administer the submaximal treadmill protocols shown in Table 6–4:

1. Heart rate should be determined the last 15 seconds of each minute of exercise (the submaximal HR should not exceed 155 beats/min).
2. Do not proceed to the next full stage of the Bruce protocol if the subject's HR exceeds 135 beats/min. For most healthy sedentary

Table 6–4. Submaximal Treadmill Test Protocols for the Estimation of Maximal Oxygen Uptake*

| | | | | Energy Cost† | |
| | | | | $\dot{V}O_2$ $(ml \cdot kg^{-1} \cdot min^{-1})$ | |
Stage	Minutes	mph	Grade (%)		METs
Bruce Protocol					
I	1–3	1.7	10	13.4	3.82
II	4–6	2.5	12	21.4	6.12
III	7–9	3.4	14	31.5	9.01
Ross Submaximal Protocol—Women					
I	1–3	3.4‡	0	14.9	4.25
II	4–6	3.4	3	18.4	5.27
III	7–9	3.4	6	22.0	6.29
IV	10–12	3.4	9	25.6	7.31
V	13–15	3.4	12	29.2	8.33
Ross Submaximal Protocol—Men					
I	1–3	3.4‡	0	14.9	4.25
II	4–6	3.4	4	19.6	5.61
III	7–9	3.4	8	24.4	6.97
IV	10–12	3.4	12	29.2	8.33
V	13–15	3.4	16	33.9	9.09

*The estimated energy cost of exercise is derived (estimated) from the last minute of a fully completed stage. To estimate $\dot{V}O_2$max, use the energy cost value and appropriate heart rate in the equation found in the text.

$$\dot{V}O_2 \ (ml \cdot kg^{-1} \cdot min^{-1}) = \left\{ [75 + (6 \times \%)] \left(\frac{mph}{60} \right) \right\} \times 3.5.[116]$$

‡A speed of 3.0 mph can be used and is especially useful for someone not accustomed to treadmill walking. The energy cost for the first stage would then be 3.75 METs.[115]

(Reprinted with permission from Baungartner, J. A., and Jackson, A. S.: **Measurement for Evaluation in Physical Education and Exercise Science.** Dubuque, IA, Wm. C. Brown, 1987. Copyright 1987, Wm. C. Brown Publishers, Dubuque, IA. All rights reserved.)

adults, an HR between 135 and 155 beats/min is reached within the first 6 minutes of exercise (stage II).

3. Do not proceed to the next full stage of the modified Balke protocol if the subject's HR exceeds 145 beats/min.

4. Once the proper HR values are determined, terminate the test and use proper cool-down procedures.

To calculate $\dot{V}O_2$max from the single-stage submaximal test, do the following:

1. Ascertain the proper energy cost and HR values determined or estimated from the submaximal test (see Table 6–4 for estimated $\dot{V}O_2$).

2. Use the following formulas* to calculate $\dot{V}O_2$max:

$$\text{Men: } \dot{V}O_2\text{max} = \dot{V}O_2\text{SM} \times \frac{(\text{HRmax} - 61)}{(\text{SM}_{HR} - 61)}$$

$$\text{Women: } \dot{V}O_2\text{max} = \dot{V}O_2\text{SM} \times \frac{(\text{HRmax} - 72)}{(\text{SM}_{HR} - 72)}$$

where SM = submaximal ($\dot{V}O_2$ or HR).

To calculate $\dot{V}O_2$max from the multistage submaximal test, do the same as for item 1 under single-stage test (see Table 6–4, modified Balke test). Then, use the following formula to calculate $\dot{V}O_2$max:

$$VO_2\text{max} = SM_2 + b\,(\text{HRmax} - HR_2)$$

$$\text{where } b = \left[\frac{(SM_2 - SM_1)}{(HR_2 - HR_1)} \right]$$

where SM_1 and SM_2 are submaximal $\dot{V}O_2$ or METs and HR_1 and HR_2 are the HR values for the two stages of the submaximal test.

Note: Either test protocol shown in Figure 6–4 can be used for the single or multistage equations in predicting $\dot{V}O_2$max. The accuracy of both equations is similar.[114] The original research of Åstrand and Rhyming[91] assumed an HRmax of 195 beats/min. They later published correction factors that accounted for differences in age.[71] Mahar and associates[114] showed that the use of 220 minus age was more accurate than the correction factor suggested by Åstrand and Rhyming.

Maximal HR can be estimated by subtracting age from 220.

Submaximal Cycle Tests. The most commonly used submaximal cycle ergometer tests include a multistage physical work

---

*These basic equations were developed by R.J. Shephard by fitting the data from the Åstrand-Rhyming nomogram.[91] Personal communication by A.S. Jackson and R.J. Shephard, 1986.[31]

capacity test developed by Sjöstrand[117] and a single-stage test by Åstrand and Ryhming.[91] Like the treadmill submaximal protocols, both tests are based on the fact that HR and $\dot{V}O_2$ are linearly related over a broad range.[71] The premise is that a younger or more fit individual has a lower submaximal steady-state HR at any given level of power output (kpm/min or watts).

The YMCAs of America have modified the Sjöstrand test by using two or three 3-minute continuous stages.[16] To administer the test properly, two HR–power-output data points are needed within a 110 to 150 beat/min range. The test can start once a participant has had a chance to become familiar with the ergometer and the proper seat height has been adjusted. The metronome should be set so that one can pedal at 50 rpm, and the test subject should be allowed to warm up by pedaling for one minute at zero resistance. Figure 6–6 can be used as a guide to set the initial and subsequent power outputs for both men and women. As shown in the directions (Fig. 6–6), if the initial power output elicits a HR of 110 beats/min or more, only one more stage is needed to complete the two plots. In most cases, the HR is lower than 110 beats/min on the initial stage; therefore, the values for the second and third stages (power outputs) are used. Each stage is timed for 3 minutes, with the HR being counted during the last half of the second and third minutes. At the end of each HR count, the scores are recorded on a form such as the one shown in Figure 6–7. The HR in the second and third minutes should not differ by more than 5 beats/min. If they do, extend the test period for an additional minute or until a stable value is obtained. When plotting the results, use the HR value for the third or final minute of each stage.

The HR is determined by measuring the length of time it takes to count 30 heart-beats. This is usually done with a stopwatch and a stethoscope. See Table 6–5 for converting HR seconds/30 beats to beats/min. Once the test is completed, a one- to two-minute recovery period of low- to zero-resistance pedaling is recommended.

The directions for calculating maximal working capacity and $\dot{V}O_2$max are shown in Figure 6–7.[16] Plot only the last two HR–power-output values determined. The lower horizontal axis shows the estimated $\dot{V}O_2$max (l/min), kcal/min, and METs for a given work load or power output. Finally, to express $\dot{V}O_2$max in ml $\cdot$ kg^{-1} $\cdot$ min^{-1}, divide the l/min value by body weight in kilograms.

Submaximal Bench Stepping Test. The prediction of $\dot{V}O_2$max also can be determined by a submaximal bench stepping test.[31, 118–121] The basic assumption of this test in regard to the linear relationship between HR and $\dot{V}O_2$ is similar to that of the submaximal treadmill and cycle tests. Given an equal amount of work to accomplish (stepping up and down on a bench at the same

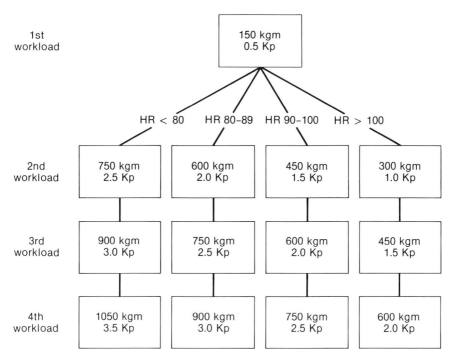

Directions:

1. Set the first workload at 150 kgm/min (0.5 Kp).
2. If the HR in the third minute is
   - less than (<) 80, set the second load at 750 kgm (2.5 Kp);
   - 80 to 89, set the second load at 600 kgm (2.0 Kp);
   - 90 to 100, set the second load at 450 kgm (1.5 Kp);
   - greater than (>) 100, set the second load at 300 kgm (1.0 Kp).
3. Set the third and fourth (if required) loads according to the loads in the columns below the second loads.

Figure 6–6. Guide for setting power outputs (workloads) for men and women on submaximal cycle ergometer test. (Reprinted with permission from Golding, L. A., Myers, C. R., and Sinning, W. E. [eds.]: Y's Way to Physical Fitness: The Complete Guide to Fitness Testing and Instruction, 3rd Ed. Champaign, IL, Human Kinetics Publishers, 1989.)

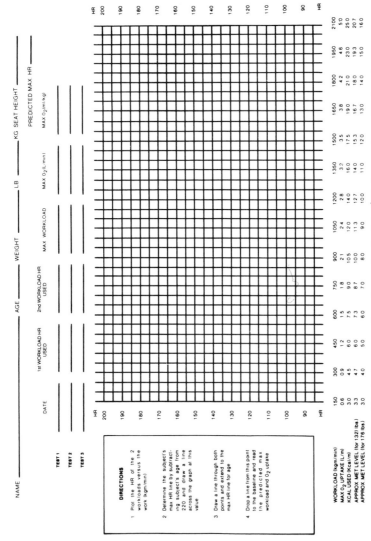

Figure 6–7. Work sheet used to plot and calculate $\dot{V}O_2$ from submaximal cycle ergometer test. (Reprinted with permission from Golding, L. A., Myers, C. R., and Sinning, W. E. [eds.]: **Y's Way to Physical Fitness: The Complete Guide to Fitness Testing and Instruction**, 3rd Ed. Champaign, IL, Human Kinetics Publishers, 1989.)

Table 6–5. Heart Rate (Beats/Min) Based on the Time to Count 30 Pulse Beats

Seconds	Per Minute	Seconds	Per Minute	Seconds	Per Minute
28.5	63	21.6	83	14.7	122
28.4	63	21.5	84	14.6	123
28.3	64	21.4	84	14.5	124
28.2	64	21.3	85	14.4	125
28.1	64	21.2	85	14.3	126
28.0	64	21.1	85	14.2	127
27.9	64	21.0	86	14.1	128
27.8	65	20.9	86	14.0	129
27.7	65	20.8	87	13.9	129
27.6	65	20.7	87	13.8	130
27.5	65	20.6	87	13.7	131
27.4	66	20.5	88	13.6	132
27.3	66	20.4	88	13.5	133
27.2	66	20.3	89	13.4	134
27.1	66	20.2	89	13.3	135
27.0	67	20.1	90	13.2	136
26.9	67	20.0	90	13.1	137
26.8	67	19.9	90	13.0	138
26.7	67	19.8	91	12.9	140
26.6	68	19.7	91	12.8	141
26.5	68	19.6	92	12.7	142
26.4	68	19.5	92	12.6	143
26.3	68	19.4	93	12.5	144
26.2	69	19.3	93	12.4	145
26.1	69	19.2	94	12.3	146
26.0	69	19.1	94	12.2	148
25.9	69	19.0	95	12.1	149
25.8	70	18.9	95	12.0	150
25.7	70	18.8	96	11.9	151
25.6	70	18.7	96	11.8	153
25.5	71	18.6	97	11.7	154
25.4	71	18.5	97	11.6	155
25.3	71	18.4	98	11.5	157
25.2	71	18.3	98	11.4	158
25.1	72	18.2	99	11.3	159
25.0	72	18.1	99	11.2	161
24.9	72	18.0	100	11.1	162
24.8	72	17.9	101	11.0	164
24.7	73	17.8	101	10.9	165
24.6	73	17.7	102	10.8	167
24.5	73	17.6	102	10.7	168
24.4	74	17.5	103	10.6	170
24.3	74	17.4	103	10.5	171
24.2	74	17.3	104	10.4	173
24.1	75	17.2	105	10.3	175
24.0	75	17.1	105	10.2	176
23.9	75	17.0	106	10.1	178
23.8	76	16.9	107	10.0	180
23.7	76	16.8	107	9.9	182
23.6	76	16.7	108	9.8	184
23.5	77	16.6	108	9.7	186
23.4	77	16.5	109	9.6	188
23.3	77	16.4	110	9.5	189
23.2	78	16.3	110	9.4	191
23.1	78	16.2	111	9.3	194
23.0	78	16.1	112	9.2	196
22.9	79	16.0	113	9.1	198
22.8	79	15.9	113	9.0	200
22.7	79	15.8	114	8.9	202
22.6	80	15.7	115	8.8	205
22.5	80	15.6	115	8.7	207
22.4	80	15.5	116	8.6	209
22.3	81	15.4	117	8.5	212
22.2	81	15.3	118	8.4	214
22.1	81	15.2	118	8.3	217
22.0	82	15.1	119	8.2	220
21.9	82	15.0	120	8.1	222
21.8	83	14.9	121	8.0	225
21.7	83	14.8	122		

rate and total time), the participant with a lower HR will be in better physical condition and therefore will have a higher $\dot{V}O_2$max.

Katch and McArdle[119] describe a submaximal bench stepping test for predicting $\dot{V}O_2$max in college-age men and women. The test is accomplished by stepping up and down on a bench 16.25 inches high (generally the height of a bleacher seat) for a total of 3 minutes. Men step at a rate of 24 steps/min and women at 22 steps/min. Again, it is best to use a metronome. On the completion of the 3-minute test, the participant remains standing while the pulse is counted for a 15-second interval, beginning 5 seconds after termination of the test. To convert the recovery HR to beats/min, the 15-second HR is multiplied by four. The equations for estimating $\dot{V}O_2$max, expressed in $ml \cdot kg^{-1} \cdot min^{-1}$, are as follows:

$$\text{Men: } \dot{V}O_2\text{max} = 111.33 - (0.42 \times \text{step test HR})$$

$$\text{Women: } \dot{V}O_2\text{max} = 65.81 - (0.1847 \times \text{step test HR})$$

A submaximal bench stepping test for healthy, middle-aged adults was developed by Kasch.[16, 120] It is a 3-minute test conducted at 24 steps/min on a bench 12 inches high. After completion of the test, the participant sits down, and the pulse is counted for a minute, beginning 5 seconds into the recovery. Norms for adult men and women[16] and police officers[122] are available.

The Canadian aerobic fitness test (CAFT), formerly called the Canadian home fitness test,[17, 18] developed by Jette and colleagues[121] and adopted as part of the Canadian Standardized Test of Fitness[6] for ages 15 to 69 years, is the best designed submaximal bench step test for varied age groups and fitness levels. The test has been used extensively in Canada, and the norms are based on the test results of thousands of participants.

To administer the test, select the proper starting stage for gender as shown:

Age	Men	Women
60–69	1	1
50–59	2	1
40–49	3	2
30–39	4	3
20–29	5	3
15–19	5	4

The test is structured so that participants start at a low level for their specific age and gender. They step at a predetermined pace following the stepping sequence as outlined in Figure 6–8. The steps are 20.3 cm in height. The stepping cadence for each stage of the test is shown:

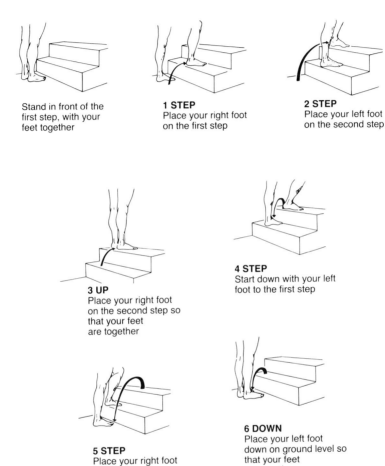

Stand in front of the first step, with your feet together

1 STEP
Place your right foot on the first step

2 STEP
Place your left foot on the second step

3 UP
Place your right foot on the second step so that your feet are together

4 STEP
Start down with your left foot to the first step

5 STEP
Place your right foot on ground level

6 DOWN
Place your left foot down on ground level so that your feet are together

Figure 6–8. Stepping sequence for the Canadian Aerobic Fitness Test. The counting sequence (cadence) is available pretaped (Fitness and Amateur Sport Canada, 365 Laurier Ave. West, Ottawa, Ontario, K1A 0X6.) The stepping cadence sounds like this: step–step up, step–step down and up–2–3, down–2–3. (Adapted from **Canadian Standardized Test of Fitness (CSTF) Operations Manual,** 3rd Ed. With permission of Fitness Canada, Fitness and Amateur Sport Canada, Ottawa, 1986.)

Stage	Men	Women
1	66	66
2	84	84
3	102	102
4	114	114
5	132	120
6	144	132
7	156	—

Each stage is 3 minutes long, with HR being counted immediately after stopping while the participant is standing. Heart rate is counted for 10 seconds immediately after stopping. Begin counting immediately after the starting command to count and stop on the stop command. The first count should be one not zero. If the predetermined HR upper limit (as shown in the following table) is not attained or exceeded, the participant performs the next stage.

Heart Rates
(beats/10 sec)

Age	*After 1st Session*	*After 2nd Session*
60–69	24	—
50–59	25	23
40–49	26	24
30–39	28	25
20–29	29	26
15–19	30	27

If the HR after the second stage is below the HR value (beats/10 sec) shown for the upper limit HR after exercise, the subject can proceed to stage 3. A subject can complete up to three stages. Upon completion of the test, a 3½-minute sitting recovery, with legs elevated if necessary, is recommended.

Sitting resting HR and BP are taken before administering the CAFT, and HR is taken at 3 to 3½ minutes and BP at ½ to 1 and 2½ to 3 minutes of recovery. The test is not recommended for use with subjects whose resting HR is above 100 beats/min and whose BP is above 150/100 mmHg. Before a subject leaves the testing site, it is recommended that the recovery HR be less than 100 beats/min and the BP be below 150/100 mmHg. When taking resting HR and BP, have subjects rest in a sitting position for 5 minutes. If they do not meet the HR and BP criteria, have them sit quietly for another 5 minutes, and repeat the test. It is recommended not to administer the CAFT to anyone who does not meet the above criteria and who is receiving medication for high BP.

To estimate $\dot{V}O_2$max from the step test results, use the following prediction equation:

$$\dot{V}O_2 \text{ max (ml} \cdot \text{kg}^{-1} \cdot \text{min}^{-1}) = 42.5 + (16.6 \times \dot{V}O_2) - (0.12 \times W) - (0.12 \times HR) - (0.24 \times A)$$

where $\dot{V}O_2$ = the average oxygen cost of the last completed exercise stage in l/min (Table 6–6);

W = the body weight in kilograms;

HR = the heart rate after the final stage of stepping in beats/min;

A = the participant's age in years.

Although the CAFT has been used successfully, the authors mention several limitations of the test.[6] Maximal oxygen uptake is underestimated in fit participants, women 20 to 29 years of age, and for heavy individuals. Maximal oxygen uptake is overestimated in poorly fit participants.

Running Field Tests. The field type of test was designed to estimate $\dot{V}O_2$max in large groups of healthy young men and women. A high correlation between the laboratory-determined $\dot{V}O_2$max and the distance run was first reported by Balke[27] (15-minute run) and later popularized by Cooper[123, 124] (12-minute run and 1.5-mile run). For many years, the national test for cardiorespiratory endurance used with school children was the 600-yard run test developed by the American Alliance for Health, Physical Education, Recreation, and Dance (AAHPERD).[125] It was subsequently shown that run tests below a mile (approximately 9 minutes) had low correlations with laboratory-determined $\dot{V}O_2$max and moderate to high correlations above this distance.[31, 126] Thus, in 1981, AAHPERD published their *Health Related Physical Fitness Test Manual,* which recommended a one-mile or 9-minute walk-run for children 12 years old and under and a 1.5-mile or 12-minute walk-run for

Table 6–6. Energy Requirements in l $O_2 \cdot \text{min}^{-1}$ of Different Stages of Canadian Aerobic Fitness Test

Stage	Men	Women
1	1.1391	0.9390
2	1.3466	1.0484
3	1.6250	1.3213
4	1.8255	1.4925
5	2.0066	1.6267
6	2.3453	1.7867
7	2.7657	—

(Reprinted with permission from Jette, M., Campbell, J., Mongeon, J., Routhier, R.: The Canadian home fitness test as a predictor of aerobic capacity. **Can. Med. Assoc. J.** 114:680–682, 1976.)

children in junior and senior high school grades (13 years old and above).[68] More recently the AAHPERD *Physical Best* program recommends the use of the one-mile walk-run test for ages 5 to 18 years.[127, 128] A 0.5-mile run test is offered as an option for ages 5 to 9 years, and the 1.5-mile or 12-minute run test is recommended as an optional test to be used by the older students. Again, as mentioned previously, the validity of a one-mile test is questionable as the speed gets below 9 minutes.

The most widely used field tests (schools, universities, and armed forces) are the 12-minute and 1.5-mile runs. The two tests have a very high intercorrelation, and because the 1.5-mile run test is easier to administer, it is preferred.

Like other unmonitored tests, the running field test should not be used as a diagnostic tool and should be administered only to healthy, young persons. An exception to this would be its use with trained middle-aged participants who have already been thoroughly evaluated for heart disease and potential risk. Best results are found when participants have had a few weeks of preliminary training. This allows time for some adaptation to training and practice in pacing oneself. The test is normally administered on a smooth, level surface (track) and is performed in running shoes. Table 6–3 shows the estimation of $\dot{V}O_2$max based on the time to run 1.5 miles.

Walking Field Test. The advent of a one-mile walk test, developed in conjunction with the Rockport Walking Institute, has provided a field test to estimate $\dot{V}O_2$max from a broader range of the adult population.[25] The study determined $\dot{V}O_2$max on a treadmill in 343 healthy adults (168 men; 175 women) who were between 30 and 69 years of age. Subjects also performed a minimum of two one-mile track walks at their fastest speed. The following generalized equation for men and women was developed to predict $\dot{V}O_2$max in $l \cdot min^{-1}$ (n = 174):

$$\dot{V}O_2max = 6.952 + (0.0091 \times W) - (0.0257 \times Age) + (0.5955 \times Sex) - (0.2240 \times TI) - (0.0115 \times HR_{1-4})$$

where W = weight (lbs);
       Age is rounded to the nearest year;
       Sex = 1 if male and 0 if female;
       TI = track walk time;
       HR_{1-4} = HR beats/min during last lap of test;
       r = 0.93, with SEE = 0.325 L/min.

A cross-validation of the equation (n = 169) resulted in r = 0.92, with SEE = $0.355\ l \cdot m^{-1}$ Cross-validation results of equations for men and women separately were r = $0.84 \pm 4.4\ ml \cdot kg^{-1} \cdot min^{-1}$

for men and 0.86 ± 3.6 ml • kg^{-1} • min^{-1} for women. Equations by decade (30 to 39, 40 to 49, 50 to 59, and 60 to 69 years) showed correlations ranging from 0.74 to 0.90 and SEE ranging from 2.4 to 5.2 ml • kg^{-1} • min^{-1}. More recently, the equation was cross-validated with 70- to 79-year-olds.[129] It was also found that counting the pulse for 15 seconds starting 5 seconds after completion of the walk test, instead of counting the pulse during the last segment of the test, was equally as effective in estimating $\dot{V}O_2$max.[130] Thus, from a practical standpoint, recovery HR would be easier to attain and can be substituted in the above equation. The Rockport Walking Institute has developed normative fitness charts based on age, HR, and time on the one-mile walk test and are available upon request (P.O. Box 480, Marlboro, MA 01752).[131, 132]

Interpretation of Graded Exercise Test Results

The interpretation of GXT results are discussed in relation to the prediction of $\dot{V}O_2$max (functional capacity), knowledge of level of cardiorespiratory fitness, and the determination of medical status of participants entering the health enhancement, preventive, or rehabilitation programs.

AEROBIC CAPACITY

To determine the level of aerobic fitness, three sets of norms are available in Appendix A.*

The advantage of these standards compared with others is that they are age-specific by decade and include a large cell size for each age classification. The data were from generally healthy young people and middle-aged and older adults. Although the values for $\dot{V}O_2$max from the three sets of norms were collected from different tests, maximal treadmill testing at the Cooper Clinic, a submaximal cycle ergometer test from the YMCA and a submaximal bench stepping test from the Canadian Fitness Survey, with subsequent predictions of $\dot{V}O_2$max, show similar results.

Which of the three sets of norms would be best to use is difficult to say. The Cooper Clinic and YMCA data were taken from mainly Caucasian middle to upper class individuals. The Canadian test was administered to mainly Caucasians but included more blue

---

*Tables A–1 to A-12, Cooper Clinic Data, calculated update provided by S. Blair and B. Barlow, Institute for Aerobics Research, Dallas, TX, January, 1989; A–13 to A–24, YMCA Data;[16] and A–25 to A–28, Canada Fitness Survey Data.[6]

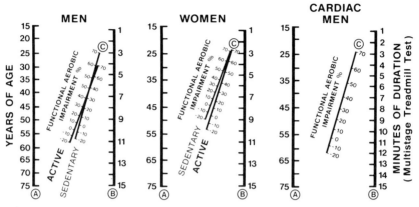

Figure 6–9. Nomograms for evaluating functional aerobic impairment (FAI) of men, women, and cardiac men according to age and by duration of exercise on Bruce protocol for sedentary and active groups. To find FAI, apply a straight edge to age and duration and read the intercepts on the diagonal. (Reprinted with permission from Bruce, R. L., Kusumi, F., and Hosmer, D.: Maximal oxygen intake and nomographic assessment of functional aerobic impairment in cardiovascular disease. **Am. Heart J.** 85:545–562, 1973.)

collar workers. The advantage of the Cooper Clinic norms is that data were collected on approximately 40,000 individuals and determined under better standardized conditions (one laboratory) in which quality control was easier to monitor. However, inspection of the body fat data shows the Cooper Clinic population to be leaner than expected and compared with their 1978 norms. The YMCA norms are based on approximately 22,000 tests administered in 180 YMCAs throughout the United States.*

Figure 6–9 illustrates another popular method of classifying men and women of various ages.[29] The functional aerobic impairment (FAI) scale was developed from treadmill performance time on the Bruce test and distinguishes between sedentary, active, and cardiac populations. In contrast to the Cooper Clinic, YMCA, and Canadian norms, much of the data reported by Bruce come from a hospital setting wherein many more persons are evaluated because of potential CAD. In addition, the FAI is applicable only to the Bruce test.

The clinical classification scale as it relates to various GXT protocols was developed by the American Heart Association (see Table 6–7).[85] Although widely used by clinicians, its generally broad categories make it less precise in determining fitness status.

---

*(Personal communication of L. Golding, University of Nevada, January 1989.)

Table 6–7. Clinical Classification as It Relates to Various Exercise Stages of Commonly Used Protocols

Functional Class	Clinical Status	O₂ Reqmt's ml·kg⁻¹·min⁻¹	Step Test — Nagle, Balke, Naughton* 2-min stages 30 steps/min (Step height increased 4 cm q 2 min) Height (cm)	Treadmill Tests — Bruce‡ 3-min stages mph	% gr	Kattus‡ 3-min stages mph	% gr	Balke§ % grade at 3.5 mph	Balke§ % grade at 3 mph	Bicycle Ergometer§ For 70 kg body weight kgm/min
		56.0								
		52.5								
Normal and I	Physically Active Subjects	49.0				4	22	26		
		45.5	40	4.2	16	4	18	24		1500
		42.0	36					22	22.5	1350
		38.5	32	3.4	14	4	14	20	20.0	1200
	Sedentary Healthy	35.0	28					18	17.5	1050
		31.5	24	2.5	12			16	15.0	900
		28.0	20			4	10	14	12.5	750
II	Diseased, Recovered	24.5	16	1.7	10	3	10	12	10.0	600
		21.0	12			2	10	10	7.5	450
		17.5	8					8	5.0	300
III	Symptomatic Patients	14.0	4					6	2.5	
		10.5						4	0.0	150
IV		7.0						2		
		3.5								

Oxygen requirements increase with work loads from bottom of chart to top in various exercise tests of the step, treadmill, and cycle ergometer types.

*Nagle, F. S., Balke, B., and Naughton, J. P.[73]

‡Bruce, R. A.[29]

‡Kattus, A. A., Jorgensen, C. R., Worden, R. E., and Alvaro, A. B.[133]

§Fox, S. M., Naughton, J. P., and Haskell, W. L.[134]

(Reprinted with permission from **Exercise Testing and Training of Apparently Healthy Individuals: A Handbook for Physicians.** Dallas, American Heart Association, 1972.)

Because norms are population-specific, the scale that most represents the participants tested should be used.

The fitness classifications shown in Table 6–3 are not to be confused with normative data. The categories developed in this table put potential participants who are interested in becoming involved in an aerobic exercise program into homogeneous subgroupings. This should help facilitate the physician or program director in determining the exercise prescription. The fitness classifications shown in Table 6–3 match up with the variety of recommended 6-week starter and 20-week training regimens described in Chapter 7.

The meaning of $\dot{V}O_2$max standards for various groups (sedentary, active, and athletic), the variability of the measure (sex, heredity, age, and so forth), and expected training responses are reviewed in Chapter 3. These factors should be taken into account when interpreting test results.

PREDICTION OF VO₂max

As mentioned earlier, $\dot{V}O_2$max can be predicted with relative accuracy from performance time and standard submaximal work load/power output tests. Maximal performance tests usually yield higher predictive scores (r = 0.75 to 0.95, SEE ± 2.5 to 4 ml $\cdot$ kg^{-1} $\cdot$ min^{-1}) than do submaximal tests (r = 0.65 to 0.75, SEE ± 4 to 5 ml $\cdot$ kg^{-1} $\cdot$ min^{-1}).[31] Laboratory-controlled maximal tests using performance time on a treadmill show the highest correlation with laboratory-determined $\dot{V}O_2$max (r = approximately 0.9, SEE = 2.5 to 4 ml $\cdot$ kg^{-1} $\cdot$ min^{-1}).[29, 65, 66] Factors that significantly affect the results of laboratory performance tests are population specificity of equations, familiarity with treadmill and test procedures (habituation), hanging onto the handrails, and inappropriate endpoints for test termination.

Bruce and associates[29] and others[37, 65, 135] have shown that the prediction of $\dot{V}O_2$max from standardized tests is population-specific. This is based on the statistical premise that a prediction equation best predicts (highest correlation and lowest standard error) at the mean value of the population used.[31, 136] If data are curvilinear, then gross prediction errors are made on participants who deviate significantly from the mean of the population from which the equation was derived (Fig. 6–10). For example, equations developed on average sedentary men or women underestimate $\dot{V}O_2$max of highly active and elite endurance athletes and overpredict cardiac patients and persons of low fitness. This regression effect toward the mean is common among tests and is discussed again under body composition evaluation.[31, 136]

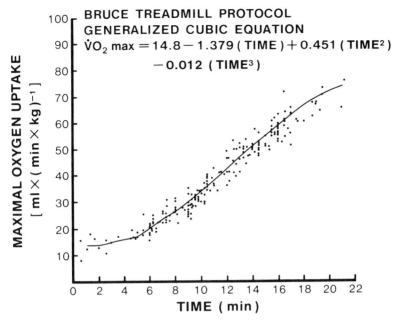

Figure 6–10. Data show the curvilinear relationship between measured $\dot{V}O_2$max to treadmill performance of persons of varied abilities (n = 200). The generalized cubic equation derived from the Bruce protocol[29] shows an r = 0.98 ± 3.35 ml · kg^{-1} · min^{-1}.[135] Treadmill time is expressed in minutes. (Published with permission from Foster, C., et al.: Generalized equations for predicting functional capacity from treadmill performance. **Am. Heart J.** 107:1229–1234, 1984.)

Population-specific equations for predicting $\dot{V}O_2$max from treadmill performance time are available for middle-aged active and sedentary men and women for the Bruce test[29, 37, 65, 66] and for cardiac patients for the Bruce test.[29]

More recently, Foster and associates[135] (see Fig. 6–10 for the Bruce protocol) developed a generalized equation for the Bruce and modified Naughton protocols that can be used for active and sedentary men and women cardiac patients. The prediction equation for the Naughton protocol is as follows:

$$\dot{V}O_2max = 1.61 \times \text{treadmill time (min)} + 3.60$$
$$r = 0.97, SEE = \pm 2.60.^{137}$$

The modification of the Naughton protocol included 2-minute stages. Using one generalized equation has the advantage of eliminating the judgmental factor of which equation to use for an individual and of having a slightly lower standard error of measurement. Other equations are available for predicting $\dot{V}O_2$max for the Balke,[37, 65, 66, 85] Ellestad,[36, 65] and Naughton[37, 78, 85] protocols. The treadmill times and estimation of $\dot{V}O_2$max shown for the various protocols in Table 6–3 are based on the results of various prediction equations. They have been cross-validated with a varied population of patients and elite, active, and sedentary young and middle-aged populations (unpublished data, M.L. Pollock). Although fewer data are available for the elderly populations, Table 6–3 also has been validated for use with active master runners.

Another important factor related to using population-specific prediction equations for estimated $\dot{V}O_2$max is their ability to predict training changes accurately. Figure 6–11 shows data from a 16-week training study conducted on cardiac patients.[138] The amount of change in $\dot{V}O_2$max was similar for actual measured $\dot{V}O_2$ compared with that predicted by equation 3 (Fig. 6–11), which was derived from cardiac patients. The other equations (1, 2, 4, and 5

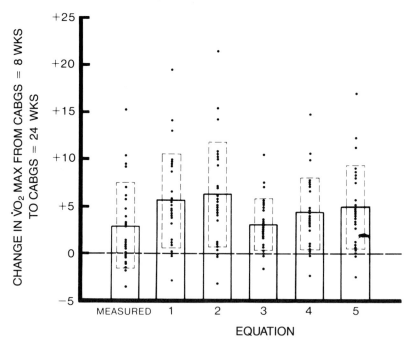

Figure 6–11. The actual measured change in $\dot{V}O_2$max (left bar) is shown for coronary artery bypass graft surgery (CABGS) patients after 16 weeks of aerobic training.[138] The data shown for equations 1 and 2 are from Pollock, M. L., et al.,[65] on healthy sedentary and active individuals, and equations 3 to 5 are from Bruce, R. A., et al.,[29] on cardiac patients (3), and sedentary (4) and active (5) healthy men. Notice all equations that were derived from noncardiac populations overestimate the actual change in $\dot{V}O_2$max. (Data from Foster, C., et al.: Prediction of oxygen uptake during exercise testing in cardiac patients and healthy volunteers. **J. Cardiac Rehabil.** 4:537–542, 1984.)

in Fig. 6–11), which were derived from healthy, sedentary, and active populations, consistently overpredicted the actual amount of $\dot{V}O_2$max change.[138]

Some clinicians have used steady-state $\dot{V}O_2$ values at various standard work loads to estimate $\dot{V}O_2$max.[26] Using this technique can also lead to gross errors of estimation.[138] For the normal population, it has been shown that $\dot{V}O_2$ often plateaus (depending upon the protocol used, 50 to 80 percent of the time)[65] from one to three minutes before the end of the test.[72, 139] Foster and colleagues[138] showed that during the clearly submaximal portions of the Bruce protocol, both cardiac and normal subjects accurately follow the estimated steady-state $\dot{V}O_2$ curve for each work load. In contrast, within 3 minutes from test termination (volitional maximum), the pattern deviated; i.e., predicted $\dot{V}O_2$max was significantly greater than the actually measured $\dot{V}O_2$max. This overprediction of $\dot{V}O_2$max was particularly evident when equations developed for normal subjects were used for cardiac patients. The measured $\dot{V}O_2$ versus steady-state $\dot{V}O_2$ values as tabulated for uphill walking by the ACSM[10] are compared in Figure 6–12 for healthy volunteers

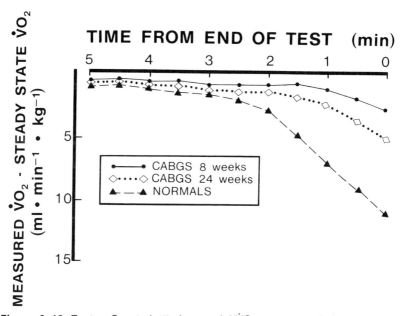

Figure 6–12. Foster, C., et al.,[138] show serial $\dot{V}O_2$ responses during the last 5 minutes of exercise on Bruce protocol for patients recovering from coronary artery bypass graft surgery (CABGS) and for healthy volunteers. See text for a detailed explanation of figure. (Reprinted with permission from Foster, C., et al.: Prediction of oxygen uptake during exercise testing in cardiac patients and healthy volunteers. **J. Cardiac Rehabil.** 4:537–542, 1984.)

and cardiac patients.[138] The pattern of response shows a progressive difference in measured $\dot{V}O_2$ versus predicted steady-state $\dot{V}O_2$ as subjects get closer to $\dot{V}O_2$max. Therefore, if steady-state $\dot{V}O_2$ values are used to predict $\dot{V}O_2$max, backing off 2 to 4 minutes from the endpoint may be necessary. Protocols that have abrupt increases in $\dot{V}O_2$ from stage to stage (Bruce or Ellestad) have greater potential error when steady-state values are used for predicting $\dot{V}O_2$max than do protocols that have smaller incremental increases (Balke, Naughton).

Habituation and hanging onto the handrails are two important factors that significantly affect prediction of $\dot{V}O_2$max from performance time.[33, 35–37, 60–63] Froelicher and colleagues[32] found treadmill performance to improve significantly when subjects were tested three times, a week apart on three different treadmill protocols. Although laboratory measurement of $\dot{V}O_2$max did not change from week to week, treadmill time did. In this study, the use of treadmill time to predict $\dot{V}O_2$max would have produced a 5 to 6 ml $\cdot$ kg^{-1} $\cdot$ min^{-1} increase in $\dot{V}O_2$max. Although not supported by the Froelicher and colleagues[32] study, other investigations suggest that one practice period should be sufficient to eliminate this prediction error.[65, 140]

Although holding onto the handrails may have little significant effect on the diagnostic aspects of the GXT, its use invalidates any prediction of aerobic capacity from treadmill performance time.[60–63] Zeimetz and colleagues[62] demonstrated an overprediction error of up to 3.2 METs with holding onto the handrails. There was also a significant reduction in HR and $\dot{V}O_2$ at standard submaximal work loads. Therefore, if actual $\dot{V}O_2$max is not measured and aerobic capacity is being estimated, holding onto the handrails should be avoided.

Whether actually measured or predicted from maximal performance time, $\dot{V}O_2$max is most accurately assessed when participants go to volitional maximum. In addition to significant clinical signs and symptoms, maximal endpoints include the following: plateauing of $\dot{V}O_2$ with an increase in work load, RER above 1.0, blood lactate levels above 90 mg/100 ml, HR approaching or above age-predicted maximum, signs of exercise intolerance (fatigue, staggering, inability to keep up with work load, and facial pallor), and RPE above 18 or 19.[13, 36, 37, 56, 59, 71, 72, 139, 141] Although more difficult to measure at peak exercise, systolic BP often decreases at maximal exercise.[36] Thus, unless a standard submaximal or maximal endpoint is used, measuring or predicting $\dot{V}O_2$max becomes less accurate, and interpretation of serial results may become impossible. Although HR associated with a standard work load is often acceptable for comparing serial results, in itself HR is usually a poor criterion to use as an endpoint for maximal GXT.

As mentioned earlier, the prediction of $\dot{V}O_2$max by the time taken to run or walk a certain distance (one to two miles) or by the distance covered in 9 to 12 minutes has a correlation with laboratory-determined $\dot{V}O_2$max of 0.5 to 0.91 (average r = 0.75 to 0.85). A summary of these studies is tabulated by Baumgartner and Jackson.[31] They go on to mention that much of the variability related to the results from walk-run tests as compared with treadmill tests relates to the size and variance of the samples used; age, maturity, and motivation of samples; prior practice in pacing; and running experience.

Cooper[142] recommends that middle-aged beginners need approximately 6 weeks of preliminary training before taking the 12-minute or 1.5-mile tests. High school and college students and military recruits probably need less preparation for these tests.

RATING OF PERCEIVED EXERTION (RPE) SCALE

The RPE scale was first conceived and introduced by Borg.[143, 144] The original scale has a 15-grade category ranging from 6 to 20, with a descriptive verbal anchor at every odd number (Fig. 6–13, column A). More recently, Borg has recommended different terminology for describing the various anchor points (column B).[146] Borg's newer 10-grade category scale was designed with ratio properties (column C).

The rating of perceived exertion and HR are linearly related to each other and to work intensity across a variety of exercise modalities and conditions.[102, 144, 145, 147–154] The rating of perceived exertion also relates well to various physiological factors: a multiple correlation of 0.85 was found with $\dot{V}_E$, HR, lactate levels, and $\dot{V}O_2$.[155] (Note that only individual correlations are found in this reference. Multiple correlations are available from authors.)

The original concept was developed from young adults; addition of a zero to each of the points in the scale would reflect the HR value under various levels of work intensity. For example, 6 would become 60 and represent HR at rest, and 19 and 20 would represent HRmax (190 to 200 beats/min).[143, 144] When the scale was applied to persons of various ages, it was found that the same linear relationship with work intensity existed at all ages, but the HR was consistently lower at each older age increment used.[144] When subjects were placed on atropine or practolol, the HR was significantly increased or decreased in relation to the control test, but the HR values under these conditions remained linear and parallel with increased intensity of exercise.[150] Another study using propranolol showed the same results as with practolol.[102, 140] In all cases (age differences, drug effects on HR, obese versus lean subjects),[102, 140, 144, 145, 147–150, 152–154] when RPE was expressed in terms of relative work (percentage of $\dot{V}O_2$max or percentage of HRmax reserve), the RPE values were similar. Thus, when the RPE scale is used under a variety of conditions as described previously, the use of the RPE scale under its original conception (RPE of 15 = HR of 150 beats/min, and so on) is not valid. The scale is valid, though, in relation to its various anchor points (see Fig. 6–13) and when HR is expressed relative to a percentage of maximum.[102, 141, 147–154]

The importance of the RPE scale is its strong relationship to factors indicating relative fatigue. In this regard, the scale has been used for approximately 30 years in exercise testing laboratories. It has become more popular in the clinical setting during the past 5 to 10 years.[156] Its use in exercise prescription is detailed in Chapters 7 and 8.

As described previously, the RPE scale has been shown to be a valid indicator of the level of physical exertion (relative fatigue). It

| | 15-Grade Scale | | 10-Grade Scale | |
	A	*B*	*C*	
6		(No exertion at all)	0	Nothing at all
7	Very, very light	(Extremely light)	0.5	Very, very weak (just noticeable)
8			1	Very weak
9	Very light	(Very light)	2	Weak (light)
10			3	Moderate
11	Fairly light	(Light)	4	Somewhat strong
12			5	Strong (heavy)
13	Somewhat hard	(Somewhat hard)	6	
14			7	Very strong
15	Hard	(Hard–heavy)	8	
16			9	
17	Very hard	(Very hard)	10	Very, very strong (almost max)
18				
19	Very, very hard	(Extremely hard)	•	Maximal
20		(Maximal exertion)		

Figure 6–13. The rating of perceived exertion (RPE) scales developed by Borg.[144–146] Columns A and B refer to the anchor points for the original 15-grade category scale of RPE. Column C refers to the anchor points for the newer 10-grade category scale with ratio properties. Anchor points shown in column B are Borg's latest terminology used for describing the 15-grade scale.[146]

has also been shown to be reliable[144, 147] and thus can be used effectively in repeat testing. For example, if a patient rates the endpoint of a GXT 18 on one occasion, the 18 on subsequent tests should be interpreted the same way relative to the patient's feelings of fatigue. This has important implications for GXT when lactate levels, $\dot{V}O_2$, and $\dot{V}_E$ are not measured. The rating of perceived exertion gives the tester an objective indicator through which to compare the relative degree of fatigue attained from test to test.[145] Thus, if aerobic capacity and treadmill performance significantly increased or decreased and the endpoint RPE remained the same between test results, the tests could then be interpreted as representing a true change in cardiorespiratory fitness or medical status and not a reflection of whether the patient pushed as hard. Knowing the RPE is also helpful to the clinician in judging when the patient may want to terminate the test.

Few persons rate maximum at 20, with 17 to 19 being selected most often.[102, 140, 141] Pollock and associates[141] found that young, healthy subjects rated maximum at 19, middle-aged healthy subjects at 18, and cardiac patients at 17.

Although the previous information shows the value of the RPE scale, it must be interpreted in the proper context. First, there are under- and overraters, and it has been estimated that about 5 to 10 percent of the population cannot use the scale with any accuracy.[157] Use of proper instructions is important. Morgan[157] has pointed out that different psychological states can also affect RPE ratings. When the Borg scale is first introduced, the use of the following written instructions can be helpful:

> **You are now going to take part in a graded exercise test. You will be walking or running on the treadmill while we are measuring various physiological functions. We also want you to try to estimate how hard you feel the work is; that is, we want you to rate the degree of perceived exertion you feel. By perceived exertion we mean the total amount of exertion and physical fatigue. Don't concern yourself with any one factor such as leg pain, shortness of breath, or work grade, but try to concentrate on your total, inner feeling of exertion. Try to estimate as honestly and objectively as possible. Don't underestimate the degree of exertion you feel, but don't overestimate it either. Just try to estimate as accurately as possible.***

Borg[146] offers the following set of instructions to be read to or explained to the participant before GXT or training:

> **During the exercise we want you to rate your perception of exertion. We want you to use this rating scale where 6 means no exertion at**

---

*Provided by William Morgan, Ed.D., University of Wisconsin, Madison, WI. Published with permission.

all and 20 means a maximal exertion. 9 is a very light exercise, like walking slowly for some minutes (for healthy people). 13 on the scale is a somewhat heavy exercise but it still feels fine, and you should not have any problems to continue exercising. When you come to 17, "very hard," it is really very strenuous; you can still go on, but you have to push yourself very much. 19 on the scale is an extremely strenuous exercise. For most people this is an exercise as strenuous as they have ever experienced before.

Try to appraise your feeling of exertion as honestly as possible. Don't underestimate it, but don't overestimate it either. Some people are a bit insensitive or want to be "brave" and rate too low. Don't do that but try to feel your exertion as you perceive it. Don't bother about how heavy the load is physically or what the exercise objectively might be. We are only interested in your own feeling of effort and exertion. Look at the scale and the wordings and then give us a number. You can equally well give us an even as an odd number.

The written instructions can then be reinforced verbally. It is advisable to remind participants not to focus on any one problem but rather on general fatigue. For patients with angina, claudication, orthopedic problems, and similar conditions, rating their specific problem separately is helpful. It is also helpful to remind the participant of the various anchor points listed on the scale: 6 or 7 is resting, 13 to 14 is moderately difficult, 15 to 16 is hard but tolerable, and most persons rate maximum between 17 and 20. The same set of instructions can be used with the 0-to-10 scale (see Fig. 6–13) by adjusting the numbers appropriately.

Participants tend to rate treadmill and cycle ergometer exercise approximately the same.[148, 153] If relative work is taken into account, arm ergometer activity is rated similarly to leg work, i.e., percentage of $\dot{V}O_2$max or HR on each respective test mode.[102, 149, 158]

The Borg 15-point scale is not linear in relation to equal increments of increased intensity.[143–145] The scale is rather flat through a rating of 10 and then becomes curvilinear.[144, 145] Above 15 on the scale, it takes very little added intensity to increase the RPE rating. Many participants do not discriminate well at the lower end of the scale. Smutok and coworkers[159] suggested that RPE was accurate to use in exercise prescription at running speed or at an HR above 150 beats/min (80 percent of HRmax) but was inaccurate and unreliable at slower speeds, such as are used in walking programs. Contrary results have been reported by Gutmann and coworkers[160] and Pollock and coworkers[102]—i.e., patients were able to discriminate accurately at 11 to 13 on the RPE scale— and in a review by Birk and Birk[161] with a wider variety of subjects. The difference in results may be related to the subjects in the latter studies having had multiple practice periods in using the scale before data collection.

As mentioned earlier and shown in Figure 6–13, Borg[145] has published a new 10-grade category scale for differential use that has the positive attributes of a general-ratio scale. This scale is linear in relation to categories and increased intensity and has the advantage of expressing relative fatigue according to their quantitative meaning.[145] For example, the rating of 4 as shown in Figure 6–13, 10-grade scale, is twice as intense as the rating of 2. What scale should be used? It appears that both scales can be used effectively in the research and in the clinical settings, thus, it becomes a personal preference. Borg[145] states that no scale is perfect for all situations and favors the continued use of the original 15-grade category scale. Borg suggests that the newer category scale may be more suitable for use when other subjective symptoms need to be assessed and monitored, such as aches and pain and breathing difficulties. The authors also favor the use of the 15-grade category scale and have found it to be valuable in assessing and monitoring local pain and fatigue and dyspnea associated with physical exercise.

Although most research data and the clinical use of the RPE scale has been with running, walking, cycling, and arm ergometry, some evidence now supports its use with lifting and strength tasks and resistance training exercise.[162, 163] Kraemer and associates[163] found a correlation of 0.84 between lactate levels and RPE in response to heavy resistance exercise with short rest periods. During this high-intensity training session (10 exercise stations), HR rose from approximately 60 beats/min at rest to 180 beats/min after the first exercise session and remained at that level after each subsequent exercise. In contrast, both lactate levels and RPE rose steadily with each bout of exercise. More data are necessary to validate the full physiological meaning of resistance and strength training in relation to a variety of subjects, exercise modalities, and training sequences. Until such information is available, the authors recommend its use in regard to these types of programs.

A review of more recent advances in the study and clinical use of RPE is available.[145, 151, 152, 156, 161, 164, 165] In light of all the discussion concerning the RPE scale, it should not be used or interpreted in a vacuum. It is not a perfect scale and should be used in conjunction with common sense and other pertinent clinical, psychological, and physiological information. Borg's summarization of this point follows:[145]

In defense of the use of perceived exertion it may be said that there is little evidence that a certain heart rate is a better indicator of "dangerous strain" than a certain perceived exertion. On any given day one may run and achieve a heart rate of 150 and feel "fine" with

an RPE of 13, while on another day the same exertion may cause the runner to feel "bad" with an RPE of 17 as a result of physical and emotional negative factors.

The elevated RPE value may be used equally with heart rate in determining a "risk factor." Neither a single RPE value nor a heart rate measure may be used alone as an accurate indicator of "dangerous strain." They complement each other.

A "perfect" or "excellent" indicator of "dangerous strain" must involve an integration of all important risk factors, such as arrhythmias, blood pressure elevations, S-T depressions, body temperature changes, blood lactate levels, and hormonal excretions. A single, heart rate must be used in relation to the other strain variables and understood to be just one factor in a complicated pattern of interacting factors. A patient's perceived exertion is considered in exercise prescription because it is related closely to the heart rate, but it also integrates some other important strain variables.

SAFETY OF THE GRADED EXERCISE TEST

The most quoted study on the risk of a cardiovascular event associated with a GXT was the report of Rochmis and Blackburn in 1971.[166] Their survey of 73 medical centers included results from 173,000 GXTs. The overall mortality rate from these centers was one death per 10,000 tests, and the rate of serious cardiac complications (morbidity and mortality) was 4 per 10,000 tests. Other studies or surveys have shown similar results as Rochmis and Blackburn but, like the original study, do not differentiate among different patient types, type of tests, and endpoints (maximal or submaximal). Bruce and McDonough[167] reported a morbidity risk of one per 3,000 for maximal tests and 1 in 15,000 for submaximal tests. They reported no deaths in 6,000 maximal tests and 4 deaths in 102,000 submaximal tests (one per 25,500 tests).

More recent surveys or studies with patient populations or with a high percentage of subjects who are being screened for CAD show similar cardiovascular events (morbidity) associated with GXT as do the earlier studies.[77, 169-171] The striking difference with the more recent studies is the lower mortality rates.[77, 169-171] For example, Stuart and Ellestad,[77] in a survey of 1,375 centers (514,448 GXTs), found only 0.5 deaths per 10,000 tests, with a morbidity rate of 8.3 per 10,000 tests. Scherer and Kaltenbach[168] reported no deaths or morbidity in 353,638 GXTs completed on "sports persons" and one death per 42,000 tests and one morbid event per 7,400 tests with cardiac patients. Atterhog and colleagues[169] and Cahalin and colleagues[171] reported a mortality rate of 0.4 and 0.9 per 10,000 tests and a morbidity rate of 5.2 and 3.8 per 10,000 tests, respectively.

Data for clearly healthy populations or centers in which most subjects are not patients with suspected cardiovascular disease show significantly less morbidity and mortality associated with GXT. Most recently, Gibbons and colleagues[172] have reported the incidence rate on 71,914 SL-GXTs conducted at the Cooper Clinic, Dallas, Texas, from 1971 through 1987. The overall cardiac complication rate was 0.8 complications per 10,000 tests. Only six complications, including one death, were reported during this time period, with five of the six patients having a cardiac history. Further, they have had no complications in the past 10 years in 45,000 SL-GXTs. Thus, it is quite clear that the safety of GXTs has improved over the years. Ellestad[36] concluded that:

> **Even in the face of an enormous increase in volume, the mortality from stress testing has decreased at least 50 percent, and possibly more. It would seem that the risks of serious complications in stress testing are reasonable, and when using established techniques with continuous monitoring, they can be greatly minimized.**

DRUGS: EXERCISE TESTING AND TRAINING

Most patients with cardiovascular and pulmonary disease are taking medications. For the most part, medications are not contraindicative for GXT or training and often are beneficial and enhance working capacity. Van Camp[173] reviewed and tabulated the major medications and drugs that are used by subjects involved in GXT and exercise training programs and their effects on HR, BP, ECG and working capacity (Table 6–8). Lowenthal and Kendrick[174] and Lowenthal and coworkers[175] have extensive reviews on the effects of drugs and drug interactions and their relationship with the acute and chronic effects of exercise.

Of all the drugs, beta-adrenergic blockers are the most discussed in relation to exercise testing and training.[176–179] Wilmore[178] and Van Baak[178a] reviewed the advantages and disadvantages of the types of beta-blockade used and its effects on exercise testing and training. It appears that the beta-selective blockers (B_1, cardioselective) have advantages over the nonselective types. In general, B_1-selective blockers have less effect on ventilation and HRmax and thus cause smaller reductions in $\dot{V}O_2$max and working capacity than beta-blocking nonselective drugs. The effect of exercise training is also less attenuated with B_1 selective blockers. Much of the controversy reported on the effect of beta-adrenergic blockade on both acute and chronic exercise results from the varied doses of blockade used (Fig. 6–14), types of drugs, subject population (angina-limited, healthy adult, athlete), and duration and intensity of training.[176–179] Refer to review articles for details.

Text continued on page 301

Table 6–8. Effects of Medications on Heart Rate, Blood Pressure, Electrocardiographic Findings, and Exercise Capacity

Medications	Heart Rate		Blood Pressure (Rest [R] and Exercise [E])	ECG		Exercise Capacity
	Rest	Exercise		Rest	Exercise	
Beta blockers (including labetalol)	↓*	↓	↓	↓ HR*	↓ ischemia†	↑ in patients with angina; ↓ or ↔ in patients without angina
Nitrates	↑	↑ or ↔	↓ (R) ↓ or ↔ (E)	↑ HR	↑ or ↔ HR ↓ ischemia†	↑ in patients with angina; ↔ or ↓ in patients without angina; ↑ or ↔ in patients with congestive heart failure (CHF)
Calcium channel blockers						
Nifedipine	↑	↑	↓	↑ HR	↑↓ HR ↓ ischemia†	↑ in patients with angina; ↔ in patients without angina
Diltiazem	↓	↓	↓	↓ HR	↓ HR ↓ ischemia†	↑ in patients with angina; ↔ in patients without angina
Verapamil	↓	↓	↓	↓ HR	↓ HR ↓ ischemia†	↑ in patients with angina; ↔ in patients without angina
Digitalis	↓ in patients with atrial fibrillation and possibly CHF. Not significantly altered in patients with sinus rhythm	↔	↔	May produce nonspecific S–T–T-wave changes	May produce S–T–segment depression	Improved only in patients with atrial fibrillation or in patients with CHF
Diuretics	↔	↔	↔ or ↓	↔	May cause premature ventricular contractions (PVCs) and false-positive test results if hypokalemia occurs	↔, except possibly in patients with CHF (see text)

Vasodilators						
Nonadrenergic	↑ or ↔	↑ or ↔	→	↑ or ↔ HR	↑ or ↔ HR	↔, except ↑ or ↔ in patients with CHF
α-Adrenergic blockers	↔	↔	→	↔	↔	↔
Antiadrenergic agents without selective blockade of peripheral receptors	↓ or ↔	↓ or ↔	→	↓ or ↔ HR	↓ or ↔ HR	↔
Antiarrhythmic agents						
Class I						
Quinidine	↑ or ↔	↑ or ↔	↑ or ↔ (R) ↔ (E)	May prolong QRS and Q-T intervals	Quinidine may cause false-negative test results.	↔
Disopyramide						
Procainamide	↔	↔	↔	May prolong QRS and Q-T intervals	Procainamide may cause false-positive test results.	↔
Phenytoin						
Tocainide						
Mexiletine						
Encainide						
Flecainide						
Class II Beta blockers	(see previous entry)	(see previous entry)				
Class III Amiodarone	→	→	↔	↔	↔	↔
Class IV Calcium channel blockers	(see previous entry)	(see previous entry)				
Bronchodilators						
Methylxanthines	↑ or ↔	↑ or ↔	↑, ↔, or ↓	↑ or ↔ HR; may produce PVCs	↑ or ↔ HR; may produce PVCs	Bronchodilators ↑ exercise capacity in patients limited by bronchospasm.
Sympathomimetic agents	↑ or ↔	↑ or ↔	↑, ↔, or ↓	↑ or ↔ HR	↑ or ↔ HR	
Cromolyn sodium	↔	↔	↔	↔	↔	
Corticosteroids	↔	↔	↔	↔	↔	

Table continued on following page

297

Table 6–8. Effects of Medications on Heart Rate, Blood Pressure, Electrocardiographic Findings, and Exercise Capacity *Continued*

Medications	Heart Rate		Blood Pressure (Rest [R] and Exercise [E])	ECG		Exercise Capacity
	Rest	Exercise		Rest	Exercise	
Hyperlipidemic agents						↔
Clofibrate may provoke arrhythmias and angina in patients with prior myocardial infarction. Dextrothyroxine may ↑ HR and BP at rest and during exercise, provoke arrhythmias, and worsen myocardial ischemia and angina. Nicotinic acid may ↓ BP. Probucol may cause Q-T interval prolongation. All other hyperlipidemic agents have no effect on HR, BP, and ECG.						
Psychotropic medications						
Minor tranquilizers						↔
Antidepressants	↑ or ↔	↑ or ↔	↓ or ↔ or ↔	(see text)	May cause false-positive test results	
May ↓ HR and BP by controlling anxiety. No other effects.						
Major tranquilizers	↑ or ↔	↑ or ↔	↓ or ↔	(see text)	May cause false-positive or false-negative test results	
Lithium	↔	↔	↔	May cause T-wave changes and arrhythmias	May cause T-wave changes and arrhythmias	
Nicotine	↑ or ↔	↑ or ↔	↑	↑ or ↔ HR; may provoke ischemia, arrhythmias	↑ or ↔ HR; may provoke ischemia, arrhythmias	↔, except ↑ or ↔ in patients with angina; ↔

Medications	Rest HR	Rest BP / notes	Exercise HR / notes	Exercise (cont.)	Maximal Exercise Capacity
Antihistamines	↔	↔	↔	↔	↔
Cold medications with sympathomimetic agents	Effects similar to those described in *Sympathomimetic agents*, although magnitude of effects is usually diminished				↔
Thyroid medications Only levothyroxine	↑	↑	↑ HR; provoke arrhythmias; ↑ ischemia	↑ HR; provoke arrhythmias; ↑ ischemia	↔, unless angina worsened
Alcohol	↔	Chronic use may have role in ↑ BP	May provoke arrhythmias	May provoke arrhythmias	↔
Hypoglycemic agents Insulin and oral agents	↔	↔	↔	↔	↔
Dipyridamole	↔	↔	↔	↔	↔
Anticoagulants	↔	↔	↔	↔	↔
Antigout medications	↔	↔	↔	↔	↔
Antiplatelet medications	↔	↔	↔	↔	↔
Pentoxifylline	↔	↔	↔	↔	↑ or ↔ in patients limited by intermittent claudication

↑ = increase, ↔ = no effect, ↓ = decrease.
*Beta blockers with intrinsic sympathomimetic activity lower resting HR only slightly.
†May prevent or delay myocardial ischemia.

(Reprinted with permission from Van Camp, S. P.: Pharmacologic factors in exercise and exercise testing. In Blair, S. N., Painter, P., Pate, R. R., Smith, L. K., and Taylor, C. B. [eds.]: **Resource Manual for Guidelines for Exercise Testing and Prescription.** Philadelphia, Lea & Febiger, 1988, pp. 135–154.)

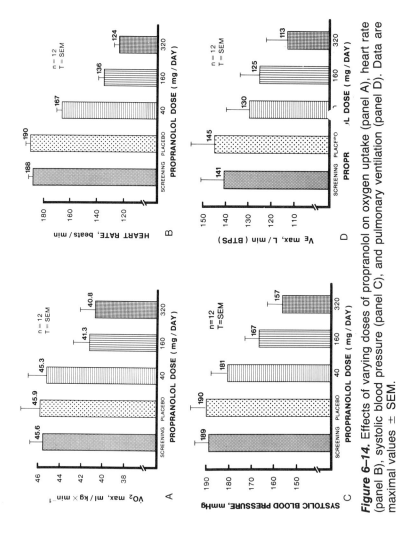

Figure 6-14. Effects of varying doses of propranolol on oxygen uptake (panel A), heart rate (panel B), systolic blood pressure (panel C), and pulmonary ventilation (panel D). Data are maximal values ± SEM.

An example from one of these problems, Figure 6–14 shows the dose-response effect of propranolol on $\dot{V}O_2$max (panel A), HRmax (panel B), systolic BPmax (panel C), and $\dot{V}_E$max (panel D) for 12 healthy volunteers.[140, 179] The screening test was an initial GXT given to subjects upon entering the study. The other four GXTs were administered randomly, 2 weeks apart, with propranolol or a placebo dosage taken for 4 days before each test. Dosage was disguised in white opaque capsules so that both subjects and investigators did not know the contents. The results clearly show a dose response in relation to maximal exercise with a moderate clinical dose, 40 mg/day of propranolol, significantly reducing HRmax and systolic BPmax but not effecting $\dot{V}O_2$max and treadmill performance. In all cases, RPEmax was similar (about 19). From a clinical standpoint, resting HR and BP showed a dose-response reduction plateauing at the 160 mg/day dosage.

For information on exercise prescription for patients on beta-adrenergic blockade, see Chapter 8. In general, because the relationship between percentage of HRmax reserve and percentage of $\dot{V}O_2$max are similar during submaximal exercise for patients on or off beta-blocking drugs, the determination of target HR by percentage of HR from symptom-limited maximum (as described in Chapter 7) can be used. Figure 6–15 shows the dose-response relationship between HR (panel A), $\dot{V}O_2$ (panel B), RPE (panel C), and oxygen pulse (panel D) and exercise time on a treadmill from 12 volunteers on varying doses of propranolol.[140, 179] The exercise intensity shown in Figure 6–15 was submaximal. An increase in stroke volume (and oxygen extraction), reflective of the increase in oxygen pulse, compensates for the lower HR to keep $\dot{V}O_2$ (cardiac output) constant at submaximal levels of exercise. The relationship between $\dot{V}O_2$ and RPE with exercise time are similar over varying doses of propranolol. Thus, by calculating the percentage of HRmax reserve over the range of 50 to 85 percent, as generally prescribed for most patients, gives the appropriate prescription.[102, 105, 141] The calculated prescription is based on the GXT results with the patient on the required dosage.

Another important factor regarding the use of beta-adrenergic blockers is their potential deleterious effect on thermoregulation in patients during exercise training.[180, 181] The problem appears to be mainly with the beta blocker nonselective drugs, which cause an accelerated sweat rate that could lead to dehydration.[180] Gordon[180] recommends the need for patients taking beta-adrenergic blockers to adhere strictly to a fluid replacement regimen during exercise training. Heat regulation is normally not a problem during the shorter time span of the GXT.

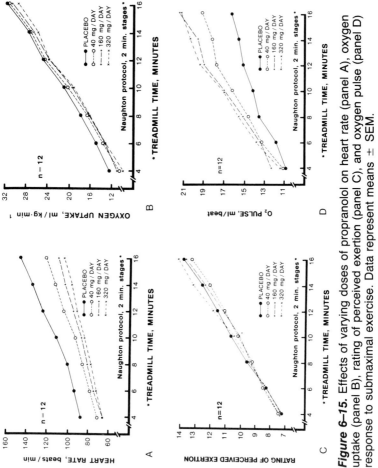

Figure 6-15. Effects of varying doses of propranolol on heart rate (panel A), oxygen uptake (panel B), rating of perceived exertion (panel C), and oxygen pulse (panel D) response to submaximal exercise. Data represent means ± SEM.

It is important for the exercise test technologist and exercise specialists to be familiar with the various drugs shown in Table 6–8 and their effect on acute (GXT) and chronic (training) exercise. The exercise and rehabilitation team should be familiar with the side effects associated with drugs so that they can be reported to the primary physician. One of the purposes of the GXT and monitored exercise program is to help the primary physician evaluate the effect of the patient's drug regimen.

A final point of importance to note concerning drug therapy relates to the timing in which medications are taken. All drugs generally have certain half-lives, and the peak effect of various drugs differ. Thus, it is important to be aware of these factors, and the timing of the GXT and training sessions should be consistent in respect to time of drug administration.

Preparation for Exercise Testing for Diagnostic Purposes

The diagnostic GXT is usually performed with a multiple-lead ECG system.[36,37] As shown from Table 6–9, approximately 70 to 89 percent of the abnormal S-T–segment responses to exercise can be picked up by lead V_5 alone.[182] It appears that the addition of at least one precordial (horizontal) lead (V_1 to V_3) and an inferior (vertical) lead (II, III, or V_F) adds significantly to the diagnosis.

Figure 6–16 shows the Mason-Likar 12-lead ECG system, and Figure 6–17 illustrates a 3-lead system popularized by Ellestad.[36] Each of these systems has been popularly used and is well accepted. In comparison to the standard 12-lead system, which uses the conventional ankle and wrist attachments, placing the limb leads

Table 6–9. Six Series of Patients Studied with Multilead Exercise Tests Evaluating Relative Yield of Abnormal Responses in Leads Other Than V_5

Study	V_5 Alone	Other Leads Alone
Blackburn and Katigbak[183]	89%	4% (aV_F), 2% (II), 1% (V_3), 2% (V_4), 2% (V_6)
Mason and associates[184]	70%	7% (II, III), 3.6% (V_3), 7% (V_4), 12.5% (V_6)
Phibbs and Buckels[185]		
Series A	85.5%	85.5% (II, aV_F, III) 4% (V_6)
Series B	79%	15% (II, aV_F, III) 3% (V_6), 2% (V_4). One each in I, V_1, and V_{2-4}
Robertson and associates[186]	75%	10% (II, aV_F, III), 5% (V_4), 5% (V_6), 5% (mixed)
Tucker and associates[187]	70%	17% (aV_F), 13% (other)

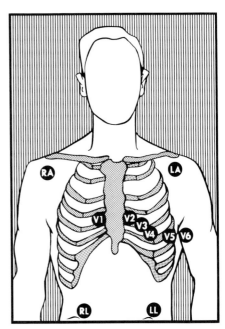

Figure 6–16. The Mason-Likar 12-lead exercise ECG lead system. (Reproduced with permission from Froelicher, V. F.: **Exercise and the Heart: Clinical Concepts,** 2nd Ed. Chicago, Year Book Medical Publishers, 1987.)

at the shoulders and base of the torso can eliminate most of the movement artifact found during the GXT. Although the modified electrode placement systems offer an ECG pattern similar to that of the conventional lead system, they display a more rightward axis of the ECG, and the QRS vectors are directed more inferiorly, posteriorly, and rightward.[182a] Thus, in the initial screening, a standard 12-lead ECG using the conventional limb leads should be taken before attaching the limb leads to the torso. Caution should be taken if the limb leads, as shown in Figure 6–16, are moved more onto the abdomen and chest. It may eliminate additional movement artifact, but it will further distort the ECG.[37, 182a]

For the most part, standard commercial ECG recorders offer acceptable frequency responses to obtain ECGs of diagnostic quality (0 to 100 Hz). Alternation of the 25 to 45 Hz frequency response is the most common cause of the distortion of the S-T segment.[37] See the American Heart Association's standards for ECG recording equipment and Froelicher[37,89] for more details concerning proper frequency responses, ECG distortion, and calibration checking of ECG equipment.

Advances in the manufacturing of electrodes and cable connectors for GXT have helped reduce movement artifact. Both nondisposable and disposable electrodes can be used. Silverplated or silver–silver chloride crystal pellets are used as electrode materials.

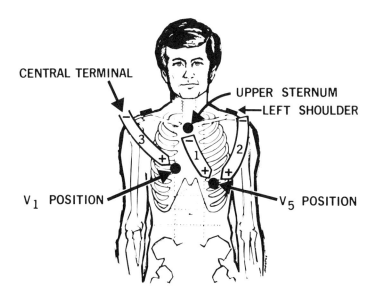

CENTRAL TERMINAL

UPPER STERNUM
LEFT SHOULDER

V₁ POSITION

V₅ POSITION

1. BIPOLAR — STERNUM TO V_5 (CM$_5$)
2. BIPOLAR — LEFT SHOULDER TO V_5 (VERTICAL)
3. CENTRAL TERMINAL TO V_1 (HORIZONTAL)

Figure 6–17. A 3-lead ECG monitoring system described and used by Ellestad.[36] It shows the location of the 2 bipolar electrode systems and the V_1 attachment. This system provides not only the most sensitive single monitoring lead (CM$_5$) but a vertical and horizontal lead system as well. (Reprinted with permission from Ellestad, M. S.: **Stress Testing Principles and Practices,** 3rd Ed. Philadelphia, F. A. Davis, 1986.)

Nondisposable electrodes are recessed and have to be filled with electrode paste, whereas disposable electrodes are pregelled. The disposable electrodes are more convenient but are significantly more expensive. To obtain a good skin-to-electrode contact, the outer epidermal layer of skin must be removed. This can be accomplished by the use of an emery cloth, making light abrasions with a stick or hand-held drill. In hairy people, the area of electrode placement must first be shaved. Usually the patient is placed in the supine position, the anatomical landmarks for electrode placement are noted (marked), the skin is cleansed with an alcohol-saturated gauze pad, the epidermal layer of skin is removed, and the electrodes are firmly placed. Do not underestimate the importance of proper skin preparation. The use of an alternating current (AC) impedance meter (ohmmeter) aids in evaluating skin resistance. A force of less than 5,000 ohms is recommended, and each electrode is tested against a common electrode. Although more expensive, a drill-type applicator with a built-in impedance meter has been developed for electrode application (Quickprep, Quinton Instrument Co., Seattle, WA). The electrode has an abrasive center that is automatically spun until the proper skin impedance is determined.

Once the electrodes are in place, the BP cuff is attached. Baseline ECG tracings are determined in the supine, sitting, and standing positions. Another tracing is recorded after 30 seconds of hyperventilation. Because of an occasional problem with hypotension (faintness), hyperventilation should be done in the sitting position. Changes in ECG or BP caused by orthostasis and hyperventilation should be noted before beginning the test.[36, 37]

Diagnostic Aspects of Graded Exercise Testing

This section covers some of the basic aspects of GXT and its diagnostic value. A more detailed description of the medical aspects of the ECG,[3, 10, 20, 21, 36, 37, 182–199a] radionuclide angiography,[37, 200–205] and thallium scintigraphy[37, 205–207] is found elsewhere. See Figure A–6, Appendix A, for an example of a GXT data collection form. The guidelines for exercise testing established by a joint task force of the American College of Cardiology and the American Heart Association are important for the clinician to review.[194] The statement is valuable in attempting to clarify questions concerning indications for exercise testing and discussing the issues regarding the value of the GXT with different patient populations.

Many aspects of the GXT have been shown to be important for diagnostic and prognostic purposes. Significant S-T–segment depression or elevation, abnormal HR and BP response to exercise, angina pectoris, dysrhythmia, and poor effort tolerance ($\dot{V}O_2$max) have been shown to be of significant value in predicting future cardiac events.[36, 37, 189, 199, 199b] Significant S-T–segment depression has a high correlation with myocardial ischemia; usually, a minimum of 1.5 to 2 mm of upsloping and 1 mm of flat or downsloping S-T–segment depression, 0.08 seconds from the J point, is considered significant.[36, 37] Ellestad[36] has recommended several criteria for determining significant S-T–segment depression with GXT, depending on resting S-T–T configuration, exercise or postexercise S-T configuration, and S-T–segment depression and point of measurement. Table 6–10 outlines these specific criteria. It should be noted that for the normal recording speed of 25 mm/sec and 1 cm deflection with 1 mV of electrical impulse, each small 1 mm square of the ECG paper represents 0.04 seconds horizontally and 0.10 mV

Table 6–10. Criteria for Significant S-T–Segment Depression with Maximal Exercise as Recommended by Ellestad

Resting S-T–T Configuration	Exercise or Postexercise S-T Configuration	S-T Depression and Point of Measurement
Normal	Horizontal	1.0 mm at 60 msec from J-point
	Upsloping	1.5 mm at 80 msec from J-point
	Downsloping	1.0 mm more depressed than at rest
Flat or sagging S-T and T	Horizontal	1.0 mm more depressed than at rest
	Upsloping	1.5 mm more depressed than at rest at 80 msec from J-point
	Downsloping	1.0 mm more depressed than at rest
Inverted T	Horizontal	1.5 mm at 60 msec from J-point
	Upsloping	1.5 mm at 80 msec from J-point
	Downsloping	1.5 mm at 20 msec from J-point

Note that these current criteria are slightly different depending on the configuration of the resting S-T segment and T-wave.

(Reprinted with permission from Ellestad, M.S.: **Stress Testing Principles and Practices**, 3rd Ed. Philadelphia, F.A. Davis Co., 1986.)

vertically. Figure 6–18 shows a normal (left panel) and an abnormal (right panel) ECG. Figure 6–19 (upper panel) shows an example of significant upsloping S-T–segment depression, and Figure 6–20 (lower panel) shows nonsignificant upsloping S-T–segment depression. Figure 6–19 (lower panel) shows an example of significant downsloping S-T–segment depression and Figure 6–20 (middle panel) shows significant horizontal S-T–segment depression. Other ECG responses to GXT that are associated with myocardial ischemia are S-T–segment elevation,[196] T-wave inversion, U-wave inversion (mainly found during early recovery period), increased R-wave amplitude, and loss of Q-wave.[10, 36, 37] The magnitude of S-T–segment change from rest (at least 3 to 4 mm), how early it is precipitated, and how long it persists are directly related to the severity of disease.[36, 37, 194]

The exercise test has been shown to be a useful and reliable technique in eliciting arrhythmias, evaluating drug efficacy, and determining toxic drug effects.[208] There are different classification systems and degrees of significance used for rating dysrhythmias.[10, 36, 37, 208–213] Significant or complex dysrhythmias usually include the following: exercise induced frequent unifocal (more than 10 beats/min or greater than 30 percent of total beats) or multifocal (more than 4 beats/min) premature ventricular contractions (PVCs), ventricular couplets (more than one or two consecutive PVCs), R-on-T ventricular extrasystoles (early premature contraction on T-wave), ventricular tachycardia (three or more consecutive PVCs), atrial tachycardia or fibrillation, left or right bundle branch block, and second or third-degree heart block.[10, 36, 37]

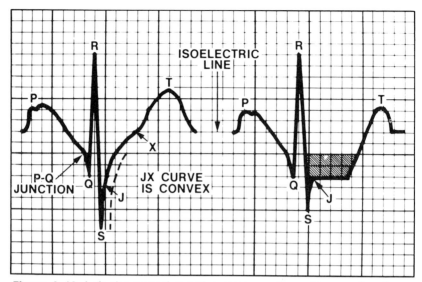

Figure 6–18. Left, the normal exercise electrocardiographic complex. It can be noted that the P-Q segment is deflected below the isoelectric line. This point is considered to be a baseline for determining S-T–segment abnormalities. Right, a horizontal S-T–segment depression of 2.0 mm as measured from the P-Q segment. (Reprinted with permission from Ellestad, M. S.: **Stress Testing Principles and Practices,** 3rd Ed. Philadelphia, F. A. Davis, Co., 1986.)

Figure 6–19 shows an example of a single PVC (lower panel). Figure 6–20 illustrates a multifocal PVC (middle panel), ventricular couplet (upper panel), and ventricular tachycardia (lower panel). When referring to the significance of dysrhythmia in regard to sudden death, Lown and Wolf[210] have developed the grading system shown in Table 6–11. Grades are designated according to severity of risk, with grades 4 and 5 considered most significant. Controversy

Table 6–11. The Lown and Wolf Grading System

Lown Grade	Definition
0	No PVCs
1	Fewer than 30 PVCs/hr
2	30 or more PVCs/hr
3	Multiform PVCs
4A	Paired PVCs
4B	Ventricular tachycardia
5	R-on-T PVCs

(Data taken from Lown, B.: Sudden cardiac death: the major challenge confronting contemporary cardiology. **Am. J. Cardiol.** *43*:313–328, 1979; Lown, B., and Wolf, M.: Approaches to sudden death from coronary heart disease. **Circulation** *44*:130–142, 1971.)

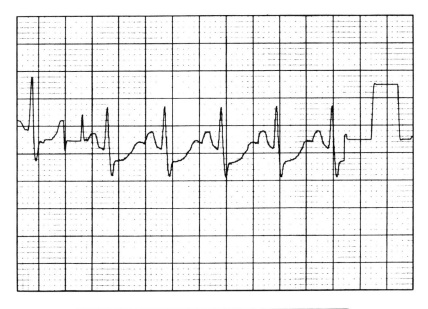

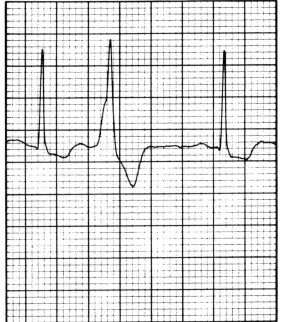

Figure 6–19. The upper panel shows an example of 2 mm upsloping S-T–segment depression and the lower panel shows 1.6 mm downsloping S-T–segment depression. The lower panel also shows an example of a single premature ventricular contraction.

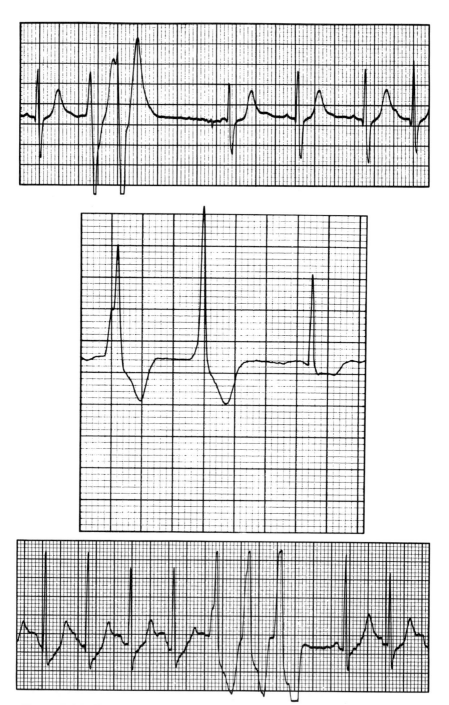

Figure 6–20. The upper panel shows an example of a ventricular couplet, the middle panel a multifocal premature ventricular contraction, and the lower panel a ventricular tachycardia. The middle panel also shows an example of 2 mm horizontal S-T–segment depression.

exists over the use of this system.[212] In addition, electrophysiologists find it difficult to agree on any one system. See Akhtar, Wolf, and Denker[213] for further details on dysrhythmias and sudden death. Whatever the system used, it is agreed that patients with significant (complex) dysrhythmias and left ventricular dysfunction (an ejection fraction of less than 0.50) are at greater risk for sudden death than patients with less complex dysrhythmias or left ventricular dysfunction alone.

Heart rate and systolic BP rise linearly with increased levels of exercise, and diastolic BP should decrease slightly or may remain rather constant.[71] Froelicher[37] and Ellestad[36] find a wide variation in HR and systolic BP responses to exercise. The standard deviation for HRmax is approximately ± 12 beats/min.[37, 214] It has been suggested that the average HR and systolic BP response to exercise is approximately 8 to 10 beats/min and 7 to 10 mmHg, respectively, for each 1 MET increase in work load.[26] These standards were developed from the data collected on average men and are not relevant to elite endurance athletes. Subsequent data gathered on women show an 11 to 13 beat/min rise in HR and a 5 to 6 mmHg increase in systolic BP per 1 MET increase in work load.[66] Although the HR response per MET is less for trained than for sedentary persons, not much difference is found between groups for rises in systolic BP.[65, 66] Cardiac patients and patients on beta-blocking drugs have a blunted HR and systolic BP response to increased exercise. Heart rate increased between 5 and 7 beats/min per MET (see Fig. 8–7 for HR data on patients soon after CABG surgery).[215] For patients not on beta-blocking medication, the blunted HR response to exercise for cardiac patients persists for approximately 3 to 6 months.[216] If a patient is apprehensive or unfamiliar with the GXT procedure, an artificially high HR and systolic BP may be present initially. Under these conditions, a slight fall in these values may occur early in the test.[33, 36]

A chronotropic (very low HR) response to GXT in untrained individuals reflects an abnormal response to exercise and has significant prognostic value.[36, 37] Usually, depending on the person's age, the HRmax should reach a minimum of 130 to 150 beats/min. Do not look at HR alone for diagnosis. Pollock tested a highly fit master runner (52 years of age) who had an HRmax of 138 beats/min. He had a good HR reserve, a resting HR of 35 beats/min, and a $\dot{V}O_2$max of 53 ml $\cdot$ kg^{-1} $\cdot$ min^{-1} (unpublished data from author). When maximal effort is approached, the HR and systolic BP responses level off.[71] At maximal effort, systolic BP may begin to fall but should rebound within 30 to 60 seconds of recovery.[36] Systolic BP for highly trained individuals may return to near preexercise levels within one to two minutes of recovery.

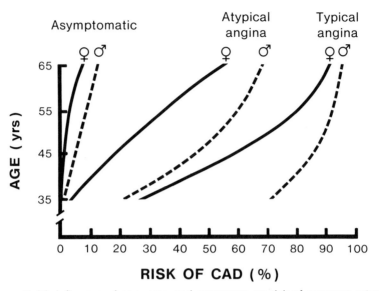

Figure 6–21. Influence of age, sex, and symptoms on risk of coronary artery disease (CAD) (derived from data of Diamond, G. A., and Forrester, J. S.[20]). (Reprinted with permission from Epstein, S. E.: Implications of probability analysis on the strategy used for noninvasive detection of coronary artery disease. **Am. J. Cardiol.** 46:491–499, 1980.)

A drop in systolic BP during the submaximal portion of the GXT (both at steady state and with increased work load) is clearly an abnormal response. A systolic BP response above 250 mmHg has been suggested as an endpoint for GXT,[10] but values of 250 to 280 mmHg have been recorded without incidence.[37] Bruce and associates[3] have shown that a maximal systolic BP response of less than 130 mmHg, along with cardiomegaly or a functional capacity of less than 4 METs, significantly increased the annual morbidity and mortality rate in the Seattle Heart Watch project.

Development of angina pectoris during exercise is the most significant finding associated with ischemia (CAD).[36, 37] Approximately 90 percent of patients with angina have been shown to have significant CAD by angiography (Fig. 6–21).[21, 37]

Predictive Value of the Graded Exercise Test

The prognostic and diagnostic value of the GXT depends not only on the various abnormal findings of the GXT as described in the previous sections but also on the pretest likelihood or prevalence of CAD of the population tested. The Bayes theorem states that

Table 6–12. Relation of Prevalence of a Disease and Predictive Value
of a Test*

Actual Disease Prevalence (%)	Predictive Value of a Positive Test (%)	Predictive Value of a Negative Test (%)
1	16.1	99.9
2	27.9	99.9
5	50.0	99.7
10	67.9	99.4
20	82.6	98.7
50	95.0	95.0
75	98.3	83.7
100	100.0	—

*Sensitivity and specificity rates each equal 95%.
(From Vecchio, T. H.: Predictive value of a single diagnostic test in unselected populations. **N. Engl. J. Med.** 274:1171–1177, 1966. Reprinted with permission of the **N. Engl. J. Med.**)

"the odds of a patient having the disease after a test will be the product of the odds before the test and the odds that the test provided true results."[37] For example, Table 6–12 shows the relation of disease prevalence in regard to the prediction value of a positive (abnormal) or negative (normal) test result.[217]

To explain the Bayes theorem more clearly, the definitions that are used to demonstrate the diagnostic value of a test have been described.[20, 21, 36, 37, 217] In Table 6–13, Froelicher[37] gives the definitions for sensitivity, specificity, relative risk, and the predictive

Table 6–13. Definitions and Calculation of Terms Used to Demonstrate the
Diagnostic Value of a Test

$$\text{Sensitivity} = \frac{\text{TP}}{\text{TP} + \text{FN}} \times 100 \qquad \text{Relative risk} = \frac{\dfrac{\text{TP}}{\text{TP} + \text{FP}}}{\dfrac{\text{FN}}{\text{TN} + \text{FN}}}$$

$$\text{Specificity} = \frac{\text{TN}}{\text{FP} + \text{TN}} \times 100 \qquad \genfrac{}{}{0pt}{}{\text{Predictive value}}{\text{of abnormal test}} = \frac{\text{TP}}{\text{TP} + \text{FP}} \times 100$$

Predictive value of an abnormal response is the percentage of individuals with an abnormal test who have disease.

Relative risk, or risk ratio, is the relative rate of occurrence of a disease in the group with an abnormal test compared with those with a normal test.

TP = true positives, or those with abnormal test results and disease; FN = false negatives, or those with normal test results and with disease; TN = true negatives, or those with normal test results and no disease; FP = false positives, or those with abnormal test results and no disease.

(Reproduced with permission from Froelicher, V. F.; **Exercise and the Heart: Clinical Concepts**, 2nd Ed. Chicago, Year Book Medical Publishers, 1987.)

value of a test. The terms sensitivity and specificity are commonly used to determine how valid a test is in differentiating between patients with or without CAD. Sensitivity of a test refers to the percentage of patients with disease who have an abnormal test result. Specificity of a test refers to the percentage of participants without disease who have a normal test result. The problem with diagnostic testing is that no test is ever perfect and must be interpreted in both the context of the test results (post-test likelihood of disease) and the population from which the patient is being tested (pretest likelihood of disease). Froelicher[37] best describes the problem of overlap among tests (measurement values) to predict CAD with groups with and without disease. Figure 6–22 shows two bell-shaped curves illustrating the distribution of persons with (C) and without (A) CAD. The optimal test (B) would be able to attain the best separation of the two curves without much overlap. Unfortunately most tests used to diagnose CAD have varying degrees of overlap. Froelicher[37] further illustrates that the problem in predicting CAD from various tests (including the exercise ECG) is that if the criterion value used to predict CAD is established too far to the right (Fig. 6–22)—e.g., 2 mm of S-T–segment depression—in order to identify nearly all the normals as being free of disease (giving the test a high specificity), then a substantial number of those with disease are called normal. In contrast, if the criterion value used is far to the left—e.g., 0.5 mm of S-T–segment depression—it will identify almost all of those with disease as being abnormal, giving the test a high sensitivity. In the latter case, though, many normals would be classified abnormal. Sensitivity and specificity are inversely related, and thus, a criterion should be set that offers the best predictive accuracy.[37]

Epstein,[21] using the data of Diamond and Forrester,[20] showed

Figure 6–22. Bell-shaped curves that illustrate the distribution of individuals with test results expressed as continuous variables. The optimal test (B) separates the normal (A) and diseased (C) groups, which have little overlap. (Reproduced with permission from Froelicher, V. F.: **Exercise and the Heart: Clinical Concepts,** 2nd Ed. Chicago, Year Book Medical Publishers, 1987.)

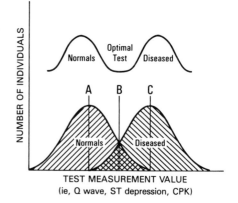

how age, symptoms, and risk factors are used to determine the pretest likelihood of having CAD. Figure 6–21 shows the risk of CAD in relation to age, sex, and angina pectoris. Note that for both atypical and typical angina, diagnosis and determination of risk are significantly more difficult in women. The same is true for women when the results of the GXT (S-T–segment change) and testing with radionuclides (static and dynamic imaging) are used.

Epstein[21] illustrates well that once the pretest likelihood of disease and the results from various tests are available (post-test likelihood of disease), then a family of curves can be drawn to estimate the likelihood of disease. The use of intercepting lines based on the appropriate sensitivity and specificity permits a revised (post-test) determination of likelihood of disease. Figure 6–23 illustrates the likelihood of CAD with increased S-T–segment depression, and Figure 6–24 is based on the ECG results of a GXT (ECG EX) plus thallium perfusion scanning (TL SCAN) and radionuclide cineangiography (RN CINE). Thus, it is easy to surmise from these figures that increased S-T–segment depression and the addition of TL SCAN and RN CINE increase the likelihood of correctly categorizing patients in regard to the probability of having

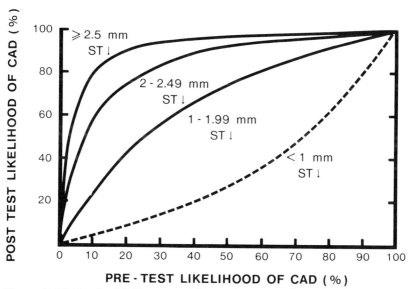

Figure 6–23. Family of S-T–segment depression curves (based on data derived from Diamond, G. A., and Forrester, J. S.[20]) and likelihood of coronary artery disease (CAD). ST ↓ = S-T–segment depression. (Reprinted with permission from Epstein, S. E.: Implications of probability analysis on the strategy used in noninvasive detection of coronary artery disease. **Am. J. Cardiol.** 46:491–499, 1980.)

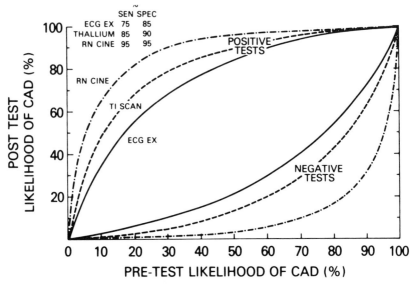

Figure 6–24. Probability of coronary artery disease (CAD). Comparison of electrocardiographic exercise testing (ECG EX), thallium perfusion scanning (TI SCAN), and radionuclide cineangiography (RN CINE). (Sensitivity [SEB] and specificity [SPEC] values are approximations derived from published series.) (Reprinted with permission from Epstein, S. E.: Implications of probability analysis on the strategy used in noninvasive detection of coronary artery disease. **Am. J. Cardiol.** 46:491–499, 1980.)

disease. Although most research supports the value of Bayesian theory applied to GXT (diagnosis and prognosis),[20, 21] some potential pitfalls have been identified by Hlatky and associates;[218] the main issue is they feel that clinical factors such as age, gender, and anginal symptoms can affect sensitivity and specificity, independent of any relationship with disease severity. They go on to suggest that a full understanding of the GXT as a diagnostic tool will not be complete until populations of old, middle-aged, and young men and women are tested who have a variety of symptom types and severities; presence or absence of prior MI; one-, two-, or three-vessel disease; and high or low ejection fractions.

For those not familiar with nuclear cardiology, two of the noninvasive procedures used to evaluate cardiac function are briefly described.[37, 205] As mentioned previously, they include TL SCAN and RN CINE. The TL SCAN is usually performed in conjunction with a GXT. In this case, an intravenous line is placed into the right arm before the test, and the GXT proceeds as previously described. During the last minute of exercise, approximately 15 mCI of [201]thallium is injected intravenously. After an abbreviated recovery (usually less than 5 minutes), the patient is immediately placed under a gamma camera, and images are acquired in the anterior, 45-degree left anterior oblique, and left lateral positions or in the 70-degree left anterior oblique position. The measurements are repeated approximately 4 hours later. The technique is based on the premise that the potassium analog ^{201}thallium goes where capillary perfusion (blood flow) is adequate to avoid ischemia. This generally depends on two factors, capillary perfusion and cell viability. Necrotic or scar tissue and ischemic areas will not perfuse, whereas viable tissue will (Fig. 6–25). Thus, by evaluating the immediate postexercise TL SCAN and comparing it with the resting values (4 hours after exercise), normal, scarred, and ischemic areas may be differentiated.

The RN CINE evaluates the dynamic action of the heart.[37, 205] Although different techniques may be used (gated or first pass), both derive an outer perimeter of the left ventricular chamber during systole (end-systolic volume) and diastole (end-diastolic volume) (Fig. 6–26). The test is performed with a patient seated or supine, with exercise performed on a modified cycle ergometer. Patients exercise with a gamma camera placed against the chest, and a radionuclide (e.g., ^{99m}technetium) is introduced into the venous system (usually through the antecubital vein). The scintillation camera picks up the counts as the radioactive materials pass

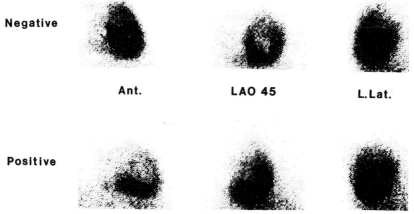

Negative

Ant.   LAO 45   L.Lat.

Positive

Figure 6–25. A normal (upper panel) and an abnormal (lower panel) thallium scintigram. The normal scan reveals a relatively homogeneous distribution of the indicator, whereas the abnormal study reveals an anteroseptal defect seen best in the anterior and LAO views. (Reprinted with permission from Schmidt, D. H., and Port, S.: The clinical and research application of nuclear cardiology. In Pollock, M. L., and Schmidt, D. H. [eds.]: **Heart Disease and Rehabilitation,** 2nd Ed. New York, Churchill Livingstone, 1986, pp. 149–166.)

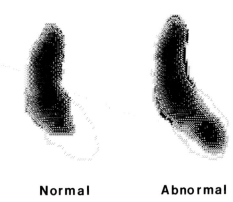

Normal   **Abnormal**

Figure 6–26. Radionuclide angiograms done in the right anterior oblique position. A normal study (left) and an abnormal study (right) are shown. Wall motion is represented by the distance between the end-diastolic perimeter and the end-systolic image. (Reprinted with permission from Schmidt, D. H., and Port, S.: The clinical and research application of nuclear cardiology. In Pollock, M. L., and Schmidt, D. H. [eds.]: **Heart Disease and Rehabilitation,** 2nd Ed. New York, Churchill Livingstone, 1986, pp. 149–166.)

through the heart. The RN CINE method is particularly good for determination of ejection fraction and regional wall motion. See Schmidt and Port[205] and Froelicher[37] for more details concerning methodology and interpretation of radionuclide procedures.

More recently, exercise echocardiography is becoming more popular as a diagnostic tool to detect CAD.[37, 219, 220] Two-dimensional echocardiography is a practical means of assessing cardiac function and, in particular, regional left ventricular function. Feigenbaum (presentation at the Indiana Heart Institute, September, 1988) stated that with the multiple tomographic views available, every segment of the left ventricular cavity can be examined from two different dimensions. He felt that with the newer computer technology, technically satisfactory exercise echocardiograms are attainable in over 90 percent of patients. Although the technique still has problems its comparable accuracy with that of nuclear tests gives it many advantages to the patient (no radiation or intravenous injections.)

Clearly the optimal exercise test of the future will include all aspects of the SL-GXT as described earlier, with the assessment of oxygen consumption and various ventilatory gas exchange measurements,[37, 59, 221] ECG, and evaluation of cardiac function all in one test.[36, 37] Froelicher[37] points out how modern computer technology has improved the ECG data gathering process and has provided the clinician with a more noise- and artifact-free ECG image. He also reviews some of the newer computer methods for evaluating S-T–segment change.

Body Composition

This section deals with the various techniques used for measuring body composition. Both laboratory and field techniques are described and illustrated. Determination of ideal weights and interpretation of results are discussed.

MEASUREMENT

Many methods are currently available for estimating body density (percentage of body fat).[222] The most common are the underwater weighing, volume displacement, radiographic analysis, [40]potassium, isotopic dilution, and ultrasound techniques. More recently, electrical conductance, computerized tomography, and magnetic resonance imaging have become more popular.[222, 223] Behnke and Wilmore[222] and Forbes[223] describe the principles and methodologies of these techniques. Because of time, equipment, and space requirements, these methods are not generally used in clinical practice. Anthropometric measures (skinfold fat and body circumference and diameter measures) are more practical for use in a clinical or nonlaboratory setting.[30, 222, 225]

UNDERWATER WEIGHING

Principle, Equations, and Measurement Errors. Of the various laboratory techniques used for determining body density, only the underwater weighing method is described here. This technique is the most widely used laboratory procedure for measuring body density. The underwater weighing technique is based on Archimedes' principle. It utilizes the "basic physical principle that a body immersed in a fluid is acted on by a buoyancy force, which is evidenced by a loss of weight equal to the weight of the displaced fluid."[222] In other words, an object placed in water must be buoyed up by a counterforce that equals the weight of the water it displaces. The density of bone and muscle tissue (1.2 to 3.0) is higher than that of water, whereas fat (0.90) is less dense than water.[222, 226] Therefore, a person with proportionately more bone and muscle mass for the same total body weight weighs more in water and thus has a higher body density (lower percentage of body fat). This was illustrated in Figure 2–1.

To determine body density from underwater weighing, the following equation has been derived:[222, 226, 228]

$$D_b = \frac{W_a}{\dfrac{(W_a - W_w)}{D_w} - (RV + 100 \text{ ml})}$$

where D_b = body density;
W_a = body weight out of the water;
W_w = weight in the water;
D_w = density of water;
RV = residual volume.

The 100 ml is the estimated air volume of the gastrointestinal tract. Although this volume can fluctuate, Buskirk[228] has suggested the use of a constant correction factor.

The other body gas volume that is needed to calculate body density is residual volume (RV). The RV is the amount of air left in the lungs after a maximal expiration. Residual volume is normally measured by an open circuit nitrogen washout technique or by a closed circuit oxygen or helium dilution method.[222] Residual volume can also be estimated by average population values based upon age, sex, and height[229] or by an estimated percentage of the vital capacity (approximately 25 to 30 percent).[230] If the RV of a large population were measured by the three methods (actual percent measurement; value based on age, sex, and height; or value based on a percentage of vital capacity), RV would vary little among them.[231] Wilmore[231] showed that the difference in mean body density calculated among groups using actual and estimated values for RV was less than 0.001 g/ml. Thus, for screening purposes or when measuring large groups, the estimation of RV would be an acceptable technique. However, RV is quite variable at any given age, height, or vital capacity and may result in errors of up to 5 percent of body fat (see example in Table 6–14). Therefore, for individual analysis and counseling, the actual measured RV is recommended.[222, 231, 232]

When determining body density, if an estimation of RV is used, the following equations developed by Goldman and Becklake[229] are recommended:

Men:

RV = 0.017 (age in years) + 0.06858 (height in inches) − 3.477

Women:

RV = 0.009 (age in years) + 0.08128 (height in inches) − 3.9

Table 6–14. The Effect of Errors in Residual Volume (RV), Scale Weight in the Water (W_w), and Body Weight Out of the Water (W_a) on Determination of Body Density (D_b) from Underwater Weighing

Measure	Actual*	Errors†		
		1	*2*	*3*
RV (L)	1.200	1.400	1.700	2.200
D_b (g/cc)	1.0605	1.0631	1.0669	1.0734
Fat (%)	16.74	15.63	13.95	11.16
W_w (kg)	4.24	4.29	4.34	4.44
D_b (g/cc)	1.0605	1.0612	1.0618	1.0631
Fat (%)	16.74	16.46	16.18	15.62
W_a (kg)	88.70	88.80	89.20	89.70
D_b (g/cc)	1.0605	1.0605	1.0601	1.0598
Fat (%)	16.74	16.78	16.91	17.09

*Actual values are from Figure 6–27.
†Each error for D_b and percent fat is calculated with the other two variables from the actual values.

The density of water also has to be accounted for in the equation to determine body density. Water density varies with temperature and requires a standard conversion factor.[228] Table 6–15 lists water density at various common water temperatures from 23°C to 37°C.[232] For subject comfort, measuring underwater weight at temperatures between 32°C and 35°C is recommended. Although water density is important to determine, its slight variation within the temperature range used for underwater weighing makes its effect negligible on the error of measurement within the calculation of body density.

Figure 6–27 is an example of a body composition and pulmonary function form used to record data for determining body density by underwater weighing. The form shows actual values of a 20-year-old man. Residual volume was measured twice outside the water, with the subject in a sitting position. Two values are determined for verification purposes. If repeat values differ by more than 100 ml, then a third measure should be taken. The amount of

Table 6–15. Conversion Chart for Determining Water Density (D_w) at Various Water Temperatures (W Temp)

W Temp (°C)	D_w	W Temp (°C)	D_w
23	0.997569	31	0.995372
24	0.997327	32	0.995057
25	0.997075	33	0.994734
26	0.996814	34	0.994403
27	0.996544	35	0.994063
28	0.996264	36	0.993716
29	0.995976	37	0.993360
30	0.995678		

accuracy that is acceptable when determining RV depends upon the equipment and technique used and the purpose of the test (screening or research). For calculation purposes, the RV values listed in Figure 6–27 were averaged.

BODY COMPOSITION AND PULMONARY FUNCTION

Name:				Date:	10/5/82

Age: 20	Body Wt: 88.70 X kg	Ht: 177.8 X cm	Bar. Pr.	746.1
	_lb	_ in		

Group:			Sex: M

	Trial 1	Trial 2		Trial 1	Trial 2
PF			Temp	22.0	22.0
$FEV_{1.0}$			Volume I	6.91	7.05
VC			E_{N2}	0.073	0.069
$(FEV_{1.0}/VC)\cdot 100$			I_{N2}	0.003	0.002
$FEV_{2.0}$			A_{iN2}	0.771	0.769
$FEV_{3.0}$			A_{fN2}	.079	.072
MVV			DS	.09	.09
Temp. (°C)			PREDICTED RV	.	.
			CALCULATED RV	1.225	1.174
			AVERAGE RV =	1.200	

UNDERWATER WEIGHT

Trial	Wt (kg)	Temp. (°C)	Trial	Wt (kg)	Temp. (°C)
①	12.96	34.0			
2	13.00	34.0			
3	13.02	34.0			
4	13.08	34.0			
5	13.06	34.0			
⑥	13.08	34.0			
⑦	13.08	34.0			
⑧	13.06	34.0			
⑨					
10					

Chair and belt wt.	8.84*		Chair and belt wt.		
Db	1.0605		Db		
Calculated % fat (Siri)	16.74		Calculated % fat (Siri)		

*To be subtracted from the underwater weight to derive the net underwater weight of the subject.

Figure 6–27. Body composition and pulmonary function form used in determining body density by underwater weighing. (Courtesy of The Human Performance Laboratory, Mount Sinai Medical Center, Milwaukee, WI.)

To determine underwater weighing, multiple (6 to 10) trials are recommended.[234] As shown with the data in Figure 6–27, there is a learning curve. When the data level off and remain so, even with continued encouragement from the tester, the test can be terminated. What criteria should be used in picking the actual underwater weight? Behnke and Wilmore[222] have used the following method: (1) select the highest observed weight if it is obtained more than once; (2) if criterion 1 is not met, select the second highest weight if it is observed more than once; (3) if criteria 1 and 2 are not met, select the third highest measure. With the data in Figure 6–27, trials 6 and 7 were used in the calculation of body density. Although it is apparent from the subject's data in Figure 6–27 that he leveled off after trial 4, additional trials were determined to verify his best effort.

What is meant by the chair and belt weight shown in Figure 6–27? This is simply the weight of the chain, chair, weight belt, and other equipment that is subtracted from the total observed weight (Fig. 6–28). This measure is usually obtained after the

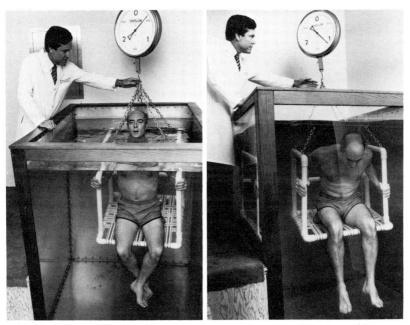

Figure 6–28. The right panel shows the subject seated in the underwater weighing tank. The left panel shows the subject placing his head underwater and being measured for underwater weight. The above tank is 4 × 5 × 5 feet. It is constructed of ¼-inch stainless steel bottom and sides with two sides of ¾-inch plexiglas. The tank has its own filtering and heating system. The chair is constructed from 2-inch PVC pipe. (Photographs by Wendy V. Watriss 1985. Published with permission.)

underwater weight is determined, with the chair lowered to the level at which the underwater weight was observed. For the calculation of underwater weight from the data in Figure 6–27, 8.84 kg (chair and weight belt) is subtracted from 13.08 kg (total weight observed).

As an example of calculating body density by underwater weighing, the subject's data shown in Figure 6–27 are substituted into the equation used to derive body density:

$$D_b = \frac{88.70}{\dfrac{(88.7 - 4.24)}{0.994} - (1.20 + 0.100)}$$

$$D_b = 1.0605$$

Percentage of fat is usually predicted from one of the two following equations:

Brozek and associates:[226]

$$\% \text{ body fat} = \left[\left(\frac{4.570}{D_b} \right) - 4.142 \right] \times 100$$

Siri:[235]

$$\% \text{ body fat} = \left[\left(\frac{4.950}{D_b} \right) - 4.500 \right] \times 100$$

Both equations are based on the general assumption that various body components—e.g., muscle, bone, and fat—are of a constant density and that total body water is of a constant nature. Both percentage of body fat equations correlate highly ($r = 0.995$ to 0.999) and give similar mean values.[222] With the body density value determined from the subject in Figure 6–27 (1.0605), percentage of body fat values calculated by the Siri and Brozek equations are 16.74 percent and 16.71 percent, respectively. The method is accurate only to the first decimal, so essentially both equations gave identical values. Thus, either equation is recommended for use, but consistency with the use of a particular equation should be maintained. When comparing percentage of body fat results (norms, research studies), the equation used to derive the comparative data should be known. The percentage of body fat norms shown in Appendix A, Tables A–1 to A–12, were derived from the Siri equation.

Although Brozek and Siri equations are universally accepted, they are not without problems. Both equations were based on the results of direct compositional analysis through dissection of fresh human cadavers.[222, 223] Only a few cadavers were used, and they did not represent a distribution of the normal population. All assumptions of compositional analysis used to derive the percentage of fat equations have not been validated on children, youth, and the elderly. Lohman[236–237a] and others[68, 222, 238, 239] have discussed the problems of using percentage of body fat equations with youth and children. Bone density is less during this period of life, and total body water is higher (see Fig. 2–2).[223, 237, 237a, 240] It must be noted here that new equations for predicting percentage of body fat from body density in children and youth have been developed by Slaughter and colleagues[237b] and look promising for general use. The authors have attempted to account for differences in bone density and total body water (FFW) as described by Lohman.[236, 237]

After 40 to 50 years of age for women and 50 years of age for men, bone density decreases.[223, 241, 242] Loss of muscle mass is also evident in the elderly.[223] Because of this problem, percentage of body fat equations are not valid for use in children and youth up to 16 or 17 years of age and are questionable for use in the elderly. Because of this invalidity, the new *Health Related Physical Fitness Test Manual*[68, 127] developed by AAHPRD for use with school children and youth aged 6 to 18 years uses the sum of two or three skinfold fat measures for body fat analysis and comparison and does not make a conversion to percentage of body fat.

Martin and colleagues[243, 243a] have completed extensive dissections of 12 male and 13 female adult cadavers. Their data show a significant variance among cadavers for the various body components. These data could well lead to more refined equations for predicting percentage of body fat in adults.

In regard to potential errors in determining body density from the underwater weighing technique, RV, scale weight (W_w), and body weight (W_a) are critical factors. Table 6–14 shows body density and percentage of body fat calculated from the actual RV, scale weight, and body weight shown in Figure 6–27. To determine the potential error of each of the three factors on the calculation of body density, the following additions were made to the actual values: RV, 200, 500, and 1,000 ml; W_w, 50, 100, and 200 g; and W_a, 100, 500, and 1,000 g, respectively. The ramifications of each error factor are discussed separately.

The errors related to actually measuring or estimating RV from age and height or from vital capacity were discussed earlier. As shown in Table 6–14, errors in RV can make a dramatic difference in the results. A 2.0 to 5.5 percent units error in body fat was found with 500 to 1,000 ml differences in estimating RV. Another potential error in measuring RV is whether the measure is actually determined in the water at the time of the underwater weighing or separately, out of the water. Although 200 to 300 ml differences in RV have been reported between the two methods, if care is taken to have the subject exhale fully and replicate the body position for the measurements (sitting and so on), the error is probably smaller.[222, 244] Nevertheless, even if a 200 ml difference is found, only an approximate 1 percent error in body fat is found (Table 6–14). This error is certainly acceptable for clinical and research purposes, and if replicated consistently, it is adequate for serial analysis, i.e., RV should be a constant error in one direction.

As part of an eight-center research project, a subject visited each laboratory within a 2-week period for assessment of body composition. The purpose of the visit was to standardize testing procedures and determine interlab variation among measures. All laboratories had experienced investigators and determined body density using the underwater weighing technique. Four of the laboratories measured RV while the subject was out of the water, and four measured it while he was in the water as part of the procedure. Among laboratories, body weight varied from 77.4 to 78.3 kg ($\bar{X}$ = 77.9 ± 0.35 kg), body density from 1.0717 to 1.0761 g/ml ($\bar{X}$ = 1.0733 ± 0.00136 g/ml), RV from 1.00 to 1.44 l ($\bar{X}$ = 1.22 ± 0.13 l), and percent fat from 10.0 to 11.9 ($\bar{X}$ = 11.2 ± 0.6%). As can be seen, variation among laboratories was small, and there was no mean difference in body density and percent fat between laboratories who measured RV in the water as compared with those who measured it out of the water.*

Normally, an error of 50 g or more in underwater scale weight would be unusual; therefore, the error associated with an incorrect underwater weight should be less than 0.5 percent fat (see Table 6–14). Scales not being calibrated, subjects being unable to coordinate the underwater weighing procedure, and oscillations created by water movement are the most common problems associated with reading the scale weight. Periodic calibration of the scale with known weights can easily correct the first problem, and multiple practice trials can correct the second. A stable, comfortable chair aids in increasing the subject's ability to minimize underwater motion (see Fig. 6–28). Water oscillations are more problematic in large bodies of water (swimming pools) than in smaller tanks. Having the subject move slowly in the water and be relaxed in the chair seat, as well as the use of a weighted belt, enhances the accuracy in reading the scale. Usually some oscillation is present, but interpolation should be within 20 to 60 g and rarely more than 100 g. If a small water tank is used and techniques are adequate,

---

*Unpublished data from T. Lohman, University of Arizona, Tucson, December 1987.

the scale stylus should have imperceptible movement in approximately 50 percent of adult subjects.

Body weight can be quite variable and changes with time of day, dietary pattern, state of hydration, and illness. Best results are obtained in the morning, before breakfast and exercise. A scale graduated to 100 g increments is quite satisfactory for use in this procedure and would account for a very small error of measurement (see Table 6–14). Excessive hydration or dehydration (caused by exercise, sauna, diarrhea, or menstruation) can have a significant effect on body density.[41] For example, a 2 to 3 kg weight gain or loss would cause a 0.75- to 1.0-percent change in the percentage of body fat.

The scale used in Figure 6–28 is a 15 kg scale, calibrated in 20 g increments. This type of scale or a 9 kg (10 g increments) scale is adequate for use with the underwater weighing procedure. In the figure, the scale is attached to a quarter-ton hoist. The hoist is helpful in adjusting the seat height to the proper level. In the same figure, the technician is helping to hold (stabilize) the scale when the subject is hyperventilating (before going under the water), placing his head underwater, and bringing his head out of the water. This helps to keep the subject from accidentally swallowing water and reduces water oscillations during the procedure. The hand is removed from the scale (chain) once the subject is in position and stable underwater.

Using a strain gauge or load cell that is directly connected to a recorder is a more sophisticated (and expensive) technique in measuring the underwater weight. In this case, the chair can still be suspended from the ceiling or set directly on the load cells. Although the use of a load cell system makes the measurement more objective and has the advantage of supplying a permanent record of the procedure, it has not been shown to be more accurate with experienced technicians.[245] Fahey and Schroeder,[245] using trained subjects and trained technicians, showed a mean of 2.30 ± 0.48 kg versus 2.29 ± 0.45 kg (not significant) when comparing the load cell and autopsy scale methods, respectively. Fluctuations in the readings were less with the load cell system and thus may be a better system for use with less experienced technicians.

Procedure. The underwater weighing procedure can be accomplished in almost any body of fresh water that is at least 3 to 4 feet deep. Water tanks may be as diverse as an Olympic-size swimming pool, a small framed crib that is placed in a swimming pool (decreases water turbulence),[234] a wine vat, a 120-gallon gas drum, a canvas bag, a specially built small swimming pool, or a stainless-steel or fiberglass-enforced tank. With this in mind, the cost can vary from almost nothing to 10,000 to 15,000 dollars. A tank no smaller than 4 feet by 4 feet by 4 feet is recommended. A 5-foot depth has been helpful in testing subjects over 6 feet 8 inches in height. A water heater and filtering system are recommended. In addition, an easily accessible emergency water drainage system should be built in. If possible, the tank should be recessed into the floor, or if not possible, a platform should be built on at least one side so that the top of the tank is about waist high and the weight scale is approximately at eye level (see Fig. 6–28).

The underwater weighing procedure can also be performed with the subject in the standing or prone position. Different specifications for tank size are needed for other body positions.

For best results, instructions to and preparation of the subject before underwater weighing are important. A normal diet, drinking, and exercise pattern is recommended. Subjects should avoid foods that can cause excessive amounts of gas to develop in the gastrointestinal tract. Situations that cause unusual hydration or dehydration should be avoided. There should be no eating or smoking for at least 2 to 3 hours before testing. If eating is necessary before testing, just a moderate portion is recommended.

Men should be measured in the nude or in a supporter or swimming brief. Women should wear a two-piece tank suit or bikini type of bathing suit. A regular two-piece bathing suit can be acceptable for use, but more caution is needed to avoid air trapping. Air trapping from a bathing suit (top or bottom) can lead to a significant error in measuring underwater weight.

Before beginning the procedure, subjects should be asked to void their bladder and defecate. Once this has been accomplished, body weight should be measured. If anthropometric measures are to be taken, they should be done next, followed by the underwater weighing. Doing the underwater weighing procedure first and then having the subject dry off changes the texture of the skin and thus may influence the skinfold fat measurement.

The underwater weighing procedure described is with the tank and accessory apparatus shown in Figure 6–28. After subjects are standing in the tank and before they sit on the chair (water about chest depth), have them slowly rub their hands over the surface of all body parts, stirring the water as little as possible, to help eliminate air bubbles attached to the skin. Start with one foot and leg and then the other, culminating with dipping the head under the water and rubbing the shoulders and head. Wiggling the top and bottom of the swim suit helps release any trapped air. Once this has been completed, take the weight belt and secure it around the waist. A scuba type of weight belt with approximately 3 to 5 kg of weight attached is satisfactory. The subject then sits on the chair and assumes a comfortable position. The seat height is then adjusted to bring the chin or mouth to water level.

Explain the total procedure, and use the first trial as a talk-through rehearsal. Have the subject do the following:

1. Hyperventilate five to six times and expel most of the air while in the upright position.
2. Continue to expel air from the lungs, and slowly lower the head under the water until the top of the head clears the surface. If the head is not completely submerged, the technician should tap the top of the subject's head until it does clear the surface.
3. Place hands on top of the thighs, and relax once all of the air has been forcefully expelled. Often an imbalance (counter balance or rocking motion) is experienced (unsteadiness in water) if the subject pulls self down by holding on to the knees or chair.
4. Lift the head back out of the water when the measurement has been determined. Knocking on the side of the tank can generally be used as a signal to come up.
5. Repeat the procedure six to ten times. A critique and review of problems between trials improves accuracy. Brief rest periods may be necessary if the subject gets tired.

A few subjects may have to use a nose clip during the underwater weighing procedure. It should be noted that a few individuals may not be able to complete the procedure satisfactorily (approximately 1 to 2 percent). Patience and making the subject feel comfortable in the water are key factors. For beginners, the RV procedure may take 10 to 15 minutes, and the underwater weighing, 20 to 30 minutes. As mentioned earlier, RV measurement is repeated at least one time.

ANTHROPOMETRIC MEASURES

Anthropometry is the science that deals with the measurement of size, weight, and proportions of the human body. In the areas of body composition, measurement, exercise science, and sports medicine, skinfold fat, circumferences, and body diameter measures have been utilized.[222, 223, 225, 240, 241] As mentioned earlier in the book and in this section, anthropometric measures are used to predict body density and percentage of body fat. In some cases and in particular with school children (although the new prediction equations of Slaughter and colleagues[237b] seem promising), the sum of skinfold measures should be used. In addition, various individual skinfold fat and circumference measures, when taken serially over weeks or months, can demonstrate a shift in body composition. For example, the gluteal and waist circumference measures are excellent in showing reductions in body fat with aerobic training, and biceps circumference increases with strength training.

Although the aforementioned laboratory methods of assessing body density are considered most accurate, they are often not practical for the clinical setting or for mass testing. Anthropometric measurement estimates of body composition correlates well with the underwater weighing method and has several advantages: the necessary equipment is inexpensive and needs little or no space, and the measures can be obtained easily and quickly.[222] The results from many studies using skinfold fat or combinations of skinfold fat, circumferences, and diameters are shown in Table 6–16. These data represent studies conducted on both men and women and on persons of various ages and body fatness (density). In addition, see Table 6–17 for comparisons of correlations of various anthropometric measures with body density.[30]

In general, the results show that the correlations for predicting body density from height and weight are below 0.6, from the best combination of height and weight indices, e.g., the Body Mass Index (BMI),[246] 0.65 to 0.7, and from multiple regression equations using a combination of skinfolds or skinfold, circumference, and diameter measures at or above 0.8.[30, 31]

The first body composition regression equations using anthropometric techniques were published in 1951 by Brozek and Keys,[247] who used skinfolds to estimate body density for young and middle-aged men. In the early 1960's, Sloan and associates[267] and Young and associates[269, 270] published similar equations for women of selected age groups. These equations were developed by using various combinations of skinfold fat measurements. From the middle 1960's to the 1970's, numerous researchers published additional equations for women and men (see Table 6–16). The objective of this research was to produce more accurate prediction equations. In addition to skinfold measurements, several body circumferences and, in some instances, bone diameters were used as independent variables. During this era, electronic computers and stepwise multiple regression computer programs became readily available to researchers. This increased computing capacity made it easier to analyze a large number of variables and select the combination of anthropometric variables that produced the highest multiple correlation. The equations consisting of skinfolds, circumferences, and diameters were more accurate than the earlier equations using only skinfolds; this was especially true for women and middle-aged men.[259, 265]

The research leading to the development of population-specific equations has shown that age and gender are important sources of body density variation. Body density differences between men and women can largely be traced to essential fat variance.[222] In addition, population-specific equations for gender have been important be-

Table 6–16. Means and Standard Deviations of Hydrostatically Determined Body Density and Concurrent Validity of Regression Equations for Men and Women

Source	Sample		Body Density		Regression Analysis	
	Age*	n	$\bar{x}$	s	R	SE
Men						
Brozek and Keys	20.3	133	1.077	0.014	0.88	0.007
(1951)[247]	45–55	122	1.055	0.012	0.74	0.009
Cureton et al. (1975)[248]	8–11	49	1.053	0.013	0.77	0.008
Durnin and Rahaman	18–33	60	1.068	0.013	0.84	0.007
(1967)[249]	12–15	48	1.063	0.012	0.76	0.008
Durnin and Wormsley	17–19	24	1.066	0.016	†	0.007
(1974)[250]	20–29	92	1.064	0.016	†	0.008
	30–39	34	1.046	0.012	†	0.009
	40–49	35	1.043	0.015	†	0.008
	50–68	24	1.036	0.018	†	0.009
Forsyth and Sinning (1973)[251]	19–29	50	1.072	0.010	0.84	0.006
Haisman (1970)[252]	22–26	55	1.070	0.010	0.78	0.006
Harsha et al. (1978)[253]	6–16	79‡	1.046	0.018	0.84	0.010
	6–16	49§	1.055	0.020	0.90	0.009
Jackson and Pollock (1978)[254]	18–61	308	1.059	0.018	0.92	0.007
Katch and McArdle (1973)[255]	19.3	53	1.065	0.014	0.89	0.007
Katch and Michael (1969)[256]	17.0	40	1.076	0.013	0.89	0.006
Parizkova (1961)[257]	9–12	57	†	†	0.92	0.011
Pascale et al. (1956)[258]	22.1	88	1.068	0.012	0.86	0.006
Pollock et al. (1976)[259]	18–22	95	1.068	0.014	0.87	0.007
	40–55	84	1.043	0.013	0.84	0.007
Sloan (1967)[260]	18–26	50	1.075	0.015	0.85	0.008
Wilmore and Behnke (1969)[261]	16–36	133	1.066	0.013	0.87	0.006
Wright and Wilmore (1974)[262]	27.8	297	1.061	0.014	0.86	0.007
Women						
Durnin and Rahaman	18–29	45	1.044	0.014	0.78	0.010
(1967)[249]	13–16	38	1.045	0.011	0.78	0.008
Durnin and Wormsley	16–19	29	1.040	0.017	†	0.009
(1974)[250]	20–29	100	1.034	0.021	†	0.011
	30–39	58	1.025	0.020	†	0.013
	40–49	48	1.020	0.016	†	0.011
	50–68	37	1.013	0.016	†	0.008
Harsha et al. (1978)[253]	6–16	52‡	1.033	0.016	0.85	0.008
	6–16	39§	1.041	0.019	0.90	0.008
Jackson et al. (1980)[263]	18–55	249	1.044	0.016	0.87	0.008
Katch and McArdle (1973)[255]	20.3	69	1.039	0.015	0.84	0.009
Katch and Michael (1968)[264]	19–23	64	1.049	0.011	0.70	0.008
Parizkova (1961)[257]	9–12	56	†	†	0.81	0.012
	13–16	62	†	†	0.82	0.010

Table continued on following page

Table 6–16. Means and Standard Deviations of Hydrostatically Determined Body Density and Concurrent Validity of Regression Equations for Men and Women *Continued*

Source	Sample		Body Density		Regression Analysis	
	*Age**	*n*	$\bar{x}$	*s*	*R*	*SE*
Pollock et al. (1975)[265]	18–22	83	1.043	0.014	0.84	0.008
	33–50	60	1.032	0.015	0.89	0.007
Sinning (1978)[266]	17–23	44	1.064	0.010	0.81	0.006
Sloan et al. (1962)[267]	20.2	50	1.047	0.012	0.74	0.008
Wilmore and Behnke (1970)[268]	21.4	128	1.041	0.010	0.76	0.007
Young (1964)[269]	53.0	62	1.020	0.014	0.84	0.008
Young et al. (1962)[270]	17–27	94	1.034	0.009	0.69	0.007

*Age is expressed as the mean or range.
†Data not available.
‡White.
§Black.
(From Baumgartner, J. A., and Jackson, A. S.: **Measurement and Evaluation in Physical Education and Exercise Science,** 3rd Ed., Copyright 1987, Wm. C. Brown Publishers, Dubuque, IA. All rights reserved. Reprinted with permission.)

cause of the differences in subcutaneous fat distribution for men and women.[271] Bone density changes are related to aging; bone density increases up to age 20 and decreases after age 50.[223, 236, 241, 242] Lohman[236] showed how the relationship between body density and subcutaneous fat is affected by gender and age. Using published

Table 6–17. Correlation Between Hydrostatically Determined Body Density (D_b) and Anthropometric Variables

Anthropometric Variable	Women (n = 249)			Men (n = 308)		
	r	*SE (D_b)*	*SE (%F)*	*r*	*SE (D_b)*	*SE (% F)*
Age	−0.35	0.015	6.7	−0.38	0.017	7.4
Height	−0.08	0.016	7.2	0.01	0.018	8.0
Weight	−0.63	0.012	5.6	−0.62	0.014	6.3
Body Mass Index*	−0.70	0.011	5.1	−0.69	0.013	5.8
Sum of seven skinfolds	−0.85	0.008	3.8	−0.88	0.009	3.8
Sum of Three I†	−0.84	0.009	3.9	−0.89	0.008	3.6
Sum of Three II‡	−0.83	0.009	4.0	−0.86	0.009	4.1

*Body Mass Index = Wt/Ht^2, where weight is in kilograms and height in meters.
†Sum of three skinfold fat measures: women = triceps, suprailium, and thigh; men = chest, abdomen, and thigh.
‡Sum of three skinfold fat measures: women = triceps, abdomen, and suprailium; men = chest, triceps, and subscapula.
(From Pollock, M. I., Schmidt, D. H., and Jackson, A. S.: Measurement of cardiorespiratory fitness and body composition in the clinical setting. **Compr. Ther.** 6:12–27, 1980. Published with permission of The Laux Company, Inc., Harvard, MA.)

data involving men and women who varied in age,[259, 265] Lohman examined skinfold thickness with body density adjusted to 1.050 g/ ml (21.4 percent fat [Siri equation]). With this common body density, the skinfold thicknesses of women were lower than those of men, and older subjects had less subcutaneous fat than their younger counterparts. Since skinfold thickness is the primary variable used in body density equations, the analysis by Lohman showed that equations developed on one group are biased when applied to subjects who differ in gender, age, and fatness. Equations developed on younger subjects overestimate the body density of older subjects. Using gender-specific equations and applying them to the opposite sex produce a constant prediction error of about 0.025 g/ml (11 percent fat).[236] The findings from the research on population-specific equations show that gender, age, and degree of fatness need to be considered when estimating body density from anthropometric variables.[236, 250, 271–273]

Not only are the population-specific equations sensitive to differences in age, gender, and degree of fatness, but they are also subject to error regarding a basic assumption that hydrostatically determined body density is linearly related to skinfold fat. Figure 6–29 clearly shows that the latter relationship is curvilinear rather than linear.[254] This means that population-specific equations predict most accurately at the mean of the population in which the data were collected and the equation developed. As subjects differ from the mean, the standard error of measurement increases significantly.[272] This concept is diagrammatically shown in Figure 6–30.

Development of Generalized Equations for Predicting Body Density from Anthropometric Measures. The more recent trend has been to develop generalized rather than population-specific equations. These specific equations provide valid estimates with subjects representative of defined populations. Durnin and Wormersley[250] were the first to consider the generalized approach. They published equations with a common slope but adjusted the intercept to account for aging. More recently, Jackson and Pollock published generalized equations for adult men[254] and women.[263] Their research was an extension of the Durnin and Wormersley work and was designed to further overcome some of the limitations of population-specific equations. The newer generalized equations by Jackson and Pollock added age in the prediction equation to account for potential changes in the ratio of internal to external fat and bone density. The generalized equations of Jackson and Pollock have been cross-validated by other investigators.[274–280]

Tables 6–17 and 6–18 illustrate the differences in the prediction accuracy of body density and percentage of body fat using the best body height and weight index, the BMI, and linear and curvilinear equations. The data were from 249 women, 18 to 55 years of age (an average of 31.4 years), who ranged from 4 to 44 percent fat (an average of 24.1 percent), and from 308 men, 18 to 61 years of age (an average of 32.6 years), who ranged from 1 to 33 percent fat (an average of 17.7 percent).[30] The zero-order correlations and standard errors of measurement between selected anthropometric variables and body density determined by underwater weighing are shown in Table 6–17. Height was the only variable not related to body density. The BMI had only a slightly better correlation than did body weight alone. The sum of skinfold fat measures represented the highest correlations. In addition, the correlation between the various combinations of the sum of three skinfold measures exceeded 0.97.[30, 254, 272, 273] Certain circumference measures, such as gluteal (buttocks) for women, show slightly higher correlations in combination with skinfolds.[263] Inclusion of circumference measures in the prediction equations shown in Table 6–18 was of minimal additional value. The sum of skinfolds provides a more representative sample of subcutaneous body fat and is more highly correlated with body density than are individual sites.

It should be noted that the use of the quadratic component and age in the generalized equation shown in Table 6–18 did not increase the correlation substantially over the linear equation shown in Table 6–17. The value of the generalized equations over the linear equations is that they minimize large prediction errors that occur at the extremes of the body density distribution. This is shown in Figures 6–29 and 6–30.

It is important to recognize that every measurement method has defined sources of error. Bakker and Struikenkamp[281] have raised this issue with hydrostatically determined measures of lean body weight and have demonstrated that the method had defined degrees of inaccuracy. Lohman[236] has estimated the standard error for hydrostatically determined percentage of body fat of specific populations to be 2.7 percent. Since error variances are uncorrelated, it means that the generalized equations add only about 1 percent to the measurement error of percentage of body fat.

To determine body density from anthropometric measures, select an equation from Table 6–18. Once body density is found, convert to percentage of body fat in the same manner as was described for underwater weighing, i.e., use either the Siri or the Brozek equation.

For ease of determination, actual calculated percentages of body fat using age and the sum of triceps, suprailium, and thigh skinfolds for women and the sum of chest, abdomen, and thigh skinfolds for men are shown in Tables 6–19 and 6–20, respec-

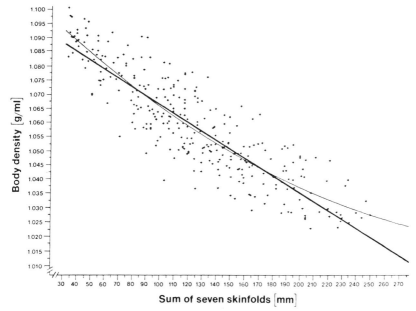

Figure 6–29. Scattergram of body density and the sum of 7 skinfolds, with the linear and quadratic regression lines for adult men age 18 to 61 years. (From Jackson, A. S., and Pollock, M. L.: Generalized equations for predicting body density in men. **Br. J. Nutr.** 40:497–504, 1978. Reprinted with permission of Cambridge University Press.)

tively.[30] For example, if the sum of three skinfolds for a 35-year-old woman was 63 mm, her percentage of body fat would be 25.5 percent, and if a 50-year-old man had 60 mm, he would be 20.0 percent fat. Using age and the same sum of three skinfolds for men

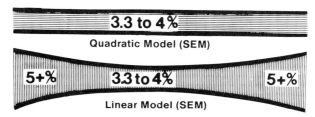

Figure 6–30. The figure diagrammatically illustrates the differences of the standard error of measurement (SEM) for predicting percentage of body fat (body density) using the linear and quadratic regression models. Note that the SEM are similar at the population means but vary significantly away from the mean for the linear model. The linear model tends to underestimate body density in lean subjects and overestimate it in fatter than average subjects. (Reprinted with permission from Jackson, A. S., and Pollock, M. L.: Steps toward the development of generalized equations for predicting body composition of adults. **Can. J. Appl. Sport Sci.** 7:189–196, 1982.)

Table 6–18. Generalized Regression Equations for Predicting Body Density (D_b) for Adult Women and Men

Variables	Regression Equation	r	SE (D_b)	SE (% F)
	Adult Women			
Σ 7, Age	$D_b = 1.0970 - 0.00046971\ (X_1) + 0.00000056$ $(X_1)^2 - 0.00012828\ (X_6)$	0.85	0.008	3.8
Σ 3, Age	$D_b = 1.0994921 - 0.0009929\ (X_2) + 0.0000023$ $(X_2)^2 - 0.0001392\ (X_6)$	0.84	0.009	3.9
Σ 3, Age	$D_b = 1.089733 - 0.0009245\ (X_5) + 0.0000025$ $(X_5)^2 - 0.0000979\ (X_6)$	0.83	0.009	3.9
	Adult Men			
Σ 7, Age	$D_b = 1.11200000 - 0.00043499\ (X_1) +$ $0.00000055\ (X_1)^2 - 0.00028826\ (X_6)$	0.90	0.008	3.5
Σ 3, Age	$D_b = 1.1093800 - 0.0008267\ (X_3) + 0.0000016$ $(X_3)^2 - 0.0002574\ (X_6)$	0.91	0.008	3.4
Σ 3, Age	$D_b = 1.1125025 - 0.0013125\ (X_4) + 0.0000055$ $(X_4)^2 - 0.0002440\ (X_6)$	0.89	0.008	3.6

X_1 = Sum of seven skinfolds (mm); X_2 = sum of triceps, suprailium, and thigh skinfolds (mm); X_3 = sum of chest, abdomen, and thigh skinfolds (mm); X_4 = sum of chest, triceps, and subscapular skinfolds (mm); X_5 = sum of triceps, suprailium, and abdomen skinfolds (mm); X_6 = age in years.

(From Pollock, M. L., Schmidt, D. H., and Jackson, A. S.: Measurement of cardiorespiratory fitness and body composition in the clinical setting. **Compr. Ther.** 6:12–7, 1980. Published with permission of The Laux Company, Inc. Harvard, MA.)

and women, as shown in Tables 6–19 and 6–20, Baun and associates[282] developed a nomogram for estimating percentage of body fat. Because thigh skinfolds are difficult for some technicians to measure, other equations not using thigh skinfolds are available.[16, 30, 283] For women, the triceps, abdomen, and suprailium are used, and for men, the triceps, chest, and subscapula are used[283] (see Appendix A, Tables A–29 and A–30). Other charts are available for women for the sum of four skinfolds (abdomen, suprailium, triceps, and thigh) and for men for the sum of four skinfolds (abdomen, suprailium, triceps, and thigh) and the sum of three skinfolds (abdomen, suprailium, and triceps).[16] Charts for the sum of seven skinfolds (chest, triceps, axilla, subscapula, suprailium, abdomen, and thigh) for both men and women are available from one of the authors (Pollock) by request.

If fat calipers are not available, a relatively accurate estimation of percentage of body fat has been developed from circumference measures.[119] Katch and McArdle[119] have used the following circumference measures for young women (abdomen, right thigh, and right forearm), older women (abdomen, right thigh, and right calf), young men (right upper arm, abdomen, and right forearm), and older men (buttocks, abdomen, and right forearm) to estimate the percentage of body fat (see their publication for conversion charts to predict body fat).

Table 6–19. Percentage of Body Fat Estimation for Women from Age and Triceps, Suprailium, and Thigh Skinfolds*

Sum of Skinfolds (mm)	Under 22	23 to 27	28 to 32	33 to 37	38 to 42	43 to 47	48 to 52	53 to 57	Over 58
23–25	9.7	9.9	10.2	10.4	10.7	10.9	11.2	11.4	11.7
26–28	11.0	11.2	11.5	11.7	12.0	12.3	12.5	12.7	13.0
29–31	12.3	12.5	12.8	13.0	13.3	13.5	13.8	14.0	14.3
32–34	13.6	13.8	14.0	14.3	14.5	14.8	15.0	15.3	15.5
35–37	14.8	15.0	15.3	15.5	15.8	16.0	16.3	16.5	16.8
38–40	16.0	16.3	16.5	16.7	17.0	17.2	17.5	17.7	18.0
41–43	17.2	17.4	17.7	17.9	18.2	18.4	18.7	18.9	19.2
44–46	18.3	18.6	18.8	19.1	19.3	19.6	19.8	20.1	20.3
47–49	19.5	19.7	20.0	20.2	20.5	20.7	21.0	21.2	21.5
50–52	20.6	20.8	21.1	21.3	21.6	21.8	22.1	22.3	22.6
53–55	21.7	21.9	22.1	22.4	22.6	22.9	23.1	23.4	23.6
56–58	22.7	23.0	23.2	23.4	23.7	23.9	24.2	24.4	24.7
59–61	23.7	24.0	24.2	24.5	24.7	25.0	25.2	25.5	25.7
62–64	24.7	25.0	25.2	25.5	25.7	26.0	26.7	26.4	26.7
65–67	25.7	25.9	26.2	26.4	26.7	26.9	27.2	27.4	27.7
68–70	26.6	26.9	27.1	27.4	27.6	27.9	28.1	28.4	28.6
71–73	27.5	37.8	28.0	28.3	28.5	28.8	28.0	29.3	29.5
74–76	28.4	28.7	28.9	29.2	29.4	29.7	29.9	30.2	30.4
77–79	29.3	29.5	29.8	30.0	30.3	30.5	30.8	31.0	31.3
80–82	30.1	30.4	30.6	30.9	31.1	31.4	31.6	31.9	32.1
83–85	30.9	31.2	31.4	31.7	31.9	32.2	32.4	32.7	32.9
86–88	31.7	32.0	32.2	32.5	32.7	32.9	33.2	33.4	33.7
89–91	32.5	32.7	33.0	33.2	33.5	33.7	33.9	34.2	34.4
92–94	33.2	33.4	33.7	33.9	34.2	34.4	34.7	34.9	35.2
95–97	33.9	34.1	34.4	34.6	34.9	35.1	35.4	35.6	35.9
98–100	34.6	34.8	35.1	35.3	35.5	35.8	36.0	36.3	36.5
101–103	35.3	35.4	35.7	35.9	36.2	36.4	36.7	36.9	37.2
104–106	35.8	36.1	36.3	36.6	36.8	37.1	37.3	37.5	37.8
107–109	36.4	36.7	36.9	37.1	37.4	37.6	37.9	38.1	38.4
110–112	37.0	37.2	37.5	37.7	38.0	38.2	38.5	38.7	38.9
113–115	37.5	37.8	38.0	38.2	38.5	38.7	39.0	39.2	39.5
116–118	38.0	38.3	38.5	38.8	39.0	39.3	39.5	39.7	40.0
119–121	38.5	38.7	39.0	39.2	39.5	39.7	40.0	40.2	40.5
122–124	39.0	39.2	39.4	39.7	39.9	40.2	40.4	40.7	40.9
125–127	39.4	39.6	39.9	40.1	40.4	40.6	40.9	41.1	41.4
128–130	39.8	40.0	40.3	40.5	40.8	41.0	41.3	41.5	41.8

*Percentage of fat calculated by the formula of Siri: percentage of fat = $[(4.95/D_b) = 4.5] \times 100$, where D_b = body density.

(From Pollock, M. L., Schmidt, D. H., and Jackson, A. S.: Measurement of cardiorespiratory fitness and body composition in the clinical setting. **Compr. Ther.** 6:12–27, 1980. Published with permission of The Laux Company, Inc., Harvard, MA.)

Table 6–20. Percentage of Body Fat Estimation for Men from Age and the Sum of Chest, Abdominal, and Thigh Skinfolds*

Sum of Skinfolds (mm)	Age to the Last Year							
	Under *22*	*23 to 27*	*28 to 32*	*33 to 37*	*38 to 42*	*43 to 47*	*48 to 52*	*53 to 57*	*Over 57*
8–10	1.3	1.8	2.3	2.9	3.4	3.9	4.5	5.0	5.5
11–13	2.2	2.8	3.3	3.9	4.4	4.9	5.5	6.0	6.5
14–16	3.2	3.8	4.3	4.8	5.4	5.9	6.4	7.0	7.5
17–19	4.2	4.7	5.3	5.8	6.3	6.9	7.4	8.0	8.5
20–22	5.1	5.7	6.2	6.8	7.3	7.9	8.4	8.9	9.5
23–25	6.1	6.6	7.2	7.7	8.3	8.8	9.4	9.9	10.5
26–28	7.0	7.6	8.1	8.7	9.2	9.8	10.3	10.9	11.4
29–31	8.0	8.5	9.1	9.6	10.2	10.7	11.3	11.8	12.4
32–34	8.9	9.4	10.0	10.5	11.1	11.6	12.2	12.8	13.3
35–37	9.8	10.4	10.9	11.5	12.0	12.6	13.1	13.7	14.3
38–40	10.7	11.3	11.8	12.4	12.9	13.5	14.1	14.6	15.2
41–43	11.6	12.2	12.7	13.3	13.8	14.4	15.0	15.5	16.1
44–46	12.5	13.1	13.6	14.2	14.7	15.3	15.9	16.4	17.0
47–49	13.4	13.9	14.5	15.1	15.6	16.2	16.8	17.3	17.9
50–52	14.3	14.8	15.4	15.9	16.5	17.1	17.6	18.2	18.8
53–55	15.1	15.7	16.2	16.8	17.4	17.9	18.5	19.1	19.7
56–58	16.0	16.5	17.1	17.7	18.2	18.8	19.4	20.0	20.5
59–61	16.9	17.4	17.9	18.5	19.1	19.7	20.2	20.8	21.4
62–64	17.6	18.2	18.8	19.4	19.9	20.5	21.1	21.7	22.2
65–67	18.5	19.0	19.6	20.2	20.8	21.3	21.9	22.5	23.1
68–70	19.3	19.9	20.4	21.0	21.6	22.2	22.7	23.3	23.9
71–73	20.1	20.7	21.2	21.8	22.4	23.0	23.6	24.1	24.7
74–76	20.9	21.5	22.0	22.6	23.2	23.8	24.4	25.0	25.5
77–79	21.7	22.2	22.8	23.4	24.0	24.6	25.2	25.8	26.3
80–82	22.4	23.0	23.6	24.2	24.8	25.4	25.9	26.5	27.1
83–85	23.2	23.8	24.4	25.0	25.5	26.1	26.7	27.3	27.9
86–88	24.0	24.5	25.1	25.7	26.3	26.9	27.5	28.1	28.7
89–91	24.7	25.3	25.9	26.5	27.1	27.6	28.2	28.8	29.4
92–94	25.4	26.0	26.6	27.2	27.8	28.4	29.0	29.6	30.2
95–97	26.1	26.7	27.3	27.9	28.5	29.1	29.7	30.3	30.9
98–100	26.9	27.4	28.0	28.6	29.2	29.8	30.4	31.0	31.6
101–103	27.5	28.1	28.7	29.3	29.9	30.5	31.1	31.7	32.3
104–106	28.2	28.8	29.4	30.0	30.6	31.2	31.8	32.4	33.0
107–109	28.9	29.5	30.1	30.7	31.3	31.9	32.5	33.1	33.7
110–112	29.6	30.2	30.8	31.4	32.0	32.6	33.2	33.8	34.4
113–115	30.2	30.8	31.4	32.0	32.6	33.2	33.8	34.5	35.1
116–118	30.9	31.5	32.1	32.7	33.3	33.9	34.5	35.1	35.7
119–121	31.5	32.1	32.7	33.3	33.9	34.5	35.1	35.7	36.4
122–124	32.1	32.7	33.3	33.9	34.5	35.1	35.8	36.4	37.0
125–127	32.7	33.3	33.9	34.5	35.1	35.8	36.4	37.0	37.6

*Percentage of fat calculated by the formula of Siri: percentage of fat = [4.95/D_b − 4.5] × 100, where D_b = body density.

(From Pollock, M. L., Schmidt, D. H., and Jackson, A. S.: Measurement of cardiorespiratory fitness and body composition in the clinical setting. **Compr. Ther.** 6:12–27, 1980. Published with permission of The Laux Company, Inc., Harvard, MA.)

Measurement of Anthropometric Indices. A description of anatomical landmarks and measurements of skinfold fat, circumference, and diameter measures follows.

Skinfold Fat

Chest: a diagonal fold taken one half of the distance between the anterior axillary line and the nipple for men and one third of the distance from the anterior axillary line and the equivalent position for women (Fig. 6–31).

Axilla: a vertical fold on the midaxillary line at the level of the xiphoid process of the sternum (Fig. 6–32).

Triceps: a vertical fold on the posterior midline of the upper arm (over triceps muscle), halfway between the acromion and olecranon processes; the elbow should be extended and relaxed (Fig. 6–33).

Subscapular: a fold taken on a diagonal line coming from the vertebral border to 1 to 2 cm from the inferior angle of the scapula (Fig. 6–33).

Abdominal: a vertical fold taken at a lateral distance of approximately 2 cm from the umbilicus (Fig. 6–34).

Suprailium: a diagonal fold above the crest of the ilium at the spot where an imaginary line would come down from the anterior axillary line (Fig. 6–34). It should be noted that some recommend that the measure be taken more laterally at the midaxillary line.[222, 225] Data for the generalized equations of Jackson and Pollock[254, 263] were determined at the anterior axillary line. This difference in sites may result in a 3 to 6 mm skinfold fat difference, with the anterior site being smaller.

Thigh: a vertical fold on the anterior aspect of the thigh, midway between the inguinal crease and the proximal border of the patella (Fig. 6–34). To help locate the inguinal crease have the subject flex the hip. The proximal reference point is located on the inguinal crease at the midpoint of the long axis of the thigh.

Circumference Measures

Shoulder: taken in the horizontal plane at the maximal circumference of the shoulders at the level of the greatest lateral protrusion of the deltoid muscles.

Chest: taken in the horizontal plane at the fourth costosternal joints during mid–tidal volume. The fourth costosternal joints are generally located on a flat surface above the nipples (in men).

Abdominal: taken in a horizontal plane at the smallest circumference in the abdominal region, generally 2 to 4 inches above the umbilicus.

Waist: taken in the horizontal plane at the level of the umbilicus.

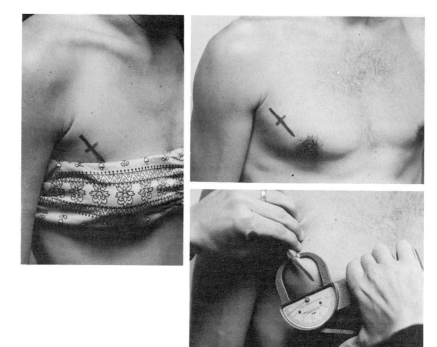

Figure 6–31. Chest skinfold fat site for men and women. (From Pollock, M. L., Schmidt, D. H., and Jackson, A. S.: Measurement of cardiorespiratory fitness and body composition in the clinical setting. **Compr. Ther.** 6:12–27, 1980. Published with permission of The Laux Company, Inc., Harvard, MA.)

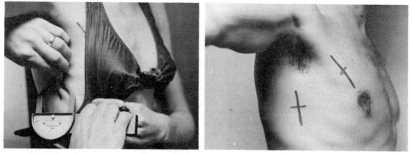

Figure 6–32. Axilla skinfold fat site. (From Pollock, M. L., Schmidt, D. H., and Jackson, A. S.: Measurement of cardiorespiratory fitness and body composition in the clinical setting. **Compr. Ther.** 6:12–27, 1980. Published with permission of The Laux Company, Inc., Harvard, MA.)

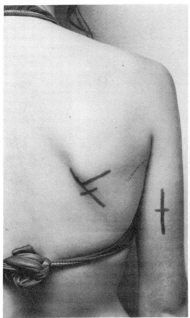

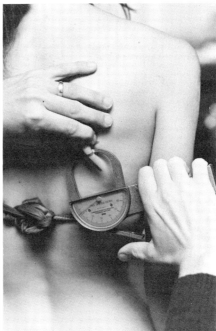

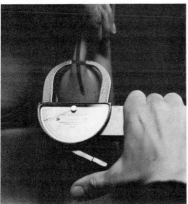

Figure 6–33. Triceps and subscapular skinfold fat sites. (From Pollock, M. L., Schmidt, D. H., and Jackson, A. S.: Measurement of cardiorespiratory fitness and body composition in the clinical setting. **Compr. Ther.**. 6:12–27, 1980. Published with permission of The Laux Company Inc., Harvard, MA.)

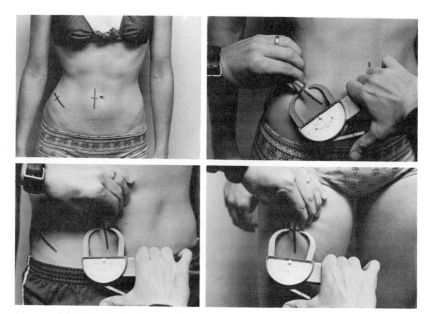

Figure 6–34. Abdominal, suprailium, and front thigh skinfold fat sites. (From Pollock, M. L., Schmidt, D. H., and Jackson, A. S.: Measurement of cardiorespiratory fitness and body composition in the clinical setting. **Compr. Ther.** 6:12–27, 1980. Published with permission of the Laux Company, Inc., Harvard, MA.)

Gluteal: taken in the horizontal plane at the largest circumference around the buttocks. Subjects stand with feet together and gluteals tensed (Fig. 6–35).

Thigh: taken in the horizontal plane just below the gluteal fold or maximal thigh girth. Thigh flexed.

Calf: taken in the horizontal plane at the maximal girth of the calf, with muscle tensed.

Ankle: taken in the horizontal plane at the smallest point above the malleoli.

Arm: taken at maximal girth of the midarm when flexed to the greatest angle, with the underlying muscles fully contracted.

Forearm: taken at the largest circumference, with the forearm parallel to the floor, the elbow joint at a 90-degree angle, the hand in the supinated position, and the muscles flexed.

Wrist: taken over the styloid process of the radius and ulna with the arm extended in front of the body and the fist loosely clenched, relaxed, and pronated.

Diameter Measures

Shoulder: distance between the outermost protrusions of the shoulder (deltoid muscles).

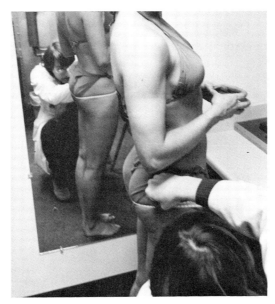

Figure 6–35. Measuring gluteal circumference with a 2 m steel tape. Mirror in background assists the technician in adjusting tape at the proper level.

Biacromial: distance between the most lateral projections of the acromial processes.

Chest: arms abducted slightly for placement of the anthropometer at the level of the xiphoid process.

Bi-iliac: distance between the most lateral projections of the iliac crests.

Bitrochanteric: distance between the most lateral projections of the greater trochanters.

Knee: 45-degree angle measurement at the smallest width of the knee, which is taken with the right foot on a small stool so that the knee is flexed at a 90-degree angle.

Wrist: distance between the radial and ulna styloid processes.

An example of a data collection form used for recording anthropometric measures is shown in Figure A–7, Appendix A.

A caliper that is accurately calibrated and has a constant pressure of 10 g/mm^2 throughout the full range of the caliper opening is recommended for taking skinfold fat measures. Caliper specifications and recommended standards for measurement are well documented.[222, 225, 284–286]

Recent data have suggested that the use of cheaper calipers often gives results similar to those achieved with the recommended constant-pressure type of calipers.[287–289] Although this may be true, more information is needed regarding long-term use (durability), quality control, and so on. Some evidence suggests that even the highly recommended calipers may give different results. Lohman and colleagues[289] found that the Lange caliper yielded higher values than the Harpenden caliper. Although experienced technicians collected the data, none had equal experience in using both calipers; thus, a bias may have been present. More recently, Gruber and colleagues[290] confirmed the finding of Lohman and colleagues[289] and found that the Harpenden caliper gave a 10 percent lower value than the Lange. In general, it appears that a variety of calipers may be satisfactorily used, but because of possible differences among them, use of the caliper with which the data for the specific body density equation were developed is recommended. The Lange caliper was used for the equations developed by Jackson and Pollock.[254, 263]

The accuracy of predicting body density from skinfold fat measures is subject to large intertester error.[291] A difference of as much as 12 mm on one skinfold fat site and up to 3 percent in body fat can be noted even by experienced testers.[292] When testers practice together and take care to standardize their testing procedures, however, intertester error usually results in less than a 1 percent fat calculated error.[291–294] A review suggests that the largest error found among investigators results from the nonstandardization of sites and differences in selecting a skinfold site.[291] When procedures are standardized, measurement error for skinfold fat appears to be more related to the size of the skinfold than to the specific site or gender. Pollock, Jackson, and Graves[294] found a consistent 10-percent error of measure among skinfold sites for both men and women. The average error for the 68 subjects for skinfold thicknesses of 10, 20, 30, and 40 mm was 1.3, 2.3, 3.2, and 4.2 mm, respectively. The error of measurement included both day-to-day variation as well as intertester differences. For the same amount of skinfold thickness, the suprailium site had the largest error among seven skinfolds.

The development of a standardization manual for assessing anthropometric measures was a result of the Airlie Consensus Conference in 1986. The reference manual included input from 41 experts from various disciplines and includes a comprehensive description of over 40 anthropometric measures.[225] It is thought that this standardization of procedures will be used across disciplines and provides more exacting methodology to reduce intertester error of measurement.

A flexible steel tape is generally used for taking circumference measures. The tape should be approximately 2 meters in length and should be easily retractable. A sliding broad-breadth caliper (anthropometer) is used for assessing diameters. Usually circumference and diameter measures are recorded to the nearest 0.1 cm. Further discussion of procedures and description of sites of anthropometric measures are provided by Behnke and Wilmore,[222] Lohman, Roche, and Martorell,[225] and Hertzberg and associates.[284]

In measuring skinfold fat, the skinfold is grasped firmly by the thumb and index finger; the caliper is perpendicular to the fold at approximately 1 cm (¼ to ½ inch) from the thumb and index finger.[222, 225] Then, while maintaining a grasp of the skinfold, allow the caliper grip to be released so that the full tension is exerted on the skinfold. In grasping the skinfold, the pads at the tip of the thumb and index finger are used. Testers should trim their nails. The dial is read to the nearest 0.5 mm (Lange) or 0.1 mm (Harpenden) approximately 1 to 2 seconds after the grip has been released. A minimum of two measurements should be taken at each site. If the repeated measurement varies by more than 1 mm, a third should be taken. If consecutive fatfold measurements become increasingly smaller, the fat is being compressed; this occurs mainly with fleshy subjects. If this occurs, the tester should proceed to the next site and return to the troubled spot after finishing the other measurements; the final value is the average of the two that seem to represent the skinfold fat site best. It is better to take measurements when the skin is dry because it is more difficult to get a good grasp of the skinfold when the skin is moist or wet. Practice is necessary to grasp the same size of skinfold consistently at exactly the same location every time. Most skinfold fat equations or sums of skinfold norms are based on taking measurements on the right side of the body.

BIOELECTRICAL IMPEDANCE

An easy-to-operate, reliable, and portable bioelectrical impedance (BIA) meter has recently been developed and has potential for widespread use for estimating body composition in the clinical setting. The method is based on the principle that a resistance to a mild electrical current is inversely related to total body water and electrolyte distribution. Lukaski[224] states that "the hypothesis that bioelectrical impedance measurements can be used to determine fat-free mass (FFM) is based upon the principle that the impedance of a geometrical system is related to conductor length and configuration, its cross-sectional area, and signal frequency." Since the fat-free mass contains almost all the water and electrolytes of the body, conductivity is greater in it than in fat mass. In theory, therefore, the magnitude of an impedance measurement enables a differentiation of fat-free mass and fat mass.

The BIA technique requires the careful placement of four electrodes on the supine subject in well-defined sites. A low-level, undetectable, excitation current is introduced at a frequency of 50 kHz, which is passed from the source electrode to the sensing electrode. The voltage drop detected by the sensing electrode is recorded to the nearest ohm.

The problem with the BIA procedure is that it has produced mixed results in the literature.[295-304] Lukaski and associates[295] reported r = 0.88 ± 3.1% and r = 0.93 ± 2.7% for prediction of body fat in women and men, respectively. This was not confirmed by Segal and colleagues[296] or Jackson, Pollock, and Graves.[298] The latter study using the Lukaski equations showed r = 0.76 ± 4.7% and r = 0.71 ± 4.6% for predicting body fat in women and men, respectively. This study also showed that the BMI accounted for most of the variance in the BIA equation. More recently, in an eight-university study, Lohman[299] showed r = 0.59 ± 3.1% and r = 0.75 ± 3.8% for young women and men. In the Lohman study,[299] the standard error of measures was comparable with what is reported for the skinfold technique. The correlation coefficients were most likely affected by the homogeneous sample used in the study.

There appears to be a general consensus that more data are needed on a more varied population, as well as refinement of prediction equations and further cross-validation, before widespread application can be recommended.[300-305] Although the BIA meter is significantly more expensive than skinfold fat calipers, its potential for reducing intertester error is promising. Even so, at best the accuracy of the BIA technique is equivalent to that of anthropometric methods.[305]

CALCULATION OF DESIRED/TARGET WEIGHT

Desired, or target, weight is described in Chapter 2. If 23 percent fat for women and 16 percent fat for men are used as the desired body fat standards, then the following equations can be used:

$$\text{Women: desired weight} = \frac{[\text{weight} - (\text{weight} \times \% \text{ fat})/100]}{0.77}$$

$$\text{Men: desired weight} = \frac{[\text{weight} - (\text{weight} \times \% \text{ fat})/100]}{0.84}$$

For example, a 35-year-old man who is 23 percent fat and weighs 210 pounds would have to reduce to 192.5 pounds to attain his goal of 16 percent fat. A 45-year-old woman who is 28 percent fat and weighs 145 pounds would have to reduce to 135.6 pounds to attain her desired goal of 23 percent fat. For ease in computation of desired weight based on 23 percent fat for women and 16 percent fat for men, see Tables A–31 and A–32, Appendix A.

The numerator of these two formulas is derived by subtracting the fat weight from the total body weight, leaving the fat-free weight. The denominator adds back the desired amount of fat weight to the fat-free weight. If another desired weight (percentage fat goal) is wanted, simply change the fraction value in the denominator to represent the new function of fat-free weight desired. This technique for estimating desirable weight is not without error, and it is suggested that 2 pounds be added and subtracted from the desired weight to provide a desired weight range. For the preceding examples, this would mean 190.5 to 194.5 pounds for the man and 133.6 to 137.6 for the woman.

Although these desired weight formulas are useful in working with people and giving them objective goals for fat and weight loss, they have certain limitations. Weight loss depends on caloric intake and expenditure, but diet and exercise affect body composition differently.[306, 307] When weight loss comes from diet alone, both fat and lean tissue are reduced, whereas exercise alone increases, maintains, or attenuates the loss of fat-free weight and reduces body fat. Therefore, the accuracy of the desired weight formulas depends on how weight and fat are lost. Periodic checks of body composition during the weight reduction program help refine estimations.

Estimating body composition in the obese population has been difficult. The authors generally recommend the BMI for use in the obese population. More recently, Weltman and associates[308, 309] have developed prediction equations for estimating body composition in adult obese men and women:[308, 309]

Men: % fat = 0.31457 (mean Abd) − 0.10969 (Wt) + 10.8336
$$(r = 0.54, \text{SEE} = 2.88\%)$$

Women: % fat = 0.11077 (mean Abd) − 0.17666 (Ht) + 0.14354
(Wt) + 51.03301
$$(r = 0.76, \text{SEE} = 2.9\%)$$

where mean Abd = the average of two circumferences of the abdomen as described by Behnke and Wilmore,[222]
Wt = weight,
Ht = height.

Although more cross-validation of these equations is necessary before full acceptance can occur, they appear to be an improvement over using just the BMI.

Normative data on skinfolds and other anthropometric measures are available for school children and youth 6 to 17 years of age and adults up to 79 years of age through the National Center for Health Statistics.[310] Normative data for skinfold fat of school children and youth are also available elsewhere.[68, 311] Percentile rankings for percentage of fat and for chest, abdomen, suprailium, axilla, triceps, subscapula, and front thigh skinfolds are available for both men and women from 18 to 65+ years of age in *The Y's Way to Physical Fitness.*[16]

Muscular Strength and Endurance, and Flexibility

STRENGTH

As mentioned in Chapter 5, strength relates to both dynamic and static contractions. Strength testing has usually been conducted by the use of weights (free standing or various apparatus), dynamometers, cable tensiometers (static), isokinetic devices, and elaborately designed force transducers and recorders.[312–315] A thorough description of these methods and discussion concerning reliability and validity can be found in Chapter 5 and in several texts.[13, 31, 312–315] Elaborate strength and endurance type of equipment can be expensive and may not always provide a substantial improvement in measurement accuracy. For the purpose of this section, only the field tests listed in Table 6–2 are described in detail. More sophisticated testing of muscular strength and endurance and the testing of athletes are described by Berger,[314] Wilmore and Costill,[312] and MacDougall, Wenger, and Green.[13] See Jones and associates[315] and Chapter 7 for information on the testing of the lumbar spine.

Strength can be easily assessed by the one-repetition maximum test (1-RM).[31, 314] The basic muscle or muscle group to be tested is selected, then the individual is given a series of trials to determine the greatest weight that can be lifted only once for that particular lift. This test is conducted largely through trial and error when subjects are inexperienced in lifting weights. The subject starts with a weight that can be lifted comfortably, then weight is added progressively until the weight can be lifted correctly just one time. If this weight can be lifted more than once, more weight needs to be added until a true 1-RM is reached.

If one test only is to be selected, use the 1-RM bench press. Berger[314, 316] showed moderately high intercorrelations between back hyperextension, bench press, standing military press, sit-up, squat, upright rowing, and curl exercises. Using 174 college-age men, he found that the best single lifts for predicting total dynamic strength (sum of 1-RM of seven exercises listed previously) were bench press (r = 0.84) and standing military press (r = 0.87). For safety and administrative purposes, the 1-RM bench press was selected for use.

Although the bench press can be used for assessing strength, test batteries usually select three or four exercises that represent the body's major muscle groups. Tables 6–21 and 6–22 are norms for the 1-RM bench press and 1-RM leg press for men and women from 20 to 60+ years of age. These tests were performed on Universal Gym equipment, and the methods are described by Jackson, Watkins, and Patton.[317] As mentioned previously, the 1-RM bench press is recommended as an indicator for upper body strength, and the leg press is a good indicator for lower body strength.[317] To use the norms properly, strength in pounds is divided by body weight. Although strength requirements differ for each sport or activity, or even for position or event within each sport, these were developed for the average person who is training mainly for general fitness purposes. Specific standards for each sport have yet to be developed.

The bench press test recommended by the YMCA combines muscular strength and endurance.[16] In their test, women use a 35-pound barbell weight and men an 80-pound weight. This test has limitations in that it is a test of endurance for the stronger participants and a test of strength for the weaker individuals. The norms listed in Appendix A, Tables A–13 to A–24, are bench press repetitions to maximum with the weights prescribed above.

Table 6–21. Standard Values for Bench Press Strength in 1-RM lbs/lb of Body Weight

| | Age (yr) | | | | |
Rating	*20–29*	*30–39*	*40–49*	*50–59*	*60+*
Men					
Excellent	>1.26	>1.08	>0.97	>0.86	>0.78
Good	1.17–1.25	1.01–1.07	0.91–0.96	0.81–0.85	0.74–0.77
Average	0.97–1.16	0.86–1.00	0.78–0.90	0.70–0.80	0.64–0.73
Fair	0.88–0.96	0.79–0.85	0.72–0.77	0.65–0.69	0.60–0.63
Poor	<0.87	<0.78	<.071	<0.64	<0.59
Women					
Excellent	>0.78	>0.66	>0.61	>0.54	>0.55
Good	0.72–0.77	0.62–0.65	0.57–0.60	0.51–0.53	0.51–0.54
Average	0.59–0.71	0.53–0.61	0.48–0.56	0.43–0.50	0.41–0.50
Fair	0.53–0.58	0.49–0.52	0.44–0.47	0.40–0.42	0.37–0.40
Poor	<0.52	<0.48	<0.43	<0.39	<0.36

(Reprinted with permission from The Institute for Aerobics Research: **1985 Physical Fitness Norms.** [Unpublished Data.] Dallas, TX, 1985.)

Table 6–22. Standard Values for Upper Leg Press Strength in 1-RM lbs/lb of Body Weight

Rating	Age (yr)				
	20–29	*30–39*	*40–49*	*50–59*	*60+*
Men					
Excellent	>2.08	>1.88	>1.76	>1.66	>1.56
Good	2.00–2.07	1.80–1.87	1.70–1.75	1.60–1.65	1.50–1.55
Average	1.83–1.99	1.63–1.79	1.56–1.69	1.46–1.59	1.37–1.49
Fair	1.65–1.82	1.55–1.62	1.50–1.55	1.40–1.45	1.31–1.36
Poor	<1.64	<1.54	<1.49	<1.39	<1.30
Women					
Excellent	>1.63	>1.42	>1.32	>1.26	>1.15
Good	1.54–1.62	1.35–1.41	1.26–1.31	1.13–1.25	1.08–1.14
Average	1.35–1.53	1.20–1.34	1.12–1.25	0.99–1.12	0.92–1.07
Fair	1.26–1.34	1.13–1.19	1.06–1.11	0.86–0.98	0.85–0.91
Poor	<1.25	<1.12	<1.05	<0.85	<0.84

(Reprinted with permission from The Institute for Aerobics Research: **1985 Physical Fitness Norms.** [Unpublished Data.] Dallas, TX, 1985.)

MUSCULAR ENDURANCE

Muscular endurance has been measured in a number of different ways, including the greatest number of sit-ups that can be performed in a fixed period of time (usually 30 seconds or a minute) or the maximal number of push-ups, pull-ups, or bar dips that can be performed continuously in an indefinite time period.[16, 31, 312, 314] Many of these tests penalize the participant who has long legs, long arms, or a heavy body weight. To eliminate this, a concept has evolved that uses a fixed percentage of the individual's body weight as the resistance; the individual lifts this as many times as possible until he or she reaches the point of fatigue or exhaustion.[314] Firm guidelines have yet to be established with regard to what the actual fixed percentages of the individual's body weight should be for each of the muscle groups tested. In fact, it is debatable whether the weight used in the test should be a fixed percentage of the individual's body weight or a fixed percentage of the individual's 1-RM, or absolute strength. As an example, if the endurance test for the bench press movement was conducted using 50 percent of the individual's body weight as the resistance, the 180-pound man would be asked to lift 90 pounds as many times as he could. A strong man of this body weight would be able to lift this 90-pound weight 20 or more times, whereas the relatively weak man who weighs 180 pounds may not be able to lift the 90-pound weight even one single repetition, i.e., the designated weight exceeds his 1-RM. (This further illustrates the limitation of the YMCA's recommended bench press test as described earlier.) In this case, the test for muscular endurance would be highly dependent on strength. To isolate muscular endurance as a pure component, where the test is not as dependent on the individual's strength, it is advocated that the test battery be established on the basis of the individual's strength, not body weight.

Two tests that have been traditionally used to measure muscular endurance are the push-up and sit-up tests to assess upper body (triceps, anterior deltoids, and pectoralis major) and abdominal muscular endurance, respectively.[6, 16, 31, 68, 125, 127, 128] The push-up test is administered with the individual in the standard "up" position for a full push-up (Fig. 6–36). Participants lower themselves down until the chest touches the floor, keeping the back straight, and then raising back to the up position. The maximal number of correctly completed push-ups is counted. Norms for push-ups are shown in Appendix A, Table A–28. These standards are listed relative to age and sex. Women can perform this test from the knee-supported position (Fig. 6–37).[6, 31, 125]

In the sit-up test, individuals start by lying on their back, knees bent, feet flat on the floor, with heels between 12 and 18 inches from the buttocks. Hands should be interlocked behind the neck. The tester holds the person's feet down. The individual performs as many correct sit-ups (Fig. 6–38) as possible in 60-seconds. Elbows should be touched to the knees in the up position,

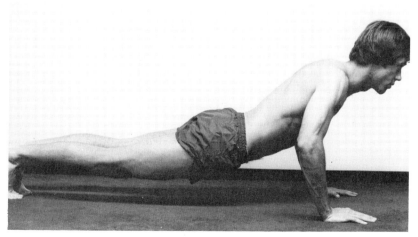

Figure 6–36. Standard or full push-up. Recommended for men; the method is compatible with norms for men listed in Appendix A, Table A–26. (Reprinted with permission from Pollock, M. L., Wilmore, J. H., and Fox, S. M.: **Health and Fitness Through Physical Activity.** New York, copyright John Wiley and Sons, 1978.)

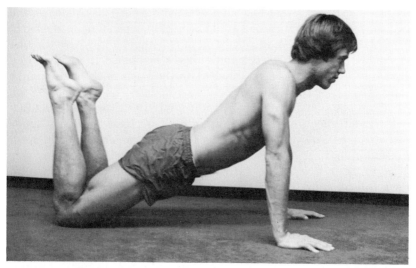

Figure 6–37. Modified knee push-up. Recommended for women; the method is compatible with norms for women listed in Appendix A, Table A–26. (Reprinted with permission from Pollock, M. L., Wilmore, J. H., and Fox, S. M.: **Health and Fitness Through Physical Activity.** New York, copyright John Wiley and Sons, 1978.)

and this must be followed by a complete return to the full lying position before starting the next sit-up. The total number of sit-ups performed in 60 seconds is recorded and compared with Tables A–13 to A–24 or A–27, Appendix A, which lists standards relative to age and sex. Data and standards for school children 5 to 17 years of age are also available.[31, 68, 127, 311] Method of hand placement for the sit-up test varies among testing agencies, thus check procedures carefully before using norms. Tests for school children usually place hands and arms across the chest rather than behind the head for sit-ups.

FLEXIBILITY

Probably the most accurate tests of flexibility currently available are those that assess the actual range of motion of the various joints. Although this is easily accomplished by instruments such as the Leighton Flexometer[318] and the electrogoniometer,[319] these pieces of equipment are not readily available.[31] See MacDougall, Wenger, and Green[13] and Wilmore and Costill[312] for more specific recommendations for testing the flexibility of various joints.

Since flexibility is specific to each joint, no generalized flexibility test is available.[31] Because the emphasis of this book is on adult

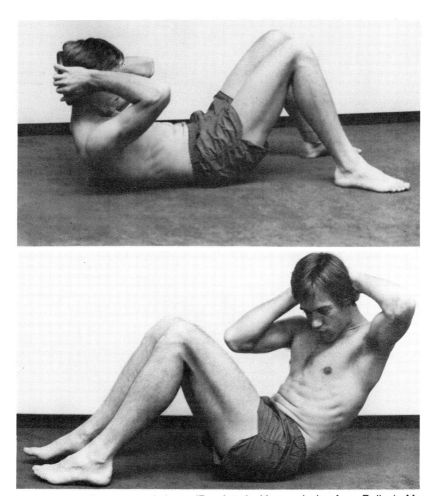

Figure 6–38. Sixty-second sit-up. (Reprinted with permission from Pollock, M. L., Wilmore, J. H ., and Fox, S. M.: **Health and Fitness Through Physical Activity.** New York, copyright John Wiley and Sons, 1978.)

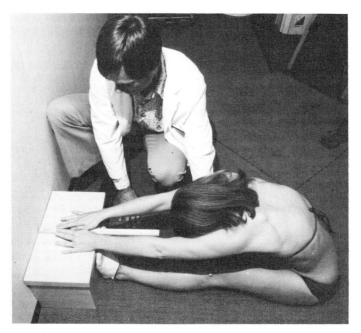

Figure 6–39. The Sit and Reach Test (trunk forward flexion) to determine flexibility of the low back and posterior thigh muscles. (Reprinted with permission from Pollock, M. L., Wilmore, J. H., and Fox, S. M.: **Health and Fitness Through Physical Activity.** New York, copyright John Wiley and Sons, 1978.)

physical fitness and related health aspects, lower back flexibility is mentioned here. As stated earlier, low back pain and disability are prevalent among men and women in the adult population.[315, 320] Much of this problem is related to the lack of flexibility in the back of the legs (hamstrings), hips, and lower back.[320, 321] To measure this capability, a simple field test called the Sit and Reach Test can be used (Fig. 6–39).

In the Sit and Reach Test, the individual sits with the legs extended directly in front of him or her and the knees pressed against the floor. The feet are placed against a board that is attached to a yardstick, with the 15-inch mark (YMCA test) placed at the point where the foot contacts the block (it should be noted that for the Sit and Reach Test as described by the Canadian Standardized Test of Fitness, Appendix A, Table A–26, the ruler is placed at the 26 cm mark).[6] The individual puts the index fingers of both hands together and reaches forward slowly as far as possible. The distance reached is noted on the yardstick and recorded. The knees must be kept in contact with the floor, and bouncing is discouraged. A short warm-up of four to six stretches is recommended before starting the test. Norms based on men and women of various ages are shown in Appendix A, Tables A–13 to A–24 and A–26. Norms for school children and youths 5 to 17 years of age are also available.[68, 127] Obviously, the Sit and Reach Test is influenced by the length of the arms and legs of the individual, in addition to flexibility.

SUMMARY

This chapter has presented an explanation and discussion of many of the factors involved in a comprehensive medical screening and physical fitness examination. In the first portion of the chapter, risk factors related to coronary artery disease and a coronary risk factor profile chart were shown. Within this profile chart, risk is estimated to be high or low. The established risk factor charts should be used as education tools, and their limitations with regard to validity should be understood.

Next, tests to evaluate cardiorespiratory fitness, body composition (leanness-fatness), strength, muscular endurance, and flexibility were described. The recommended tests were graded with regard to their sophistication and feasibility.

An important aspect of this chapter is its ability to explain to the participants how to assess their health and fitness status properly and safely. This information should give participants a secure basis for initiating an exercise program at the proper level or for monitoring the progress of the exercise program. To aid in evaluation of physical fitness, norm tables that are specific to age and sex were presented.

References

1. Hurst, W.J.: **The Heart,** 6th Ed. New York, McGraw-Hill, 1986.
2. Braunwald, E.: **Heart Disease: A Textbook of Cardiovascular Medicine,** 3rd Ed. Philadelphia, W.B. Saunders Co., 1988.
3. Bruce, R.A., DeRouen, T.A., and Hossack, K.F.: Value of maximal exercise tests in the risk assessment of primary coronary heart disease events in healthy men. Five years' experience of the Seattle heart watch study. **Am. J. Cardiol.** 46:371–378, 1980.
4. Chisholm, D.M., Collis, M.L., Kulak, L.L., Davenport, W., and Gruber, N.: Physical activity readiness. **Br. Col. Med. J.** 17:375–378, 1975.
5. Jette, M.: The standardized test of fitness in occupational health: a pilot project. **Can. J. Public Health** 69:431–438, 1978.
6. Government of Canada: **Fitness and Amateur Sports: Canadian Standardized Test of Fitness (CSTF) Operations Manual,** 3rd Ed. Ottawa, Minister of State, FAS 73–78, 1986.
7. Herbert, D.L., and Herbert, W.G.: **Legal Aspects of Preventive and Reha-**

bilitative **Exercise Programs.** Canton, OH, Professional and Executive Reports and Publications, 1985.

8. Herbert, W.G., and Herbert, D.L.: Legal considerations. In Blair, S. N., Painter, P., Pate, R. R., Smith, L.K., and Taylor, C. B. (eds.): **Resource Manual for Guidelines for Exercise Testing and Exercise Prescription.** Philadelphia, Lea & Febiger, 1988, pp. 395–399.
9. Policy Statement Regarding the Use of Human Subjects and Informed Consent. **Med. Sci. Sports Exerc.** 21:v, 1989.
10. American College of Sports Medicine: **Guidelines for Graded Exercise Testing and Exercise Prescription,** 3rd Ed. Philadelphia, Lea & Febiger, 1986.
11. Ellestad, M.H., Blomqvist, C.G., and Naughton, J.P.: Standards for adult exercise testing laboratories. **Circulation** 59:421a–430a, 1979.
12. Fry, G., and Berra, K.: **YMCArdiac Therapy.** Chicago, National Council of the YMCA, 1981.
13. MacDougall, J. D., Wenger, H. A., and Green, H. J. (eds.): Canadian Association of Sport Sciences: **Physiological Testing of the Elite Athlete.** Ottawa, Mutual Press Limited, 1982.
14. Howley, E.T., and Franks, B.D.: **Health/Fitness Instructors Handbook.** Champaign, IL, Human Kinetics Publishers, 1986.
15. Fardy, P.S., Yankowitz, F.G., and Wilson, P.K.: **Cardiac Rehabilitation, Adult Fitness, and Exercise Testing,** 2nd Ed. Philadelphia, Lea & Febiger, 1988.
16. Golding, L.A., Meyers, C.R., and Sinning, W.E.: **Y's Way to Physical Fitness: The Complete Guide to Fitness Testing and Instruction,** 3rd Ed. Champaign, IL, Human Kinetics Publishers, 1989.
17. Shephard, R.J.: The current status of the Canadian home fitness test. **Br. J. Sports Med.** 14:114–125, 1980.
18. Shephard, R.J., Bailey, D.A., and Mirwald, R.L.: Development of the Canadian home fitness test. **Can. Med. Assoc. J.** 114:675–679, 1976.
19. The National Heart, Lung, and Blood Institute: **Exercise and Your Heart.** Washington, D.C., U.S. Government Printing Office, 726–248, 1981.
20. Diamond, G.A., and Forrester, J.S.: Analysis of probability as an aid in the clinical diagnosis of coronary-artery disease. **N. Engl. J. Med.** 300:1350–1358, 1979.
21. Epstein, S.E.: Implications of probability analysis on the strategy used for noninvasive detection of coronary-artery disease. **Am. J. Cardiol.** 46:491–499, 1980.
22. Kannel, W.B., McGee, D., and Gordon, T.: A general cardiovascular risk profile: the Framingham study. **Am. J. Cardiol.** 38:46–51, 1976.
23. Kannel, W.B.: Contributions of the Framingham study to the conquest of coronary artery disease. **Am. J. Cardiol.** 62:1109–1112, 1988.
24. American Heart Association: **Coronary Risk Handbook.** Dallas, American Heart Association, 1973.
25. Kline, G.M., Porcari, J.P., Hintermeister, R., Freedson, P.S., Ward, A., McCarron, R.F., Ross, J., and Rippe, J.M.: Estimation of $\dot{V}O_2$max from a one-mile track walk, gender, age, and body weight. **Med. Sci. Sports Exerc.** 19:253–259, 1987.
26. American Heart Association: **Exercise Testing and Training of Individuals with Heart Disease or at High Risk for its Development: A Handbook for Physicians.** Dallas, American Heart Association, 1975.
27. Balke, B.: **A Simple Field Test for the Assessment of Physical Fitness.** CARI Report 63-6. Oklahoma City, Civil Aeromedical Research Institute, Federal Aviation Agency, 1963.
28. Cooper, K.H.: Correlation between field and treadmill testing as a means of assessing maximal oxygen intake. **JAMA** 203:201–204, 1968.
29. Bruce, R.A., Kusumi, F., and Hosmer, D.: Maximal oxygen intake and nomographic assessment of functional aerobic impairment in cardiovascular disease. **Am. Heart J.** 85:545–562, 1973.

30. Pollock, M.L., Schmidt, D.H., and Jackson, A.S.: Measurement of cardiorespiratory fitness and body composition in the clinical setting. **Compr. Ther.** 6:12–27, 1980.

31. Baumgartner, J.A., and Jackson, A.S.: **Measurement for Evaluation in Physical Education and Exercise Science,** 3rd Ed. Dubuque, IA, William C. Brown Co., 1987.

32. Froelicher, V.F., Brammel, H., Davis, G., Noguera, I., Stewart, A., and Lancaster, M.C.: A comparison of reproducibility and physiologic response to three maximal treadmill exercise protocols. **Chest** 65:512–517, 1974.

33. Taylor, H.L., Wang, Y., Rowell, L., and Blomqvist, G.: The standardization and interpretation of submaximal and maximal tests of working capacity. **Pediatrics** 32:703–722, 1963.

34. American College of Sports Medicine: Directory of Preventive and Rehabilitative Programs for Graduate Study. Unpublished, 1983.

35. Taylor, H.L., Haskell, W., Fox, S.M., and Blackburn, H.: Exercise tests: a summary of procedures and concepts of stress testing for cardiovascular diagnosis and function evaluation. In Blackburn, H. (ed.): **Measurement in Exercise Electrocardiography.** Springfield, IL, Charles C Thomas, 1969, 259–305.

36. Ellestad, M.S.: **Stress Testing Principles and Practice,** 3rd Ed. Philadelphia, F.A. Davis Co., 1986.

37. Froelicher, V.F.: **Exercise and the Heart: Clinical Concepts,** 2nd Ed. Chicago, Year Book Medical Publishers, 1987.

38. **Lipid Research Clinics Manual of Laboratory Operations, Vol. 1. Lipid and Lipoprotein Analysis.** HEW Publication No. N1H75-628. Washington, D.C., U.S. Government Printing Office, 1974.

39. Dufaux, B., Assmann, G., Order, U., Hoederath, A., and Hollman, W.: Plasma lipoproteins, hormones, and energy substrates during the first days after prolonged exercise. **Int. J. Sports Med.** 2:256–260, 1981.

40. Buskirk, E.R., Iampietro, P.F., and Bass, D.E.: Work performance after dehydration: effects of physical conditioning and heat acclimation. **J. Appl. Physiol.** 12:189–194, 1958.

41. Girandola, R.N., Wiswell, R.A., and Romero, G.: Body composition changes resulting from fluid ingestion and dehydration. **Res. Q.** 48:299–303, 1977.

42. Aronow, W.S., Cassidy, J., Vangrow, J.S., March, H., Kern, J.C., Goldsmith, J.R., Khemka, M., Pagano, J., and Vawter, M.: Effect of cigarette smoking and breathing carbon monoxide on cardiovascular hemodynamics in anginal patients. **Circulation** 50:340–347, 1974.

43. Ward, A., and Morgan, W.P.: Adherence patterns of healthy men and women enrolled in an adult exercise program. **J. Cardiac Rehabil.** 4:143–152, 1984.

44. Dishman, R.K. (ed.): **Exercise Adherence: Its Impact on Public Health.** Champaign, IL, Human Kinetics Books, 1988.

45. American Heart Association: **Recommendations for Human Blood Pressure Determination by Sphygmomanometers.** Dallas, American Heart Association, 1987.

46. American Heart Association of Wisconsin: **Blood Pressure Measurement Education Program.** Milwaukee, AHA/Wisconsin Affiliate, 1981.

47. Souchek, J., Stamler, J., Dyer, A.R., Oglesby, P., and Lepper, M.H.: The value of two or three versus single reading of blood pressure at first visit. **J. Chron. Dis.** 32:197–210, 1979.

48. National High Blood Pressure Education Program, National Heart, Lung, and Blood Institute: The 1988 report of the Joint National Committee on Detection, Evaluation, and Treatment of High Blood Pressure. **Arch. Int. Med.** 148:1023–1038, 1988.

49. Dishinger, P., and DuChane, A.G.: Quality control aspects of blood pressure measurements in the multiple risk factor intervention trial. **Control. Clin. Trials** 7:1375–1575, 1986.

50. Pickering, T.G., James, G.D., Boddie, C., Harshfield, G.A., Blank, S., and Laragh, J.H.: How common is white coat hypertension? **JAMA** 259:225–228, 1988.

51. Lind, A.R., and McNicol, G.W.: Muscular factors that determine the cardio-vascular responses to sustained and rhythmic exercise. **Can. Med. Assoc. J.** 96:706–713, 1967.

52. Bezucha, G.R., Lenser, M.C., Hanson, P.G., and Nagle, F.J.: Comparison of hemodynamic responses to static and dynamic exercise. **J. Appl. Physiol.** 53:1589–1593, 1982.

53. MacDougall, J.D., Tuxen, D., Sale, D.G., Moroz, J.R., and Sutton, J.R.: Arterial blood pressure response to heavy resistance exercise. **J. Appl. Physiol.** 58:785–790, 1985.

54. American Heart Association: **Physician's Cholesterol Education Handbook.** Dallas, American Heart Association, 1988.

55. Clecman, J.I., and Lenfant, C.: New guidelines for the treatment of high blood cholesterol in adults from the National Cholesterol Education Program. **Circulation** 76:960–962, 1987.

56. Consolazio, F.C., Johnson, R.E., and Pecora, L.J.: **Physiological Measurements of Metabolic Function in Man.** New York, McGraw-Hill, 1963.

57. Wilmore, J.H., and Costill, D.L.: Semiautomated systems approach to the assessment of oxygen uptake during exercise. **J. Appl. Physiol.** 36:618–620, 1974.

58. Wilmore, J.H., Davis, J.A., and Norton, A.C.: An automated system for assessing metabolic and respiratory function during exercise. **J. Appl. Physiol.** 40:619–624, 1976.

59. Wasserman, K., Hansen, J.E., Sue, D.Y., and Whipp, B.J.: **Principles of Exercise Testing and Interpretation.** Philadelphia, Lea & Febiger, 1987.

60. Ragg, K.E., Murray, T.F., Karbonit, L.M., and Jump, D.A.: Errors in predicting functional capacity from a treadmill exercise stress test. **Am. Heart J.** 100:581–583, 1980.

61. Haskell, W.L., Savin, W., Oldridge, N., and DeBusk, R.: Factors influencing estimated oxygen uptake during exercise testing soon after myocardial infarction. **Am. J. Cardiol.** 50:299–304, 1982.

62. Zeimetz, G.A., McNeil, J.F., Hall, J.R., and Moss, R.F.: Quantifiable changes in oxygen uptake, heart rate, and time to target heart rate, when hand support is allowed during treadmill exercise. **J. Cardiopul. Rehabil.** 5:525–530, 1985.

63. McConnell, T.R., and Clark, B.A.: Prediction of maximal oxygen consumption during handrail-supported treadmill exercise. **J. Cardiopul. Rehabil.** 7:324–331, 1987.

64. Wyndham, C.H.: Submaximal tests for estimating maximum oxygen intake. **Can. Med. Assoc. J.** 96:736–745, 1967.

65. Pollock, M.L., Bohannon, R.L., Cooper, K.H., Ayres, J.J., Ward, A., White, S.R., and Linnerud, A.C.: A comparative analysis of four protocols for maximal treadmill stress testing. **Am. Heart J.** 92:39–46, 1976.

66. Pollock, M.L., Foster, C., Schmidt, D., Hellman, C., Linnerud, A.C., and Ward, A.: Comparative analysis of physiologic responses to three different maximal graded exercise test protocols in healthy women. **Am. Heart J.** 103:363–373, 1982.

67. Price, C.S., Pollock, M.L., Gettman, L.R., and Kent, D.A.: **Physical Fitness Programs for Law Enforcement Officers: A Manual for Police Administrators.** Washington, D.C., U.S. Government Printing Office, 1977.

68. American Alliance for Health, Physical Education, Recreation, and Dance: **Health Related Physical Fitness Test Manual.** Reston, VA, AAHPERD, 1981.

69. Drews, F.R., Bedynek, J.L., Rushatz, A.S., and Emerson, J.B.: **Individual Fitness Handbook.** Carlisle Barracks, PA, U.S. Army War College, 1983.

70. Haskell, W.L., and DeBusk, R.: Cardiovascular responses to repeated treadmill exercise testing soon after myocardial infarction. **Circulation** 60:1247–1251, 1979.

71. Åstrand, P.O., and Rodahl, K.: **Textbook of Work Physiology,** 3rd Ed. New York, McGraw-Hill, 1986.

72. Mitchell, J.H., Sproule, B.J., and Chapman, C.B.: The physiological meaning of the maximal oxygen intake test. **J. Clin. Invest.** 37:538–547, 1958.

73. Nagle, F.S., Balke, B., and Naughton, J.P.: Gradational step tests for assessing work capacity. **J. Appl. Physiol.** 20:745–748, 1965.
74. Balke, B., and Ware, R.: An experimental study of physical fitness of Air Force personnel. **U.S. Armed Forces Med. J.** 10:675–688, 1959.
75. Blomqvist, C.G.: Exercise testing in rheumatic heart disease. **Cardiovasc. Clin.** 5:267–287, 1973.
76. James, F.W., Blomqvist, C.G., Freed, M.D., Miller, W.W., Moller, J.H., Nugent, E.W., Riopel, D.A., Strong, W.B., and Wessel, H.U.: Standards for exercise testing in the pediatric age group. **Circulation** 66:1377a–1397a, 1982.
77. Stuart, R.J., and Ellestad, M.H.: National survey of exercise stress testing facilities. **Chest** 77:94–97, 1980.
78. Naughton, J.P., and Haider, R.: Methods of exercise testing. In Naughton, J.P., Hellerstein, H.K., and Mohler, L.C. (eds.): **Exercise Testing and Exercise Training in Coronary Heart Disease.** New York, Academic Press, 1973, pp. 79–91.
79. Holland, G.J., Weber, F., Heng, M.K., Reese, S.S., Marin, J.J., Vincent, W.J., Mayers, M.M., Hoffman, J.J., and Caston, A.L.: Maximal steptreadmill exercise and treadmill exercise by patients with coronary heart disease: a comparison. **J. Cardiopul. Rehabil.** 8:58–68, 1988.
80. Pollock, M.L., Miller, H.S., Linnerud, A.C., Royster, C.L., Smith, W.E., and Sonner, W.H.: Physiological findings in well-trained middle-aged American men. **Br. J. Sports Med.** 7:222–229, 1973.
81. Pollock, M.L.: Submaximal and maximal working capacity of elite distance runners. Part I: cardiorespiratory aspects. **Ann. N.Y. Acad. Sci.** 301:310–322, 1977.
82. Pate, R.R., Sparling, P.B., Wilson, G.E., Cureton, K.J., and Miller, B.J.: Cardiorespiratory and metabolic responses to submaximal and maximal exercise in elite women distance runners. **Int. J. Sports Med.** 8(Suppl.):91–95, 1987.
83. Starling, M.R., Crawford, M.H., and O'Rourke, R.A.: Superiority of selected treadmill exercise protocols predischarge and six weeks postinfarction for detecting ischemic abnormalities. **Am. Heart J.** 104:1054–1060, 1982.
84. Lerman, J., Bruce, R.A., Sivarajan, E., Pettet, G.E.M., and Trimble, S.: Low-level dynamic exercises for earlier cardiac rehabilitation: aerobic and hemodynamic responses. **Arch. Phys. Med. Rehabil.** 57:355–360, 1976.
85. American Heart Association: **Exercise Testing and Training of Apparently Healthy Individuals: A Handbook for Physicians.** Dallas, American Heart Association, 1972.
86. Schauer, J.E., and Hanson, P.: Usefulness of a branching treadmill protocol for evaluation of cardiac functional capacity. **Am. J. Cardiol.** 60:1373–1377, 1987.
87. Adams, W.C., McHenry, M.M., and Bernauer, E.M.: Multistage treadmill walking performance and associated cardiorespiratory responses of middle-aged men. **Clin. Sci.** 42:355–370, 1972.
88. Wilmore, J.H., Constable, S.H., Stanforth, P.R., Buono, M.J., Tsao, Y.W., Roby, F.B., Lowdon, B.J., and Ratliff, R.A.: Mechanical and physiological calibration of four cycle ergometers. **Med. Sci. Sports Exerc.** 14:322–325, 1982.
89. Hellerstein, H.K.: Specifications for exercise testing equipment. **Circulation** 59:849a–854a, 1979.
90. Howley, E.T.: The exercise testing laboratory. In Blair, S.N., Painter, P., Pate, R.R., Smith, L.K., and Taylor, C.B.: **Resource Manual for Guidelines for Exercise Testing and Prescription.** Philadelphia, Lea & Febiger, 1988, pp. 406–413.
91. Åstrand, P.O., and Ryhming, I.A.: Nomogram for calculation of aerobic capacity from pulse rate during submaximal work. **J. Appl. Physiol.** 7:218–221, 1954.
92. Faria, I.E., and Cavanagh, P.R.: **The Physiology and Biomechanics of Cycling.** New York, John Wiley and Sons, 1978.
93. Hermansen, L., and Saltin, B.: Oxygen uptake during maximal treadmill and bicycle exercise. **J. Appl. Physiol.** 26:31–37, 1969.

94. Faulkner, J.A., Roberts, D.E., Elk, R.L., and Conway, J.: Cardiovascular response to submaximal and maximal effort cycling and running. **J. Appl. Physiol.** 30:457–461, 1971.

95. Pollock, M.L., Dimmick, J., Miller, H.S., Kendrick, Z., and Linnerud, A.C.: Effects of mode of training on cardiovascular function and body composition of adult men. **Med. Sci. Sports** 7:139–145, 1975.

96. Pels, A.E., Pollock, M.L., Lemberger, K., Dohmeir, T., and Oehrlein, B.: Training and testing specificity using a stationary cycle, motor driven treadmill and leg press apparatus. (Abstr.) **Med. Sci. Sports Exerc.** 17:248, 1985.

97. Åstrand, P.O., and Saltin, B.: Maximal oxygen uptake and heart rate in various types of muscular activity. **J. Appl. Physiol.** 16:977–981, 1961.

98. Sawka, M.N., Foley, M.E., Pimental, N.A., Tomer, M.M., and Pandolf, K.B.: Determination of maximal aerobic power during upper-body exercise. **J. Appl. Physiol.** 54:113–117, 1983.

99. Pollock, M.L., Miller, H.S., Linnerud, A.C., Laughridge, E., Coleman, E., and Alexander, E.: Arm pedaling as an endurance training regimen for the disabled. **Arch. Phys. Med. Rehabil.** 55:418–424, 1974.

100. Franklin, B.A.: Exercise testing, training and arm ergometry. **Sports Med.** 2:100–119, 1985.

101. McCarthy, C.E., Balady, G.J., Green, A.M.: Cost effective modification of a supine exercise bicycle for arm ergometry. **J. Nucl. Med. Tech.** 14:135–137, 1986.

102. Pollock, M.L., Jackson, A.S., and Foster, C.: The use of the perception scale for exercise prescription. In Borg, G., and Ottoson, D. (eds.): **The Perception of Exertion in Physical Work.** London, MacMillan Press, 1986, pp. 161–176.

103. Balady, G.J., Weiner, D.A., McCabe, C.H., and Ryan, T.J.: Value of arm exercise testing in detecting coronary artery disease. **Am. J. Cardiol.** 55:37–39, 1985.

104. Balady, G.J., Weiner, D.A., Rothendler, J.A., and Ryan, T.J.: Arm exercise–thalium imaging testing for detection of coronary artery disease. **J. Am. Coll. Cardiol.** 9:84–88, 1987.

105. Pollock, M.L., Pels, A.E., Foster, C., and Ward, A.: Exercise prescription for rehabilitation of the cardiac patient. In Pollock, M. L., and Schmidt, D.H. (eds.): **Heart Disease and Rehabilitation,** 2nd Ed. New York, Churchill Livingstone, 1986, pp. 477–516.

106. Glaser, R.M., Sawka, M.N., Brune, M.F., and Wilde, S.W.: Physiological responses to maximal effort wheelchair and arm crank ergometry. **J. Appl. Physiol.** 48:1060–1064, 1980.

107. Markiewicz, W., Houston, N., and DeBusk, R.: A comparison of static and dynamic exercise soon after myocardial infarction. **Israel J. Med. Sci.** 15:894–897, 1979.

108. DeBusk, R.F., Valdez, R., Houston, N., and Haskell, W.: Cardiovascular responses to dynamic and static effort soon after myocardial infarction. Application to occupational work assessment. **Circulation** 58:368–375, 1978.

109. Van Loan, M.D., McCluer, S., Loftin, J.M., and Boileau, R.A.: Comparison of physiological responses to maximal arm exercise among able-bodied, paraplegics and quadriplegics. **Paraplegia** 25:397–405, 1987.

110. Glaser, R.M., Sawka, M.N., Brune, M.F., and Wilde, S.W.: Physiological responses to maximal effort wheelchair and arm ergometry. **J. Appl. Physiol.** 48:1060–1064, 1980.

111. Pitetti, K.H., Snell, P.G., and Gundersen-Stray, J.: Maximal response of wheelchair-confined subjects to four types of arm exercise. **Arch. Phys. Med. Rehabil.** 68:10–13, 1987.

112. Golding, L.A., Horvat, M.A., Horvat–Beutal, T., and McConnell, T.J.: A graded exercise test protocol for spinal cord injured individuals. **J. Cardiopul. Rehabil.** 6:362–367, 1986.

113. Dreisinger, T.E., and Londeree, B.R.: Wheelchair exercise: a review. **Paraplegia** 20:20–34, 1982.

114. Mahar, M., Jackson, A.S., Ross, A.M., Pivarnik, J.M., and Pollock, M.L.:

Predictive accuracy of single and double stage submax treadmill work for estimating aerobic capacity. (Abstr.) **Med. Sci. Sports Exerc.** 17:206–207, 1985.

115. Ross, R.M.: **Understand Exercise.** Houston, TX, Cardio-Stress, 1984.

116. Ross, R.M., and Jackson, A.S.: Development and validation of total work equations for estimating the energy cost of walking. **J. Cardiopul. Rehabil.** 6:182–192, 1986.

117. Sjöstrand, T.: Changes in respiratory organs of workmen at an ore melting works. **Acta Med. Scand.** (Suppl.) 196:687–695, 1947.

118. Kurucz, R.L., Fox, E.L., and Mathews, D.K.: Construction of a submaximal cardiovascular step test. **Res. Q.** 40:115–122, 1969.

119. Katch, F.I., and McArdle, W.D.: **Nutrition, Weight Control, and Exercise,** 3rd Ed. Philadelphia, Lea & Febiger, 1988.

120. Kasch, F.W., and Boyer, J.L.: **Adult Fitness Principles and Practice.** San Diego, San Diego State College, 1968.

121. Jette, M., Campbell, J., Mongeon, J., and Routhier, R.: The Canadian home fitness test as a predictor of aerobic capacity. **Can. Med. Assoc. J.** 114:680–682, 1976.

122. Price, C., Pollock, M.L., Gettman, L.R., and Kent, D.A.: **Physical Fitness Programs for Law Enforcement Officers: A Manual for Police Administrators.** Washington, D.C., U.S. Government Printing Office, No. 027-000-00671-0, 1978.

123. Cooper, K.H.: **Aerobics.** New York, M. Evans and Co., 1968.

124. Cooper, M., and Cooper, K.H.: **Aerobics for Women.** New York, M. Evans and Co., 1972.

125. American Alliance for Health, Physical Education, and Recreation: **AAHPER Youth Fitness Test Manual.** Washington, D.C., AAHPER, 1958.

126. Ribisl, P.M., and Kachadorian, W.A.: Maximal oxygen intake prediction in young and middle-aged males. **J. Sports Med. Phys. Fitness** 9:17–22, 1969.

127. American Alliance for Health, Physical Education, Recreation, and Dance: **Physical Best.** Reston, VA, AAHPERD, 1988.

128. McSwegan, P., Pemberton, C., Petray, C., and Going, S.: **Physical Best: The AAHPERD Guide to Physical Fitness Education and Assessment.** Reston, VA, AAHPERD, 1989.

129. O'Hanley, S., Ward, A., McCarron, R., Wilkie, S., and Rippe, J.: Validation of a one-mile walk test in 70 to 79 year olds. Submitted for publication, 1989.

130. Wilkie, S.A., O'Hanley, S.A., Ward, A., Zwiren, L., Freedson, P.S., Crawford, B., Kleinerman, J., and Rippe, J.M.: Estimation of $\dot{V}O_2$max using recovery heart rate in the one-mile walk equation. Submitted for publication, 1989.

131. The Rockport Walking Institute: **Rockport Fitness Walking Test.** Marlboro, MA, The Rockport Co., 1986.

132. Rippe, J.M., Ward, A., Porcari, J.P., and Freedson, P.S.: Walking for health and fitness. **JAMA** 259:2720–2724, 1988.

133. Kattus, A.A., Jorgensen, C.R., Worden, R.E., and Alvaro, A.B.: S-T segment depression with near-maximal exercise in detection of preclinical coronary heart disease. **Circulation** 41:585–595, 1971.

134. Fox, S.M., Naughton, J.P., and Haskell, W.L.: Physical activity and the prevention of coronary heart disease. **Ann. Clin. Res.** 3:404–416, 1971.

135. Foster, C., Jackson, A.S., Pollock, M.L., Taylor, M.M., Hare, J., Sennett, S.M., Rod, J.L., Sarwar, M., and Schmidt, D.H.: Generalized equations for predicting functional capacity from treadmill performance. **Am. Heart J.** 107:1229–1234, 1984.

136. Cohen, J., and Cohen, P.: **Applied Multiple Regression/Correlation Analysis for the Behavioral Sciences.** New York, John Wiley and Sons, 1975.

137. Foster, C., Pollock, M.L., Rod, J.L., Dymond, D.S., Wible, G., and Schmidt, D.H. Evaluation of functional capacity during exercise radionuclide angiography. **Cardiology** 70:85–93, 1983.

138. Foster, C., Hare, J., Taylor, M., Goldstein, T., Anholm, J., and Pollock, M.L.: Prediction of oxygen uptake during exercise testing in cardiac patients and healthy volunteers. **J. Cardiac Rehabil.** 4:537–542, 1984.

139. Taylor, H.L., Buskirk, E., and Henschel, A.: Maximal oxygen intake as an objective measure of cardiorespiratory performance. **J. Appl. Physiol.** 8:77–83, 1955.
140. Pollock, M.L., Foster, C., Rod, J., Stoiber, J., Hare, J., Schmidt, D.H.: Effects of propranolol dosage on the response to submaximal and maximal exercise. (Abstr.) **Am. J. Cardiol.** 49:1000, 1982.
141. Pollock, M.L., Foster, C., Rod, J.L., and Wible, G.: Comparison of methods for determining exercise training intensity for cardiac patients and healthy adults. In Kellerman, J.J. (ed.): **Comprehensive Cardiac Rehabilitation.** Basel, S. Karger, 1982, pp. 129–133.
142. Cooper, K.H.: **The Aerobics Way.** New York, M. Evans and Co., 1977.
143. Borg, G.: **Physical Performance and Perceived Exertion.** Lund, Sweden, Gleerup, 1962, pp. 1–63.
144. Borg, G.: Subjective effort in relation to physical performance and working capacity. In Pick, H.L., Jr. (ed.): **Psychology: From Research to Practice.** New York, Plenum Publishing, 1978, pp. 333–361.
145. Borg, G.A.V.: Psychophysical bases of perceived exertion. **Med. Sci. Sports Exerc.** 14:377–381, 1982.
146. Borg, G.: **An Introduction to Borg's RPE—Scale.** Ithaca, NY, Mouvement Publications, 1985.
147. Skinner, J.S., Hutsler, R., Bergsteinova, V., and Buskirk, E.R.: The validity and reliability of a rating scale of perceived exertion. **Med. Sci. Sports** 5:94–96, 1973.
148. Skinner, J.S., Hutsler, R., Bergsteinova, V., and Buskirk, E.R.: Perception of effort during different types of exercise and under different environmental conditions. **Med. Sci. Sports** 5:110–115, 1973.
149. Sargeant, A.J., and Davies, C.T.M.: Perceived exertion during rhythmic exercise involving different muscle masses. **J. Hum. Ergol.** 2:3–11, 1973.
150. Davies, C.T.M., and Sargeant, A.J.: The effects of atropine and practolol on the perception of exertion during treadmill exercise. **Ergonomics** 22:1141–1146, 1979.
151. Pandolf, K.B.: Differentiated ratings of perceived exertion during physical exercise. **Med. Sci. Sports. Exerc.** 14:397–405, 1982.
152. Borg, G., and Ottoson, D. (eds.): **The Perception of Exertion in Physical Work.** London, MacMillan Press, 1986.
153. Borg, G., Van Den Berg, M., Hassman, P., Keijser, L., and Tanaka, S.: Relationships between perceived exertion, HR and HLa in cycling, running, and walking. **Scand. J. Sports Sci.** 9:69–77, 1987.
154. Onodera, K., and Miyashita, M.: A study on Japanese scale for rating of perceived exertion in endurance exercise. **Jpn. J. Phys. Educ.** 21:191–203, 1976.
155. Morgan, W.P., and Pollock, M.L.: Psychologic characterization of the elite distance runner. **Ann. N.Y. Acad. Sci.** 301:382–403, 1977.
156. Noble, B.J.: Clinical applications of perceived exertion. **Med. Sci. Sports Exerc.** 14:406–411, 1982.
157. Morgan, W.P.: Psychophysiology of self-awareness during vigorous physical activity. **Res. Q. Exerc. Sport** 52:385–427, 1981.
158. Borg, G., Hassmen, P., and Lagerstrom, M.: Perceived exertion related to heart rate and blood lactate during arm and leg exercise. **Eur. J. Appl. Physiol.** 65:679–685, 1987.
159. Smutok, M.A., Skrinar, G.S., and Pandolf, K.B.: Exercise intensity: subjective regulation by perceived exertion. **Arch. Phys. Med. Rehabil.** 61:569–574, 1980.
160. Gutmann, M.C., Squires, R.W., Pollock, M.L., Foster, C., and Anholm, J.: Perceived exertion–heart rate relationship during exercise testing and training in cardiac patients. **J. Cardiac Rehabil.** 1:52–59, 1981.
161. Birk, T.J., and Birk, C.A.: Use of ratings of perceived exertion for exercise prescription. **Sports Med.** 4:1–8, 1987.
162. Jackson, A.S., and Osburn, H.G.: **Validity of Isometric Strength Tests for**

Predicting Performance in Underground Coal Mining Tasks. Houston, TX, Employment Services, Shell Oil Co., 1983.

163. Kraemer, W.J., Noble, B.J., Clark, M.J., and Calver, B.W.: Physiologic responses to heavy-resistance exercise with very short rest periods. **Int. J. Sports Med.** 8:247–252, 1987.

164. Cafarelli, E.: Peripheral contributions to the perception of effort. **Med. Sci. Sports Exerc.** 14:382–389, 1982.

165. Robertson, R.J.: Central signals of perceived exertion during dynamic exercise. **Med. Sci. Sports Exerc.** 14:390–396, 1982.

166. Rochmis, P., and Blackburn, H.: Exercise tests: a survey of procedures, safety, and litigation experience in approximately 170,000 tests. **JAMA** 217:1061–1068, 1971.

167. Bruce, R.A., and McDonough, J.R.: Maximal exercise testing in assessing cardiovascular function. **J. S. Carolina Med. Assoc.** 65 (Suppl. I):26–33, 1969.

168. Scherer, D., and Kaltenbach, M.: Frequency of life-threatening complications associated with stress testing. **Dtsch. Med. Wochenschr.** 104:1161–1165, 1979.

169. Atterhog, J.H., Jonsson, B., and Samuelson, R.: Exercise testing: a prospective study of complication rates. **Am. Heart J.** 98:572–579, 1979.

170. Sheffield, L.T., Haskell, W., Heiss, G., Kioschos, M., Leon, A., Roitman, D., and Schrott, H.: Safety of exercise testing volunteer subjects: the lipid research clinics prevalence study experience. **J. Cardiac Rehabil.** 2:395–400, 1982.

171. Cahalin, L.P., Blessey, R.L., Kimmer, D., and Simard, M: The safety of exercise testing performed independently by physical therapists. **J. Cardiopul. Rehabil.** 7:269–276, 1987.

172. Gibbons, L., Blair, S.N., Kohl, H.W., and Cooper, K.: The safety of maximal exercise testing. **JAMA** in press.

173. Van Camp, S.P.: Pharmacologic factors in exercise and exercise testing. In Blair, S. N., Painter, P., Pate, R. R., Smith, L. K., and Taylor, C. B. (eds.): **Resources Manual for Guidelines for Exercise Testing and Exercise Prescription.** Philadelphia, Lea & Febiger, 1988, pp. 135–152.

174. Lowenthal, D.T., and Kendrick, Z.V.: Drug-exercise interactions. **Ann. Rev. Pharmacol. Toxicol.** 25:275–305, 1985.

175. Lowenthal, D.T., Kendrick, Z.V., Chase, R., Paran, E., and Permutter, G.: Cardiovascular drugs and exercise. In Pandolf, K. B. (ed.): **Exercise and Sport Sciences Reviews.** New York, Macmillan Publishing Co., 1987, pp. 67–94.

176. Harrison, D.C. (ed.): Beta blockers and exercise: a symposium. **Am. J. Cardiol.** 55:1D–171D, 1985.

177. Blood, S.M., and Ades, P.A.: Effects of beta-adrenergic blockade on exercise conditioning in coronary patients: a review. **J. Cardiopul. Rehabil.** 8:141–144, 1988.

178. Wilmore, J.H.: Exercise testing, training, and beta-adrenergic blockade. **Phys. Sportsmed.** 16:45–51, 1988.

178a. Van Baak, M.A.: Beta–adrenoceptor blockade and exercise on update. **Sports Med.** 4:209–225, 1988.

179. Pollock, M.L., Foster, C., Rod, J., Stoiber, J., Hare, J., and Schmidt, D.H.: Acute and chronic responses to exercise in patients treated with beta blockers. **Ann. Clin. Res.** in press, 1990.

180. Gordon, N.F.: Effect of selective and non-selective beta-adrenoceptor blockade on thermo-regulation during prolonged exercise in the heat. **Am. J. Cardiol.** 55:74D–78D, 1985.

181. Gordon, N.F., Myburgh, D.P., Schwellnus, M.P., and Van Rensburg, J.P.: Effect of beta-blockade on exercise core temperature in coronary artery disease patients. **Med. Sci. Sports Exerc.** 19:591–596, 1987.

182. Koppes, G., McKiernan, T., Bassan, M., and Froelicher, V.F.: Treadmill exercise testing. **Curr. Probl. Cardiol.** 7:1–44, 1977.

182a. Sevilla, D.C., Dohrmann, M.L., Somelofski, C.A., Wawrzynski, R.P., Wagner,

N.B., and Wagner, G.S.: Invalidation of the resting electrocardiogram obtained via exercise electrode sites as a standard 12-lead recording. **Am. J. Cardiol.** 63:35–39, 1989.

183. Blackburn, H., and Katigbak, R.: What electrocardiographic leads to take after exercise? **Am. Heart J.** 67:184–191, 1963.

184. Mason, R.E., Likar, I., Biern, R.O., and Ross, R.S.: Multiple-lead exercise electrocardiography. Experience in 107 normal subjects and 67 patients with angina pectoris, and comparison with coronary cinearteriography in 84 patients. **Circulation** 36:517–525, 1967.

185. Phibbs, B., and Buckels, L.: Comparative yield of ECG leads in multistage stress testing. **Am. Heart J.** 90:275–281, 1975.

186. Robertson, D., Kostuk, W.J., and Ahuja, S.P.: The localization of coronary artery stenosis of 12 lead ECG response to graded exercise test: support for intercoronary steal. **Am. Heart J.** 91:437–444, 1976.

187. Tucker, S.C., Kemp, V.E., Holland, W.E., and Horgan, J.H.: Multiple lead ECG submaximal treadmill exercise tests in angiographically documented coronary heart disease. **Angiology** 27:149–155, 1976.

188. Bruce, R.A., DeRouen, T.A., and Hammermeister, K.E.: Noninvasive screening criteria for enhanced 4 year survival after aortocoronary bypass surgery. **Circulation** 60:638–646, 1979.

189. McNeer, J.F., Margolis, J.E., Lee, K.L., Kisslo, J.A., Peter, R.H., Kong, Y., Behar, V.S., Wallace, A.G., McCants, C.B., and Rosati, R.A.: The role of the exercise test in the evaluation of patients for ischemic heart disease. **Circulation** 57:64–70, 1978.

190. McHenry, P.L., and Morris, S.N.: Exercise electrocardiography—current state of the art. In Schlanti, R.C., and Hurst, J.W. (eds.): **Advances in Electrocardiography,** Vol. 2. New York, Grune & Stratton, 1976, pp. 265–304.

191. Chaitman, B.R., and Hanson, J.S.: Comparative sensitivity and specificity of exercise electrocardiographic lead systems. **Am. J. Cardiol.** 47:1335–1349, 1981.

192. Simoons, M.L., and Block, P.: Toward the optimal lead system and optimal criteria for exercise electrocardiography. **Am. J. Cardiol.** 47:1366–1374, 1981.

193. Weiner, D.A., McCabe, C.H., and Ryan, T.J.: Identification of patients with left main and three vessel coronary disease with clinical and exercise test variables. **Am. J. Cardiol.** 46:21–27, 1980.

194. American College of Cardiology/American Heart Association Task Force on Assessment of Cardiovascular Procedures (Subcommittee on Exercise Testing): Guidelines for exercise testing. **J. Am. Coll. Cardiol.** 8:725–738, 1986.

195. Rautaharju, P.M., Prineas, R.J., Eifler, W.J., Furberg, C.D., Neaton, J.D., Crow, R.S., Stamler, J., and Culter, J.A.: Prognostic value of exercise electrocardiogram in men at high risk of future coronary heart disease: multiple risk factor intervention trial experience. **J. Am. Coll. Cardiol.** 8:1–10, 1986.

196. Bruce, R.A., and Fisher, L.D.: Unusual prognostic significance of exercise-induced ST elevation in coronary patients. **J. Electrocardiol.** 20(Suppl.):84–88, 1987.

197. Dubach, P., Froelicher, V.F., Klein, J., Oakes, D., Grover-McKay, M., and Friis, R.: Exercise-induced hypotension in a male population: criteria, causes, and prognosis. **Circulation** 78:1380–1387, 1988.

198. Weiner, D.A., Ryan, T.J., McCabe, C.H., Ny, G., Chaitman, B.R., Sheffield, L.T., Tristani, F.E., and Fisher, L.D.: Risk of developing an acute myocardial infarction and sudden coronary death in patients with exercise-induced silent myocardial ischemia. A report from the coronary artery surgery study (CASS) registry. **Am. J. Cardiol.** 62:1155–1158, 1988.

199. Froelicher, V.F., Duarte, G.M., Oakes, D.F., Klein, J., Dubach, P.A., and Janosi, A.: The prognostic value of the exercise test. **Disease-a-Month** 34:681–735, 1988.

199a. Bruce, R.A.: Improvements in exercise electrocardiography. **Circulation** 79:458–459, 1989.

199b. Mark, D.B., Hlatky, M.A., Harrell, F.E., Lee, K.L., Califf, R.M., and Pryor,

D.B.: Exercise treadmill score for predicting prognosis in coronary artery disease. **Ann. Intern. Med.** 106:793–800, 1987.

200. Ritchie, J.L., Zaret, B.L., Strauss, H.W., Pitt, B., Berman, D.S., Shelbert, H.R., Ashburn, W.L., Berger, H.J., and Hamilton, G.W.: Myocardial imaging with thallium-201: a multicenter study in patients with angina pectoris or acute myocardial infarction. **Am. J. Cardiol.** 42:345–350, 1978.

201. Borer, J.S., Bacharach, S.L., Green, M.V., Kent, K.M., Epstein, S.E., and Johnston, G.S.: Real-time radionuclide cineangiography in the noninvasive evaluation of global and regional left ventricular function at rest and during exercise in patients with coronary artery disease. **N. Engl. J. Med.** 296:839–844, 1977.

202. Iskandrian, A.S., Hakki, A.H., DePace, N.L., Manno, B., and Segal, B.L.: Evaluation of left ventricular function by radionuclide angiography during exercise in normal subjects and in patients with chronic coronary heart disease. **J. Am. Coll. Cardiol.** 1:1518–1529, 1983.

203. Port, S., Cobb, R.R., Coleman, R.E., and Jones, R.H.: Effect of age on the response of the left ventricular ejection fraction to exercise. **N. Engl. J. Med.** 303:1133–1137, 1980.

204. Jones, R.H., McEwan, P., Newman, G.E., Port, S., Rerych, S.K., Scholz, P.M., Upton, M.T., Peter, C.A., Austin, E.H., Leong, K., Gibbons, R.J., Cobb, F.R., Coleman, R.E., and Sabiston, D. C., Jr.: Accuracy of diagnosis of coronary artery disease by radionuclide measurement of left ventricular function during rest and exercise. **Circulation** 64:586–601, 1981.

205. Schmidt, D.H., and Port, S.: The clinical and research application of nuclear cardiology. In Pollock, M.L., and Schmidt, D.H. (eds.): **Heart Disease and Rehabilitation,** 2nd Ed. New York, Churchill Livingstone, 1986, pp. 149–166.

206. Kaul, S., Lilly, D.R., Gascho, J.A., Watson, D.D., Gibson, R.S., Oliner, C.A., Ryan, J.M., and Beller, G.A.: Prognostic utility of the exercise thallium-201 test in ambulatory patients with chest pain: comparison with cardiac catheterization. **Circulation** 77:745–758, 1988.

207. Iskandrian, A.S., Heo, J., DeCoskey, D., Askenase, A., and Segal, B.: Use of thallium-201 imaging for risk stratification of elderly patients with coronary artery disease. **Am. J. Cardiol.** 61:269–272, 1988.

208. Podrid, P.J., Vendilli, F.J., Levine, P.A., and Klein, M.D.: The role of exercise testing in evaluation of arrhythmias. **Am. J. Cardiol.** 62:24H–33H, 1988.

209. Lown, B.: Sudden cardiac death: the major challenge confronting contemporary cardiology. **Am. J. Cardiol.** 43:313–328, 1979.

210. Lown, B., and Wolf, M.: Approaches to sudden death from coronary heart disease. **Circulation** 44:130–142, 1971.

211. DeMaria, A.N., Zakauddin, V., Amsterdam, E.A., Mason, D.T., and Massumi, R.A.: Disturbances of cardiac rhythm and conduction induced by exercise, diagnostic, prognostic and therapeutic implications. **Am. J. Cardiol.** 33:732–736, 1974.

212. Bigger, J.T., and Weld, F.M.: Shortcomings of the Iowa grading system for observational or experimental studies in ischemic heart disease. **Am. Heart J.** 100:1081–1088, 1980.

213. Akhtar, M., Wolf, F., and Denker, S.: Sudden cardiac death. In Pollock, M.L., and Schmidt, D.H. (eds.): **Heart Disease Rehabilitation,** 2nd Ed. New York, Churchill Livingstone, 1986, pp. 115–130.

214. Cooper, K.H., Purdy, J.G., White, S.R., Pollock, M.L., and Linnerud, A.C.: Age-fitness adjusted maximal heart rates. In Brunner, D., and Jokl, E. (eds.): **Medicine and Sport, Vol. 10: The Role of Exercise in Internal Medicine.** Basel, S. Karger, 1977, pp. 78–88.

215. Rod, J.L., Squires, R.W., Pollock, M.L., Foster, C., and Schmidt, D.H.: Symptom-limited graded exercise testing soon after myocardial revascularization surgery. **J. Cardiac Rehabil.** 2:199–205, 1982.

216. Powles, A.C.P., Sutton, J.R., Wicks, J.R., Oldridge, N.B., and Jones, N.L.: Reduced heart rate response to exercise in ischemic heart disease: the fallacy of the target heart rate in exercise testing. **Med. Sci. Sport** 11:227–233, 1979.

217. Vecchio, T.H.: Predictive value of a single diagnostic test in unselected populations. **N. Engl. J. Med.** 274:1171–1177, 1966.
218. Hlatky, M.A., Mark, D.B., Harrell, F.E., Lee, K.L., Califf, R.M., and Pryor, D.B.: Rethinking sensitivity and specificity. **Am. J. Cardiol.** 59:1195–1198, 1987.
219. Ryan, T., Vasey, C.G., Presti, C.F., O'Donnell, J.A., Feigenbaum, H., and Armstrong, W.: Exercise echocardiography: detection of coronary artery disease in patients with normal left ventricular wall motion at rest. **J. Am. Coll. Cardiol.** 11:993–999, 1988.
220. Richards, K.L.: Exercise echocardiography. **J. Am. Coll. Cardiol.** 11:1000–1001, 1988.
221. Cohn, J.N. (ed.): Quantitative exercise testing for the cardiac patient: the value of monitoring gas exchange. **Circulation** 76 (Suppl. VI):1–58, 1987.
222. Behnke, A.R., and Wilmore, J.H.: **Evaluation and Regulation of Body Build and Composition.** Englewood Cliffs, NJ, Prentice-Hall, 1974.
223. Forbes, G.B.: **Human Body Composition: Growth, Aging, Nutrition, and Activity.** New York, Springer-Verlag, 1987.
224. Lukaski, H.C.: Methods for the assessment of human body composition: traditional and new. **Am. J. Clin. Nutr.** 46:537–556, 1987.
225. Lohman, T.G., Roche, A.F., and Martorell, R. (eds.): **Anthropometric Standardization Reference Manual.** Champaign, IL, Human Kinetics Books, 1988.
226. Brozek, J., Grande, F., Anderson, T., and Keys, A.: Densitometric analysis of body composition: revision of some quantitative assumptions. **Ann. N.Y. Acad. Sci.** 110:113–140, 1963.
227. Goldman, R.F., and Buskirk, E.R.: Body volume measurement by underwater weighing: description of a method. In Brozek, J., and Henschel, A. (eds.): **Techniques for Measuring Body Composition.** Washington, D.C., National Academy of Sciences, 1961, pp. 78–89.
228. Buskirk, E.R.: Underwater weighing and body density: a review of procedures. In Brozek, J., and Henschel, A. (eds.): **Techniques for Measuring Body Composition.** Washington, D.C., National Academy of Sciences, 1961, pp. 90–105.
229. Goldman, H.I., and Becklace, M.R.: Respiratory function tests: normal values of medium altitudes and the prediction of normal results. **Am. Rev. Tuber. Respir. Dis.** 79:457–467, 1959.
230. **Clinical Spirometry.** Braintree, MA, W.C. Collins, 1967.
231. Wilmore, J.H.: The use of actual, predicted and constant residual volumes in the assessment of body composition by underwater weighing. **Med. Sci. Sports** 1:87–90, 1969.
232. Katch, F.I., and Katch, V.L.: Measurement and prediction errors in body composition assessment and the search for a perfect prediction equation. **Res. Q. Exerc. Sport** 51:249–260, 1980.
233. Weast, R.C. (editor-in-chief): **Handbook of Chemistry and Physics,** 50th Ed. Cleveland, The Chemical Rubber Co., 1969.
234. Katch, F.I.: Apparent body density and variability during underwater weighing. **Res. Q.** 39:993–999, 1968.
235. Siri, W.E.: Body composition from fluid spaces and density. In Brozek, J., and Henschel, A. (eds.): **Techniques for Measuring Body Composition.** Washington, D.C., National Academy of Science, 1961, pp. 223–244.
236. Lohman, T.G.: Skinfolds and body density and their relation to body fatness: a review. **Hum. Biol.** 53:181–225, 1981.
237. Lohman, T.G.: Applicability of body composition techniques and constants for children and youth. In Pandolf, K.B. (ed.): **Exercise and Sport Sciences Reviews.** New York, Macmillan Publishing Co., 1986, pp. 325–357.
237a. Lohman, T.G.: Assessment of body composition in children. **Pediatr. Exerc. Sci.** 1:19–30, 1989.
237b. Slaughter, M.H., Lohman, T.G., Boileau, R.A., Horswill, C.A., Stillman, R.J., Van Loan, M.D., and Bemben, D.A.: Skinfold equations for estimation of body fatness in children and youth. **Hum. Biol.** in press.

238. Wormersley, J., Durnin, J.V.G.A., Boddy, K., and Mahaffy, M.: Influence of muscular development obesity and age on the fat-free mass of adults. **J. Appl. Physiol.** 41:223–229, 1976.

239. Garn, S.M.: Some pitfalls in the quantification of body composition. **Ann. N.Y. Acad. Sci.** 110:171–174, 1963.

240. Lohman, T.G.: Body composition methodology in sports medicine. **Phys. Sportsmed.** 10:47–58, 1982.

241. Cureton, T.K.: **Physical Fitness Appraisal and Guidance.** St. Louis, C.V. Mosby Co., 1947.

242. Garn, S.M.: Adult bone loss, fracture epidemiology and nutritional implications. **Nutrition** 27:107–115, 1973.

243. Martin, A.D.: **An Anatomical Basis for Assessing Human Body Composition: Evidence from 25 Dissections.** Doctoral Thesis, Simon Fraser University, Barnaby, British Columbia, Canada, 1984.

243a. Clarys, J.P., Martin, A.D., and Drinkwater, D.T.: Gross tissue weights in human body by cadaver dissection. **Hum. Biol.** 56:459–473, 1984.

244. Craig, A.B., and Ware, D.E.: Effect of immersion in water on vital capacity and residual volume of lungs. **J. Appl. Physiol.** 23:423–425, 1967.

245. Fahey, T.D., and Schroeder, R.: A load-cell system for hydrostatic weighing. **Res. Q.** 49:85–87, 1978.

246. Keys, A., Fidanza, F., Karvonen, M.J., Kimura, N., and Taylor, H.L.: Indices of relative weight and obesity. **J. Chronic Dis.** 25:329–343, 1972.

247. Brozek, J., and Keys, A.: The evaluation of leanness-fatness in man: norms and intercorrelations. **Br. J. Nutr.** 5:194–206, 1951.

248. Cureton, K.J., Boileau, R.A., and Lohman, T.G.: A comparison of densitometric, potassium 40 and skinfold estimates of body composition in prepubescent boys. **Hum. Biol.** 47:321–336, 1975.

249. Durnin, J.V.G.A., and Rahaman, M.M.: The assessment of the amount of fat in the human body from measurements of skinfold thickness. **Br. J. Nutr.** 21:681–689, 1967.

250. Durnin, J.V.G.A., and Wormersley, J.: Body fat assessed from total body density and its estimation from skinfold thickness: measurements on 481 men and women aged from 16 to 72 years. **Br. J. Nutr.** 32:77–92, 1974.

251. Forsyth, M.L., and Sinning, W.E.: The anthropometric estimation of body density and lean body weight of male athletes. **Med. Sci. Sports** 5:174–180, 1973.

252. Haisman, M.F.: The assessment of body fat content in young men from measurements of body density and skinfold thickness. **Hum. Biol.** 42:679–688, 1970.

253. Harsha, D.W., Fredrichs, R.R., and Berenson, G.S.: Densitometry and anthropometry of black and white children. **Hum. Biol.** 50:261–280, 1978.

254. Jackson, A.S., and Pollock, M.L.: Generalized equations for predicting body density of men. **Br. J. Nutr.** 40:497–504, 1978.

255. Katch, F.I., and McArdle, W.D.: Prediction of body density from simple anthropometric measurements in college age women and men. **Hum. Biol.** 45:445–454, 1973.

256. Katch, F.I., and Michael, E.D.: Densitometric validation of six skinfold formulas to predict body density and percent fat of 17 year old boys. **Res. Q.** 40:712–716, 1969.

257. Parizkova, J.: Total body fat and skinfold thicknesses in children. **Metabolism** 10:794–807, 1961.

258. Pascale, L., Grossman, M., Sloane, H., and Frankel, T.: Correlations between thickness of skinfolds and body density in 88 soldiers. **Hum. Biol.** 28:165–176, 1956.

259. Pollock, M.L., Hickman, T., Kendrick, Z., Jackson, A., Linnerud, A.C., and Dawson, G.: Prediction of body density in young and middle-aged men. **J. Appl. Physiol.** 40:300–304, 1976.

260. Sloan, A.W.: Estimation of body fat in young men. **J. Appl. Physiol.** 23:311–315, 1967.

261. Wilmore, J.H., and Behnke, A.R.: An anthropometric estimation of body density and lean body weight in young men. **J. Appl. Physiol.** 27:25–31, 1969.
262. Wright, H.F., and Wilmore, J.H.: Estimation of relative body fat and lean body weight in a United States Marine Corps population. **Aerospace Med.** 45:301–306, 1974.
263. Jackson, A.S., Pollock, M.L., and Ward, A.: Generalized equations for predicting body density of women. **Med. Sci. Sports Exerc.** 12:175–182, 1980.
264. Katch, F.I., and Michael, E.D.: Prediction of body density from skinfold and girth measurement of college females. **J. Appl. Physiol.** 25:92–94, 1968.
265. Pollock, M.L., Laughridge, E., Coleman, B., Linnerud, A.C., and Jackson, A.: Prediction of body density in young and middle-aged women. **J. Appl. Physiol.** 38:745–749, 1975.
266. Sinning, W.E.: Anthropometric estimation of body density, fat and lean body weight in women gymnasts. **Med. Sci. Sports** 10:243–249, 1978.
267. Sloan, A.W., Burt, J.J., and Blyth, C.S.: Estimation of body fat in young women. **J. Appl. Physiol.** 17:967–970, 1962.
268. Wilmore, J.H., and Behnke, A.R.: An anthropometric estimation of body density and lean body weight in young women. **Am. J. Clin. Nutr.** 23:267–274, 1970.
269. Young, C.M.: Prediction of specific gravity and body fatness in older women. **J. Am. Diet. Assoc.** 45:333–338, 1964.
270. Young, C.M., Martin, M., Tensuan, R., and Blondin, J.: Predicting specific gravity and body fatness in young women. **J. Am. Diet. Assoc.** 40:102–107, 1962.
271. Parizkova, J.: **Body Fat and Physical Fitness.** The Hague, Martinus Nijhoff b.v., 1977.
272. Jackson, A.S., and Pollock, M.L.: Steps toward the development of generalized equations for predicting body composition in adults. **Can. J. Appl. Sport. Sci.** 7:189–196, 1982.
273. Jackson, A.S., and Pollock, M.L.: Factor analysis and multivariate scaling of anthropometric variables for the assessment of body composition. **Med. Sci. Sports** 8:196–203, 1976.
274. Sinning, W.E., and Wilson, J.R.: Validity of generalized equations for body composition analysis in women athletes. **Res. Q.** 55:153–160, 1984.
275. Smith, J.F., and Mansfield, E.R.: Body composition prediction in university football players. **Med. Sci. Sports Exerc.** 16:398–405, 1984.
276. Bulbulian, R.: The influence of somatotype on anthropometric prediction of body composition in young women. **Med. Sci. Sports Exerc.** 16:389–397, 1984.
277. Thorland, W.G., Johnson, G.O., Tharp, G.D., Fagot, T.G., and Hammer, R.W.: Validity of anthropometric equations for the estimation of body density in adolescent athletes. **Med. Sci. Sports Exerc.** 16:77–81, 1984.
278. Scherf, J., Franklin, B.A., Lucas, C.P., Stevenson, D., and Ruberfire, M.: Validity of skinfold thickness measures of formerly obese adults. **Am. J. Clin. Nutr.** 43:128–135, 1986.
279. Latin, R.W.: Percent body fat determinations by body impedance analysis and skinfold measurements. **Fit. Business** 2:24–27, 1987.
280. Jackson, A.S., Pollock, M.L., Graves, J.E., and Mahar, M.T.: Reliability and validity of bioelectrical impedance in determining body composition. **J. Appl. Physiol.** 64:529–534, 1988.
281. Bakker, H.K., and Struikenkamp, R.S.: Biological variability and lean body mass estimates. **Hum. Biol.** 49:187–202, 1977.
282. Baun, W.B., Baun, M.R., and Raven, P.B.: A nomogram for the estimate of percent body fat from generalized equations. **Res. Q. Exerc. Sport** 52:380–384, 1981.
283. Jackson, A.S., and Pollock, M.L.: Practical assessment of body composition. **Phys. Sportsmed.** 13:76–90, 1985.
284. Hertzberg, H.T.E., Churchill, E., Dupertuis, C.W., White, R.M., and Damon, A.: **Anthropometric Survey of Turkey, Greece, and Italy.** New York, Macmillan, 1963.

285. Keys, A: Recommendations concerning body measurements for the characterization of nutritional status. **Hum. Biol.** 28:111–123, 1956.
286. Edwards, D.A.W., Hammond, W.H., Healy, M.J.R., Tanner, J.M., and Whitehouse, R.H.: Design and accuracy of calipers for measuring subcutaneous tissue thickness. **Br. J. Nutr.** 9:133–143, 1955.
287. Leger, L.A., Lambert, J., and Martin, P.: Validity of plastic skinfold caliper measurements. **Hum. Biol.** 54:667–675, 1982.
288. Hawkins, J.D.: An analysis of selected skinfold measuring instruments. **JOPERD** 54:25–27, 1983.
289. Lohman, T.G., Pollock, M.L., Slaughter, M.H., Brandon, L.J., and Boileau, R.A.: Methodological factors and the prediction of body fat in female athletes. **Med. Sci. Sports Exerc.** 16:92–96, 1984.
290. Gruber, J.J., Pollock, M.L., Graves, J.E., Colvin, A.B., Braith, R.W.: Comparison of Harpenden and Lange calipers in predicting body composition. **Res. Q.** in press.
291. Pollock, M.L., and Jackson, A.S.: Research progress in validation of clinical methods of assessing body composition. **Med. Sci. Sports Exerc.** 16:606–613, 1984.
292. Lohman, T.G., Wilmore, J.H., and Massey, B.H.: **Interinvestigator Reliability of Skinfolds. AAHPERD Research Abstracts.** Washington, D.C., AAHPERD, 1979, p. 102.
293. Jackson, A.S., Pollock, M.L., and Gettman, L.R.: Intertester reliability of selected skinfold and circumference measurements and percent fat estimate. **Res. Q.** 49:546–551, 1978.
294. Pollock, M.L., Jackson, A.S., and Graves, J.E.: Analysis of measurement error related to skinfold site, quantity of skinfold, and sex. **Med. Sci. Sports Exerc.** 18(Suppl.):532, 1986.
295. Lukaski, H.C., Bolonchuk, W.W., Hall, C.B., and Siders, W.A.: Validation of tetrapolar bioelectrical impedance method to assess human body composition. **J. Appl. Physiol.** 60:1327–1332, 1986.
296. Segal, K.R., Gutin, B., Presta, E., Wang, J., and Van Itallie, T.B. Estimation of human body composition by electrical impedance methods: a comparative study. **J. Appl. Physiol.** 58:1565–1571, 1985.
297. Graves, J.E., Pollock, M.L., Colvin, A.B., Van Loan, M., and Lohman, T.G.: Comparison of different bioelectrical impedance analyzers in prediction of body composition. **Am. J. Hum. Biol.** in press.
298. Jackson, A.S., Pollock, M.L., Graves, J.E., and Mahar, M.: Comparison of the reliability and validity of total body bioelectrical impedance and anthropometry in determining body composition. **J. Appl. Physiol.** 62:529–534, 1988.
299. Lohman, T.G.: Preliminary results from the 1986 Valhalla interlaboratory investigation on bioelectrical impedance. Unpublished data, 1988.
300. Katch, F.I.: Assessment of lean body tissues by radiography and by bioelectric impedance. In Roche, A.S. (ed.): **Body Composition Assessments and Use in Adults, Report of the 6th Ross Conference on Medical Research.** Columbus, Ohio, 1985.
301. Guo, S., Roche, A.F., Chumlea, W.C., Miles, D.S., and Pohlman, R.L.: Body composition predictions from bioelectric impedance. **Hum. Biol.** 59:221–233, 1987.
302. Van Loan, M., and Mayolin, P.: Bioelectrical impedance analysis: is it a reliable estimator of lean body mass and total body water? **Hum. Biol.** 59:299–309, 1987.
303. Chumlea, W.C., Baumgartner, R.N., and Roche, A.F.: Specific resistivity used to estimate fat-free mass from segmental body measures of bioelectrical impedance. **Am. J. Clin. Nutr.** 48:7–15, 1988.
304. Khaled, M.A., McCutcheon, M.J., Reddy, S., Pearman, P.L., Hunter, G.R., and Weinsier, R.L. Electrical impedance in assessing human body composition: the BIA method. **Am. J. Clin. Nutr.** 47:789–792, 1988.
305. Malina, R.M.: Bioelectric methods for estimating body composition: an overview and discussion. **Hum. Biol.** 59:329–335, 1987.

306. Zuti, W.B., and Golding, L.A.: Comparing diet and exercise as weight reduction tools. **Phys. Sportsmed.** 4:49–53, 1976.
307. Pavlon, K.N., Steffee, W.P., Lerman, R.H., and Burrows, B.A.: Effects of dieting and exercise on lean body mass, oxygen uptake, and strength. **Med. Sci. Sports Exerc.** 17:466–471, 1985.
308. Weltman, A., Seip, R.L., and Tran, Z.V.: Practical assessment of body composition in adult obese males. **Hum. Biol.** 59:523–535, 1987.
309. Weltman, A., Levine, S., Seip, R.L., and Tran, Z.V.: Accurate assessment of body composition in obese females. **Am. J. Clin. Nutr.** 48:1179–1183, 1988.
310. Johnston, F.E., Hamill, D.V., and Lemeshow, S.: **Skinfold Thickness of Children 6–11 Years—United States** (series II No. 120, 1972), **Skinfold Thickness of Youth 12–17 Years** (series II No. 132, 1974), and **Skinfolds, Body Girths, Biacromial Diameter, and Selected Anthropometric Indices of Adults** (series II, No. 35, 1970). U.S. National Center for Health Statistics, HEW. Washington, D.C., U.S. Government Printing Office.
311. **Manitoba Physical Fitness Performance Test Manual and Fitness Objectives.** Winnipeg, Manitoba Department of Education, 1977.
312. Wilmore, J.H., and Costill, D.L.: **Training for Sport and Activity—The Physiological Basis of the Conditioning Process,** 3rd Ed. Dubuque, IA, William C. Brown Publishers, 1988.
313. Clarke, H.H.: **Muscular Strength and Endurance in Man.** Englewood Cliffs, NJ, Prentice-Hall, 1966.
314. Berger, R.A.: **Applied Exercise Physiology.** Philadelphia, Lea & Febiger, 1982.
315. Jones, A., Pollock, M.L., Graves, J., Fulton, M., Jones, W., MacMillan, M., Baldwin, D., and Cirulli, J.: **Safe and Specific Testing and Rehabilitative Exercise for the Muscles of the Lumbar Spine.** Santa Barbara, CA, Sequoia Communications, 1988.
316. Berger, R.A.: Classification of students on the basis of strength. **Res. Q.** 34:514–515, 1963.
317. Jackson, A., Watkins, M., and Patton, R.: A factor analysis of twelve selected maximal isotonic strength performances on the Universal Gym. **Med. Sci. Sports Exerc.** 12:274–277, 1980.
318. Leighton, J.: An instrument and technique for the measurement of joint motion. **Arch. Phys. Med. Rehabil.** 36:571–578, 1955.
319. Adrian, M.J.: An introduction to electrogoniometry. In **Kinesiology Review.** Washington, D.C., American Association of Health, Physical Education and Recreation, 1968.
320. Kraus, H.: **Clinical Treatment of Back and Neck Pain.** New York, McGraw-Hill, 1970.
321. Melleby, A.: **The Y's Way to a Healthy Back.** Piscataway, NJ, New Century Publishers, 1982.

7

PRESCRIBING EXERCISE FOR THE APPARENTLY HEALTHY

GUIDELINES AND PRELIMINARY CONSIDERATIONS

A clear understanding of a person's needs, medical history, and present medical and physiological status is necessary in order to prescribe exercise safely and adequately. People vary greatly in status of health and fitness, structure, age, motivation, and needs; therefore, the individual approach to exercise prescription is recommended.

The needs and goals of elementary school children, college athletes, middle-aged men and women, and cardiac patients clearly differ. For example, an athlete often must get into condition quickly for a competition. In this case, many safeguards concerning intensity and progression of exercise are not closely followed. Although the abrupt approach is followed in certain instances, its general use is not recommended. The initial experience with exercise training should be of low to moderate intensity and slow to moderate progression that allows for gradual adaptation.[1-5] Experience has shown that the abrupt approach to training can result in discouraging future motivation for participation in endurance or other activities. Improper advice or prescription also can lead to undue muscle or joint strain or soreness, other orthopedic problems, excessive fatigue, and risk of precipitating a heart attack (which is rare and occurs mainly with middle-aged and older participants).[6, 7] Most incidents have occurred because of the lack of appropriate medical evaluation and clearance, incorrect exercise prescription, inadequate supervision, or an extreme climatic condition such as excessive heat and humidity or severe cold.[6-15] A more thorough discussion of the risk of cardiovascular events or sudden death associated with physical activity programs is provided in Chapter 8 for both noncardiac and cardiac adults (also see Fig. 8–1).

Although many of the suggestions and guidelines for exercise prescription are similar for both apparently healthy and diseased patients, this chapter focuses on exercise programs for the apparently healthy. Chapter 8 is devoted to exercise prescription for the diseased patient.

The following guidelines are suggested in the exercise prescription process:

Preliminary Suggestions

1. Have adequate medical information available to assess health status properly. This includes a medical history and risk factor analysis and possibly a physical examination and laboratory tests. See Chapter 6 for more details on evaluation before beginning an exercise program.
2. Know the individual's present status of physical fitness and exercise habits.
3. Know the individual's needs, interests, and objectives for being in an exercise program.
4. Set realistic short-term and long-term goals.
5. Give advice on proper attire and equipment for an exercise program (see Chapter 9).

Suggestions for Initial Phases of an Exercise Program

1. Properly educate the participant in the principles of exercise, exercise prescription, and methods of monitoring and recording exercise experiences.
2. Give adequate leadership and direction in the early stages of the exercise program to ensure proper implementation and progression. Exercise prescription is an art and takes years of experience to develop and perfect. Computers may generate a nice package program—but they lack the ability to sense individual differences among like participants that need to be considered for proper and adequate programming.
3. Remember that education, motivation, and leadership are the keys to a successful exercise program.
4. In general, slower is better than faster, low intensity better than high, and above all "more" is not always better.

Long-Term Suggestions

1. Follow-up evaluations are desirable for reassessing individual status, physical fitness, and exercise prescription.

2. Follow-up evaluations are also important in the education and motivation processes.
3. For long-term adherence, caution participants regarding the factors that cause or are associated with dropping out of programs. Staying injury free, keeping volume and intensity of effort in the proper perspective (moderate), and setting realistic goals that do not take too much time (usually no more than 60 minutes per day) are just a few to consider.

The program is prescribed as soon as the health and fitness status and needs and objectives of the participants are determined. From this information, as well as from knowledge of the participants' activity interests and available time, the desired type and quantity of exercise may be determined. It is important for the initial exercise experience to be enjoyable, refreshing, and not too demanding either physiologically or in terms of time. The slow, gradual approach to initiating an exercise program helps cultivate a more positive attitude toward physical activity and enhance the probability of long-term adherence. In addition, as discusssed in Chapter 3, if the prescribed program is too demanding, adherence is not as likely.[16–19] More details regarding program adherence are discussed in Chapter 9.

The importance of a well-rounded exercise program should be emphasized. The well-rounded program includes aerobic activities for developing and maintaining cardiorespiratory fitness and proper weight control, strength and muscular endurance activities, and flexibility exercises. Specificity of exercise training is an important concept to consider when prescribing exercise. As emphasized in Chapters 3 and 5, no one activity gives a participant total fitness. Strength and muscular endurance exercises are recommended to help maintain proper muscle tone and bone integrity and to protect against injury and low back pain. Flexibility exercises are important for developing and maintaining joint range of motion and should be practiced often.[20, 21] Reduced flexibility can lead to poor posture, fatigue, and injury.[1] An endurance activity such as jogging can reduce the flexibility of the extensor muscles of the hip, thigh, and leg. A combination of these tight extensor muscles, plus strong flexor muscles of the anterior thigh and hip, and weak abdominal muscles is associated with low back, hamstring, calf muscle, or Achilles tendon problems.

The authors' experience has been that once individuals get started in a program, if strength, muscular endurance, and flexibility activities are not stressed, they tend to be forgotten. In addition, with the emphasis placed on the aerobic phase of the program, the participant may get the impression that the other activities are secondary and only necessary if there is enough time. For example, a few years ago, one of the authors integrated the Cooper point system into his adult fitness program. Cooper[2] had set up an elaborate point system that gave participants points for doing aerobic exercises. Points were based on the intensity and duration of the activity. In essence, an individual received points for expending kilocalories. Because little or no points were awarded for doing strength (calisthenics and weight training) and flexibility exercises, participants began to equate this with a lack of importance. Cooper himself feels that a well-rounded program is vital and that it is unfortunate if some have misinterpreted this fact from his books.[2, 22] Another important example relates to the findings of the authors' 10-year follow-up study on Master runners and walkers.[23] As mentioned in Chapter 3, when training remained constant over this time, maximal oxygen uptake ($\dot{V}O_2max$) did not decline. Body weight was down slightly and body fat increased 1 to 2 percent. An important finding of this study was that the athletes lost an average of 4 pounds of fat-free weight (FFW). As shown in Chapter 4, usually FFW is maintained in short-term experiments in which aerobic activities are emphasized. These short-term studies also reveal modest reductions in body weight and fat. The loss in FFW appeared to be related to the type of training in which the subjects were participating. Most just ran or walked, with some stretching and very little strength training. The anthropometric results showed a significant reduction in arm circumference, while thigh circumference remained constant. Only three of the 24 athletes participated regularly in weight training exercise, and one was also an avid cross-country skier in the winter months. The significant aspect here was that the three who included a well-rounded program into their training regimens maintained their FFW. Thus it is important for the practitioner to continue to prescribe exercise with emphasis on a well-rounded program.[25]

An adequate program stressing the various components of physical fitness can be designed for a 60-minute period. For most individuals, a program lasting more than 60 minutes may become a deterrent for long-term continuation. The four main components of an exercise program include warm-up, muscle-conditioning, aerobic, and cool-down periods. Table 7–1 gives a suggested time frame for each component. The variability of each time frame—in particular, the muscle-conditioning and aerobic periods—depends on the individual's health and fitness status and personal needs and goals. For example, if the program was being designed for police officers or fire fighters, the muscle-conditioning period would become more important, and a minimum of 20 minutes would be recommended

Table 7–1. Components of a Training Program

Components	Activities	Recommended Time
Warm-up	Stretching, low-level calisthenics, walking	10 minutes
Muscular conditioning	Calisthenics, weight training, pulley weights	15–30 minutes
Aerobics	Fast walk, jog-run, swim, bicycle, cross-country skiing, vigorous games, dancing, stair stepping	20–50 minutes
Cool-down	Walking, stretching	5–10 minutes

for that component alone.[24] Depending on intensity, the aerobic period would be 20 to 30 minutes in duration. In contrast, a healthy but overweight 48-year-old executive would probably start out with 15 to 20 minutes of strength activities and an aerobic period of 30 to 45 minutes. Initially, the sedentary executive will emphasize stretching and low-level muscle-conditioning exercises. The aerobic activity would be of low-to-moderate intensity, probably of an interval type stressing a combination of walking and jogging or slow and fast walking.

EXERCISE PRESCRIPTION FOR CARDIORESPIRATORY ENDURANCE AND WEIGHT REDUCTION

The research findings reported in Chapters 3 and 4 described the amount of work considered necessary to develop and maintain an optimal level of cardiorespiratory endurance and an optimal weight. Within certain limits, the total energy cost of a training regimen is the most important factor in the development of cardiorespiratory endurance and in weight reduction and control. For most people, this energy cost amounts to approximately 900 to 1,500 kcal per week or 300 to 500 kcal per exercise session.[22, 25, 27] Table 7–2 summarizes the optimal frequency, intensity, and duration of training needed to attain a certain level of energy expenditure and gives general recommendations for exercise prescription.[26, 27] These recommendations are designed for the general population and not for highly trained endurance athletes or persons in poor health.

Frequency

Exercise should be performed on a regular basis 3 to 5 days per week. Although programs of sufficient intensity and duration

Table 7–2. Recommendations for Exercise Prescription

1. Frequency	3 to 5 days per week
2. Intensity	60 to 90 percent of maximal heart rate (HRmax)
	50 to 85 percent of maximal oxygen uptake or HRmax reserve
3. Duration	20 to 60 minutes (continuous)
4. Mode-activity	Walking-hiking, running-jogging, cycling-bicycling, cross-country skiing, dance, rope skipping, rowing, stair climbing, swimming, skating, and various endurance game activities
5. Resistance training	8 to 10 exercises (1 set per exercise of 8 to 12 repetitions) that condition the major muscle groups at least 2 days per week
6. Initial level of fitness	High = higher work load
	Low = lower work load

(Adapted from the American College of Sports Medicine: Position statement on the recommended quantity and quality of exercise for developing and maintaining fitness in healthy adults. **Med. Sci. Sports** 10:vii–x, 1978. Revised and will be published in **Med. Sci. Sports Exerc.** in late 1989 or early 1990).

produce some cardiorespiratory improvements with a frequency of fewer than 3 days per week, little or no loss of body weight or fat is found.[28] In addition, improvement in cardiorespiratory endurance is only minimal to modest in programs of fewer that 3 days per week (usually less than 10 percent). Participants in one- or two-days-per-week programs often complain that the workout sessions are too intermittent and break the continuity of the training regimen. Another commonly heard complaint is: "It seemed as though I was starting anew each time I came out." The authors' experience has shown that feelings such as these often lead to dropping out of a program. Under unusual conditions, if time and available facilities are important considerations, then one- or two-days-per-week regimens, while not desirable, are acceptable and may serve a temporary purpose.[28–30] As mentioned in Chapters 3 and 5, reduced training frequency or duration for up to 10 to 15 weeks has shown little effect on cardiorespiratory fitness, body composition, and strength maintenance if intensity of training is maintained.[29, 30] The practical implication here is that when you are ill or busier than usual at work, backing off on your frequency and duration of exercise training is appropriate, but if possible, do not stop altogether.

Conditioning every other day is most frequently recommended when an endurance exercise regimen is initiated. Daily, vigorous exercise often becomes too demanding initially and does not allow enough rest time between workouts for the musculoskeletal system to adapt properly. This is particularly true with high-impact activities such as running or aerobic dance.[16, 31] This nonadaptive state generally leads to undesirable muscle soreness, fatigue, and possible injury. This guideline may seem to contradict the research findings reported in Chapter 3. However, the data from young men running 30 minutes, 5 days per week, or 45 minutes, 3 days per week, showed that they incurred injuries at a significantly higher rate than those who were on 3-days-per-week programs of 15- and 30-minute durations.[16] In fact, the men in the 3-days-per-week programs had little or no injury problems. Most of the injuries that did occur concerned problems of the knee, anterior leg, shin, ankle, or foot.

Persons who are at a low level of fitness and whose initial programs are restricted to 5 to 15 minutes per session may want to exercise twice each day and often every day.[27, 32, 33] An example of this special condition is a person who is placed into a walking program of low-to-moderate intensity and short duration. In this case, a person may adapt better to shorter but more frequent exercise sessions. Another substitute for exercising every other day is to alternate the regular exercise session with days of milder activity. For persons who are initiating a jog-walk program, stretching and moderate warm-up exercises (calisthenics) for 10 to 15 minutes followed by a continuous walk for 20 to 30 minutes on alternate days are recommended.

Participants can begin to increase their frequency of training to a daily basis after several weeks or months of conditioning. The point in time at which this increase in frequency can be accommodated properly is an individual matter and is dependent upon age, initial level of fitness, intensity of training, and whether the participant is free from excessive soreness or injury. Also, high-impact activities are associated with greater numbers of injury and thus should be avoided on a daily basis. Generally, persons who are older, overweight, and lower in fitness are more prone to musculoskeletal problems. For weight reduction programs, 4 to 5 days per week of training are generally better than three.[26, 33] The key is to alternate high- and low-intensity training sessions to allow time for adaptation and to avoid high-impact activities. Generally, persons who are out of shape and overweight will be involved in low-intensity programs, so the added frequency and duration will be necessary to expend enough kilocalories.

Intensity and Duration

Although intensity and duration are separate entities, it is difficult to discuss intensity without mentioning its interaction with duration. As noted in Chapter 3, exercise regimens of low intensity (less kcal/min of expenditure) but with a long duration produced improvements similar to those of the high-intensity and short-duration regimens; the total kilocalories expenditures were approximately equal for both programs. The caloric difference between running a mile in 8 minutes and running a mile in 9 minutes is minimal;[34] therefore, running a little extra time at a slower pace will offset the extra kilocalories burned at the faster pace.[27, 35] Although the caloric cost of running a mile does not differ much for the running speeds that are used in adult fitness programs, the caloric cost of walking a mile is significantly less than that of running a mile.[36–39] Margaria and associates[39] found that the difference may be as great as 50 percent lower for walking; the average being about 30 percent lower.[37, 38] This has important implications for exercise prescription, because many participants are not capable of or do not desire to train at the higher intensity levels that are associated with run-jog programs. Thus, the time adjustments to provide an adequate level of total energy expenditure in walking programs are important. For example, Santiago and associates[40] compared the effects of walking training versus running training when caloric cost was similar between groups. The walkers exercised at 71 percent of maximal heart rate (HRmax) for 53 minutes, and the joggers trained at 84 percent of HRmax for 34 minutes. The findings showed similar improvements in $\dot{V}O_2max$. The important concept is that as long as the intensity is above the minimal threshold level and a certain amount of total work is completed in an exercise session, the manner in which the end result is accomplished can vary.[22, 27, 35, 40–42]

The above-mentioned concept has important implications for exercise prescription for adults, and it should be remembered that low-to-moderate-intensity, long-duration types of programs are generally recommended for beginners. This recommendation is particularly appropriate for those showing a low functional capacity or who are obese, are hypertensive or have heart disease. The important point is to prescribe a regimen at a low-to-moderate intensity so that the participant can accomplish a sufficient amount of work. Initially, the prescription may call for a moderate-to-brisk walk for 20 to 30 minutes.

Table 7–2 outlines a certain minimal threshold of intensity that is necessary for improving cardiorespiratory function. As was mentioned in Chapter 3, programs of an intensity of less than 50 percent of HRmax reserve often produce improvement in persons with low initial levels of fitness. These persons generally qualify for fitness classifications 1 to 3, as listed in Table 6–3. Special starter programs of less than 50-percent intensity may be recommended for these individuals. In addition, for weight control purposes, all expended kilocalories are important. Whether they are above or below the minimal threshold does not matter.

The training duration will vary from day to day and from activity to activity. The important factor is to design a program that meets the criteria for improving and maintaining a sufficient level of physical fitness, i.e., is enjoyable (tolerable), and that fits into the participant's time demands. It should be rewarding to the participant—preferably, it should be fun.

The level of training intensity that can be tolerated varies greatly, depending on status of fitness and health, age, experience, and general ability. Long-distance runners may tolerate 2 to 3 hours of continuous running at 80 to 90 percent of maximum capacity, but most beginners cannot perform a continuous effort at this level for more than a few minutes. For beginners to accomplish 20 to 30 minutes of continuous training, they must choose the proper intensity level. The proper intensity level for beginners ranges from 50 to 75 percent of HRmax reserve (moderate to brisk walking programs) to 75 to 85 percent of HRmax reserve for jogging (some poorly fit participants may increase their HR to above 75 percent HRmax reserve with brisk walking). The latter program is generally interspersed with bouts of walking, with peak intensity occurring during jogging. Most persons in fitness categories 1 and 2 (Table 6–3) will start with a walking program, and those in categories 3 and above can begin with a combination walk-jog routine.

The walk-jog routine, or low- and moderate-intensity periods of work if another mode of activity is being performed, will have a peak intensity of 85 to 90 percent of maximum and a low intensity of 50 to 65 percent. The average intensity level will range between 70 and 80 percent of HRmax reserve. Experience has shown that an intensity level of 45 to 60 percent of HRmax reserve can be tolerated comfortably for 20 to 30 minutes by most persons and can be classified as light-to-moderate-intensity training. Intensity levels ranging from 50 to 74 percent are considered as moderate, 75 to 84 percent of HRmax reserve as heavy to hard, and those 85 percent and above of HRmax reserve as very heavy to hard. See Table 3–3 for classification of exercise training intensity. The results of the initial graded exercise test (GXT) are important in placing the participant at a correct and safe level of intensity.

Upon initiating an endurance training regimen, most participants notice the training effect rather quickly. They usually experience the ability to perform more total work in subsequent exercise sessions. The increased total work is a result of the ability of the participant to increase the training duration or to tolerate a greater intensity or both. The increased higher average intensity found as an adaptation to aerobic training is a function of a higher peak intensity level or an increase in the ratio of high to low bouts of work or both. For example, a participant in a walk-jog routine can tolerate longer periods of jogging interspersed with shorter periods of walking. As these adaptations to training occur, changes in the exercise prescription are recommended. Periodic re-evaluations (initially, 3 to 6 months) help in determining a new status of physical fitness, in enhancing motivation, and in facilitating proper exercise prescription.

Estimation of Exercise Intensity

How is a participant's exercise intensity determined and how can it be estimated during an exercise session? The three most popular ways in which training intensity is estimated are as follows: metabolic ($\dot{V}O_2$ or METs),[4, 43, 44] HR (beats/min),[43-47] and rating of perceived exertion (RPE).[43, 47-52] Metabolic determination of training intensity is accomplished by measuring the participant's $\dot{V}O_2$max (aerobic capacity) during a GXT or by some other indirect method as described in Chapter 6. The training intensity is usually calculated between 50 and 85 percent of maximal aerobic capacity ($\dot{V}O_2$ or METs).[43, 44, 47] As mentioned earlier, 50 percent of maximum ($\dot{V}O_2$max, METs, or HRmax reserve) relates to the minimal threshold for improving cardiorespiratory fitness, and 85 percent represents the upper limit at which most participants tolerate aerobic training.[26, 27, 43] A specified percentage of maximal limit recommended for training is called the "target rate," and when an upper and lower limit range is specified, it is called the "training zone."

As shown in Figure 3–11, HR and oxygen uptake have a linear relationship during exercise.[54] Because of the impracticality of routinely measuring oxygen uptake and the ease with which HR can be measured, the HR standard is recommended for general use. Maximal HR can be determined (1) by using the highest HR found on a GXT, (2) after a difficult bout of endurance exercise (for example, an all-out run), (3) by subtracting current age in years from 220,[44] or (4) by referring to the population-, sex-, and age-specific norms shown in Appendix A, Tables A–1 to A–12. The first method of estimating HRmax is preferred because there is considerable individual variation even for the same sex and age.[55-58] In addition, HR is usually attained while qualified personnel are evaluating the performance of a participant. The second method is to count the HR after an all-out 12-minute run or similar endurance field test (1.5-mile run). This type of test is not recommended for beginners or persons at a high risk of coronary heart disease.[2, 22, 43] The third and fourth methods of determining HRmax are the least accurate but may be used for a rough approximation. The inaccuracy of the third and fourth methods stems from a variability of HRmax at any given age (standard deviation of 12 beats/min).[55–58] For example, the HRmax of a man 50 years of age averages approximately 170 beats/min, but presumably healthy individuals may have rates ranging from below 140 to over 200 beats/min.

There has been much discussion as to possible differences in HRmax between men and women, between fit and unfit individuals, and with various ergometers, such as treadmill, stationary cycle, or swim tests. Hakki and colleagues,[58] in a brief review, suggested that the HRmax of women was significantly lower than that of men, particularly at the older ages. They recommended subtracting age from 220 for predicting HRmax for women but subtracting half of age from 205 for men.

In the most comprehensive review to date, Londeree and Moeschberger[57] combined HRmax data from 23,000 different subjects ranging from 5 to 81 years of age. They found that age in itself accounted for 70 to 75 percent of the variance in HRmax. Their data analysis showed no difference in HRmax for sex or race. Maximal HR was slightly lower on the cycle ergometer than on a treadmill, the difference being small at the younger ages and increased with age. The greater difference between apparatus with age was thought to be associated with local muscle fatigue and weaker leg muscles specific to the cycle ergometer test. Maximal HR was also shown to be considerably lower with swimming as compared with treadmill use (14 beats/min). Their analysis showed that in cross-sectional studies, active subjects had lower HRmax at the younger ages and higher at the older ages. The weaker musculature found in the legs of older sedentary versus active individuals may account for this difference. They concluded from their analysis and review that "even with all factors accounted for, the 95-percent confidence interval of individual HRmax was about 45 beats/min."

Thus, these data show the inaccuracies of estimating HRmax from age alone. Without the actual measurement of HRmax, the practitioner must be aware of its general variation within the population and the added variation resulting from apparatus or protocol, status of health, fitness, and medications. The effects of medications on HRmax are discussed in Chapter 8.

Table 7–3. Recommended Training Zone
for Exercise Prescription for Fitness

Oxygen uptake, HRmax reserve	50%	⟶	85%
Heart rate	60%	⟶	90%
RPE*	12–13	⟶	15–16
	Somewhat hard		Hard/heavy

*Rating of Perceived Exertion, Borg Scale.[48]

The RPE scale that was described in Figure 6–13 also relates well to oxygen uptake and HR.[47–52, 59–61] The training zone for RPE and how it relates to oxygen uptake and percentage of HRmax reserve are shown in Table 7–3. More precisely, 50 to 60 percent of the HRmax reserve corresponds to an RPE of 12 to 13, and 85 percent corresponds to a rating of 15 to 16.[47, 52, 59, 60]

There are three primary methods of calculating target HR. Method I represents the percentage of the HRmax calculated from zero to peak HR (percent HRmax). Method II represents the percent difference between resting and maximal HR added to the resting HR. As mentioned earlier, this technique was first described by Karvonen and colleagues[46] and is called percentage of HRmax reserve. See Figure 7–1 for an example of calculating the target

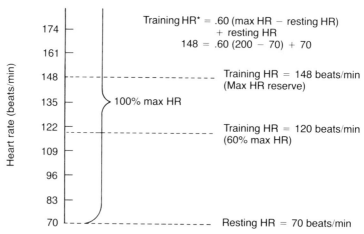

Figure 7–1. Formula for determination of 60% of maximum heart rate reserve. Also shown is an example of the calculation of target heart rate at 60% of maximum.

*Karvonen, M., et al.[46]

(Reprinted with permission from Pollock, M. L., Wilmore, J. H., and Fox, S. M.: **Health and Fitness Through Physical Activity.** New York, copyright John Wiley and Sons, 1978.)

HR at 60 percent of HRmax reserve. Method III represents the HR at a specified percentage of $\dot{V}O_2$max (percentage of maximal METs).

Method I, percentage of HRmax, is easier to calculate than the percentage of HRmax reserve method. All three techniques are acceptable for use in determining the target HR or training zone or both, but Method I yields a significantly lower HR value. Table 7–4 compares the training HRs calculated according to these three most used methods.[32] Data from ten healthy adults and ten cardiac patients were used to make these calculations. The table shows that the target HRs for both healthy adults and cardiac patients, calculated at 70 and 85 percent of HRmax reserve and maximal METs achieved on the GXT, are in close agreement. The target HR of healthy adults calculated by the percentage of HRmax method was approximately 25 and 13 beats/min (10 to 15 percent) lower than that calculated by the other two methods at 70 and 85 percent of maximum, respectively. For cardiac patients, the difference in HR is approximately 20 and 11 beats/min, respectively. The difference between these methods has been discussed by Davis and Convertino[45] (young, healthy adults) and Kaufmann and Kasch* (middle-aged adults), who showed that percentage of HRmax reserve correlated closely with actual METs determined on a GXT.

---

*Unpublished data, San Diego State University, 1975.

Table 7–4. Comparison of Training Heart Rate Calculated as a Percentage of Maximum Heart Rate, Percentage of Maximum Heart Rate Reserve, and Heart Rate at a Percentage of Maximum METs

		Methods		
Group	Intensity (%)	% HRmax	% HRmax Reserve	% Max METs (HR)
Healthy adults* (n = 10)	70	130.1 ± 7.5	154.0 ± 8.6	158.9 ± 9.0
	85	158.3 ± 9.1	170.2 ± 9.6	174.3 ± 11.4
Cardiac patients† (n = 10)	70	106.9 ± 14.8	131.2 ± 19.0	126.1 ± 20.5
	85	129.8 ± 18.2	141.8 ± 20.3	139.9 ± 22.8

*Data calculated on men 36.2 years (± 3.2); standing resting heart rate, 78.7 beats/min (± 12.6); maximal heart rate, 186.2 beats/min (± 11.0); and maximal capacity of 11.9 METs (± 1.5).

†Data calculated on cardiac patients (seven CABG and three MI) 9 weeks postevent. Age, 50.8 years (± 8.3); standing resting heart rate, 81.0 beats/min (± 17.7); maximal heart rate, 152.7 beats/min (± 21.5); and maximal capacity of 9.8 METs (± 2.4).

(Reprinted with permission from Pollock, M. L., Pels, A., Foster, C., and Ward, A.: Exercise prescription for rehabilitation of the cardiac patient. In Pollock, M. L., and Schmidt, D. H. (eds.): **Heart Disease and Rehabilitation,** 2nd Ed. New York, copyright John Wiley and Sons, 1986, pp. 417–516.)

Our experience with a few coronary artery bypass surgery patients with high resting HRs has shown a target HR lower than resting HR when calculated by the percent HRmax method.

The matter of simplicity is important, but conceptually the percent HRmax method (Method I) does not make sense. To illustrate this, the data for one of the authors' patients is shown in Figure 7–2.[61] The GXT results are from a 55-year old cardiac patient who had an exercise capacity of 7 METs, an HRmax of 155 beats/min, and a resting HR of 65 beats/min. Conceptually the percent HRmax method projects the resting HR to begin at zero, and as can be seen in Figure 7–2, at rest the patient is already at 42 percent of HRmax. Because of the large disparity between the two HR techniques in determining training intensity, both methods were compared using the RPE scale.[47] Three diverse groups were tested: young, healthy adults ($\bar{x}$ = 28 years, n = 51); healthy adults older than 40 years of age ($\bar{x}$ = 54 years, n = 42); and cardiac patients ($\bar{x}$ = 54 years, n = 48). Figure 7–3 plots the HR results calculated by the percentage of HRmax and percentage of HRmax reserve techniques, at 60, 70, and 85 percent of maximum versus the RPE rating. Method II, percentage of HRmax reserve, clearly shows a more consistent pattern among groups and makes more sense relative to the RPE scale. Because most patients in an inpatient exercise setting rate ambulatory training at 11 to 12[62, 63] and outpatients rate it at 12 to 13 on the RPE scale,[61] the percentage

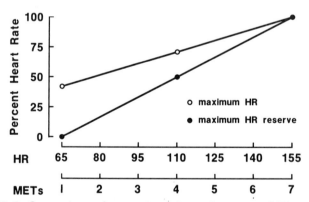

Figure 7–2. Comparison of percent maximum heart rate (HR) and percent maximum HR reserve during a symptom-limited graded exercise test. The test data were collected on a 55-year-old cardiac patient who had a 7-MET capacity, a resting HR of 65 beats/min, and a maximum HR of 155 beats/min. Note that at rest the patient is already at 42% of his maximum HR. (Reprinted with permission from Metier, C. P., Pollock, M. L., Graves, J E.: Exercise prescription for the coronary artery bypass surgery patient. **J. Cardiopul. Rehabil.** 6:236–242, 1986.)

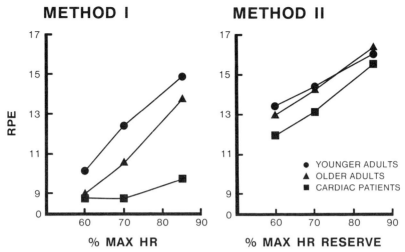

Figure 7–3. Relationship between heart rate (HR) and perceived exertion (RPE) with two methods of calculating training heart rate. Percent maximum HR (method I) was calculated on the basis of the percentage of the difference between zero and peak HR attained. Percent maximum HR reserve (method II) was calculated according to Karvonen, M., et al.[46] and represents the percent difference between the resting and maximum HR added to the resting HR. (Reprinted with permission from Pollock, M. L., Foster, C., Rod, J. L., and Wible, G.: Comparison of methods for determining exercise training intensity for cardiac patients and healthy adults. In Kellermann, J. J. (ed.): **Comprehensive Cardiac Rehabilitation.** Basel, S. Karger, 1982, pp. 129–133.)

of HRmax method seems too conservative.[32, 43, 61] Even with the above-mentioned limitations of the percent HRmax method, many clinicians prefer its use. Thus, if it is used, it has been recommended to add 10 to 15 percent to the training HR.[32, 43, 47, 61]

The variability of resting HR that is mentioned as a criticism when used with the HRmax reserve technique is valid. Thus, multiple readings of resting HR on different days under standardized conditions add to the accuracy of the method. On the other hand, a 10 beat/min error in resting heart rate only affects the HRmax reserve value by 2 to 3 percent. Also, when using HR range rather than target HR, you protect against this type of error.

How and when should HR be counted? Resting HR is less variable in the morning, before rising.[64] Change in posture from lying to standing, smoking, eating, emotional stress, and similar activities significantly increase resting and submaximal HR.[64] Maximal HR is not affected by these factors.[64] In order to estimate the target HR, resting HR should be counted for 30 seconds while the subject is in a comfortable, quiet, sitting position. Because resting HR decreases with training, it should be periodically re-evaluated.

Taking the average HR on two or three mornings is the best way to estimate resting HR.

Beta-adrenergic–blocking drugs significantly lower both resting and maximal HR.[65, 66] Thus, when medications are changed, both resting and maximal HR should be re-evaluated under the same conditions in which the participant will be exercising. More detailed information concerning the exercise prescription with patients on beta-adrenergic–blocking drugs is found in Chapter 8.

Estimating exercise HR during training is usually accomplished by counting the pulse rate with the palpation technique immediately after exercise is stopped.[43, 67, 68] This is performed by placing the tips of the first two fingers lightly on the carotid artery, or on the radial artery, or by placing the heel of the hand over the left side of the chest (at the apex of the heart) and by counting the pulsations.[5] If the carotid artery is used, caution must be taken not to apply too much pressure. Excessive pressure on the carotid artery may cause the HR to slow down by reflex action.[69] Pulsations at the apex of the heart are normally felt only after vigorous exercise. Participants should experiment to see which technique is best for them. A few persons will not be able to count the pulse at any site and will need to resort to the use of a stethoscope.

White[70] found that counting the pulse by the carotid artery technique significantly reduced the immediate postexercise HR. He questioned its use for estimating training intensity. These results have not been replicated in subsequent investigations.[71–73]

Thus, the use of the immediate postexercise carotid pulse for estimating training HR has been shown to be valid for both cardiac patients and healthy subjects. Its use with those few patients who are hypersensitive to the baroreceptor response is not recommended.

Heart rate begins to decelerate soon after cessation of exercise (usually after only 15 seconds); therefore, the count should begin as soon as possible.[67, 74] It is recommended that one count the pulse for 10 seconds and complete it within 15 seconds after cessation of exercise. Only 2 to 4 seconds are needed to position the hand or fingers properly and to feel the heartbeat rhythm. Thus, by counting beats per 10 seconds, it is possible to complete the count within 15 seconds and to avoid errors resulting from the deceleration of the heartbeat.[68]

A wristwatch, wall clock, or stopwatch can be used for determining HR; however, a stopwatch is the most accurate. The stopwatch facilitates starting the count more quickly as well as enhances general counting accuracy. After establishing the HR rhythm, the count can start on a full beat, with the first count being zero (it can start this way only when a stopwatch is being used). If the count does not end on an even beat, then one half a beat is added to the last full count. This counting detail is important with the 10-second technique because each one-beat error in counting results in a 6 beat/min error.

Another HR counting procedure that can be used satisfactorily is to count beats per 15 seconds. This method has some advantages: counting the heart rate over a longer time span can reduce the errors in counting, and multiplying the counted value by four to get beats per minute is easier for the beginner. The disadvantage is the possible 5- to 10-percent error that may occur with the added counting time.[67, 74]

Each of the techniques requires some experimentation and practice to ensure proficiency. Table 7–5 is a conversion chart for transforming raw HR data to beats per minute.

Table 7–5. Conversion Chart for Transforming Heart Rate Counted for 10 or 15 Seconds to Beats/Min

Beats/10 Sec	Beats/Min	Beats/15 Sec	Beats/Min
15	90	23	92
16	96	24	96
17	102	25	100
18	108	26	104
19	114	27	108
20	120	28	112
21	126	29	116
22	132	30	120
23	138	31	124
24	144	32	128
25	150	33	132
26	156	34	136
27	162	35	140
28	168	36	144
29	174	37	148
30	180	38	152
31	186	39	156
32	192	40	160
33	198	41	164
34	204	42	168
		43	172
		44	176
		45	180
		46	184
		47	188
		48	192
		49	196
		50	200
		51	204

(Reprinted with permission from Pollock, M. L., Wilmore, J. H., and Fox, S. M.: **Health and Fitness Through Physical Activity.** New York, copyright John Wiley and Sons, 1978.)

USE OF RATING OF PERCEIVED EXERTION AS AN ADJUNCT TO HEART RATE IN MONITORING TRAINING

The validity and use of the RPE scale for GXT is described in Chapter 6. The use of the scale is an important adjunct to HR for monitoring intensity of training.[47–52, 59] As mentioned in Chapter 6, RPE correlates highly with HR, pulmonary ventilation, and lactic acid build-up.[48] Thus, like HR, RPE will increase at standard work loads under hot environmental conditions or when going uphill and will decrease under cooler climatic conditions or when going downhill. It also decreases in proportion to HR when adaptation to training occurs.[75]

For participants who do not have heart disease, the use of HR for monitoring training intensity may become laborious and unnecessary. When a training program is initiated, the use of both HR and RPE is recommended. The use of HR illustrates to the participants where they are relative to the training zone. Knowledge of both HR and RPE allows the exerciser to develop a more precise individual relationship between the two indicators. Once this individual relationship is determined, a participant can usually estimate training HR rather accurately by knowing RPE.[76] The obvious advantage of RPE at this stage of training is that training intensity can be accurately and continuously monitored throughout the total session without stopping. Knowledge of RPE informs the exercise leader of how the participant is adjusting to the exercise program and when further progression in training should occur.

Because the RPE is a good general indicator of fatigue, it can be used to estimate the intensity of non–steady-state training sessions. This includes many of the game type of activities listed in Table 7–6. For example, the kilocalorie-per-minute expenditure for racquetball is listed at 10 to 15 (8 to 12 METs). How would a participant determine what value to use? The authors recommend that for a moderate, a moderate to hard, and a very hard workout, the RPEs of 12 to 13, 14 to 15, and 16 to 17, respectively, be used to estimate the severity of a training session. In this case, 12 to 13 would represent 10 kcal/min, 14 to 15 would represent 12.5 kcal/min, and 16 to 17 would represent 15 kcal/min. The estimation of severity of training may vary depending on the participant's level of fitness.

The relationship of RPE to HR, $\dot{V}O_2$, blood lactic acid, and pulmonary ventilation is different between intermittent and steady-state activity and aerobic and anaerobic training, and its validity has been established with only aerobic steady-state exercise. More

Table 7–6. Energy Cost of Various Activities*

Activity	Kilocalories† (kcal/min)	METs‡	Oxygen Uptake (ml · kg⁻¹ · min⁻¹)
Archery	3.7–5	3–4	10.5–14
Backpacking	6–13.5	5–11	17.5–38.5
Badminton	5–11	4–9	14–31.5
Basketball			
Nongame	3.7–11	3–9	10.5–31.5
Game	8.5–15	7–12	24.5–42
Bed exercise (arm movement, supine or sitting)	1.1–2.5	1–2	3.5–7
Bench stepping (see Table 6–5)			
Bicycling			
Recreation/transportation	3.7–10	3–8	10.5–28
Stationary (see Table 6–4)			
Bowling	2.5–5	2–4	7–14
Canoeing (rowing and kayaking)	3.7–10	3–8	10.5–28
Calisthenics	3.7–10	3–8	10.5–28
Dancing			
Social and square	3.7–8.5	3–7	10.5–24.5
Aerobic	7.5–11	6–9	21–31.5
Fencing	7.5–12	6–10	21–35
Fishing			
Bank, boat, or ice	2.5–5	2–4	7–14
Stream, wading	6–7.5	5–6	17.5–21
Football (touch)	7.5–12	6–10	21–35
Golf			
Using power cart	2.5–3.7	2–3	7–10.5
Walking, carrying bag, or pulling cart	5–8.5	4–7	14–24.5
Handball	10–15	8–12	28–42
Hiking (cross-country)	3.7–8.5	3–7	10.5–24.5
Horseback riding	3.7–10	3–8	10.5–28
Horseshoe pitching	2.5–3.7	2–3	7–10.5
Hunting, walking			
Small game	3.7–8.5	3–7	10.5–24.5
Big game	3.7–17	3–14	10.5–49
Jogging (see Table 7–9)			
Mountain climbing	6–12	5–10	17.5–35
Paddleball/racquet	10–15	8–12	28–42
Rope skipping	10–14	8–12	28–42
Sailing	2.5–6	2–5	7–17.5
Scuba diving	6–12	5–10	17.5–35
Shuffleboard	2.5–3.7	2–3	7–10.5
Skating (ice or roller)	6–10	5–8	17.5–28
Skiing (snow)			
Downhill	6–10	5–8	17.5–28
Cross-country	7.5–15	6–12	21–42
Skiing (water)	6–8.5	5–7	17.5–24.5
Snow shoeing	8.5–17	7–14	24.5–49
Squash	10–15	8–12	28–42
Soccer	6–15	5–12	17.5–42
Softball	3.7–7.5	3–6	10.5–21
Stair-climbing	5–10	4–8	14–28

Table continued on following page

Table 7–6. Energy Cost of Various Activities* *Continued*

Activity	Kilocalories† (kcal/min)	METs‡	Oxygen Uptake (ml · kg⁻¹ · min⁻¹)
Swimming	5–10	4–8	14–28
Table tennis	3.7–6	3–5	10.5–17.5
Tennis	5–11	4–9	14–31.5
Volleyball	3.7–7.5	3–6	10.5–21
Walking (see Table 7–9)			
Weight training			
Circuit	10	8.2	28

*Energy cost values based on an individual of 154 pounds of body weight (70 kg).

†kcal: a unit of measure based upon heat production. One kcal equals approximately 200 ml of oxygen consumed.

‡MET: basal oxygen rquirement of the body sitting quietly. One MET equals 3.5 ml · kg⁻¹ · min⁻¹ of oxygen consumed.

(Modified with permission from Pollock, M. L., Wilmore, J. H., and Fox, S. M.: Health and Fitness Through Physical Activity. New York, copyright © John Wiley and Sons, 1978.)

recently, some data exist validating the use of the RPE scale with heavy strength and lifting tasks.[77, 78] As stated in Chapter 6, more information is still necessary before the full physiological interpretation of RPE and heavy to moderate levels of strength and lifting exercise can be determined. Even so, because how one perceives the intensity of effort is important and relates to adherence to exercise regimens, the authors have all participants rate their training regardless of whether the activity is considered steady state (aerobic or anaerobic).

MODE OF ACTIVITY

Many types of activities can provide adequate stimulation for improving cardiorespiratory function. Chapter 3 emphasizes that the total energy cost of a program is important and that as long as various activities are of sufficient intensity and duration, the training effect will occur. In addition, activities of similar energy requirements provide similar training effects.[22, 79–81] In choosing the proper mode of training, the participant should be familiar with the variety of activities that are available. Table 7–6 categorizes activities by their kilocalorie cost, METs, and $\dot{V}O_2$. An activity will vary in intensity depending on the enthusiasm and skill level of the participant as well as on the type of activity. For example, tennis singles are significantly more demanding than doubles; thus, a range of energy cost values is listed in the table. Also a skilled player would be able to expend more energy in a given time than an unskilled player.

As mentioned in Chapter 3 and shown in Table 3–3, physical activity can be classified in terms relative to the individual. It was also mentioned that exercise intensity can be expressed in terms of its absolute relation to the activity itself. The latter has been shown to be not very practical in prescribing exercise training for both cardiac and noncardiac participants. In absolute terms, generally, an activity that expends fewer than 5 kcal/min (less than 3.5 METs) is classified as low intensity and is not recommended for use in exercise regimens that are designed to develop cardiorespiratory fitness and reduce body weight. An exception to this would be for a person with a functional capacity below 6 METs. These persons can often improve their functional capacity with low-intensity work but should be encouraged to increase the duration of effort. Except for persons of extremely high or low functional capacities, activities that expend 5 to 10 kcal/min (4 to 8 METs) are considered of moderate intensity; activities from 10 to 14 kcal/min (8 to 12 METs), moderate to high intensity; and activities greater than 14 kcal/min (12 METs), high intensity. These classifications are based upon exercising continuously for up to 60 minutes and for participants of average fitness. It must be noted again that even though it is interesting to understand the general classification of work intensity as described in absolute terms, intensity expressed in relative values is what is recommended for use in adult fitness and cardiopulmonary rehabilitation programs. See Chapter 3 for more information on classification of intensity of work and the rationale for use of relative work in exercise prescription.

When choosing the proper activity, the participant should take into account level of fitness, health status, physical activity interests, availability of equipment and facilities, geographical location, and climate.[5, 43, 44, 82] The deconditioned adult should be involved initially in several weeks or months of moderate activity that does not require competition or extreme starting and stopping movements.[82] Under the latter conditions, many participants tend to overdo it and become unduly stiff and sore, fatigued, or injured. Since the joints and muscular system are not adequately developed in a beginner to handle such demands, the participant is vulnerable to injury. The need to get in shape to play games is true in most cases. Persons whose screening tests have indicated major cardiovascular problems should avoid highly competitive activities. It is important not to exceed the safe limit of exercise. The starter programs outlined later in the chapter are recommended for beginners. (For more specific information concerning cardiac rehabilitation and other special patient populations, see Chapter 8.)

Participation in a variety of activities is recommended and can be accomplished by interchanging some of the various activities listed in Table 7–6. Choosing different activities may keep a participant interested in endurance exercise over a long-term period. For example, one might jog 30 minutes on Monday and Thursday and play racquetball or basketball on Tuesday and Friday. The important factor is for the person to participate in these activities frequently and with sufficient intensity and duration.[27]

Although this discussion emphasized the variety of activities available for developing and maintaining cardiorespiratory endurance, this type of activity is only part of a total, well-rounded program.[1, 3, 5, 82] Endurance activities are of paramount importance, but adequate flexibility and muscular strength and endurance have equal importance and add to a balanced physical fitness program.[1, 3, 5, 43, 82]

Emphasis on Low-Impact Activities

Because of the strong relationship between high-impact activities and injuries, low-impact activities should be emphasized for many beginners and persons susceptible to orthopedic injury.[16, 19, 83–85] Participants who are older or overweight and postmenopausal women are more susceptible to orthopedic injury with high-impact activities. The data presented in Table 7–7 show the difference in injury rates of participants of various ages engaged in a 5- to 6-month training program of walking and walking-jogging conducted for 30 to 40 minutes, 3 (walking-jogging) to 4 (walking) days per week.[16, 86–88] All subjects were healthy, sedentary volunteers. In the

Table 7–7. Comparison of Injuries by Age*

Study	n	Age Range (yr)	Mode	Injuries (%)
Pollock et al., 1977	50	20–35	W/J	18
Pollock et al., 1976	22	49–65	W/J	41
Pollock et al., unpublished	14	70–79	W/J	57
Pollock et al., 1971	19	40–56	W	12

*All programs were conducted with healthy, previously sedentary individuals. Except for Pollock (1971), all programs had a walk/jog (W/J) component to them. The 1971 study included only walking (W) as the mode of training. Injuries mainly occurred in the foot, ankle, leg, or knee and were associated with nonparticipation for at least one week.

(Reprinted with permission from Pollock, M. L.: Exercise prescriptions for the elderly. In W. W. Spirduso and H. Eckert (eds.): **Physical Activity and Aging**. Human Kinetics Publishers, Champaign, IL, 1989, pp. 163–174.)

earlier experiments,[16, 87] training began with equal amounts of walking and jogging and progressed to more continuous jogging as adaptation to training occurred. In the authors' recent investigation,[88] jogging was not introduced until after 3 months of moderately paced walking (50 to 60 percent HRmax reserve, RPE of 11 to 12) to fast walking (60 to 70 percent HRmax reserve, RPE of 12 to 13) training. It is obvious from Table 7–7 that injuries are related to age and the high-impact forces that are produced with jogging. It was surprising that even after 3 months of preliminary training, the injury rate would be so high when the 70-year-old subjects began to walk-jog. The injuries occurred immediately during the first weeks of walking-jogging and, in all cases but one, were resolved within 2 to 3 weeks. During recovery from injury, the subjects continued to train but at a slower pace on a stationary cycle or by slow walking on a treadmill. One woman had a stress fracture of the tibia and could not continue in the study. Eventually, all of the 70- to 79-year-old subjects could get their training heart rate to 75 to 85 percent of HRmax reserve (RPE of 14 to 15). The injured subjects continued to walk on the treadmill at an elevation that elicited the desired heart rate response. The total group had a 22-percent increase in VO_2max;[89] thus, with these healthy 70-year-olds, the prescribed program (walking-jogging) was limited not by their cardiorespiratory system (capacity) but by their musculoskeletal system (orthopedic limitations).

Table 7–8 lists commonly used high- and low-impact activities for developing and maintaining aerobic endurance. The big distinction among activities is whether or not they cause high-impact forces on the joints. Any activity that has a running or jumping component is considered a high-impact type of activity. The inclusion of high-impact and high-intensity activities into a program in combination with high frequency and duration, increases the injury rate exponentially.[16, 19, 83, 85, 90, 91] Thus, when one is considering an

Table 7–8. Commonly Used High-Impact and Low-Impact Activities for Aerobic Endurance Training

High-Impact	Low-Impact
Jogging/Running	Walking
Basketball/Volleyball	Cycling-Bicycling
Hopping/Jumping activities	Swimming/Water activities
Rope skipping	Rowing
Aerobic dance (high-impact)	Stair climbing
	Aerobic dance (low-impact)
	Cross-country skiing

(Reprinted with permission from Pollock, M. L.: Exercise prescriptions for the elderly. In W. W. Spirduso and H. Eckert (eds.): **Physical Activity and Aging.** Human Kinetics Publishers, Champaign, IL, 1989, pp. 163–174.)

aerobic training program, activities or regimens that are associated with higher injury rates should be avoided.

PROGRAMS FOR CARDIORESPIRATORY FITNESS AND WEIGHT CONTROL

Endurance exercises develop cardiorespiratory fitness and help individuals to reduce their body weight and fat.[5, 27, 33, 92] Endurance exercises require a sustained effort, such as cross-country skiing, jogging, walking, bicycling, dancing, rope skipping, rowing, swimming, and vigorous game types of activities.

Exercise Prescription

As mentioned earlier, in order to prescribe exercise properly, it is necesary to know something about the person's health status and physical fitness level. After undergoing the physical fitness evaluation, a participant may be classified into one of eight categories of cardiorespiratory fitness. Table 6–3 shows the fitness classification scores achieved on various GXT tests. In order to be classified at the good level of cardiorespiratory fitness, a person should have a functional capacity of approximately 38 to 45 ml•kg^{-1}•min^{-1} of oxygen uptake (11 to 13 METs), depending on age.[22] Therefore, knowing the initial level of cardiorespiratory fitness helps guide the participant into the correct program.

The exercise prescription usually has three stages of progression: starter, slow progression, and maintenance (Fig. 7–4). The initial stage of training is classified as a starter program. In this phase, the exercise intensity is low and includes a lot of stretching and light calisthenics or strength training followed by aerobic exercise of low to moderate intensity. The purpose at this stage of the program is to introduce one to exercise at a low level and to allow time for proper adaptation to the initial weeks of training. If this phase is introduced correctly, the participant will experience a minimum of muscle soreness and can avoid debilitating injuries or discomfort of the knee, shin, ankle, or foot. The latter injuries are common in the initial stages of a jogging program but can be avoided if the participant takes some preliminary precautions, e.g., a good starter program, use of good training shoes, and proper warm-up and conditioning of the legs. Avoiding sharp turns and extremely hard running surfaces is also an important safeguard (see Chapter 9 for more detail). As mentioned in the previous

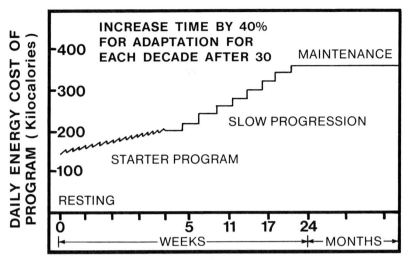

Figure 7–4. Schematic illustration for average participants of a normal progression in an aerobic training program. (Modified with permission from Pollock, M. L., Wilmore, J. H ., and Fox, S. M.: **Health and Fitness Through Physical Activity.** New York, copyright John Wiley and Sons, 1978.)

section, low-impact activities are recommended for beginner, overweight, and elderly participants.

The duration of the starter program is usually from 2 to 6 weeks but depends on the adaptation of the participant to the program. For example, a person who is classified at a poor or fair fitness level may spend as many as 4 to 6 weeks in a starter program, but for a participant scoring in the good or excellent categories, a starter program may not be necessary.

The slow progression stage of training differs from the starter phase in that the participant progresses at a more rapid rate. During this stage, the duration and intensity are increased rather consistently every one to three weeks. How well an individual adapts to the present level of training dictates the frequency and magnitude of progression. As a general rule, the older the participant and the lower the initial fitness level, the longer one takes to adapt and progress in a training regimen. Although no good data exist, the authors estimate that the adaptation to the training load takes approximately 40 percent longer for each decade in life after age 30. That is, if the progression in distance run is every 2 weeks for men of 30 to 39 years, then the interval may be 3 weeks for those of 40 to 49 years and 3.5 to 4 weeks for those who are 50 to 59 years old.

The maintenance stage of prescription usually occurs after 6 months to a year of training.[5, 22, 26, 27] At this stage, the participant has reached a satisfactory level of cardiorespiratory fitness and may no longer be interested in increasing the training load. At this point, further improvement is usually minimal, but continuing the same workout schedule (the number of miles or minutes trained per week) enables one to maintain fitness.

GENERAL GUIDELINES FOR GETTING STARTED

In designing an exercise regimen, one must select activities that can be performed on a regular basis. Generally, game types of activities are not recommended in the early stages of training. Before becoming involved in game types of activities in which running occurs, fast walking or walk-jog programs are recommended.

Table 7–6 lists the energy costs of a variety of activities commonly used in recreation and endurance fitness programs. The activities are quantified in terms of kilocalories per minute, METs, and oxygen uptake. As mentioned earlier, these values indicate the relative intensity of the effort. To determine the total kilocalorie cost of the programs, one must determine the intensity level and multiply this by the total number of minutes of participation. Because games are not played continuously with an even amount of effort, some approximation has to be made to estimate the intensity level for game types of activities. Intensity depends on how hard the game is played. As mentioned earlier, the use of the RPE scale helps in determining intensity. If the intensity is in doubt, use the average value listed for the activity in Table 7–6. For example, if handball is played for 60 minutes, then the intensity in kilocalories (12.5 kcal/min) is multiplied by the minutes played (60) to get the total kilocalorie expenditure (750). The important point here is that the participant counts only the time that was used in participation. Rest breaks and standing around do not count. For sports such as handball, racquetball, or tennis singles, cutting the total time by one half usually approximates the proper kilocalorie expenditure. Therefore, in the preceding example, 60 minutes of handball would be calculated at 12.5 kcal times 30 minutes, for a total of 375 kcal.

The energy costs of running and walking are listed in Table 7–9. An endurance training program can be designed from this table, but because of the difficulty of knowing the proper pace or sequence of progression, several programs are outlined in Tables 7–11 to 7–21. The programs include walking and running routines and are designed relative to various levels of fitness.

Table 7–9. Energy Cost of Walking and Running*

Activity	Speed mph	Min/Mile (min:sec)	Grade (%)	Kilocalories† (kcal/min)	METs‡	Oxygen Cost (ml · kg⁻¹ · min⁻¹)
Walking	2.0	30:00	0	2.5	2.0	7
	2.5	24:00	0	3.0	2.5	8.7
	3.0	20:00	0	3.7	3.0	10.5
	3.0	20:00	5	6.0	5.0	17.5
	3.0	20:00	10	8.5	7.0	24.5
	3.0	20:00	15	11.0	9.0	31.5
	3.5	17:08	0	4.2	3.5	12.3
	3.5	17:08	5	7.5	5.9	21
	3.5	17:08	10	10.0	8.3	29
	3.5	17:08	15	13.0	10.7	37.5
	3.75	16:00	0	4.9	4.0	14
	4.0	15:00	0	5.5	4.6	16.1
	4.0	15:00	5	9.0	7.3	25.6
	4.0	15:00	10	12.0	10.0	35
	4.0	15:00	15	15.6	12.8	44.8
	4.5	13:20	0	7.0	5.7	20
	5.0	12:00	0	8.3	6.9	24
Running	5.5	10:55	0	10.1	8.3	29
	6.0	10:00	0	12.0	10.0	35
	7.0	8:35	0	14.0	11.5	40.3
	8.0	7:30	0	15.6	12.8	44.8
	9.0	6:40	0	17.5	14.2	49.7
	10.0	6:00	0	19.6	16.0	56
	11.0	5:30	0	21.7	17.7	62
	12.0	5:00	0	24.5	20.0	70

*Energy cost values based on an individual of 154 pounds of body weight (70 kg).

†Kilocalorie: a unit of measure based upon heat production. One kilocalorie equals 200 ml of oxygen consumed.

‡MET: basal oxygen requirement of the body sitting quietly. One MET equals 3.5 ml · kg⁻¹ · min⁻¹ of oxygen consumed.

(Reprinted with permission from Pollock, M. L., Wilmore, J. H., and Fox, S. M.: **Health and Fitness Through Physical Activity.** New York, copyright © John Wiley and Sons, 1978.)

Although walking and running can be done in a variety of settings—e.g., running tracks, roads, parks, and shopping malls—the course should be a measured distance. This can be accomplished by the use of an odometer from an automobile or bicycle or by the use of a measured track. Training on an oval track can get boring over a long period of time but, if available, is a good way of getting started. Tracks generally have a smooth running surface and are of a known distance.

Table 7–10 helps in determining the pace for walking and running programs. Speeds range from a moderate walk (2.9 mph) to a fast run (12.5 mph). To aid in pacing, reference points of 110

Table 7–10. Pacing Chart for Walking and Running Program Conducted on Track Measured in 110-Yard Increments

Pace			Pace			Pace		
110 Yd (sec)	*440 Yd (min:sec)*	*Mph*	*110 Yd (sec)*	*440 Yd (min:sec)*	*Mph*	*110 Yd (sec)*	*440 Yd (min:sec)*	*Mph*
18	1:12	12.5	38	2:32	5.9	58	3:52	3.9
19	1:16	11.8	39	2:36	5.8	59	3:56	3.8
20	1:20	11.2	40	2:40	5.6	60	4:00	3.7
21	1:24	10.7	41	2:44	5.5	61	4:04	3.7
22	1:28	10.2	42	2:48	5.4	62	4:08	3.6
23	1:32	9.8	43	2:52	5.2	63	4:12	3.6
24	1:36	9.4	44	2:56	5.1	64	4:16	3.5
25	1:40	9.0	45	3:00	5.0	65	4:20	3.5
26	1:44	8.6	46	3:04	4.9	66	4:24	3.4
27	1:48	8.3	47	3:08	4.8	67	4:28	3.4
28	1:52	8.0	48	3:12	4.7	68	4:32	3.3
29	1:56	7.7	49	3:16	4.6	69	4:36	3.3
30	2:00	7.5	50	3:20	4.5	70	4:40	3.2
31	2:04	7.3	51	3:24	4.4	71	4:44	3.2
32	2:08	7.0	52	3:28	4.3	72	4:48	3.1
33	2:12	6.8	53	3:32	4.2	73	4:52	3.1
34	2:16	6.6	54	3:36	4.2	74	4:56	3.0
35	2:20	6.4	55	3:40	4.1	75	5:00	3.0
36	2:24	6.2	56	3:44	4.0	76	5:04	2.9
37	2:28	6.1	57	3:48	3.9	77	5:08	2.9

(Reprinted with permission from Pollock, M. L., Wilmore, J. H., and Fox, S. M.: **Health and Fitness Through Physical Activity.** New York, copyright John Wiley and Sons, 1978.)

or 440 yards are helpful. If a stopwatch or wristwatch with a 60-second sweep hand or digital display is carried, the pace can be kept very accurately during the entire training program. Monitoring of the program by pace, HR response, and RPE helps as a guide to proper initiation and progression of the training regimen.

Generally, persons scoring in fitness categories 1 and 2 should begin their endurance training by walking. The walk should be at a comfortable but brisk pace. The initial speed may range from 2.5 to 4.0 mph. Distance (or time) will be approximately 1 to 1.5 miles (20 to 30 minutes) for persons in fitness category 1 and approximately 1.5 to 2 miles (30 to 40 minutes) for individuals in fitness category 2. The reason behind this combination of walking speed and distance is to get the participant started at a comfortable pace and at the same time to keep the distance long enough so that an endurance training effect can begin to occur.

Even though the kilocalorie cost of this regimen is low (approximately 100 to 200 kcal), it allows time for adaptation of most bodily systems. Do not be concerned about not working hard enough. Time, with proper progression and adaptation, will eventually lead to the higher, more demanding levels of training. Table

7–11 outlines two examples of 6-week starter programs for walking, with Program A being recommended for persons in fitness category 1 and Program B for persons in fitness category 2. See Table 6–3 for guidelines on placement into the proper fitness category.

If one of the two examples of starter programs listed in Table 7–11 is too easy or difficult, then make an on-the-spot change in the program. Remember, the exercise prescription should be individualized. A satisfactory modification can usually be made by changing the speed or distance slightly (see Tables 7–9 and 7–10). For example, elderly or obese individuals may initially limit duration of walking to 20 to 30 minutes. Walking programs for cardiac patients are shown in Chapter 8.

The programs listed here are based upon jogging-running or walking on a relatively flat surface, at sea level, and in an average climatic condition (temperature and humidity). Further program modifications have to be taken into account when persons are exercising in moderate to extreme environmental conditions. Chapter 9 discusses these modifications in more detail. Running or walking hills also dramatically alters training pace. The use of the RPE scale helps a participant in adjusting to the proper training speed.

Once the participant has completed the 6-week starter program, then the walking program listed in Table 7–15 or the combination walk-jog program outlined in Table 7–12 can be

Table 7–11. Six-Week Starter Programs for Persons in Fitness Categories 1 and 2*

Program	Week	Pace (mph)	Distance (miles)	Time (min:sec)	Kilocalories
A	1	2.5	1.0	24:00	72
	2	3.0	1.0	20:00	74
	3	3.0	1.25	25:00	92.5
	4	3.0	1.50	30:00	111
	5	3.0	2.0	40:00	148
	6	3.5	2.0	34:16	143
B	1	3.5	2.0	34:16	143
	2	3.5	2.0	34:16	143
	3	4.0	2.0	30:00	165
	4	4.0	2.0	30:00	165
	5	4.0	2.5	37:50	206
	6	4.0	2.5	37:50	206

*Programs based upon level walking at sea level and in an average climatic condition (temperature and humidity).

(Reprinted with permission from Pollock, M. L., Wilmore, J. H., and Fox, S. M.: **Health and Fitness Through Physical Activity.** New York, copyright John Wiley and Sons, 1978.)

Table 7–12. Six-Week Starter Program for Persons in Fitness Category 3*

Program	Week	Walk Pace (mph)	Walk Distance (yd)	Walk Time (sec)	Run Pace (mph)	Run Distance (yd)	Run Time (min:sec)	Repetitions Walk	Repetitions Run	Time (min:sec)	Kilocalories	Total Miles
A	1	3.75	110	60	5.5	110	:41	16	16	26:56	188.8	2.0
	2	3.75	110	60	5.5	110	:41	16	16	26:56	188.8	2.0
	3	3.75	110	60	5.5	220	1:22	11	11	26:02	205.7	2.0
	4	3.75	110	60	5.5	220	1:22	11	11	26:02	205.7	2.0
	5	3.75	110	60	5.5	330	2:03	8	8	24:24	204.8	2.0
	6	3.75	110	60	5.5	330	2:03	8	8	24:24	204.8	2.0
B	1	3.75	110	60	6.4	110	:35	16	16	25:20	197.8	2.0
	2	3.75	110	60	6.4	110	:35	16	16	25:20	197.8	2.0
	3	3.75	110	60	6.4	220	1:10	11	11	23:50	218.0	2.0
	4	3.75	110	60	6.4	220	1:10	12	12	26:00	238.0	2.25
	5	3.75	110	60	6.4	330	1:45	9	9	24:45	245.7	2.25
	6	3.75	110	60	6.4	330	1:45	9	9	24:45	245.7	2.25

*Programs based upon level walking at sea level and in an average climatic condition (temperature and humidity). (Reprinted with permission from Pollock, M. L., Wilmore, J. H., and Fox, S. M.: **Health and Fitness Through Physical Activity.** New York, copyright John Wiley and Sons, 1978.)

Table 7–13. Six-Week Starter Program for Persons in Fitness Category 4*

Program	Week	Walk			Run			Repetitions			Kilocalories	Total Miles
		Pace (mph)	Distance (yd)	Time (sec)	Pace (mph)	Distance (yd)	Time (min:sec)	Walk	Run	Time (min:sec)		
A	1	3.75	110	60	6.8	220	1:06	11	11	23:06	218.5	2.0
	2	3.75	110	60	6.8	220	1:06	11	11	23:06	218.5	2.0
	3	3.75	110	60	6.8	330	1:39	8	8	22:12	218.7	2.0
	4	3.75	110	60	6.8	330	1:39	9	9	23:51	246.1	2.25
	5	3.75	110	60	6.8	440	2:12	8	8	23:24	248.6	2.25
	6	3.75	110	60	6.8	440	2:12	8	8	25:36	278.6	2.25
B	1	3.75	110	60	7.5	220	1:00	12	12	24:00	236.4	2.25
	2	3.75	110	60	7.5	220	1:00	12	12	24:00	236.4	2.25
	3	3.75	110	60	7.5	330	1:30	9	9	22:30	243.9	2.25
	4	3.75	110	60	7.5	330	1:30	10	10	25:00	271.0	2.25
	5	3.75	110	60	7.5	440	2:00	8	8	24:00	276.0	2.25
	6	3.75	110	60	7.5	440	2:00	8	8	24:00	276.0	2.25

*Programs based upon level walking at sea level and in an average climatic condition (temperature and humidity). (Reprinted with permission from Pollock, M. L., Wilmore, J. H., and Fox, S. M.: **Health and Fitness Through Physical Activity.** New York, copyright John Wiley and Sons, 1978.)

Table 7–14. Six-Week Starter Program for Persons in Fitness Category 5*

Program	Week	Walk Pace (mph)	Walk Distance (yd)	Walk Time (sec)	Run Pace (mph)	Run Distance (yd)	Run Time (min:sec)	Repetitions Walk	Repetitions Run	Time (min:sec)	Kilocalories	Total Miles
A	1	3.75	110	60	7.5	330	1:30	9	9	22:30	243.9	2.25
	2	3.75	110	60	7.5	330	1:30	9	9	22:30	243.9	2.25
	3	3.75	110	60	7.5	440	2:00	8	8	24:00	276.0	2.5
	4	3.75	110	60	7.5	550	2:30	7	7	24:30	293.3	2.63
	5	3.75	110	60	7.5	660	3:00	6	6	24:00	295.8	2.65
	6	3.75	110	60	7.5	880	4:00	5	5	25:00	320.5	2.81
B	1	3.75	110	60	8.0	330	1:24	9	9	21:36	240.7	2.25
	2	3.75	110	60	8.0	330	1:24	9	9	21:36	240.7	2.25
	3	3.75	110	60	8.0	440	1:52	8	8	22:56	272.1	2.5
	4	3.75	110	60	8.0	550	2:20	7	7	23:20	289.1	2.63
	5	3.75	110	60	8.0	660	2:48	6	6	22:48	291.5	2.63
	6	3.75	110	60	8.0	880	3:16	6	6	24:37	330.5	3.3

*Programs based upon level walking at sea level and in an average climatic condition (temperature and humidity). (Reprinted with permission from Pollock, M. L., Wilmore, J. H., and Fox, S. M.: **Health and Fitness Through Physical Activity.** New York, copyright John Wiley and Sons, 1978.)

Table 7–15. Twenty-Week Walking Program for Fitness Categories 2 and 3*

Week	Pace (mph)	Distance (miles)	Time (min:sec)	Kilocalories
1,2	3.75	2.5	40:00	196.0
3–5	3.75	2.75	44:00	215.6
6–8	4.0	2.75	41:15	226.9
9–12	4.0	3.0	45:00	247.5
13–16	4.25	3.0	42:21	262.0
17–20	4.25	3.25	45:53	285.4

*Programs based upon level walking at sea level and in an average climatic condition (temperature and humidity).
(Reprinted with permission from Pollock, M. L., Wilmore, J. H., and Fox, S. M.: **Health and Fitness Through Physical Activity.** New York, copyright John Wiley and Sons, 1978.)

initiated. The starter program outlined in Table 7–12 is recommended for persons scoring in fitness category 3. Tables 7–13 and 7–14 show sugggested starter programs for persons scoring in fitness categories 4 and 5. Normally, participants scoring in fitness categories above 50 ml·kg^{-1}·min^{-1} of $\dot{V}O_2$max (14 METs) are considered in excellent cardiorespiratory fitness and do not require a special starter program. Persons scoring in the excellent categories of fitness who have not been exercising on a regular basis should begin with the program outlined in Table 7–21.

WALKING

Walking is safe both from a cardiovascular risk and an orthopedic risk standpoint. In all the years the authors have been conducting endurance training programs, the best adherence has been in the walking programs.[19] This probably relates to lack of orthopedic injuries and the enjoyment and comradeship that participants receive when walking. It has also been the authors' experience that participants do not like or tolerate high-intensity training as well as that of moderate intensity.[19, 24] Coupled with the safety aspect associated with walking programs, walking is also simple in nature, which allows most people to participate. It requires little in terms of skill, facilities, and equipment. A good pair of shoes is recommended.

The scientific literature as reported in Chapters 3 and 4 shows that walking is an appropriate activity for improving aerobic fitness and body composition. The usual trade-off with walking programs as compared with jogging is that walking requires increased frequency and duration of training. Thus, the kilocalorie expenditure of 20 to 30 minutes of jogging is equal to approximately 40 to 50

Text continued on page 410

Table 7-16. Twenty-Week Walking-Jogging Program for Fitness Category 2*

Week	Walk			Run				Total Time (min:sec)	Kilocalories	Total Miles
	Pace (mph)	Distance	Time (min:sec)	Pace (mph)	Distance (yd)	Time (min:sec)	Repetitions			
1,2	4.0	2.75 mi	41:15				1	41:15	226.9	
3,4	4.25	2.75 mi	38:50				1	38:50	241.5	
5,6	4.25	3.0 mi	42:21				1	42:21	262.0	
7,8	4.5	3.0 mi	40:00				1	40:00	280.0	
9,10	4.5	3.25 mi	43:20				1	43:20	303.2	
11,12	4.0	110 yd	1:00	4.75	220	1:35	18	46:26	316.6	3.375
13,14	4.0	110 yd	1:00	4.75	330	2:22	13	43:49	307.2	3.25
15,16	4.0	110 yd	1:00	4.75	440	3:10	10/11†	44:50	321.4	3.375
17,18	4.0	110 yd	1:00	5.0	330	2:15	13	42:15	314.3	3.25
19,20	4.0	110 yr	1:00	5.0	440	3:00	10/11†	43:00	328.9	3.375

*Programs based upon level walking at sea level and in an average climatic condition (temperature and humidity).
†Ten walk, 11 run.
(Reprinted with permission from Pollock, M. L., Wilmore, J. H., and Fox, S. M.: **Health and Fitness Through Physical Activity.** New York, copyright John Wiley and Sons, 1978.)

Table 7–17. Twenty-Week Walk-Jog, Jogging Program for Fitness Category 3A*

	Walk			Run				Total Time (min:sec)	Kilocalories	Total Miles
Week	Pace (mph)	Distance (yd)	Time (sec)	Pace (mph)	Distance (yd:mi)	Time (min:sec)	Repetitions			
1,2	3.75	110	60	5.6	440:¼	2:41	8	29:26	259.9	2.5
3,4	3.75	110	60	5.6	660:	4:01	6	30:06	277.6	2.63
5,6	3.75	110	60	5.6	880:½	5:22	5	31:47	300.4	2.81
7,8	3.75	110	60	5.6	1320:¾	8:02	3	30:27	297.2	2.75
					550:	3:20	1			
9,10	3.75	110	60	5.6	1760:1	10:42	3	35:08	345.7	3.19
11,12	3.75	110	60	5.6	:1¼	13:20	2	34:08	340.6	3.13
					:½	5:22	1			
13,14	3.75	110	60	5.6	:1½	16:04	2	34:08	340.8	3.13
15,16	3.75	110	60	5.6	:2	21:24	1	33:08	335.5	3.06
					:1	10:42	1			
17,18	3.75	110		5.6	:2½	26:47	1	33:09	336.0	3.06
					:½	5:22	1			
19,20				5.6	:3	32:08	1	32:08	331.0	3.00

*Programs based upon level walking at sea level and in an average climatic condition (temperature and humidity).
(Reprinted with permission from Pollock, M. L., Wilmore, J. H., and Fox, S. M.: **Health and Fitness Through Physical Activity.** New York, copyright John Wiley and Sons, 1978.)

Table 7-18. Twenty-Week Walk-Jog, Jogging Program for Fitness Category 3B*

Week	Walk			Run				Total Time (min:sec)	Kilocalories	Total Miles
	Pace (mph)	Distance (yd)	Time (sec)	Pace (mph)	Distance (yd:mi)	Time (min:sec)	Repetitions			
1,2	3.75	110	60	6.4	440:¼	2:20	8	26:40	278.2	2.5
3,4	3.75	110	60	6.4	660:	3:30	6	27:00	298.2	2.63
5,6	3.75	110	60	6.4	880:½	4:20	5	26:40	301.7	2.81
7,8	3.75	110	60	6.4	1320:¾	7:00	3	26:55	320.7	2.75
					550:	2:55	1			
9,10	3.75	110	60	6.4	1760:1	9:24	3	29:12	365.8	3.19
11,12	3.75	110	60	6.4	:1¼	11:44	2	28:48	360.7	3.13
					:½	4:20	1			
13,14	3.75	110	60	6.4	:1½	13:44	2	28:28	356.5	3.13
15,16	3.75	110	60	6.4	:2	18:48	1	29:12	365.8	3.06
					:1	9:24	1			
17,18	3.75	110	60	6.4	:2½	23:08	1	28:28	356.4	3.06
					:½	4:20	1			
19,20				6.4	:3	28:12	1	28:12	361.0	3.00

*Programs based upon level walking at sea level and in an average climatic condition (temperature and humidity). (Reprinted with permission from Pollock, M. L., Wilmore, J. H., and Fox, S. M.: **Health and Fitness Through Physical Activity.** New York, copyright John Wiley and Sons, 1978.)

Table 7-19. Twenty-Week Walk-Jog, Jogging Program for Fitness Category 4A*

Week	Walk			Run				Total Time (min:sec)	Kilocalories	Total Miles
	Pace (mph)	Distance (yd)	time (sec)	Pace (mph)	Distance (yd:mi)	Time (min:sec)	Repetitions			
1,2	3.75	110	60	6.8	660:	3:18	6	25:48	298.7	2.63
3,4	3.75	110	60	6.8	880:½	4:24	5	27:00	323.7	2.81
5,6	3.75	110	60	6.8	1320:¾	6:36	3	25:33	321.4	2.75
					550:	2:45	1			
7,8	3.75	110	60	6.8	1760:1	8:48	3	29:24	373.7	3.19
9,10	3.75	110	60	6.8	:1¼	11:00	2	28:24	368.8	3.13
					:½	4:24	1			
11,12	3.75	110	60	6.8	:1½	13:12	2	28:24	368.8	3.13
13,14	3.75	110	60	6.8	:2	17:36	1	29:36	393.9	3.31
					:1¼	11:00	1			
15,16	3.75	110	60	6.8	:2½	22:00	1	29:36	393.9	3.31
					:¾	6:36	1			
17,18	3.75	110	60	6.8	:3¼	28:36	1	28:36	389.0	3.25
19,20				6.8	:3½	30:48	1	30:48	418.9	3.5

*Programs based upon level walking at sea level and in an average climatic condition (temperature and humidity).
(Reprinted with permission from Pollock, M. L., Wilmore, J. H., and Fox, S. M.: **Health and Fitness Through Physical Activity.** New York, copyright John Wiley and Sons, 1978.)

Table 7-20. Twenty-Week Walk-Jog, Jogging Program for Fitness Category 4B*

Week	Walk Pace (mph)	Walk Distance (yd)	Walk Time (sec)	Run Pace (mph)	Run Distance (yd:mi)	Run Time (min:sec)	Repetitions	Total Time (min:sec)	Kilocalories	Total Miles
1,2	3.75	110	60	7.5	660:	3:00	6	24:00	295.8	2.63
3,4	3.75	110	60	7.5	880:½	4:00	5	25:00	320.5	2.81
5,6	3.75	110	60	7.5	1320:¾	6:00	3	23:00	318.1	2.75
					550:	2:30	1			
7,8	3.75	110	60	7.5	1760:1	8:00	3	27:00	369.9	3.19
9,10	3.75	110	60	7.5	:1¼	10:00	2	26:00	365.0	3.13
					:½	4:00	1			
11,12	3.75	110	60	7.5	:1½	12:00	2	26:00	365.0	3.13
13,14	3.75	110	60	7.5	1:2	16:00	1	27:00	389.7	3.31
					:1¼	10:00	1			
15,16	3.75	110	60	7.5	:2½	20:00	1	27:00	289.7	3.31
					:¾	6:00	1			
17,18	3.75			7.5	:3¼	26:00	1	26:00	384.8	3.25
19,20	3.75			7.5	:3½	28:00	1	28:00	414.4	3.50

*Programs based upon level walking at sea level and in an average climatic condition (temperature and humidity).

(Reprinted with permission from Pollock, M. L., Wilmore, J. H., and Fox, S. M.: **Health and Fitness Through Physical Activity**. New York, copyright John Wiley and Sons, 1978.)

Table 7-21. Twenty-Week Walk-Jog, Jogging Program for Fitness Category 5*

Week	Walk			Run						
	Pace (mph)	Distance (yd)	Time (sec)	Pace (mph)	Distance (yd:mi)	Time (min:sec)	Repetitions	Total Time (min:sec)	Kilocalories	Total Miles
1,2	3.75	110	60	7.5	880:½	4:00	6	30:00	384.6	3.38
3,4	3.75	110	60	7.5	1320:¾	6:00	4	28:00	374.8	3.25
5,6	3.75	110	60	7.5	1760:1	8:00	3	31:00	429.1	3.69
7,8	3.75	110	60	7.5	880:½	4:00	1			
					:1½	12:00	2	30:00	424.2	3.63
					:½	4:00	1			
9,10	3.75	110	60	7.5	:2	16:00	1			
					:1½	12:00	1	30:00	424.2	3.56
11,12				7.5	:3	24:00	1	24:00	355.0	3.0
13,14				7.5	:3½	28:00	1	28:00	414.8	3.3
15,16				7.5	:4	32:00	1	32:00	473.6	4.0
17,18				7.7	:4	31:10	1	31:10	470.6	4.0
19,20				8.0	:4	30:00	1	30:00	468.0	4.0

*Programs based upon walking at sea level and in an average climatic condition (temperature and humidity).

(Reprinted with permission from Pollock, M. L., Wilmore, J. H., and Fox, S. M.: **Health and Fitness Through Physical Activity**. New York, copyright John Wiley and Sons, 1978.)

minutes of fast walking.[22, 26, 27] The authors recommend that most participants over the age of 40 years and, in particular, elderly, poorly fit, obese, hypertense, cardiac, or fragile participants begin their exercise training program with walking as their aerobic activity. Other low-impact activities such as swimming, cycling, and low-impact aerobic dance are suitable substitutes. Whether participants eventually progress to a higher intensity jogging-running type of program depends on their needs, goals, desires, health status, and level of fitness.

Information provided by the President's Council on Physical Fitness and Sports,[93] the Rockport Walking Institute,[94] and others[95–98] gives additional information concerning walking training.

USE OF HAND-HELD WEIGHTS AND OTHER WEIGHT-CARRYING ACTIVITIES

The use of weights attached to the torso, ankle, or wrists has been shown to increase the energy cost of exercise.[99–110] The amount of increase in energy cost depends upon the size of weight used, speed of the activity, where the weight is placed, and, if hand weights are used, the vigorousness, frequency, and height of the arm swing (Table 7–22).[99–111] Although weight can be used while jogging, the most common use has been in walking and low-impact aerobic dance programs. Walking with 3-pound weights on the wrist or in the hands and using an arm swing up to shoulder height increased the oxygen cost by 1 MET and the HR by approximately 10 to 12 beats/min.[107, 108] On the other hand, just holding the 1- to 3-pound weights had little benefit.[111]

Even though using a weight heavier than 3 pounds for the wrist or hands and increasing the vigor or height of the arm action increases the energy cost of the activity,[106, 110] it is also associated with a significantly greater number of orthopedic problems of the elbow joint (tennis elbow). For participants who cannot run, do not like to run, or are limited in the speed at which they can walk, the use of weights is a practical means of increasing the energy cost of the activity. If a hilly terrain or grade walking on a treadmill are not available options and a participant desires a greater increase in MET cost than shown in Table 7–22, a weighted waist belt or weighted backpack can be used.[99, 102, 109] For example, Schram and Hanson[109] evaluated the added energy cost of walking at 3.0 mph, 0-percent grade, with a 5 to 20 kg backpack. They found a linear increase in HR of 6 to 7 beats/min and in $\dot{V}O_2$ of 1.5 ml·kg^{-1}·min^{-1} at each 5 kg increment from 5 to 20 kg. The energy cost of using a backpack with 35 to 70 kg loads and at various speeds of walking was reported by Soule, Pandolf, and Goldman.[112]

Table 7–22. Comparison of Selected Studies on Energy Cost Associated with Weighted Walking

Reference	Weight (lbs)	Placement	Speed (mph)	Grade (%)	$\Delta\,\dot{V}O_2$* ($ml \cdot kg^{-1} \cdot min^{-1}$)
Graves et al.[107]	3	hands†	3.9	6.3	3.8
		wrists†	3.9	6.3	3.8
		ankles	3.9	6.3	2.4
Auble et al.[106]	3	hands†‡	3.5	level	6.9
Graves et al.[105]	1	hands†	3.7	7.9	1.9
	3	hands†	3.7	7.9	3.3
Jones et al.[103]	2.5	feet	3.5	level	1.2
			4.5	level	1.7
Zarandona et al.[104]	5	hands†	3.5	level	3.0
Soule and Goldman[101]	9	hands§	3.5	level	3.3
Schram and Hanson[109]	33	backpack	3.0	0	3.0
	44	backpack	3.0	0	4.5
Borysyk et al.[111]	1	hands§	3.0	0	1.2
	1	hands§	3.5	0	1.1
	3	hands§	3.0	0	1.7
	3	hands§	3.5	0	1.8

*Change in $\dot{V}O_2$ after the addition of weights.
†Exaggerated arm swing (to shoulder height) used.
‡Stride frequency was standardized at 120 strides/min.
§Weights held at sides or slight swing.
(Adapted from Graves, J. E., Martin, A. D., Miltenberger, L. A., and Pollock, M. L.: Physiological responses to walking with hand weights, wrist weights, and ankle weights. **Med. Sci. Sports Exerc.** 20:265–271, 1988.)

The proponents of exercising with hand-held weights list strengthening the upper body as an added benefit.[110] Although some strength benefit is certain, no documentation of this can be found.

In general, the use of weights while jogging-running or during high-impact aerobic dance is not recommended. The added weight increases the kinetic energy and impact forces on the lower extremities and spine and, thus, may cause more injury. Better documentation concerning injuries with the use of weights attached to the hands and wrists, back, or ankles and feet with various types of aerobic activity is needed.

Blood pressure responses resulting from use of hand-held weights are usually small, and thus, their general use is not contraindicated for most participants, including hypertensive patients.[105, 107, 108] More information concerning the hemodynamic responses of arm, hand grip, and leg exercise are covered in Chapter 6 for exercise testing and in Chapter 8 for exercise training of the cardiac or hypertense patient.

ARM TRAINING

In general, the principles of exercise prescription and the physiological benefits for leg training are similar for arm training or the combination of arm and leg training.[113, 114] Using the HRmax found during a treadmill GXT in prescribing arm training is not usually accurate. Both Sawka[113] and Franklin[114] found HRmax for arm testing as compared with leg testing to average 7 (96 percent) and 11 (94 percent) beats/min lower, respectively. Pollock and associates[115] found that after 20 weeks of arm training, this difference was reduced from 11 to 5 beats/min with their normal-bodied group. Maximal HR does not generally differ from treadmill HRmax when arm and leg exercise are combined.[114] Thus, the use of an HRmax determined from a treadmill GXT for exercise prescription on an arm ergometer usually overestimates the training HR.

When relative values are used based on data from each of the various GXT modes (arm, leg, or combination arm and leg ergometers), there appears to be little difference in percentage of HRmax reserve, $\dot{V}O_2$, or RPE.[50, 113, 114] Thus, if possible, it would be ideal to determine the HRmax on the ergometer or mode of testing that will be used for training. Once the HRmax from an arm GXT is determined, calculate the training HR. As mentioned previously, relative to arm testing, the training HR and RPE relationship is similar to that as determined by treadmill GXT, thus, RPE has the same meaning relative to the intensity of arm training.

Because the absolute workload or power output for arm training is significantly less than what can be used for leg training, what power output should be estimated for the initial training load? Franklin[114] has recommended a power output for arm training approximating 50 percent of the power output used for leg training. He gives the example that a subject using 300 kpm/min (50 W) for leg training would use 150 kpm/min (25 W) for arm training to get the same relative response (percentage of HRmax reserve and RPE). Figure 7–5 is from the data of Schwade, Blomqvist, and Shapiro[116] and shows the relationship of the rate-pressure product (RPP) and estimated myocardial oxygen consumption ($M\dot{V}O_2$) during arm and leg exercise. As can be seen in the table, the rise in HR and hemodynamic measures showed a twofold increase with increased power output for arm exercise as compared with leg exercise, i.e., the average RPP and $M\dot{V}O_2$ for arm exercise at 150 and 300 kpm/min were similar to that of leg exercise performed at 300 and 600 kpm/min. The data from Figure 7–5 support Franklin's recommendation for beginning arm training.

Maintenance Programs

Upon completion of the 6-week starter and 20-week training programs outlined in Tables 7–11 to 7–21, a substantial improve-

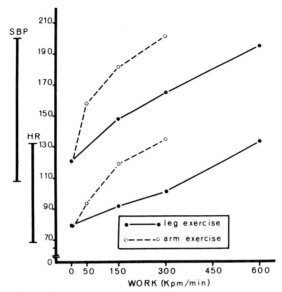

Figure 7–5. Mean heart rate-pressure product and estimated myocardial oxygen consumption (M$\dot{V}O_2$) during arm (broken line) and leg (solid line) exercise in patients with ischemic heart disease. (Data from Schwade, J., Blomqvist, C. G., and Shapiro, W.: **Am. Heart J.** 94:203–208, 1977. Figure from Franklin, B. A.: Exercise testing, training and arm ergometry. **Sports Med.** 2:100–119, 1985. Published with permission.)

ment in fitness should have been attained. To maintain fitness, a specific program should be designed that will be similar in caloric cost to the final program and that will also satisfy the needs of the participant over a long time span. For many, walking and jogging may become boring, and thus variety should be introduced into their programs. Participation in enjoyable activities is more likely to be continued.

The instructor should check over the list of activities in Table 7–6 to see which ones best meet the interests of the participants and can still give the necessary kilocalorie consumption. Fitness is not stored but must be practiced continually.[22, 27] The guidelines for frequency, intensity, and duration of training do not change and should be taken into consideration when selecting activities for participation.

If goals have not been met or if further development is required, then added caloric expenditure is needed. For example, since ideal (desired) weight may not be attained in a 20-week program, the program design should increase caloric output. Usually, added frequency of training of up to 5 or 6 days per week greatly increases the total energy expenditure. When adding frequency of training, consider low-impact activities first, otherwise the possibility for orthopedic injury will go up dramatically (see Table 7–8). The addition of one extra 400-kcal workout per week to the training regimen should remove a pound of fat every 9 weeks. If this is matched by a similar reduction in food intake, it will amount to a reduction of 12 pounds in a year.

PROGRAMS FOR MUSCULAR STRENGTH, MUSCULAR ENDURANCE, AND FLEXIBILITY

As described in Chapter 5, muscular strength and muscular endurance are developed by using the overload principle, i.e., by applying more tension on the muscle than is normally used.[56, 117–121] Muscular strength is best developed by using heavy weights (maximal or nearly maximal tension applied) with few repetitions, and muscular endurance is promoted by using lighter loads, with a greater number of repetitions.[117–123] To some extent, both strength and endurance can be developed under each condition, but each system favors a more specific type of development.[117–122]

Muscular strength and endurance can be developed by means of isometric, (static), isotonic, or isokinetic exercises (see Chapter 5 for definitions and further explanation). Although each type of training has its favorable and weak points, for healthy adults, isotonic resistance exercises are recommended for the development and maintenance of muscular strength and endurance. Resistance training for the average participant should be rhythmical, be performed at a moderate to slow speed, move through a full range of motion, and not impede normal forced breathing.

Although any magnitude of overload results in strength development, higher intensity effort at or near maximal effort gives a significantly greater effect.[117, 119, 121, 126, 127] Marcinik and colleagues[126] provide important information concerning intensity of strength training and subsequent improvement. With Navy recruits, one company (n = 41) trained by circuit weight training with two sets of 15 exercises at 70 percent of one-repetition maximum (1-RM), and another company (n = 46) trained by calisthenics. Both groups trained 3 days a week for 8 weeks, and their regimen included equal amounts of running. The circuit strength training group produced significantly greater improvements in both muscular strength and muscular endurance than did the calisthenic group. Similar results were found by Price and colleagues[24] Thus, because of its unique capability of adding intensity (weight), weight training is the superior method of increasing muscular strength and muscular endurance.

How much improvement in strength can be expected in resistance training programs? The question is difficult to answer because increases in strength related to training are affected by the participant's initial level of strength and potential for improvement.[119, 121, 128–130] For example, in one experiment, Mueller and Rohmert, as reported by deVries,[129] found increases in strength ranging from 2 to 9 percent per week, depending on initial strength levels.

Although the literature reflects a wide range of improvement in strength with resistance training programs, the average improvement for sedentary young and middle-aged men and women is 25 to 30 percent. Fleck and Kraemer,[121] in a review of 13 studies representing various forms of isotonic training, found an average improvement in bench press strength of 23.3 percent when subjects were tested on the equipment with which they were trained and 16.5 percent when tested on special isotonic or isokinetic ergometers (six studies). Fleck and Kraemer[121] also reported an average increase in leg strength of 26.6 percent when subjects were tested with the equipment with which the subjects were trained (six studies) and 21.2 percent when tested with special isotonic or isokinetic ergometers (five studies). Improvement in strength resulting from isometric training has been of the same magnitude as that found with isotonic training.[121, 124, 127, 131, 132]

When muscle groups can be properly evaluated and trained through a full range of motion, the percentage of improvement may vary greatly through the full range of motion, i.e., a greater percentage of improvement is found in the weaker portion of the range of motion.[135] Pollock and coworkers[135] have more recently reported that isolated lumbar extension strength improved 102 percent at the weakest part of the range of motion (extension) and 42 percent at its strongest point (full flexion). The magnitude of strength increase found in the lumbar extensor muscles reflected their low level of initial strength.

The principle of specificity of training is discussed in Chapter 5. Figure 5–9 shows the results of Group A, who trained the first half of the range of motion; group B, who trained the second half; group AB, who trained the full range of motion; and the control group, who did not train.[124] These results clearly show that the training result was specific to the range of motion trained, with group AB getting the best full range effect. These data are in agreement with Knapik and coworkers,[125] who observed a transfer effect of isometric strength of only 20 degrees from the specific angle trained. Thus, the need for full range of motion exercise is important for a full range effect.

Another advantage of the newer weight machines is their capability of limiting range of motion, i.e., much of the equipment can be double-pinned. This is particularly important in the elderly or in other participants who have joint problems (pain or weakness related to injury or joint disease, such as arthritis). Thus, these participants can be exercised in the part of the range of motion in which they do not experience pain or discomfort. As mentioned previously and in Chapter 5, limited range of motion exercise can still have some degree of full range effect.

In lieu of all the information reported previously, what is the resistance training program that is recommended for the average healthy adult? As mentioned in Table 7–2, the updated American College of Sports Medicine's position statement on the quantity and quality of exercise necessary for the healthy adult recommends a minimum of eight to ten exercises performed a minimum of twice a week. It is also recommended that one set of eight to twelve repetitions to fatigue is sufficient. These minimal standards for resistance training are based on two factors. First, as shown in Table 7–1, the time aspect should be considered when recommending a comprehensive, well-rounded exercise program. Second, although greater frequencies of training[118, 131, 131a] and additional sets or combinations of sets and repetitions elicit larger strength gains,[119, 121, 127, 128] the magnitude of difference is usually small. For example, Braith and associates[131] compared training 2 days per week with 3 days per week of variable resistance training for 18 weeks. The subjects performed one set of seven to ten repetitions to momentary fatigue (failure). The 2-day-per-week group showed a 21-percent increase in strength compared with a 28-percent increase in the 3-day-per-week group. In other words, 75 percent of what could be attained in a 3-day-per-week program was attained in 2 days per week. Also, the 21-percent improvement in strength found by the 2-day-per-week regimen is 70 to 80 percent of the improvement reported by other programs using additional frequencies of training and combinations of sets and repetitions.[121] In another example, Graves and associates,[124] Gettman, Ward, and Hagman,[136] Hurley and associates,[137] and Braith and associates[131] found that programs using one set to fatigue showed a greater than 25-percent increase in strength.

Thus, the sliding scale for the time components suggested for the muscular conditioning and aerobic phases of training (see Table 7–1) must be considered carefully when designing an exercise program. Certainly significant gains in strength and maintenance of strength in the major muscle groups of the body can be accomplished in 20 minutes, 2 days per week. The sliding scale shown in Table 7–1 suggests that if strength training is important for your everyday life or is a high-priority program, then a greater frequency and duration may be warranted.

Recommended Program for Developing and Maintaining Muscular Strength and Endurance

The main program recommended for the healthy adult requires the use of variable-resistance equipment. This would not have been recommended as part of the basic program 10 years ago and was not included in the first edition of this text (1984). Although calisthenics can provide enough overload to produce increases in strength and endurance in lesser fit participants, they are not as adaptable for progression and do not allow for higher levels of resistance that are necessary to attain optimal benefits. Exercise training equipment is now readily available. For the most part, compared with free weights, the newer equipment is safer to use, often protecting the lower back and forcing participants to use better form and technique. Balance and coordination are less of a problem with the machines, and some apparatus are designed to avoid hand gripping. As mentioned earlier, the hand grip can drive the blood pressure up dramatically.[123] The following basic program is recommended for most healthy adults.

Text continued on page 433

Recommended Resistance Training Program for Healthy Adults

1. LEG EXTENSION

Starting Position: Sit in machine. Place feet behind roller pad. Fasten seat belt across hips. Keep head and shoulders against seat back. Some people may need an extra back pad. Grasp handles lightly.

Movement: Straighten both legs smoothly. Pause in top position. Lower resistance slowly. Repeat.

Primary Muscle Used: Quadriceps.

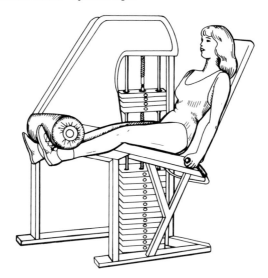

2. SIDE LEG CURL

Side Leg Curl: This machine was designed so that a participant can exercise the hamstrings and at the same time lessen compression forces on the lower back and abdomen.

Starting Position: Lie on left side facing weight stack. Slide lower legs between small roller pads. One pad should be on shins, the other on backs of ankles. Adjust large roller pad firmly against thighs. Place head in comfortable position on pad. Grasp handles lightly.

Movement: Curl legs and try to touch heels to buttocks. Pause in contracted position. Lower slowly. Repeat.

Primary Muscle Used: Hamstrings.

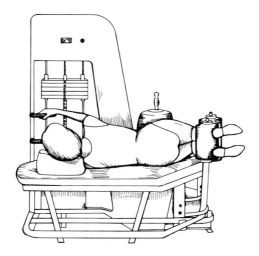

3. PULLOVER

Starting Position: Adjust seat so shoulder joints are in line with axes of cam. Assume erect position and fasten seat belt tightly. Leg press foot pedal until elbow pads are about chin level. Place elbows on pads. Hands should be open and resting on curved portion of bar.

Movement: Remove legs from pedal and slowly rotate elbows as far back as possible. Stretch. Rotate elbows down until bar touches midsection. Pause. Return slowly to stretched position. Repeat.

Primary Muscles Used: Latissimus dorsi and teres major.

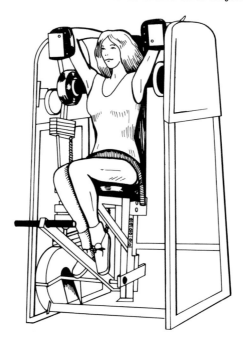

4. DUO DECLINE PRESS

Starting Position: Use foot pedal to raise handles into starting position. Grasp handles with parallel grip. Hand grips are adjustable, as is seat. Both should be adjusted to allow for greatest range of movement of weight stack. Fasten seat belt. Keep head back and torso erect.

Movement: Press bar forward in controlled fashion. Lower resistance slowly, keeping elbows wide. Stretch in bottom position then continue pressing movement. Repeat. Movement can also be performed one arm at a time or in an alternating fashion.

Primary Muscles Used: Pectoralis major, deltoids, and triceps.

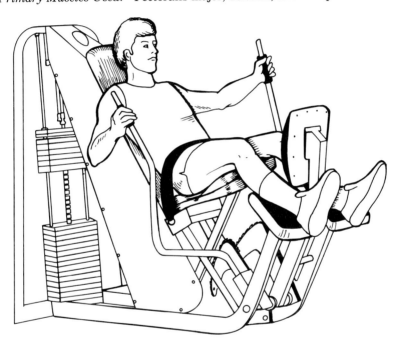

5. 10-DEGREE CHEST

Starting Position: Lie on back with head higher than hips. Adjust torso until shoulders are in line with axes of cams. Place upper arms under roller pads. Pads should be in crook of elbows.

Movement: Move both arms in rotary fashion until roller pads touch over chest. Pause. Lower slowly to starting position. Repeat.

Primary Muscle Used: Pectoralis major.

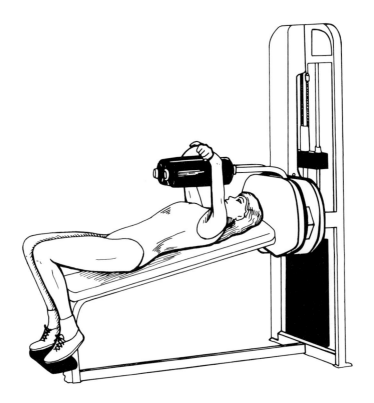

6. LATERAL RAISE

Starting Position: Adjust seat so shoulder joints are in line with axes of cams. Fasten seat belt. Grasp handles and pull back. Make sure elbows are slightly behind torso and firmly against pads.

Movement: Raise elbows smoothly until about chin level. Pause. Lower slowly to sides. Repeat.

Primary Muscle Used: Deltoids.

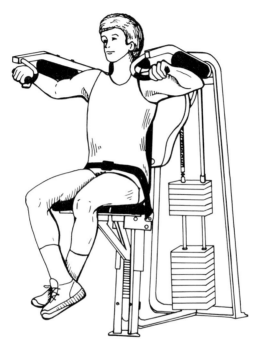

7. OVERHEAD PRESS

Starting Position: Adjust seat for greatest range of movement. Fasten seat belt. Grasp handles above shoulders.

Movement: Press handles overhead while being careful not to arch lower back. Lower resistance slowly, keeping elbows wide. Repeat.

Primary Muscles Used: Deltoids, triceps, and trapezius.

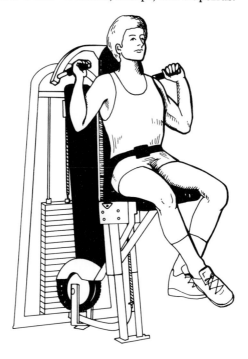

8. ROWING TORSO

Starting Position: Sit with back toward weight stack. Some individuals will need an extra pad in front. Place arms between roller pads and cross arms.

Movement: Bend arms in rowing fashion as far back as possible. Keep arms parallel to floor. Pause. Return slowly to starting position. Repeat.

Primary Muscles Used: Deltoid, rhomboid, and trapezius.

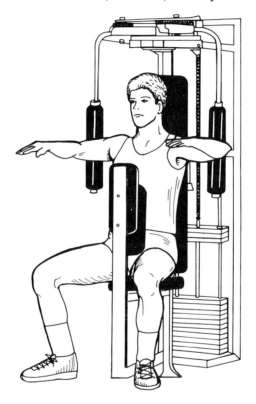

9. ABDOMINAL

Starting Position: Sit in machine with swivel pads in front of chest. Adjust seat until axis of rotation of movement arm is parallel to navel. Hook both feet under bottom roller pads. Adjust swivel pads on chest to comfortable position. Place hands over waist. Keep knees wide.

Movement: To isolate rectus abdominis muscles, keep the range of movement limited. Shorten the distance between the sternum and navel by moving forward and down. Pause in the contracted position. Return slowly to starting position. Repeat.

Primary Muscles Used: Rectus abdominis and iliopsoas.

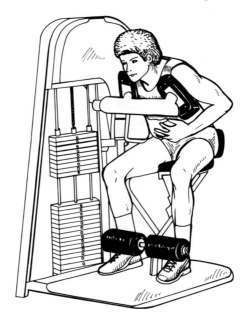

10. HIPS AND LOWER BACK

Starting Position: Enter machine from side by straddling seat. Sit on seat bottom, not angle between seat bottom and seat back. Upper back should be underneath highest roller pad. Stabilize lower body by moving thighs under bottom roller pads. Place feet firmly on platform. Fasten seat belt around hips. Interlace fingers across waist.

Movement: Move torso backward smoothly until in line with thighs. Pause in contracted position. Return slowly to starting position. Repeat.

Primary Muscles Used: Gluteal and hamstring muscles and to lesser extent the erector spinae group.

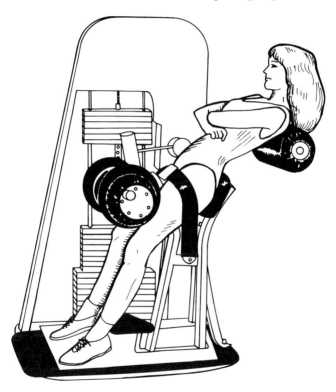

11. ROTARY TORSO

Starting Position: Face machine while standing. Weight stack should be in back and double-sided seat in front. Straddle seat on right side and cross ankles securely. Do not allow hips and legs to move with torso. Turn to right and place forearms on sides of pads. Right palm should be firmly against middle bar of movement arm.

Movement: Rotate torso from right to left by pushing with the right palm. Do not use triceps or biceps to push or pull the movement arm. Use torso rotators. Move head with torso by focusing between parallel bars of movement arm. Pause in contracted position. Rotation of torso will be less than 180 degrees. Return slowly to starting position and repeat. Straddle seat on other side of machine and reverse procedure for left-to-right torso rotation.

Primary Muscles Used: External and internal obliques.

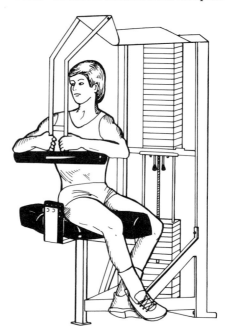

12. MULTI-BICEPS

Starting Position (both arms together): Place elbows on pad and in line with axes of cams. Adjust seat so shoulders are slightly lower than elbows. Grasp handles lightly.

Movement: Curl both handles to contracted position. Pause. Lower slowly to stretched position. Repeat.

Primary Muscles Used: Biceps.

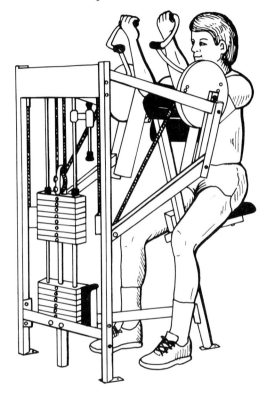

13. MULTI-TRICEPS

Starting Position (both arms together):	Adjust seat so shoulders are slightly lower than elbows. Place sides of hands on movement arms and elbows on pad in line with axes of cams.
Movement:	Straighten arms to contracted position. Pause. Lower slowly to stretched position. Repeat.
Primary Muscles Used:	Triceps.

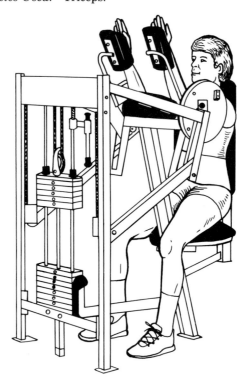

14 HIP ABDUCTION

Starting Position: Sit in machine and place legs on movement arms. Some people may require an extra back pad. Fasten seat belt. Keep head and shoulders against seat back.

Movement: Push knees and thighs laterally to widest position. Pause. Return to knee-together position. Repeat.

Primary Muscles Used: Gluteus medius and tensor fasciae latae.

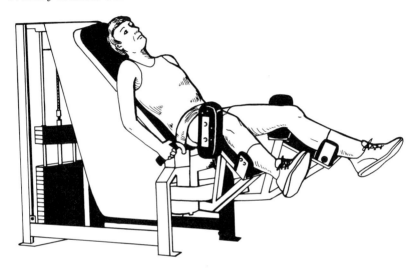

15. HIP ADDUCTION

Starting Position: Adjust lever on right side of machine for range of movement. Sit in machine and place knees and ankles on movement arms in a spread-legged position. The inner thighs and knees should be firmly against the resistance pads. Some people may need an extra back pad. Fasten seat belt. Keep head and shoulders against seat back.

Movement: Pull knees and thighs together smoothly. To isolate the adduction muscles better, keep the feet pointed inward and pull with the thighs, not the lower legs. Pause in the knee-together position. Return slowly to the stretched position. Repeat.

Primary Muscles Used: Adductor group.

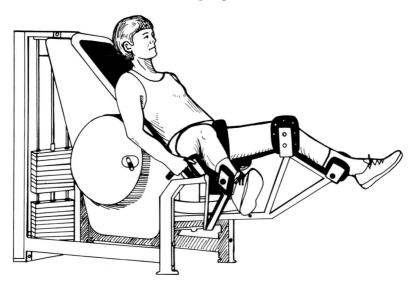

The variable resistance training program includes 15 exercises: four leg, three trunk, and eight arm and shoulder exercises. In the larger health clubs, other resistance machines are available. Also, other machines being developed and modifications of the current machines shown in exercises 1 to 15 are continually taking place; thus, the exercise specialist may choose to substitute exercises when appropriate. Ultimately, how many exercises a participant does will depend on the available time, equipment, needs and goals, and personal preference. Basic guidelines for particpating in a resistance training program as shown in exercises 1 to 15 have been described.[121, 127, 138, 139]

Frequency

The rationale for 2 or 3 days per week of training has already been mentioned. Most experts recommend a minimum of 48 hours of rest between bouts of heavy resistance exercise. If training 3 days per week, a Monday, Wednesday, and Friday or Tuesday, Thursday, and Saturday sequence works well. If training 2 days per week, a Monday or Tuesday and Thursday, Friday, or Saturday sequence is suggested. Some participants do not recover quickly from high-intensity resistance training. Thus, if recovery from resistance training is slow, less frequent training sessions may be appropriate. Once a participant gets to a certain level of strength development, will stopping for a few weeks or reducing training affect strength maintenance? Graves and associates[132] trained young men and women with bilateral knee extension exercise to volitional fatigue. Groups trained either 2 or 3 days per week for 10 or 18 weeks, followed by 12 weeks of reduced or no further training. As shown in Figure 7–6, when training was stopped, subjects lost 68 percent of their original strength gain in 12 weeks. As long as one quality training session was completed each week, training gains were maintained. Thus, periodic reduced or suspended training does not affect strength as long as one quality exercise session is performed per week. The main point here is do not stop training altogether.

Intensity

The ultimate goal for most participants is to complete eight to twelve repetitions to momentary fatigue. Usually, beginners will start with approximately 60 percent of 1-RM for the legs, 50 percent

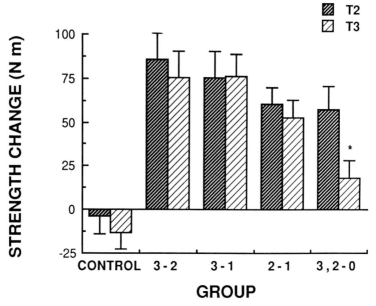

Figure 7–6. Absolute change in peak isometric strength of the knee extensors after training (T2) and 12 weeks of reduced training (T3). Groups training 3 days/wk reduced their training frequency to 2, 1, or 0 days/wk, and groups that trained 2 days/wk reduced to 1 or 0 days/wk. The control group never trained.

*p ≤ 0.01.

(Data from Graves, J. E., et al. Effects of reduced training frequency on muscular strength. **Int. J. Sports Med.** 9:316–319, 1988. Reprinted with permission.)

of 1-RM for the trunk, and 40 percent of 1-RM for the arms and shoulders. If a participant cannot complete a minimum of eight repetitions, then reduce the weight. If more than 12 repetitions can be attained, then add weight.

Duration

The time the participant has set aside for the muscular conditioning period dictates the number of exercises that can be performed during each session. By moving rapidly between exercise stations, ten to twelve exercises can be completed in 15 to 20 minutes. If training frequency is 3 days per week, then some exercises can be planned on alternate workout days. Although all four components of training (see Table 7–1) can be accomplished during each training session, performing the muscular conditioning and aerobic phases of training on different days may be less taxing and more enjoyable.

Progression

The initial weights that were suggested under intensity of training are only guestimates. If a participant is poorly fit, fragile, or elderly, starting at a lower weight may be advisable. Progression in training should also be more gradual with the poorly fit, fragile participant. To avoid undue muscle soreness, it is best to progress slowly for the first 2 to 4 weeks of training. Once the initial adaptation occurs, then going to fatigue (momentary failure) during each session at each exercise station should be the goal. When the participant can complete 12 repetitions of any exercise with good form, then add 5 percent to the training weight for the next session. Improvement usually comes quickly, 2 to 10 percent per week, depending on the participant's ability and initial level of strength. Training effects (exercise weight increases) begin to level off after the first 3 to 5 months, then, for many, the program will become one of maintenance.

Form

Good form is one of the most important aspects of training. Good form includes lifting the weight slowly and smoothly, with at least one good inspiration and expiration with each repetition. Dardin[138] and Wescott[127] recommend taking 2 seconds to raise the weight and 4 seconds to lower it. The slow movement through a full range of motion enhances good form and helps the participant avoid any jerking or throwing of the weight. The slower, smoother action helps avoid undue ballistic actions of the muscles and allows the muscle to be better trained through its full range.[140] Another important point is to have the participant exhale as the weight is lifted and inhale as it is lowered. This helps keep the glottis open during the more difficult part of the exercise and hopefully keeps intrathoracic pressures at a reasonable level.

Sequence

The order in which the previous exercises are listed is the sequence of training suggested by the authors. Obviously there are other acceptable sequences for training, but it is important to keep the order relatively constant from time to time. Fatigue develops as the participant goes through the sequence of exercise, thus, for comparative purposes (the progression and monitoring of training), the training weights used from day to day and the sequence of training should be consistent. As far as sequence of training is concerned, most experts recommend starting with the largest muscle groups first and then proceeding to the smallest. Also, many favor starting with the hip and legs first, then proceeding to the torso (shoulders) and arms, followed by the trunk (waist) and neck muscle groups.

Other Factors to Consider in Resistance Training

Record keeping is very important. Participants should use a card on which they can keep accurate records as to seat height or special machine adjustments, e.g., limiting range of motion, weight used, repetitions, RPE, and date. Records of body weight and anthropometric measures may also be included.

Whether participants complete their muscular conditioning program or aerobic program first or perform them on separate days is not important. No data suggest one sequence is better than the other. Mostly, this should be regulated by personal preference and available time. For comparative purposes though, the sequence should be kept consistent. For example, running 4 miles just before strength training reduces the amount of weight or repetitions that can be completed during resistance training and vice versa. Because of the sweating that occurs after running (aerobic phase), often it is more pleasant to be on the resistance machines first.

Lifting heavy weights can impede blood circulation and breathing, increasing blood pressure dramatically, which can be potentially dangerous for persons with high blood pressure, coronary heart disease, left ventricular dysfunction, and other circulatory problems.[100, 133, 134] In general, resistance training and maximal strength testing have been shown to be extremely safe for healthy adults, with no cardiovascular events and few injuries being reported.*

See Chapter 8 for more detailed information concerning the cardiovascular and hemodynamic responses to resistance exercise and its safety when used with cardiac patients.

---

*Pollock, M.L., and Graves, J.E., Center for Exercise Science, University of Florida, Gainesville, unpublished data, 1989; and Blair, S., Institute for Aerobics Research, Dallas, TX, personal communication, March 1988.

Because of the availability of weight training machines in most communities and their ease of adjustment and regulation of intensity (resistance), their use is generally recommended for almost all participants. How the resistance training program is applied differs among groups. Middle-aged and elderly participants use lighter weights initially and progress slower than younger or more athletic persons. Many individuals who are considered more fragile, e.g., elderly, hypertensives, or cardiac patients, generally train at a moderate intensity level.

Supplementary or Home Program Recommended for Developing and Maintaining Flexibility and Muscular Strength and Endurance

It has already been stated that the exercise prescription should include a balanced training program that comprises activities for the development and maintenance of muscular strength and endurance and of flexibility, as well as aerobic training.[1, 5, 82] It is felt that this type of training program best meets the interests and needs of the adult population.[82] As an adjunct or alternative to the previously described resistance training program, a series of stretching-calisthenic and weight training (free weights) exercises—to develop and maintain muscular strength, muscular endurance, and flexibility for most of the major muscle groups of the body—are outlined. If participants do not carry out a resistance training program as previously suggested, the following one can be used as an alternate or home program.

The stretching exercises should be included as part of the regular routine and can be incorporated into the warm-up or cooldown periods of the program. There may be some advantage to stretching at the end of the total workout (recovery phase) while the body is warm and more pliable. The muscular strength and endurance routine can be used either after the stretching routine or after the aerobic phase. Before beginning the aforementioned routines, the participants should be familiar with the described starting position, movement, and suggested repetitions. The training load has been designed to give the participant a moderate amount of muscular strength and endurance.

The exercise routines are divided into the following two categories: first, flexibility exercises (1 to 11), which include upper body, trunk, and lower back stretching (1 to 6), and hip and leg stretching (7 to 11); and second, muscular strength and endurance exercises (12 to 21). Many of the exercises have several options. In the first category (stretching exercises), some of the alternate exercises are more advanced and should be used only after the initial starter exercise has been mastered. The muscular strength and endurance exercises offer options depending on the availability of weight training equipment (free weights). Many of the calisthenic exercises for muscular strength and endurance have options that should be substituted if the participant is too weak to perform the first exercise (e.g., 14bii, negative pull-up; 15aii, modified sit-up; or 17bii, modified push-up).

In general, the same principles of exercise outlined and discussed for resistance training also hold true for the calisthenic and free-weight exercises. Good form, slow movements, rhythmical breathing, proper progression, and factors associated with frequency, intensity, and duration of training are the same. If more options or specific stretching exercises are required for the participant, see Anderson's book on stretching.[20] For the more serious weight trainer or lifter, the texts by Westcott,[127] Fleck and Kraemer,[121] Riley,[139] Darden,[138] Berger,[118] and Wilmore and Costill[119] are recommended.

Text continued on page 472

Flexibility Exercises: Upper Body, Trunk, and Lower Back Stretching Exercises*

1. TRUNK ROTATION

Purpose:	To stretch muscles of back, sides, and shoulder girdle.
Starting Position:	Stand astride with feet pointed forward; raise arms to shoulder level. May use bar over shoulders to increase stretch to deltoid and waist muscles.
Movement:	Twist trunk to right; avoid lifting heels. Repeat 3 to 4 times before twisting to left side.
Repetitions:	10

---

*(Reprinted with permission from Pollock, M.L., Wilmore, J.H., and Fox, S.M.: **Health and Fitness Through Physical Activity.** New York, copyright © John Wiley and Sons, 1978.)

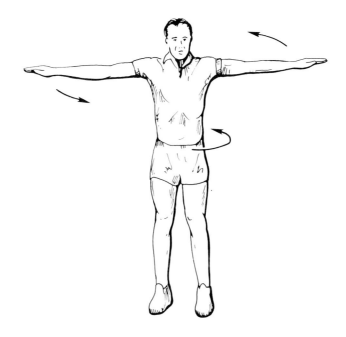

2a. DOUBLE ARM CIRCLES AND TOE RAISES

Purpose: To stretch muscles of shoulder girdle and to strengthen muscles of foot, ankle, and calf.

Starting Position: Stand with feet about 12 inches apart and arms at side.

Movement: Swing arms upward and around, making large circles. As arms are raised and crossed overhead, rise on toes. Do one half of arm circles swinging arms forward and one half by swinging them to rear.

Repetitions: 10 to 15

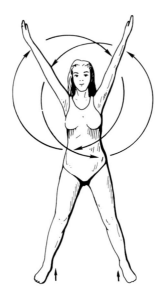

2b. SHOULDER STRETCH

Purpose: To stretch muscles of shoulder girdle.

Starting Position: Stand facing bars. Reach up and forward, grasping bar, with hands facing outward. Knees should be bent slightly.

Movement: Slowly lean forward letting chest and head hang forward (down); maintain tension on muscles for 30 to 60 seconds.

Repetitions: 1 to 2

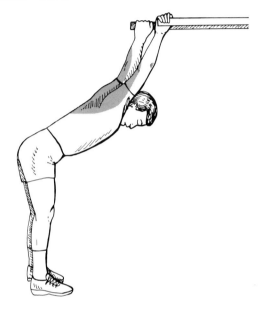

3a. FORWARD BEND

Purpose:	To stretch muscles of buttocks and posterior leg.
Starting Position:	Stand astride with hands on hips.
Movement:	Slowly bend forward to 90-degree angle; return slowly to starting position; keep back flat.
Repetitions:	10

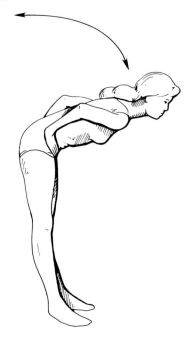

3b. ABDOMINAL CHURN

Purpose:	To stretch muscles of buttocks, abdomen, and posterior leg.
Starting Position:	Stand astride with hands on hips.
Movement:	Lower trunk sideward to left; rotate to forward position and to right; return to upright position. Repeat and reverse direction after two rotations.
Repetitions:	10

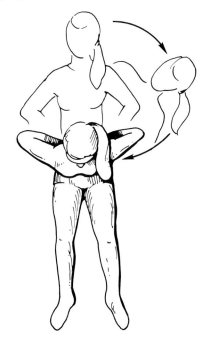

3c. BAR HANG

Purpose: To stretch muscles of arms, shoulders, back, trunk, hips, and pelvic regions. Good general body stretcher.

Starting Position: Hang from bar with arms straight.

Repetitions: 10 for up to 60 seconds

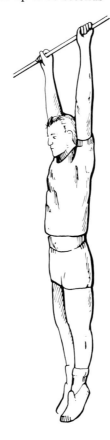

4. SHOULDER AND CHEST STRETCH

Purpose:	To stretch muscles of chest and shoulders.
Starting Position:	Stand astride or kneel with arms at shoulder level and elbows bent.
Movement:	Slowly force elbows backward and return to starting position.
Repetitions:	10 to 15

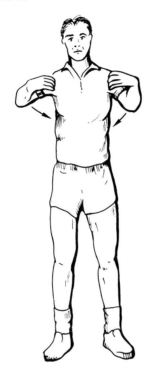

5a. LOWER BACK STRETCH

Purpose:	To stretch muscles of lower back.
Starting Position:	Crouch on hands and knees, with hands extended forward, palms face down and touching floor.
Movement:	Slowly rock back until buttocks touch heels; emphasize rounding back; return to starting position.
Repetitions:	10

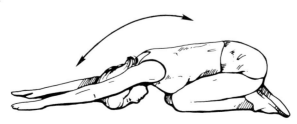

5b. ALTERNATE LOWER BACK STRETCH

Purpose:	To stretch muscles in lower back and buttocks.
Starting Position:	Lie on back with legs extended, or stand erect.
Movement:	Lift and bend one leg; grasp knee and keep opposite leg flat; pull knee to chest. Repeat with alternate leg.
Repetitions:	10

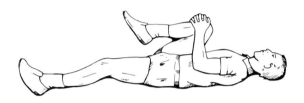

5c. ADVANCED LOWER BACK AND HAMSTRING STRETCH

Purpose:	To stretch muscles of lower back and hamstring muscles.
Starting Position:	Lie on back with legs bent.
Movement:	Keep knees together and slowly bring them over the head; straighten legs and touch the toes to floor; hold for 2 counts; return to starting position.
Repetitions:	5 to 10

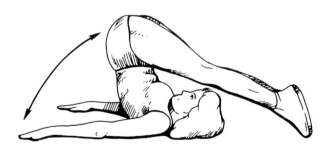

6. INVERTED STRETCH

Purpose:	To stretch and strengthen anterior hip, buttocks, and abdominal muscles.
Starting Position:	Sit with arms at side.
Movement:	Support body with heels and arms and raise trunk as high as possible.
Repetitions:	10

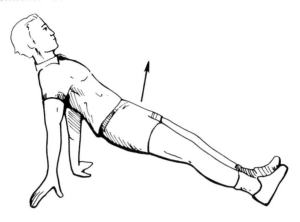

7a. FRONT LEG STRETCH

Purpose:	To stretch muscles in anterior thigh and leg. Persons with knee problems should avoid this exercise.
Starting Position:	Kneel with tops of ankles and feet flat on ground.
Movement:	Lean backward slowly; keep back straight; maintain tension on muscles for 30 to 60 seconds.
Repetitions:	1 to 2

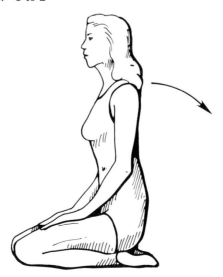

7b. FRONT LEG STRETCH

Purpose:	To stretch muscles of the anterior thigh and leg. Persons with knee problems should avoid this exercise.
Starting Position:	Kneel with feet turned outward.
Movement:	Lean backward slowly; put constant tension on muscles; use arms to control movement; hold backward position for 30 to 60 seconds.
Repetitions:	1 to 2

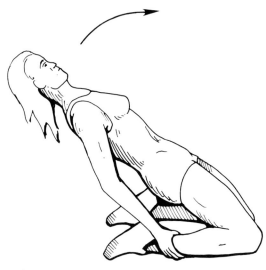

7c. ADVANCED FRONT LEG STRETCH

Purpose:	To stretch muscles of anterior thigh and hip.
Starting Position:	Lie on ground with face down, or stand erect.
Movement:	Pull ankle to hip slowly; hold for 20 to 30 seconds and release the ankle. Use same procedure for other side.
Note:	If difficulty is encountered in assuming starting position, ask for assistance.
Repetitions:	1 to 2

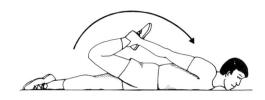

8. SIDE STRETCH

Purpose:	To stretch medial muscles of thigh and lateral muscles of trunk and thorax.
Starting Position:	Stand erect, with one arm extended upward and other relaxed at side; place feet apart at more than shoulder width.
Movement:	Bend trunk directly to right, with left arm stretching overhead; keep both feet flat. Use same procedure for other side.
Repetitions:	5 to 10

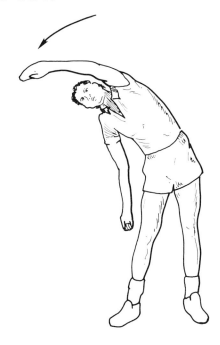

9. GROIN STRETCH

Purpose:	To stretch groin muscles.
Starting Position:	Sit with knees bent outward and bottoms of feet together.
Movement:	Grasp ankles and pull upper body as close as possible to feet. Hold stretch for 30 to 60 seconds.
Repetitions:	1 to 2

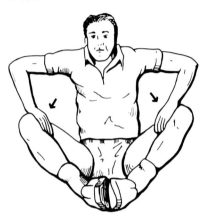

10a. HAMSTRING STRETCH, BEGINNER

Purpose:	To stretch muscles in the posterior leg and thigh.
Starting Position:	Sit on ground with one leg extended straight forward; place other leg forward, with knee bent and sole touching inner thigh of extended leg.
Movement:	Bend forward and attempt to touch head to knee; hold stretch for 30 to 60 seconds. Repeat with other leg.
Repetitions:	1 to 2

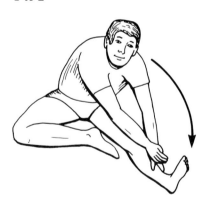

10b. HAMSTRING STRETCH, ADVANCED

Purpose:	To stretch muscles in posterior leg and thigh.
Starting Position:	Sit on ground with one leg extended straight forward; place other leg backward as in hurdler's position. Persons with knee problems should not attempt this exercise.
Movement:	Bend forward and attempt to touch head to knee; hold stretch for 30 to 60 seconds. Repeat with other leg.
Repetitions:	1 to 2

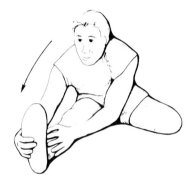

11a. CALF STRETCHER

Purpose: To stretch posterior leg and ankle muscles.

Starting Position: Stand in forward stride position with forward knee partially flexed and rear leg fully extended; keep feet pointed forward or pointed inward and heels flat on ground.

Movement: Lean trunk forward until a continuous stretch occurs in rear calf; hold stretch for 30 to 60 seconds. Repeat with other leg. To better stretch lower portion of calf muscle (soleus), repeat same movement with rear leg bent at knee.

Repetitions: 1 to 2

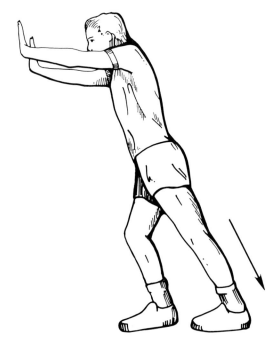

11b. CALF STRETCHER

Purpose:	To stretch posterior leg muscles.
Starting Position:	Stand in upright position with balls of feet on edge of a step.
Movement:	Slowly lower heels and hold for 30 to 60 seconds. To train calf muscles, simply raise heels and rise on toes.
Repetitions:	1 to 2 for stretching, 10 to 15 for toe raises

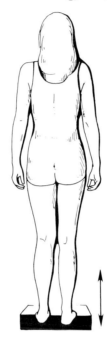

Muscular Strength and Endurance Exercises

Two options are illustrated for most of the following routines. The first option (a) utilizes weights; the second (b) stresses the same muscle group, but without utilizing weights.

12a. WEIGHT TRAINING WARM-UP

Purpose:	To utilize all major muscle groups in warm-up routine before concentrating on specific muscle groups.
Starting Position:	Place feet astride; bend knees; keep back straight; hold bar with overhand grip, hands approximately shoulder width apart (Position A).
Movement:	Straighten legs with back still straight; raise elbows to shoulder height or higher (Position B); lower elbows next to trunk and keep weight at chest level; press weight over head and fully extend arms (Position C); return weight to floor.
Repetitions:	8 to 12

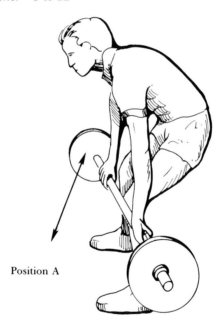

Position A

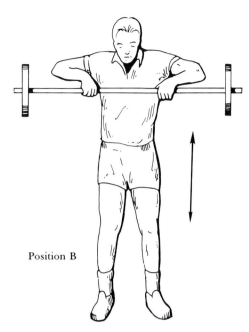

Position B

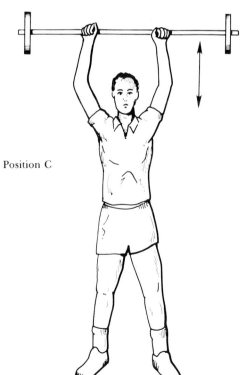

Position C

12b. JUMPING JACKS

Purpose:	To utilize all major muscle groups in warm-up routine before concentrating on specific muscle groups.
Starting Position:	Stand erect, with feet together and arms at side.
Movement:	Swing arms upward until over head and spread feet apart in one movement; in second movement, return to starting position.
Repetitions:	10 to 20

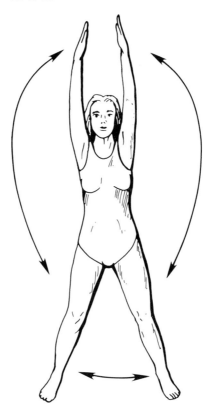

13. MILITARY PRESS

Purpose:	To strengthen shoulder, upper back, and arm muscles.
Starting Position:	Support weight at shoulder level with overhand grip.
Movement:	Push weight directly over head; keep back and knees straight; return weight slowly to starting position.
Repetitions:	8 to 12

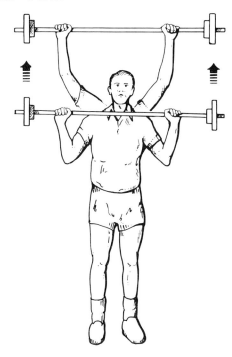

14a. CURL

Purpose:	To strengthen anterior arm muscles (biceps).
Starting Position:	Hold weight with palms-up grip; keep arms straight.
Movement:	Bend arms and bring weight up to chest; return slowly.
Repetitions:	8 to 12

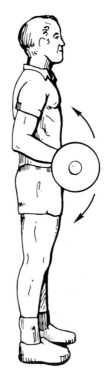

14bi. PULL-UP

Purpose:	To strengthen anterior arm, upper back, and shoulder muscles.
Starting Position:	Place hands about 18 inches apart on overhead bar with either palms-in or palms-out grip; keep arms straight in order to support body.
Movement:	Pull body up so chin comes above bar; slowly lower body to starting position.
Repetitions:	Progress to 10 to 15

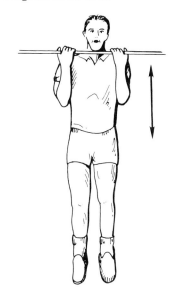

14bii. NEGATIVE PULL-UP

Purpose:	To strengthen anterior arm, upper back, and shoulder muscles.
Starting Position:	Use stool to raise body up so that chin is above bar. Use same hand position as in exercise 14bi.
Movement:	Slowly lower body until arms are straight.
Note:	This exercise is substituted for 14bi when participant cannot complete 1 pull-up.
Repetitions:	5 to 10

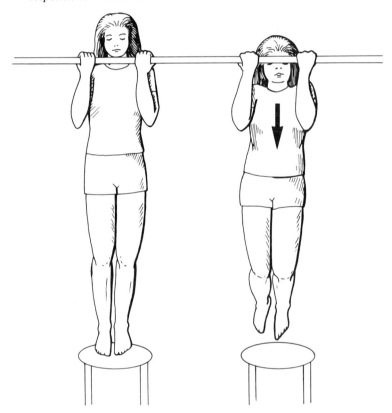

15ai. SIT-UP

Purpose:	To strengthen abdominal and hip flexor muscles.
Starting Position:	Lie on back with knees bent and hands clasped behind neck or holding weight on chest.
Movement:	Raise head and trunk to upright position; hold position for one count; slowly return to starting position. Emphasize roll-up type movement.
Repetitions:	15 to 20

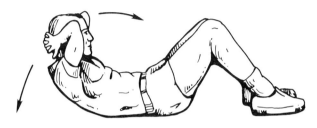

15aii. MODIFIED SIT-UP

Purpose:	To strengthen abdominal and hip flexor muscles.
Starting Position:	Lie on back with knees bent and hands resting on chest.
Movement:	Curl-up; bring shoulder blades off floor approximately 30 degrees. Hold for 1 count and slowly lower back down to starting position.
Repetitions:	10 to 20

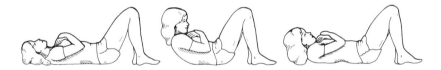

15b. LEG PULL-UP

Purpose:	To strengthen abdominal and hip flexor muscles.
Starting Position:	Hang from bar with body straight.
Movement:	Bend knees slowly; bring knees to chest; return slowly to starting position.
Repetitions:	Progress to 10 to 15

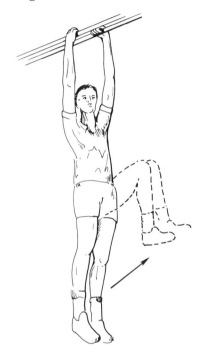

16a. BENT-OVER ROWING

Purpose:	To strengthen middle to upper back and posterior arm muscles.
Starting Position:	Stand with feet apart slightly more than shoulder width; bend forward at waist, with back straight and legs slightly bent; keep arms straight to support weight.
Movement:	Raise weight to chest and return it slowly to starting position.
Repetitions:	8 to 12

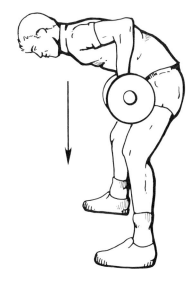

16b. PULL-UP, WIDE GRIP

Purpose:	To strengthen middle to upper back and anterior arm muscles.
Starting Position:	Place hands about 24 inches apart on overhead bar, with either palms-in or palms-out grip; hang from bar, with arms straight to support body.
Movement:	Pull body up so chin comes above bar; slowly lower body to starting position.
Repetitions:	Progress to 10 to 15

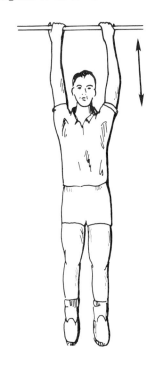

17a. SUPINE PRESS (BENCH PRESS)

Purpose:	To strengthen chest, anterior shoulder, and posterior arm muscles.
Starting Position:	Lie on back on bench 10 to 14 inches wide; use overhand grip on weight supported on standards held by two assistants; keep arms straight.
Movement:	Slowly lower weight to touch chest; raise weight until arms are straight.
Repetitions:	8 to 12

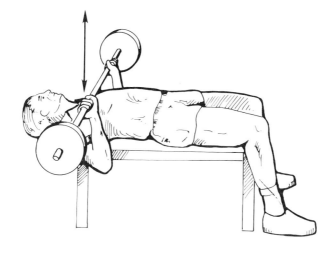

17bi. PUSH-UPS

Purpose: To strengthen chest, anterior shoulder, and posterior arm muscles.

Starting Position: Lie on stomach with hands flat on floor and positioned shoulder width apart.

Movement: Push entire body except feet and hands off the floor until arms are straight; lower body until chest touches floor.

Note: Positioning hands beyond shoulders or putting blocks beneath hands increases stretch and overload of pectoral muscles. See diagram of variation in hand placement below.

Repetitions: Progress to 20 to 30

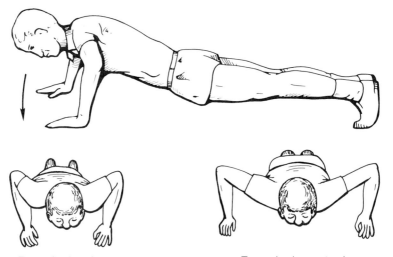

To emphasize triceps   To emphasize pectorals

17bii. MODIFIED KNEE PUSH-UPS

Purpose:	To strengthen chest, anterior shoulder, and posterior arm muscles.
Starting Position:	Lie on stomach, supporting weight with hands and knees. Hand position can be varied as described for push-up (17bi).
Movement:	Movement is the same as for push-up, except only hands and knees touch floor in up position.
Note:	Knee push-up is substituted for regular push-up when person has back problems or is too weak to do regular push-ups.
Repetitions:	Progress to 10 to 20

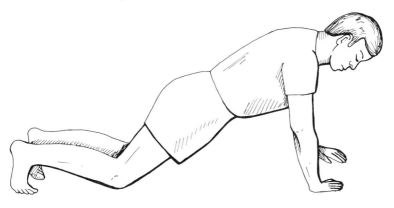

18a. DIPS

Purpose:	To strengthen triceps and anterior deltoid muscles.
Starting Position:	Arms extended fully on dip or parallel bars.
Movement:	Lower body until elbows are at 90 degree angles. Extend arms, returning to the starting position.
Repetitions:	Progress to 8 to 15

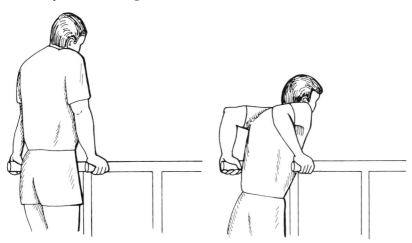

18b. SEAT DROP

Purpose:	To strengthen triceps and deltoid muscles.
Starting Position:	Use sturdy chair. Hands rest on top of chair, arms fully extended. Legs are extended forward with weight resting on heels.
Movement:	Lower body until elbows are at 90-degree angle or when buttocks touch floor. Extend arms, returning to original position.
Repetitions:	8 to 12

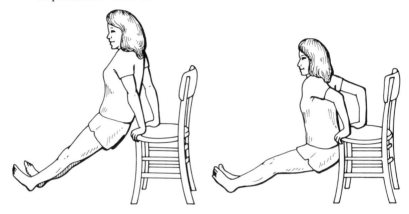

19a. BACK EXTENSION

Purpose:	To strengthen lower back muscles.
Starting Position:	Lie on bench with face down; extend body from above waist over edge of bench; strap or hold feet to other end of bench.
Movement:	Lift head and trunk; slowly lower head and trunk.
Note:	Hyperextend only slightly.
Repetitions:	Progress to 10 to 15

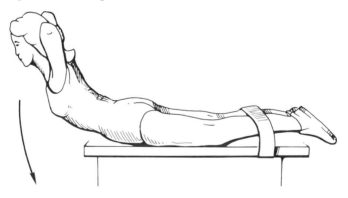

19b. BACK TIGHTENER

Purpose:	To strengthen lower back muscles.
Starting Position:	Lie on floor with face down; fold hands over lower back area.
Movement:	Raise head and chest and tense gluteal and lower back muscles.
Caution:	Hyperextend only slightly; just raise head and chest slightly off floor; concentrate mainly on tensing gluteal muscles.
Repetitions:	10 to 15

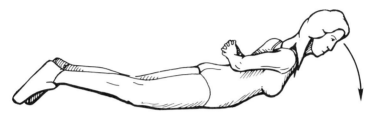

20. SQUAT

Purpose:	To strengthen anterior thigh and buttock muscles.
Starting Position:	Stand erect, with feet astride and support weight on shoulders with palms-up grip.
Movement:	Keep back straight and bend knees into squat position; return to standing position.
Note:	Do half squat if knees are weak.
Repetitions:	8 to 12

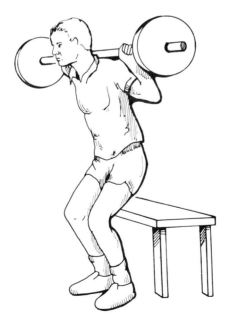

21a. HEEL RAISES (WITH WEIGHTS)

Purpose:	To strengthen calf muscles.
Starting Position:	Place feet astride and hold weight on shoulders with palms-up grip.
Movement:	Raise to toe position; lower body.
Note:	Board may be placed under toes to increase range of motion.
Repetitions:	8 to 12

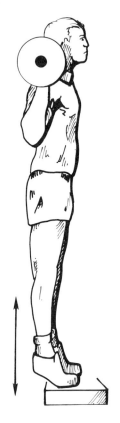

21b. HEEL RAISES

Purpose:	To strengthen calf muscles.
Starting Position:	Place feet astride and use arms for balance if necessary.
Movement:	Raise to toe position; lower body.
Note:	Board may be placed under toes to increase range of motion.
Repetitions:	10 to 15

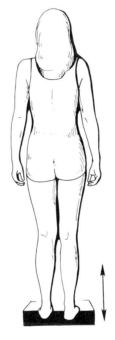

Exercise for the Lower Back

Lower back pain is one of the most common and costly medical problems in industrialized society. It has been estimated that eight of ten people will experience lower back pain sometime in their lives.[141] Melleby[142] stated that approximately 80 percent of all lumbar problems are muscular in origin, and patients suffering from chronic lower back pain are often found to have weak lumbar strength.[142–144] The use of various combinations of flexibility and strength exercise has been successful in relieving pain and symptoms of lower back problems in many whose problem is associated with muscular weakness and lack of flexibility.[145]

What exercises should be included in a back routine? First of all, if serious organic problems are suspected, the participant should get medical clearance before starting a regimen. Lower back problems are usually precipitated by an imbalance of strength and flexibility of the lower back and abdominal areas, lifting or bending from an improper position, or just plain overdoing it. Also, participants with predominantly fast twitch fibers may be unusually strong but fatigue rapidly and, thus, become vulnerable to injury in certain industrial task situations when repetitive lifting is required.[147] For more information on the cause and diagnosis of lower back problems and functional restoration for spinal disorders, see the text by Mayer and Gatchel.[148]

The following weaknesses and imbalances are often present in patients who present with lower back problems: tight hamstring and lower back muscle groups, tight hip flexor muscles, and weak abdominal and lower back muscles. Many times, these persons are generally deconditioned and overweight. Exercises that emphasize these special areas of concern include 5a, b, or c; 7a, b, or c; 10a or b, 15ai or ii; and 19a or b. The *Y's Way to a Healthy Back*[142] and the text by Mayer and Gatchel[148] are excellent resource books and describe an extensive and progressive lower back routine.

Jackson and Brown[149] have questioned the effectiveness of these various programs to benefit patients with lower back pain. The authors are particularly critical of flexion exercises as described by Williams.[150] Strengthening of abdominal muscles and in particular the oblique muscles seems important for most patients, but the flexion program in general does not meet this need. The authors emphasize the importance of aerobic exercise and lumbar extension strength. The importance of aerobic activity is related to the study of Cady and associates,[151] who found that general aerobic conditioning relieved back pain of fire-fighters. These results may be deceptive in that the fire-fighters who were in better shape were less fat (overweight) and probably in better general condition than their sedentary counterparts. Although general aerobic fitness may be a factor in combating low back pain, high-impact activities such as running, aerobic dance, and basketball, which put high compression forces on the spine, may precipitate or aggravate back problems and should be avoided.

Jackson and Brown[149] emphasize the importance of the lumbar extensor muscles and list the following rationale for their use:

1. **The spine is able to withstand greater axial compression when the normal physiological curves are maintained.**

2. **Extension unloads the disc and allows fluid influx: the disc needs low pressure to imbibe low molecular weight substances for proper nutrition.**

3. **A strong correlation exists between back muscle strength and maximal lifting loads.**

4. **Patients with chronic back pain demonstrate a significant loss of back extensor strength as compared with normal subjects.**

5. **EMG studies have demonstrated decreased extensor endurance during postural activities in patients with lower back pain.**

6. **Prolonged flexion postures are frequently associated with the onset of back pain.**

7. **In subjects who do not have back problems, trunk extensor strength exceeds flexor strength, and this normal balance should be restored.**

8. **Strong back extensors reach fatigue more slowly and are protective of the spinal ligaments in light and unloaded flexion activities.**

9. **Half of the total extensor movement is produced by the erector spinae.**

They go on to explain that the primary functions of the lumbar extensor muscles are for postural holding and eccentric control of trunk flexion; thus, it is important that these muscles are exercised regularly.

Unfortunately, until recently, technology has not allowed programs to isolate the lumbar extensor muscles so that they could be accurately evaluated or trained. Quantification of lumbar extension strength is often complicated by the involvement of the stronger gluteal and hamstring muscles. Mayer and Greenberg[152] noted that lumbar-pelvic rhythm (rotation) during lumbar testing contributed to the lumbar extension strength measure. Smidt and associates[153]

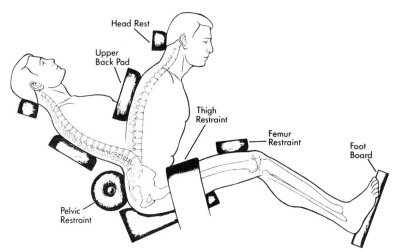

Figure 7–7. The figure shows the various restraints and pads used for pelvic stabilization and positional standardization during lumbar extension strength testing (MedX™). (From Pollock, M. L., and Graves, J. E.: New approach to low back evaluation and training. **Central Florida Phys.** 5:19–20, 1989. Reprinted with permission.)

have demonstrated the importance of stabilizing the pelvis and lower extremities to isolate the lumbar muscles during testing. Thus, effective assessment and training of the lumbar muscles require stabilization of the pelvis to isolate the lumbar extensor muscles and minimize the contribution of the hip and leg muscles. In addition, standardization of the testing and training position, correction for the influence of gravitational forces (body weight) during testing and training, and full range of motion measurement are required for accurate quantification of lumbar extension strength.[135, 147, 154] Figure 7–7 shows the schematic illustration of how a subject is secured into position for proper pelvic stabilization (MedX™ lumbar extension machine, Ocala, FL).[154a] The footboard is adjustable and pushes the femurs back into the pelvis, which is resting against the lumbar restraint pad. The femur and thigh restraints are tightened to prevent any vertical movement of the thighs or pelvis. With the thigh restraint acting as a fulcrum as the femurs are pushed up and back, the pelvis is forced back and against a specially designed lumbar pad (pelvic restraint). In this manner, the femurs are used to anchor the pelvis against the pelvic restraint for stabilization. After the subject is counterweighted to neutralize the effect of body weight, the test begins. Patients are tested isometrically through a full range of motion at 72 (full flexion), 60, 48, 36, 24, 12, and 0 degrees (full extension) of trunk flexion. The accuracy of the testing machine is extremely good, with test-retest reliability coefficients mostly above r = 0.9 and standard errors of the measures in the 5 to 10 percent range.[154] These errors of measure should be considered extremely good since Wakim and colleagues[155] showed a 5- to 10-percent day-to-day strength variation (human variation) in both men and women.

Using the new lumbar extension machine, Pollock and colleagues[135] trained 15 subjects one day a week for 10 weeks. A control group of ten subjects did not train. The unique finding of this study was the magnitude of full range of motion training responses of the isolated lumbar extensor muscles (Fig. 7–8). This increase in lumbar extension strength was particularly evident in the more extended positions, improvement in strength ranging from 102 percent (0-degree flexion) to 42 percent (72-degree flexion). The isometric strength gain in the lumbar extensor muscles in this study was greater than what has been reported in the literature for other muscle groups.

It has been demonstrated that participants who are untrained or who have a low strength level in respect to their potential to

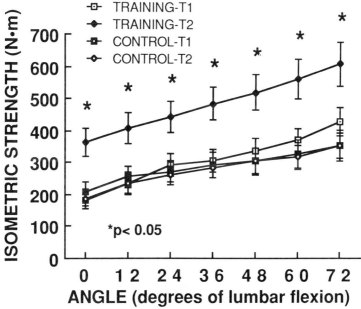

Figure 7–8. Torque (N • m) measurements for isometric strength of the lumbar extensor muscles at 0°, 12°, 24°, 36°, 48°, 60°, and 72° of lumbar flexion. T_1 and T_2 show measurements before and after 10 weeks of training, respectively. Data represent means ± SEM. (Data from Pollock, M. L., et al. Effect of resistance training on lumbar extension strength. **Am. J. Sports Med.** in press. Reprinted with permission.)

develop strength have a greater capacity to acquire strength than those who are highly trained or who are already close to their maximal potential to develop strength.[128, 130] deVries[129] and Fleck and Kraemer,[121] in recent reviews of exercise prescription for resistance training, alluded to the importance of this concept when evaluating the effectiveness of resistance training programs. Normally, it is expected that moderate to highly trained individuals will show little to no further change in strength with additional training. Subjects in the Pollock and colleagues[135] investigation were well trained and had been participating in exercise programs for a minimum of a year. Most importantly, ten of the fifteen subjects in the training group had been exercising on the Nautilus™ lower back machine on a regular basis. Thus, if the lower back extensor muscles were being adequately trained in these subjects initially, significant gains in strength would not have been expected.

The results of this study, however, identified unusually large increases in isometric lumbar extension strength and particularly in the more extended positions. Dynamic training weights also increased to a great extent (60.6 percent). How can these large gains in lumbar extension strength be explained? The most reasonable explanation is that lumbar extensor muscle strength is not normally developed or maintained with existing exercise methods. As mentioned earlier, without proper stabilization of the pelvis, the larger and stronger thigh (mainly hamstring) and gluteal muscles do most of the exercise in back extension.[147, 153, 154] This situation may be equivalent to a muscle that has been placed into a cast; it is in a state of chronic disuse, atrophies quickly, and loses its size and strength.[156–158] Thus, the lumbar extensor muscles never develop to their fullest potential and become atrophied from chronic disuse. This explains why the isolated lumbar extensor muscles have so much potential for strength development.

It is still to be determined how effective this new evaluation and training device will be in preventing and treating lower back problems. But if improving lumbar strength is an important factor in the prevention and treatment of lower back pain, then the new machine should show dramatic results.

SUMMARY

General guidelines for exercise prescription have been discussed. The exercise prescription is based upon the results from the participant's medical screening, fitness assessment, or both. A specially individualized exercise prescription based on the participant's need, interest, and physical health status has been proposed. Special recommendations concerning frequency, intensity, and duration of training have been given for beginners and advanced exercisers. Individualized 6-week starter programs and 20-week training programs for walking and jogging have also been outlined.

The total energy cost of the exercise program is the important factor in exercise prescription, and the fact that kilocalories can be expended through a variety of physical activities has been emphasized. Thus, participants should choose an activity or activities that they enjoy. The notion that exercise should be done on a regular basis has been discussed. The need for a balanced, well-rounded program has been stressed; i.e., the training regimen should include exercises for the development of muscular strength, muscular endurance, and flexibility, as well as aerobic capacity. The chapter includes special sections on the use of the rating of perceived exertion scale for monitoring training intensity, walking as an exercise program, the use of hand-held weights in exercise training, arm training, exercise for the elderly, and exercise for the lower back.

Special exercises that can be used for developing and maintaining muscular strength and endurance and flexibility were described. The exercises have been categorized in terms of the specific areas of the body that they affect and have been grouped in order of complexity. Both calisthenic exercises that need no special equipment and weight-training exercises are listed.

References

1. Cureton, T.K.: **The Physiological Effects of Exercise Programs Upon Adults.** Springfield, IL, Charles C Thomas, 1969.
2. Cooper, K.H.: **The New Aerobics.** New York, J.B. Lippincott, 1970.
3. Wilmore, J.: Individual exercise prescription. **Am. J. Cardiol.** 33:757–759, 1974.
4. Balke, B.: Prescribing physical activity. In Larson, L. (ed.): **Sports Medicine.** New York, Academic Press, 1974, pp. 505–523.
5. Pollock, M.L., Wilmore, J.H., and Fox, S.M.: **Health and Fitness Through Physical Activity.** New York, John Wiley and Sons, 1978.
6. Ragorta, M., Crabtree, J., Starner, W.Q., and Thompson, P.D.: Death during recreational exercise in the state of Rhode Island. **Med. Sci. Sports Exerc.** 16:339–342, 1984.
7. Waller, B.F.: Sudden death in middle-aged conditioned subjects: coronary atherosclerosis is the culprit. **Mayo Clin. Proc.** 62:634–636, 1987.
8. Opie, L.H.: Sudden death and sport. **Lancet** 1:263–266, 1975.
9. Gibbons, L.W., Cooper, K.H., Meyer, B.M., and Ellison, R.C.: The acute cardiac risk of strenuous exercise. **JAMA** 244:1799–1801, 1980.
10. Thompson, P.D., Funk, E.J., Carleton, R.A., and Sturner, W.Q.: Incidence of

death during jogging in Rhode Island from 1975 through 1980. **JAMA** 247:2535–2538, 1982.

11. Vander, L., Franklin, B., and Rubenfire, M.: Cardiovascular complications of recreational physical activity. **Phys. Sportsmed.** 10:89–97, 1982.

12. Hossack, K.F., and Hartwig, R.: Cardiac arrest associated with supervised cardiac rehabilitation. **J. Cardiac Rehabil.** 2:402–408, 1982.

13. Siscovick, D.S., Weiss, N.S., Fletcher, R.H., and Lasky, T.: The incidence of primary cardiac arrest during vigorous exercise. **N. Engl. J. Med.** 311:874–877, 1984.

14. Maron, B.J., Epstein, S.E., and Roberts, W.C.: Causes of sudden death in competitive athletes. **J. Am. Coll. Cardiol.** 7:204–214, 1986.

15. Van Camp, S.P., Choi, J.H.: Exercise and sudden death. **Phys. Sportsmed.** 16:49–52, 1988.

16. Pollock, M.L., Gettman, L.R., Mileses, C.A., Bah, M.D., Durstine, J.L., and Johnson, R.B.: Effects of frequency and duration of training on attrition and incidence of injury. **Med. Sci. Sports** 9:31–36, 1977.

17. Oldridge, N.B.: Adherence to adult exercise fitness programs. In Matarazzo, T.D., Weiss, S.M., Herd, J.A., Miller, N.E., and Weiss, S.M. (eds.): **Behavior Health: A Handbook of Health Enhancement and Disease Prevention.** New York, John Wiley and Sons, 1984, pp. 467–487.

18. Dishman, R.K., Sallis, J.F., and Orenstein, D.R.: The determinants of physical activity and exercise. **Pub. Health Rep.** 100:158–171, 1985.

19. Pollock, M.L.: Prescribing exercise for fitness and adherence. In Dishman, R.K. (ed.): **Exercise Adherence: Its Impact on Public Health.** Champaign, IL, Human Kinetics Books, 1988.

19a. Dishman, R.K. (ed.): **Exercise Adherence: Its Impact on Public Health.** Champaign, IL, Human Kinetics Books, 1988.

20. Anderson, B.: **Stretching.** Bolinas, CA, Shelter Publications, 1984.

21. Etnyre, B.R., and Lee, E.J.: Chronic and acute flexibility of men and women using three different stretching techniques. **Res. Q. Exerc. Sport** 59:222–228, 1988.

22. Cooper, K.H.: **The Aerobics Way.** New York, M. Evans and Co., 1977.

23. Pollock, M.L., Foster, C., Knapp, D., Rod, J.L., and Schmidt, D.H.: Effect of age and training on aerobic capacity and body composition of master athletes. **J. Appl. Physiol.** 62:725–731, 1987.

24. Price, C.S., Pollock, M.L., Gettman, L.R., and Kent, D.A.: **Physical Fitness Programs for Law Enforcement Officers: A Manual for Police Administrators.** Washington, D.C., U.S. Government Printing Office, 1977.

25. Cureton, T.K.: **Physical Fitness and Dynamic Health.** New York, The Dial Press, 1965.

26. Pollock, M.L.: How much exercise is enough? **Phys. Sportsmed.** 6:50–64, 1978.

27. American College of Sports Medicine: Position statement on the recommended quantity and quality of exercise for developing and maintaining fitness in healthy adults. **Med. Sci. Sports** 10:vii–x, 1978. (Note: revision will be published in late 1989 or early 1990.)

28. Pollock, M.L., Miller, H.S., Linnerud, A.C., and Cooper, K.H.: Frequency of training as a determinant for improvement in cardiovascular function and body composition of middle-aged men. **Arch. Phys. Med. Rehabil.** 58:141–145, 1975.

29. Hickson, R.C., Foster, C., Pollock, M.L., Galassi, T.M., and Rich, S.: Reduced training intensities and loss of aerobic power, endurance, and cardiac growth. **J. Appl. Physiol.** 58:492–499, 1985.

30. Graves, J.E., Pollock, M.L., Leggett, S.H., Braith, R.W., Carpenter, D.M., and Bishop, L.E.: Effect of reduced training frequency on muscular strength. **Int. J. Sports Med.** 9:316–319, 1988.

31. Richie, D.H., Kelso, S.F., and Bellucci, P.A.: Aerobic dance injuries: a retrospective study of instructors and participants. **Phys. Sportsmed.** 13:130–140, 1985.

32. Pollock, M.L., Pels, A.E., Foster, C., and Ward, A.: Exercise prescription for rehabilitation of the cardiac patient. In Pollock, M.L., and Schmidt, D.H. (eds.): **Heart Disease and Rehabilitation,** 2nd Ed. New York, John Wiley and Sons, 1979, pp. 413–445.

33. American College of Sports Medicine: Position statement on proper and improper weight loss programs. **Med. Sci. Sports Exerc.** 15:ix–xiii, 1983.

34. Harger, B.S., Miller, J.B., and Thomas, J.C.: The caloric cost of running. Its impact on weight reduction. **JAMA** 228:482–483, 1974.

35. Pollock, M.L., Broida, J., Kendrick, Z., Miller, H.S., Janeway, R., and Linnerud, A.C.: Effects of training two days per week at different intensities on middle-aged men. **Med. Sci. Sports** 4:192–197, 1972.

36. Dill, D.B.: Oxygen used in horizontal and grade walking and running on the treadmill. **J. Appl. Physiol.** 20:19–22, 1965.

37. Howley, E.T., and Glover, M.E.: The caloric costs of running and walking one mile for men and women. **Med. Sci. Sports** 6:235–237, 1974.

38. Fellingham, G.W., Roundy, E.S., Fisher, A.G., and Bryce, G.R.: Caloric cost of walking and running. **Med. Sci. Sports** 10:132–136, 1978.

39. Margaria, P., Cerretelli, P., Aghemo, P., and Sassi, G.: Energy cost of running. **J. Appl. Physiol.** 18:367–370, 1963.

40. Santiago, M.C., Alexander, J.F., Stull, G.A., Serfass, R.C., Hayday, A.M., and Leon, A.S.: Physiological responses of sedentary women to a 20 week conditioning program of walking or jogging. **Scand. J. Sports Sci.** 9:33–39, 1987.

41. Pollock, M.L., Gettman, L.R., Raven, P.B., Ayres, J., Bah, M., and Ward, A.: Physiological comparisons of the effects of aerobic and anaerobic training. In Price, C.S., Pollock, M.L., Gettman, L.R., Kent, D.A. (eds.): **Physical Fitness Programs for Law Enforcement Officers: A Manual for Police Administrators.** Washington, D.C., U.S. Government Printing Office, No. 027-000-00671-0, 1978.

42. Gaessner, G.A., and Rich, R.G.: Effects of high- and low-intensity exercise training on aerobic capacity and blood lipids. **Med. Sci. Sports Exerc.** 16:269–274, 1984.

43. American College of Sports Medicine: **Guidelines for Exercise Testing and Prescription,** 3rd Ed. Philadelphia, Lea & Febiger, 1986.

44. Fox, S.M., Naughton, J.P., and Gorman, P.A.: Physical activity and cardiovascular health II. The exercise prescription: intensity and duration. **Mod. Concepts Cardiovasc. Dis.** 16:21–24, 1972.

45. Davis, J.A., and Convertino, V.A.: A comparison of heart rate methods for predicting endurance training intensity. **Med. Sci. Sports** 7:295–298, 1975.

46. Karvonen, M., Kentala, K., and Musta, O.: The effects of training heart rate: a longitudinal study. **Ann. Med. Exp. Biol. Fenn.** 35:307–315, 1957.

47. Pollock, M.L., Foster, C., Rod, J.L., and Wible, G.: Comparison of methods for determining exercise training intensity for cardiac patients and healthy adults. In Kellerman, J.J. (ed.): **Comprehensive Cardiac Rehabilitation.** Basel, S. Karger, 1982, pp. 129–133.

48. Borg, G.A.V.: Psychophysical bases of perceived exertion. **Med. Sci. Sports Exerc.** 14:377–381, 1982.

49. Noble, B.J.: Clinical applications of perceived exertion. **Med. Sci. Sports Exerc.** 14:406–411, 1982.

50. Pollock, M.L., Jackson, A.S., and Foster, C.: The use of the perception scale for exercise prescription. In Borg, G., and Ottoson, D. (eds.): **The Perception of Exertion in Physical Work.** London, The MacMillan Press, 1986, pp. 161–176.

51. Borg, G., and Ottoson, D. (eds.): **The Perception of Exertion in Physical Work.** London, The MacMillan Press, 1986.

52. Birk, T.J., and Birk, C.A.: Use of ratings of perceived exertion for exercise prescription. **Sports Med.** 4:1–8, 1987.

53. Åstrand, P.O.: Measurement of maximal aerobic capacity. **Can. Med. Assoc. J.** 96:732–735, 1967.

54. Taylor, H.L., Haskell, W., Fox, S.M., and Blackburn, H.: Exercise tests: a

summary of procedures and concepts of stress testing for cardiovascular diagnosis and function evaluation. In Blackburn, H. (ed.): **Measurement in Exercise Electrocardiography.** Springfield, IL, Charles C Thomas, 1969, pp. 259–305.

55. Cooper, K.H., Purdy, J.G., White, S.R., Pollock, M.L., and Linnerud, A.C.: Age-fitness adjusted maximal heart rates. In Brunner, D., and Jokl, E. (eds.): **Medicine and Sport,** Vol. 10. The Role of Exercise in Internal Medicine. Basel, S. Karger, 1977, pp. 78–88.

56. Åstrand, P.O., and Rodahl, K.: **Textbook of Work Physiology,** 3rd Ed. New York, McGraw-Hill, 1986.

57. Londeree, B.R., and Moeschberger, M.L.: Effect of age and other factors on maximal heart rate. **Res. Q. Exerc. Sport** 53:297–304, 1982.

58. Hakki, A., Hare, T.W., Iskandrian, A.S., Lowenthal, D.T., and Segal, B.L.: Prediction of maximal heart rates in men and women. **Cardiovasc. Rev. Rep.** 4:997–999, 1983.

59. Miyashita, M., Onodera, K., and Tabata, I.: How Borg's RPE-scale has been applied to Japanese. In Borg, G., and Ottoson, D. (eds.): **The Perception of Exertion in Physical Work.** London, The MacMillan Press, 1986, pp. 27–34.

60. Pollock, M.L., and Foster, C.: Exercise prescription for participants on propranolol. (Abstr.) **J. Am. Coll. Cardiol.** 2:624, 1983.

61. Metier, C.P., Pollock, M.L., and Graves, J.E.: Exercise prescription for the coronary artery bypass graft surgery patient. **J. Cardiopul. Rehabil.** 6:236–242, 1986.

62. Faraher-Dion, W., Grevenow, P., Pollock, M.L., Squires, R.W., Foster, C., Johnson, W.D., and Schmidt, D.H.: Medical problems and physiologic responses during supervised inpatient cardiac rehabilitation: the patient after coronary artery bypass grafting. **Heart Lung** 11:248–255, 1982.

63. Silvidi, G.E., Squires, R.W., Pollock, M.L., and Foster, C.: Hemodynamic responses and medical problems associated with early exercise and ambulation in coronary artery bypass graft surgery patients. **J. Cardiac Rehabil.** 2:355–362, 1982.

64. Taylor, H.L., Wang, Y., Rowell, L., and Blomqvist, G.: The standardization and interpretation of submaximal and maximal tests of work capacity. **Pediatrics** 32:703–722, 1963.

65. Hombach, V., Braun, V., Hopp, H.W., Gil-Sanchez, D., Behrenbeck, D.W., Tauchert, M., and Hilger, H.H.: Electrophysiological effects of cardioselective and noncardioselective beta-adrenoceptor blockers with and without ISA at rest and during exercise. **Br. J. Clin. Pharmacol.** 13:285S–293S, 1982.

66. Tesch, P.A., and Kaiser, P.: Effects of beta-adrenergic blockage on O_2 uptake during submaximal and maximal exercise. **J. Appl. Physiol.** 54:901–905, 1983.

67. Cotton, F.S., and Dill, D.B.: On the relationship between the heart rate during exercise and that of immediate postexercise period. **Am. J. Physiol.** 111:554–558, 1983.

68. Pollock, M.L., Broida, J., and Kendrick, Z.: Validity of the palpation technique of heart rate determination and its estimation of training heart rate. **Res. Q.** 43:77–81, 1972.

69. Bevegard, S., and Shephard, J.T.: Circulatory effects of stimulating the carotid arterial stretch receptors in man at rest and during exercise. **J. Clin. Invest.** 45:132–142, 1966.

70. White, J.R.: EKG changes using the carotid artery for heart rate monitoring. **Med. Sci. Sports** 9:88–94, 1977.

71. Gardner, G.W., Danks, D.I., and Scharfsiein, L.: Use of carotid pulses for heart rate monitoring. (Abstr.) **Med. Sci. Sports** 11:111, 1979.

72. Oldridge, N.B., Haskell, W.L., and Single, P.: Carotid palpation, coronary heart disease and exercise rehabilitation. **Med. Sci. Sport Exerc.** 13:6–8, 1981.

73. Couldry, W., Corbin, C.B., and Wilcox, A.: Carotid vs radial pulse counts. **Phys. Sportsmed.** 10:67–72, 1982.

74. McArdale, W.D., Swiren, L., and Magel, J.R.: Validity of the postexercise heart rate as a means of estimating heart rate during work of varying intensities. **Res. Q.** 40:523–528, 1969.
75. Hartzell, A.A., Freund, B.J., Jilka, S.M., Joyner, M.J., Anderson, R.L., Ewy, G.A., and Wilmore, J.H.: The effect of beta-adrenergic blockade on ratings of perceived exertion during submaximal exercise before and following endurance training. **J. Cardiopul. Rehabil.** 6:444–456, 1986.
76. Chow, J.R., and Wilmore, J.H.: The regulation of exercise intensity by ratings of perceived exertion. **J. Cardiac Rehabil.** 4:382–387, 1984.
77. Jackson, A.S., and Osburn, H.G.: **Validity of Isometric Strength Tests for Predicting Performance in Underground Coal Mining Tasks.** Houston, TX, Employment Services, Shell Oil Company, 1983.
78. Kraemer, W.J., Noble, B.J., Clark, M.J., and Calver, B.W.: Physiological responses to heavy-resistance exercise with very short rest periods. **Int. J. Sports Med.** 8:247–252, 1987.
79. Sharkey, B.J.: Intensity and duration of training and the development of cardiorespiratory endurance. **Med. Sci. Sports** 2:197–202, 1970.
80. Pollock, M.L., Dimmick, J., Miller, H.S., Kendrick, Z., and Linnerud, A.C.: Effects of mode of training on cardiovascular function and body composition of middle-aged men. **Med. Sci. Sports** 7:139–145, 1975.
81. Pels, A.E., III, Pollock, M.L., McCole, S.D., Dohmeier, T.E., Lemberger, K.A., and Dehrlein, B.F.: Training adaptations of males and females to different exercise modes. Submitted for publication.
82. Kasch, F.W., and Boyer, J.L.: **Adult Fitness Principles and Practices.** San Diego, San Diego State College, 1968.
83. Mann, G.V., Garrett, L.H., Farhi, A., Murray, H., Billings, T.F., Shute, F., and Schwarten, S.E.: Exercise to prevent coronary heart disease. **Am. J. Med.** 46:12–27, 1969.
84. Kilbom, A., Hartley, L.H., Saltin, B., Bjure, J., Grimby, G., and Åstrand, I.: Physical training in sedentary middle-aged and older men. **Scand. J. Clin. Lab. Invest.** 24:315–322, 1969.
85. Oja, P., Teraslinna, P., Partanen, T., and Karava, R.: Feasibility of an 18 months' physical training program for middle-aged men and its effect on physical fitness. **Am. J. Pub. Health** 64:459–465, 1974.
86. Pollock, M.L., Miller, H., Janeway, R., Linnerud, A.C., Robertson, B., and Valentino, R.: Effects of walking on body composition and cardiovascular function of middle-aged men. **J. Appl. Physiol.** 30:126–130, 1971.
87. Pollock, M.L., Dawson, G.A., Miller, H.S., Jr., Ward, A., Cooper, D., Headley, W., Linnerud, A.C., and Nomeir, M.M.: Physiologic responses of men 49 to 65 years of age to endurance training. **J. Am. Geriatrics Soc.** 24:97–104, 1976.
88. Pollock, M.L., Graves, J.E., Leggett, S., Braith, R., Carroll, J., and Hagberg, J.: Injuries and adherence to aerobic and strength training exercise programs for the elderly. **Med. Sci. Sports Exerc.** 21:S59, 1989.
89. Hagberg, J.M., Graves, J.E., Limacher, M., Wood, D., Leggett, S., Cononie, C., Gruber, J., and Pollock, M.: Cardiovascular responses of 70–79 year old men and women to exercise training. **J. Appl. Physiol.** 66:2589–2594, 1989.
90. Blair, S.N., Kohl, H.W., and Goodyear, N.N.: Rates and risks for running and exercise injuries: studies in three populations. **Res. Q. Exerc. Sport** 58:221–228, 1987.
91. Powell, K.E., Kohl, H.W., Caspersen, C.J., and Blair, S.N.: An epidemiological perspective of the causes of running injuries. **Phys. Sportsmed.** 14:100–114, 1986.
92. Lampman, R.M., and Schteingart, D.E.: Moderate and extreme obesity. In Franklin, B.A., Gordon, S., and Timmis, G.C. (eds.): **Exercise in Modern Medicine.** Baltimore, Williams and Wilkins, pp. 156–174.
93. President's Council on Physical Fitness and Sports: **Walking for Exercise and Pleasure.** Washington, D.C., U.S. Government Printing Office, No. 017-001-0047-2, 1986.

94. Sweetgall, R., Rippe, J., and Katch, F.: **Rockport's Fitness Walking.** New York, The Putnam Publishing Group, 1985.
95. Walking for fitness (a round table). **Phys. Sportsmed.** 14:145–159, 1986.
96. Yanker, G.: **Sportwalking.** Chicago, Contemporary Books, 1987.
97. Editors of Consumer Guide: **Walking for Health and Fitness.** Lincolnwood, IL, Publications International, 1988.
98. Rippe, J.M., Ward, A., Porcari, J.P., and Freedson, P.S.: Walking for health and fitness. **JAMA** 259:2720–2724, 1988.
99. Goldman, R.F., and Iampietro, P.F.: Energy cost of load carriage. **J. Appl. Physiol.** 17:675–676, 1962.
100. Lind, A.R., and McNicol, G.W.: Cardiovascular responses to holding and carrying weights by hand and by shoulder harness. **J. Appl. Physiol.** 25:261–267, 1968.
101. Soule, R.G., and Goldman, R.F.: Energy cost of loads carried on the head, hands or feet. **J. Appl. Physiol.** 27:687–690, 1969.
102. Schoenfeld, Y., Udassin, R., Shapiro, Y., Birenfeld, C., Magazanik, A., and Sohar, E.: Optimal back-pack load for short distance hiking. **Arch. Phys. Med. Rehabil.** 59:281–284, 1978.
103. Jones, B.H., Toner, M.M., Daniel, W.L., and Knapik, J.J.: The energy cost and heart rate response of trained and untrained subjects walking and running in shoes and boots. **Ergonomics** 27:895–902, 1984.
104. Zarandora, J.E., Nelson, A.G., Conlee, R.K., and Fisher, A.G.: Physiological responses to hand-carried weights. **Phys. Sportsmed.** 14:113–120, 1986.
105. Graves, J.E., Pollock, M.L., Montain, S.J., Jackson, A.S., and O'Keefe, J.M.: The effect of hand-held weights on the physiological responses to walking exercise. **Med. Sci. Sports Exerc.** 19:260–265, 1987.
106. Auble, T.E., Schwartz, L., and Robertson, R.J.: Aerobic requirements for moving handweights through various ranges of motion while walking. **Phys. Sportsmed.** 15:133–140, 1987.
107. Graves, J.E., Martin, A.D., Miltenberger, L.A., and Pollock, M.L.: Physiological responses to walking with hand weights, wrist weights, and ankle weights. **Med. Sci. Sports Exerc.** 20:265–271, 1988.
108. Graves, J.E., Sagiv, M.E., Pollock, M.L., and Miltenberger, L.A.: Effect of hand-held weights and wrist weights on the metabolic and hemodynamic responses to submaximal exercise in hypertensive responders. **J. Cardiopul. Rehabil.** 8:134–140, 1988.
109. Schram, V., and Hanson, P.: Cardiovascular and metabolic responses to weight loaded walking in cardiac patients. **J. Cardiopul. Rehabil.** 8:28–32, 1988.
110. Schwartz, L.: **Heavyhands. The Ultimate Exercise.** New York, Warner Books, 1987.
111. Borysyk, L.M., Franklin, B., Gordan, S., and Timmis, G.C.: Minimal increases in aerobic requirements while walk training with hand weights. (Abstr.) **Med. Sci. Sports Exerc.** 18:598, 1986.
112. Soule, R.G., Pandolf, K.B., and Goldman, R.F.: Energy expenditure of heavy load carriage. **Ergonomics** 21:373–381, 1978.
113. Sawka, M.N.: Physiology of upper body exercise. In Pandolf, K.B. (ed.): **Exercise and Sport Sciences Reviews,** Vol. 14. New York, Macmillan, 1986, pp. 175–211.
114. Franklin, B.A.: Exercise testing, training and arm ergometry. **Sports Med.** 2:100–119, 1985.
115. Pollock, M.L., Miller, H.S., Linnerud, A.C., Laughridge, E., Coleman, E., and Alexander, E.: Arm pedaling disabled. **Arch. Phys. Med. Rehabil.** 55:418–424, 1974.
116. Schwade, J., Blomqvist, C.G., and Shapiro, W.: A comparison of response of arm and leg work in patients with ischemic heart disease. **Am. Heart J.** 94:203–208, 1977.
117. Enoka, R.M.: Muscle strength and its development: new perspectives. **Sports Med.** 6:146–168, 1988.

118. Berger, R.A.: **Applied Exercise Physiology.** Philadelphia, Lea & Febiger, 1982.
119. Wilmore, J.H., and Costill, D.L.: Training for sport and activity. **The Physiological Basis of the Conditioning Process,** 3rd Ed. Dubuque, IA, William C. Brown, 1988.
120. Rasch, P.J.: **Weight Training.** Dubuque, IA, William C. Brown, 1966.
121. Fleck, S.J., and Kraemer, W.J.: **Designing Resistance Training Programs.** Champaign, IL, Human Kinetics Books, 1987.
122. Sale, D.G.: Influence of exercise and training on motor unit activation. In Pandolf, K.B. (ed.): **Exercise and Sport Sciences Reviews,** Vol. 15. New York, Macmillan, 1987, pp. 95–152.
123. Lind, A.R., Phil, D., and McNicol, G.: Muscular factors which determine the cardiovascular responses to sustained and rhythmic exercise. **Can. Med. Assoc. J.** 96:706–713, 1967.
124. Graves, J.E., Pollock, M.L., Jones, A.E., Colvin, A.B., and Leggett, S.H.: Specificity of limited range of motion variable resistance training. **Med. Sci. Sports Exerc.** 21:84–89, 1989.
125. Knapik, J.J., Maudsley, R.H., Rammos, N.V.: Angular specificity and test mode specificity of isometric and isokinetic strength training. **J. Orthop. Sports Phys. Ther.** 5:58–65, 1983.
126. Marcinik, E.J., Hodgdon, J.A., Mittleman, U., and O'Brien, J.J.: Aerobic/calisthenic and aerobic/circuit weight training programs for Navy men: a comparative study. **Med. Sci. Sports Exerc.** 17:482–487, 1985.
127. Wescott, W.L.: **Strength Fitness: Physiological Principles and Training Techniques,** 2nd Ed. Boston, Allyn and Bacon, 1987.
128. Hettinger, T.: **Physiology of Strength.** Springfield, IL, Charles C Thomas, 1961, pp. 57–60.
129. deVries, H.A.: **Physiology of Exercise for Physical Education and Athletics,** 4th Ed. Dubuque, IA, William C. Brown, 1986.
130. Hakkinen, K.: Factors influencing trainability of muscular strength during short term and prolonged training. **Nat. Strength Condit. Assoc. J.** 7:32–34, 1985.
131. Braith, R.W., Graves, J.E., Pollock, M.L., Leggett, S.L., Carpenter, D.M., and Colvin, A.B.: Comparison of two versus three days per week of variable resistance training during 10 and 18 week programs. **Int. J. Sports Med.** in press.
131a. Gilliam, G.M.: Effects of frequency of weight training on muscle strength enhancement. J. Sports Med. 21:432–436, 1981.
132. Graves, J.E., Pollock, M.L., Leggett, S.H., et al.: Effect of reduced training frequency on muscular strength. **Int. J. Sports Med.** 9:316–319, 1988.
133. MacDougall, J.D., Tuxen, D., Sale, D.G., Moroz, J.R., and Sutton, J.R.: Arterial blood pressure response to heavy resistance exercise. **J. Appl. Physiol.** 58:785–790, 1985.
134. Haslam, D.R., McCartney, N., McKelvie, R.S., and MacDougall, J.D.: Direct measurements of arterial blood pressure during formal weightlifting in cardiac patients. **J. Cardiopul. Rehabil.** 8:213–225, 1988.
135. Pollock, M.L., Leggett, S.H., Graves, J.E., Jones, A., Fulton, M., and Cirulli, J.: Effect of resistance training on lumbar extension strength. **Am. J. Sports Med.** in press.
136. Gettman, L.R., Ward, P., and Hagman, R.D.: A comparison of combined running and weight training with circuit weight training. **Med. Sci. Sports Exerc.** 14:229–234, 1982.
137. Hurley, B.F., Seals, D.R., Ehsani, A.A., Cartier, L.J., Dalsky, G.P., Hagberg, J.M., and Holloszy, J.O.: Effects of high-intensity strength training on cardiovascular function. **Med. Sci. Sports Exerc.** 16:483–488, 1984.
138. Darden, E.: **The Nautilus Book.** Chicago, Contemporary Books, 1985.
139. Riley, D.P.: **Strength Training,** 2nd Ed. West Point, NY, Leisure Press, 1982.
140. Hubbard, A.W.: Homokinetics: muscular function in human movement. In

Johnson, W.R., and Buskirk, E.R. (eds.): **Science and Medicine of Exercise and Sports,** 2nd Ed. New York, Harper and Row, 1974, pp. 5–23.

141. Kelsey, J.L., White, A.A., Pastides, H., and Bisbee, G.E., Jr.: The impact of musculoskeletal disorders on the population of the United States. **J. Bone Joint Surg.** 61A:959–964, 1979.

142. Melleby, A.: **The Y's Way to a Healthy Back.** Piscataway, NJ, New Century Publishers, 1982.

143. Mayer, T.G., Smith, S.S., Keeley, P.T., and Mooney, V.: Quantification of lumbar function part 2: sagittal plane trunk strength in chronic low-back patients. **Spine** 10:765–772, 1985.

144. McQuade, K.J., Turner, J.A., and Buchner, D.M.: Physical fitness and low back pain: an analysis of the relationships among fitness, functional limitations, and depression. **Clin. Orthop. Rel. Res.** 223:198–204, 1988.

145. Suzuki, N., and Endo, S.: A quantitative study of trunk muscle strength and fatigability in the low-back pain syndrome. **Spine** 8:69–74, 1983.

146. Kraus, H.: **Clinical Treatment of Back and Neck Pain.** New York, McGraw-Hill, 1970.

147. Jones, A., Pollock, M., Graves, J., Fulton, M., Jones, W., MacMillan, M., Baldwin, D., and Cirulli, J.: **The Lumbar Spine.** Santa Barbara, CA, Sequoia Communications, 1988.

148. Mayer, T.G., and Gatchel, R.J.: **Functional Restoration for Spinal Disorders: The Sports Medicine Approach.** Philadelphia, Lea & Febiger, 1988.

149. Jackson, C.P., and Brown, M.D.: Analysis of current approaches and a practical guide to prescription of exercise. **Clin. Orthop. Rel. Res.** 179:46–54, 1983.

150. Williams, P.C.: **Low Back and Neck Pain: Causes and Conservative Treatment.** Springfield, IL, Charles C Thomas, 1974.

151. Cady, L.D., Bishcoff, D.P., O'Connell, E.R., Thomas, P.C., and Allan, J.K.: Strength and fitness and subsequent back injuries in fire-fighters. **J. Occup. Med.** 21:269–275, 1979.

152. Mayer, L., and Greenberg, B.: Measurements of the strength of trunk muscles. **J. Bone Joint Surg.** 4:842–856, 1942.

153. Smidt, G. Herring, T., Amundsen, L., Rogers, M., Russell, A., and Lehmann, T.: Assessment of abdominal and back extensor function: a quantitative approach and results for chronic low-back patients. **Spine** 8:211–219, 1983.

154. Graves, J.E., Pollock, M.L., Carpenter, D.M., Leggett, S.H., Jones, A., MacMillan, M., and Fulton, M.: Quantitative assessment of full range-of-motion isometric lumbar extension strength. **Spine,** in press.

154a. Pollock, M.L., and Graves, J.E.: New approach to low back evaluation and testing. **Central Florida Phys.** 5:19–20, 1989.

155. Wakim, K.G., Gersten, J.W., Elkins, E.C., and Martin, G.M.: Objective recording of muscle strength. **Arch. Phys. Med.** 31:90–100, 1950.

156. Edstrom, L.: Selective atrophy of red muscle fibers in the quadriceps in long-standing knee joint dysfunction. Injuries to the anterior cruciate ligament. **J. Neurol. Sci.** 11:551–558, 1970.

157. MacDougall, J.D., Elder, G.C.B., Sale, D.G., et al.: Effects of strength training and immobilization on human muscle fibers. **Eur. J. Appl. Physiol.** 43:25–34, 1980.

158. Lindboe, C.F., and Platou, C.S.: Disuse atrophy of human skeletal muscle. **Acta Neuropathology** 56:241–244, 1982.

8

PRESCRIBING EXERCISE FOR REHABILITATION OF THE CARDIAC PATIENT

Cardiac rehabilitation can be considered the process of restoring physical, psychological, and social functions to optimal levels in those individuals who have had prior manifestations of coronary artery disease (CAD). In the past 40 years, there has been a profound shift away from the conservative approach that discouraged anginal and heart attack patients from becoming as active as their symptoms and medical status might have permitted. Many were told to resign from their golf club, and some were advised to stop driving their cars and climbing stairs. Six weeks of bed rest after a myocardial infarction (MI) was the common standard.[1] Fortunately, many cardiologists[2-7] questioned the pessimistic and conservative approach. They demonstrated the safety of activity for the anginal patient, the early use of a bedside chair for the stabilized heart attack victim, and progressive, endurance-stimulating exercises for those whose myocardial infarcts had healed.[2-8]

Chapters 1 and 3 outline the many effects of physical activity on physiological function, risk factors associated with CAD, and morbidity and mortality. Although the benefits of cardiac rehabilitation with regard to morbidity and mortality are not fully proved but strongly suggested, the effect on quality of life is not disputed.[8-16] In addition, the concept of cardiac rehabilitation includes not only exercise but also a wide spectrum of medical, physical, and psychosocial behavioral changes. The multiple intervention approach to risk modification (smoking cessation, blood pressure [BP] and cholesterol reduction, proper diet and weight control, stress management and exercise) in cardiac rehabilitation has been supportive in favor of decreased mortality from CAD.[17-19]

Strict bed rest has been shown to have a significant detrimental effect on physiological function.[20–22] After just a few days or weeks, the patient has significantly decreased cardiorespiratory fitness, blood volume, red blood cell count, nitrogen and protein balance, strength, and flexibility and increased problems of orthostatic hypotension and thromboembolism. Early upright posture shifts, ambulation, and range-of-motion (ROM) exercise have been shown to help alleviate these problems.

In those patients who have undergone coronary artery bypass graft surgery (CABG), physical activity can help decrease postsurgical stiffness and prevent complications of postsurgical atelectasis. Other potential benefits of cardiac rehabilitation include a decrease in the incidence and severity of depression and anxiety, improved self-esteem, and a reduction in the most serious characteristics of Type-A behavior (hostility and anger).[23–29] See Kellerman,[15] Naughton, Hellerstein, and Mohler,[10] Pollock and Schmidt,[14] Krantz and Blumenthal,[28] and Froelicher[30] for reviews of the beneficial effects of early ambulation and other aspects of cardiac rehabilitation on various medical, physiological, psychological, and social factors. See Chapter 3 for physiological benefits resulting from an exercise program. In Chapter 4, the area of weight control and body composition changes with dietary and exercise training is reviewed.

RISK AND MEDICAL PROBLEMS ASSOCIATED WITH ADULT FITNESS AND CARDIAC REHABILITATION PROGRAMS

Risk of Adult Fitness Programs

Although cardiac arrest and death have occurred in cardiac rehabilitation programs, they have been infrequent.[31–37] What is the risk of fatal and nonfatal events associated with cardiac rehabilitation programs? First, as a base of comparison, what is the risk in a presumed healthy noncardiac population? Gibbons and associates[38] reported the acute cardiac risk of strenuous exercise in 2,935 men and women 13 to 76 years of age ($\bar{x}$ = 37 years) (Table 8–1). The 5.4-year follow-up period included 374,798 person-hours of exercise and 1,694,024 miles of walking and running (81 percent running). During this period, only two nonfatal cardiac events occurred. One complication occurred in a 61-year-old executive who collapsed with ventricular fibrillation (VF) during a 2-mile competitive race for which he had not adequately prepared. The other event occurred in a 35-year-old man who suffered an acute inferior

Table 8–1. Cardiovascular Complication Rates for Adult Fitness (Noncardiac) and Medically Supervised Cardiac Rehabilitation Programs in North America

	Events Per Hour	
Study	*Nonfatal*	*Fatal*
Cardiac		
Mead, 1976[32]	1/6,000	
Fletcher, 1977[33]	1/15,000	
Haskell, 1978[34]	1/34,673	1/116,402
Hossack, 1982[35]	1/14,985	
Shephard, 1983[36]	1/113,583	
Van Camp, 1986[37]	1/111,996	1/783,972
Adult Fitness		
Gibbons, 1980[38]	1/187,399	0/374,798
Vander, 1982[39]	1/887,526	1/1,124,200

MI while showering after completing a fast-paced 3-mile run. Both men had not been running regularly for 6 months before their event, and both incidents were associated with a high-intensity exercise session. No cardiac events occurred with the 1,001 women who participated in the study.

Vander, Franklin, and Rubenfire[39] surveyed 48 YMCAs and Jewish Community Centers in the United States from 1975 to 1979 and found a small risk for a cardiovascular event during recreational activities (see Table 8–1). The study represented 33,726,000 participation hours. Most fatal and nonfatal events occurred during or shortly after the more rigorous activities, e.g., racquet sports (33.9 percent) and jogging (23.5 percent), with few events occurring during walking (1.5 percent).

Thompson and colleagues[40] and others[38, 39, 41] have shown that, in the general population, the risk of precipitating a cardiovascular event (both fatal and nonfatal) during vigorous exercise is small, but during the time of exercise, the participant is at greater than normal risk. Siscovick and colleagues[41] agree with Thompson and colleagues[40] but added that even though chronic exercisers are at greater risk while participating, they are at a significantly lower total risk when nonparticipation hours are taken into account.

Important factors concerning the risk of cardiovascular events occurring in adult fitness programs are as follows:[42–45]
1. None are immune from sudden death because they are chronically active, including marathon running.
2. Most cardiovascular events occur as a result of CAD, in participants who are above 30 years of age, and from hypertrophic cardiomyopathy, anomalous origin of the left coronary artery, and other congenital defects for persons under 30 years of age.

3. Participants with previous CAD events and who are considered to be at high risk for CAD are at the greatest risk.
4. Often, prodromal symptoms, described as an onset of new symptoms or a change in health status, are present. Prodromal symptoms include chest or other pain or discomfort (neck, shoulders, arms, trunk), unusual fatigue, dyspnea, and abnormal electrocardiographic (ECG) results. Also, many affected persons had recently consulted a doctor.

The reader may want to become familiar with the facts related to the exercise-related sudden deaths of two popular exercise advocates, Jimm Fixx[46] and Pete Maravich.[45] Fixx had significant CAD, a strong family history of CAD, and during much of his life, many risk factors associated with CAD.[46] Maravich was shown to have a significant abnormality related to his coronary anatomy, which precipitated cardiac hypertrophy.[45] Both were thought to have had prodromal symptoms before their deaths. More recently, an age-group champion distance runner (aged 57 years) collapsed and died within one minute after running 3,000 meters in 10 minutes 30.2 seconds.[46a] Although he was not known to have had CAD, autopsy results showed him to have had a previous MI and significant three-vessel CAD. He had had a reported normal exercise test 22 months before his death and no reported signs or symptoms of CAD.

Risk of Cardiac Rehabilitation Programs

Table 8–1 compares the complication rates for various cardiac exercise programs. The two largest surveys are discussed in detail. First, Haskell[34] reported on the occurrence of major cardiovascular complications during exercise training in 30 cardiac rehabilitation programs in North America. The cardiac programs came from a variety of YMCA and YMHA, hospital, university, and independent medical clinics, but all were medically supervised. A physician or nurse was on site for each exercise session. The questionnaire included data from medically supervised exercise classes conducted in 103 locations with 13,570 participants who accumulated 1,629,634 patient-hours of supervised exercise. Programs accepted patients 2 to 12 weeks after the event and included an average of three exercise sessions per week, with walking, walking-jogging, running, calisthenics, and recreational games being the predominant activities. A total of 50 cardiac arrests were observed, 42 of which were successfully resuscitated and eight of which were fatal. Seven MIs were reported—five nonfatal and two fatal. Although data are not available, it stands to reason that fatal cardiac events would be significantly higher in unsupervised programs.

In the cardiac programs, 44 of the 61 major complications occurred during warm-up or cool-down, with the type of facility used not affecting the results. These results strongly suggest the need for adequate supervision during rest breaks or stops to the rest room, and a minimum of 15 to 20 minutes postexercise surveillance is necessary. The second and more recent survey was conducted by Van Camp and Peterson[37] on 51,303 patients from 142 (98-percent response rate) randomly selected outpatient cardiac rehabilitation programs in the United States. The programs surveyed included 65 percent that were administered by hospitals, 14 percent from proprietary cardiac rehabilitation centers, 8 percent from YMCArdiac therapy programs, 6 percent from free-standing independent centers, and 7 percent from university-associated centers. The survey was conducted from 1980 to 1984 and included 2,351,916 patient-hours of exercise. The results included 21 cardiac arrests in which 18 were successfully resuscitated. As shown in Table 8–1, the incidence rate for fatal and nonfatal cardiac events was extremely small and in agreement with the 1983 survey reported by Shephard.[36] Van Camp and Peterson[37] reported no significant difference in the frequency of cardiac arrests when programs were compared for size or the amount of ECG monitoring. Although not directly comparable with the earlier samples studied (lack of precise information on risk status of the various groups), it appears that cardiac rehabilitation programs are safe and have become safer with time and experience. Van Camp and Peterson[37] speculate that improved safety has stemmed from multiple factors, e.g., the identification of the higher risk patient (risk stratification), improved medications, and exercise guidelines.

Which patients are at the highest risk of having a cardiac arrest or MI? Graded exercise testing (GXT) and other noninvasive testing have shown the following factors to be related to higher risk: angina pectoris, significant S-T–segment depression or elevation from resting values, inappropriate BP response to exercise, peak heart rate (HR) of less than 120 beats/min (off drugs), significant complex arrhythmia, left ventricular dysfunction, and poor effort tolerance (less than 4 to 5 METs).[47–55a] The combination of left ventricular dysfunction (ejection fraction less than 40 percent) and significant arrhythmia greatly increases the risk of sudden cardiac death.[55a–58] As mentioned briefly in Chapter 3, Hossack and Hartwig[35] reported the results from 13 years of the CAPRI program in Seattle, Washington. During this period, 2,464 patients (80 percent men) performed 374,616 hours of supervised exercise.

Twenty-five male participants experienced VF during training, and all were successfully resuscitated. When compared with a control group of patients who did not have VF, those in the VF group had a higher aerobic capacity and more marked S-T–segment depression on a GXT (68 percent and 21 percent of the patients, respectively). The incidence of angina pectoris, exertional hypotension, and exercise-induced arrhythmias was not different between groups. Those in the VF group exceeded their upper limit prescribed training HR for 56 percent of the training sessions as compared with 24 percent for the controls. Angiography was available for 17 of the VF patients, and all had significant left main or proximal left anterior descending disease, or both. In addition, most of these incidents occurred in patients who had been in the program for more than a year. Certain abnormal responses on the GXT and exceeding one's recommended upper limit of the target HR range during training are associated with a higher risk of major cardiovascular complications.

Medical Problems Associated with Inpatient and Outpatient Cardiac Rehabilitation

As was discussed in Chapter 3 under Training with Cardiac Patients, there may be certain advantages to exercise training at higher intensities. Ehsani and colleagues[59-61] have consistently found improvement in cardiac function and concomitant reductions in angina pectoris and S-T–segment depression with high-intensity (80 to 90 percent of maximal oxygen uptake [$\dot{V}O_2$max]) training in post MI patients. Although these results are quite provocative, an extrapolation of the results of high-intensity programs to the general MI population must be taken cautiously. It is well known that high-intensity effort is associated with greater risk of precipitating a major cardiac event.[34, 35, 62, 63] The topic of exercising patients with significant S-T–segment depression requires more discussion. As mentioned by Hossack and Hartwig,[35] one of the three factors they found associated with cardiac arrest was exercise training with significant S-T–segment depression. Shephard[64] reported that five of the first seven deaths that occurred in the Ontario Exercise-Heart Collaborative Study were in patients who showed deep S-T–segment depression with exercise. Figure 8–1 diagrammatically shows the relationship between exercise intensity, improvement in $\dot{V}O_2$max, and risk of cardiovascular events. The figure shows a greater improvement in $\dot{V}O_2$max with increased intensity of training and a dramatic increase in cardiovascular events when training exceeds 85 percent of $\dot{V}O_2$max. It should be

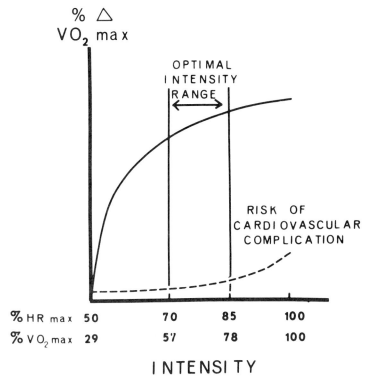

INTENSITY

Figure 8–1. The relationship between training intensity, percent change in maximum oxygen uptake ($\dot{V}O_2$max), and risk of cardiovascular complications. (From Hellerstein, H.K., and Franklin, B.A.: Exercise testing and prescription. In Wenger, N.K., and Hellerstein, H.K. (eds.): **Rehabilitation of the Coronary Patient**, 2nd Ed. New York, Churchill Livingstone, Inc., 1984, pp. 197–284. Published with permission.)

noted that Ehsani (personal communication, September, 1988) has had many patients who had significant S-T–segment depression during exercise training at a high intensity for the past 10 years without incident. He cautions that these patients received personal supervision and BP was monitored more frequently than with other patients.

This discussion has shown that exercise training in cardiac patients is generally safe, and high-risk patients can be identified with noninvasive testing. The potential for greater improvement in cardiac and cardiorespiratory function, including signs and symptoms of CAD, with high-intensity training is important, but the balance of the proper intensity of training so that the patient can receive the most benefit with the lowest risk is the primary concern of the cardiac rehabilitation specialist. There is no 100-percent solution to the problem, but the notion of risk stratification as described by DeBusk and coworkers[53] seems appropriate. The main point here is that patients should be stratified as early as possible (in most cases within 3 weeks) into low- (2 percent or less per year mortality from CAD), medium- (5 to 10 percent), and high- (greater than 10 percent) risk groups. With this stratification system, patients are triaged into programs most suited for their benefit and safety. A more detailed discussion on risk stratification comes later in this chapter.

What medical problems occur during in-hospital phase-I programs? Although the trend is to begin exercise therapy closer to the patient's event or surgery, few major complications requiring resuscitation are reported. A survey of in-hospital cardiac rehabilitation programs showed that MI patients begin treatment 2 to 4 days after the event and CABG patients, one to three days after surgery.[66] The low incidence rate is most likely due to careful patient selection and the adoption of appropriate guidelines and contraindications to exercise that are in current use.[10, 12, 14, 67] These guidelines are discussed in subsequent sections of this chapter. Even though life-threatening complications are rare, other types of major complications seem to be prevalent.

Dion and associates[66] reported medical problems associated with cardiac rehabilitation in 521 CABG patients who were 24 to 76 years of age. Ambulation and upper extremity ROM exercise began as early as 12 to 24 hours after surgery for 65 percent of the patients. Patients were treated twice daily and monitored for arrhythmia, ischemia, and BP for an average of 11 days. During the rehabilitation program, a total of 555 significant complications occurred. See Table 8–2 for a listing of these problems. Although medical complications were classified as significant, most were not considered life threatening. Approximately 25 percent of these complications were first noted by the cardiac rehabilitation staff. Medical problems that occur in the in-hospital program are associated with rehabilitation of the MI patients, who show a greater incidence of angina pectoris, ischemia, and hypotension than do CABG patients.

Many medical problems are associated with outpatient cardiac rehabilitation programs.[68, 69] Sennett and associates[68] reported medical problems that occurred in a 12-week outpatient cardiac rehabilitation program for 257 CABG patients and 108 medically treated patients (previous MI, angina pectoris, or congestive heart failure). The exercise program began with 15 minutes of warm-up, including some light strength development activity, a 30- to 45-minute aerobic period (stationary cycling, treadmill walking-jogging, and Air Dyne [arm-leg ergometer exercise]) followed by a 10-minute cool-down. Training was 3 days per week, was individ-

Table 8–2. Comparison of Medical Problems Found During Inpatient and Outpatient Cardiac Rehabilitation Programs

Medical Problem	Inpatient Surgicals (n = 521)	Outpatient Surgicals (n = 257)	Outpatient Medicals (n = 108)
Angina pectoris	4%	19%	34%
Lightheadedness	14%	24%	20%
Dyspnea	—	20%	24%
Incisional discomfort	14%	18%	0%
Claudication	3%	5%	6%
Hypotension	8%	4%	9%
Hypertension	1%	5%	5%
S-T–segment change	2%	9%	15%
Ventricular arrhythmias	44%	30%	31%
Supraventricular arrhythmias	17%	19%	14%
Frequent PVCs	6%	20%	19%
Multifocal PVCs	17%	22%	22%
Couplets	5%	22%	20%
Ventricular tachycardia	1%	12%	4%

PVCs = premature ventricular contractions.
Inpatient data from Dion and associates.[66]
Outpatient data from Sennett and associates.[68]

ualized and progressed slowly. Table 8–2 shows a comparison of medical problems found between the CABG and medical patients. Medical patients generally had more angina pectoris, S-T–segment depression, and hypotension than did CABG patients, with equal numbers of complex arrhythmias. Although incisional discomfort was prevalent for CABG patients, only 3.1 percent had sternal movement or clicking for which arm and shoulder ROM activity had to be modified. In general, these studies showed that significant medical problems exist in both inpatient and outpatient programs but are normally not life threatening. After the first month of the outpatient program, the frequency of occurrence of most medical problems declined. Many of the declines are associated with the healing process and the medical management provided the patients.

These studies emphasize the value of organized rehabilitation programs in detecting medical problems. Surveillance of this type can provide primary physicians with valuable information concerning their patients, thus allowing them to make earlier decisions about patient care.

THE NEED FOR CARDIAC REHABILITATION SERVICES

In general, the need for cardiac rehabilitation programs and the supervision of cardiac patients in their training programs is apparent.[70, 71] Questions arise, though, regarding how much supervision and how much sophisticated monitoring are necessary and for how long. The exact answers to these questions are not known, and yet they are of continuing concern to medical and health professionals, as well as third-party carriers. States vary greatly from no coverage for cardiac rehabilitation programs to almost carte blanche long-term coverage for an organized program. It appears that most state carriers and Medicaid and Medicare plans reimburse for inpatient rehabilitation and for up to 12 weeks or 36 visits of a hospital-based outpatient program. Some states also cover a medically supervised phase-III community program for up to 6 additional months. Because of the high cost of outpatient cardiac rehabilitation as it is currently practiced and the questioned need of such services for all, the current coverage as described may change. This controversy was triggered by the document published by Blue Cross/Blue Shield (BC/BS) in 1985, when they instituted their new guidelines for cardiac care. They stated that three visits for cardiac rehabilitation services are usually adequate to accomplish the education and program needs of most patients who are entering a rehabilitation program. This statement and the reaction to it stimulated the Public Health Service (PHS) through the Office of Health Technology Assessment (OHTA) to review their whole policy concerning reimbursement for cardiac rehabilitation services for Medicare and Medicaid patients.[71a] Many professional organizations, individual practitioners, and patients, as well as the authors, responded directly to the BC/BS and PHS concerning the need and value of cardiac rehabilitation services. Although the process was (is) painful, it stimulated the profession itself to respond to important issues concerning rehabilitation services, such as the safety and clinical effectiveness of programs, need for ECG monitoring, and content as well as duration of rehabilitation. Some of these problems/issues have recently been reviewed by Greenland and Chu[71b] as well as by the OHTA.[101a] The previous section and this one help clarify these issues.

When does rehabilitation end and prevention begin? In addition, should all patients be treated equally, or should stratification occur based on medical and physical status, that is, should patients who are at moderate to high risk receive more continuous ECG monitoring and their program duration be longer than that of low-risk patients? Many insurance carriers are designating an arbitrary 12-week postdischarge time as the rehabilitation period. From a physical standpoint, data support this notion and show aerobic capacity to be restored by this time.[68, 72–78] This does not mean that a patient cannot continue to improve fitness and medical- and risk-factor variables beyond this time, but by 6 to 12 weeks after discharge, most uncomplicated cardiac patients have improved their physical status enough to return to work and carry on a relatively normal lifestyle.

Need for Telemetric Monitoring: Supervised versus Unsupervised Programs

Another important aspect of the rehabilitation program revolves around the issue as to the need for formal (organized, facility oriented) programs versus informal (structured but conducted in the home environment) programs. In other words, does everyone need a formal and highly monitored program? First, a discussion of the need for sophisticated telemetric monitoring in cardiac rehabilitation seems warranted. From the previous discussion of medical problems found in formal cardiac rehabilitation programs[67, 68] and, in addition, other studies[79-84] showing complex arrhythmias during monitored outpatient rehabilitation, it is apparent that many problems exist. In particular, complex ventricular arrhythmias are prevalent in 30 to 60 percent of patients observed in these programs.[68, 69] For example, in a sample of 70 patients, Fardy and colleagues[81] found that 54 percent of their patients experienced complex arrhythmias during 12 weeks of cardiac rehabilitation. Although most of the arrhythmias were observed in the initial 7 weeks of the program, 13 percent occurred for the first time during weeks 8 to 12. The data of Sennett and associates[68] revealed fewer complex ventricular arrhythmias (30 percent) than did those of Fardy and associates but also showed that many arrhythmias persisted beyond the initial 7 weeks of the program.

Even though many potentially life-threatening arrhythmias were detected during the first 12 weeks of cardiac rehabilitation, few significant events, such as cardiac arrest, MI, or congestive heart failure, occurred. As shown in Table 8–1 and discussed earlier, the incidence rate (nonfatal and fatal) for a cardiovascular event associated with exercise rehabilitation is very low. In the two largest surveys, the difference in complication rate could not be attributed to how soon patients entered the program after their event, the type of exercise, the type of facility, or the intensity of exercise. The use of continuous ECG monitoring seemed to affect the complication rate in Haskell's survey,[34] but not in Van Camp and Peterson's.[37] Thus, one might question the need and practicality of continuous monitoring of most patients. Rubin and colleagues[85] studied risk factors and ventricular arrhythmias in 102 consecutive

CABG surgery patients with normal left ventricular function. Early 24-hour ambulatory ECG monitoring showed a 54-percent prevalence of patients with complex arrhythmias. The 16-month follow-up showed that patients with complex ventricular arrhythmias did not have a higher incidence of cardiac events than did patients without complex arrhythmias. The difficulty of treating complex arrhythmias and the lack of evidence showing that the control of arrhythmias significantly affects outcome were reviewed by Akhtar and coworkers.[58] This review lends little support to continuous monitoring of all patients.

Thus, the arbitrary monitoring by telemetry of all patients does not appear warranted. This is in agreement with a recent review by Greenland and Pomilla,[86] who concluded that only high-risk patients need the telemetric monitoring. They emphasized the point of the high cost of telemetric monitoring in cardiac rehabilitation programs and their associated low yield in improving patient safety. The American College of Cardiology recommends that only high-risk patients, estimated to be between 20 and 25 percent of rehabilitation patients, need to be monitored telemetrically.[70] They define the high-risk patient as follows:

a. **Severely depressed left ventricular function (ejection fraction under 30).**

b. **Resting complex ventricular arrhythmia (Lown type 4 or 5).**

c. **Ventricular arrhythmias appearing or increasing with exercise.**

d. **Decrease in systolic blood pressure with exercise.**

e. **Survivors of sudden cardiac death.**

f. **Patients following myocardial infarction complicated by congestive heart failure, cardiogenic shock, and/or serious ventricular arrhythmias.**

g. **Patients with severe coronary artery disease and marked exercise-induced ischemia.**

h. **Inability to self-monitor heart rate because of physical or intellectual impairment.[70]**

The term "monitoring" in cardiac rehabilitation has often been used synonymously with the act of using telemetric monitoring. A broader, more appropriate, usage of the term would include monitoring by observation and being familiar with the patient's medical history, vital signs, and daily performance including the monitoring of HR, BP, and rating of perceived exertion (RPE). Accurate record keeping is also a part of the monitoring process.

The second aspect of the question as to who needs a formal phase-II outpatient program versus an informal but structured home program is an important issue. Program length and level of monitoring are often dictated by insurance carriers. In some cases, if telemetric monitoring is not used, then coverage is not warranted. Certainly this mentality has helped stimulate the overuse of telemetric monitoring and made the cost of these programs high. On the other hand, only within the past 3 to 5 years has there been sufficient research evidence to speculate on who benefits most from formal rehabilitation programs. Most rehabilitation specialists feel that some type of formal program is necessary, but as to the extent of this program, there is a disparity of opinion. A prime example of this fact was the controversies in cardiology series presented at the thirty-fifth annual meeting of the American College of Cardiology (1986), which included the topic "Formal rehabilitation programs are not ordinarily necessary for patients recently hospitalized for acute myocardial infarction." The protagonist expert felt that only one to three formal sessions were necessary to explain the exercise plan to be used at home and to fulfill other educational needs of the patient on risk factor reduction. The antagonist expert felt a much longer period of time (8 to 12 weeks) was necessary to provide enough education and reinforcement to make behavior and life-style changes. Both experts agreed that too much unnecessary telemetric monitoring is being done in current rehabilitation programs. Just as the term "monitoring" should not be used only in the context of telemetric monitoring, a "formal" program should not infer that everyone is being monitored by telemetry.

As mentioned previously, it is really not known how much of a formal outpatient program is necessary for all patients. It is well established that low-risk MI and CABG patients can make as good an improvement in aerobic capacity by participating in a home program as they can by participating in an outpatient clinic or gymnasium program.[87-90] Also, the safety of such programs has been excellent with low-risk patients. Although equal improvements in aerobic capacity can be found in unsupervised programs as compared with supervised programs, it must be noted that this was not true in one study.[89] There was a bias in most studies in that many home programs had patients using home telephonic monitoring, provided reinforcement by periodic contact through telephone or office visits, and included only patients who completed and adhered to the home exercise program. Data from both cardiac patients and healthy adults show that adherence to home programs, both short- and long-term, is significantly affected by the amount of direct reinforcement.[89, 91-94] Strategies that require patients to keep daily records, have periodic telephone conversations with nurses or exercise specialists, and make periodic visits to their doctor or rehabilitation center improve adherence and program results. Thus, the general consensus is that home programs can be quite successful in improving aerobic capacity and are considered medically safe for low-risk patients. Home programs have been most successful when accompanied by some direct reinforcement strategy.

It appears that everyone entering a cardiac rehabilitation program needs some basic training and then can be triaged into a continued program with the proper amount and type of supervision and monitoring. The first step is to stratify patients as low, moderate, or high risk as suggested by DeBusk and coworkers (Fig. 8–2) and others.[54–57] As mentioned in Chapter 6, this can be determined within 3 to 6 weeks after the event, CABG, or valvular surgery. The patient's hospital course (signs and symptoms, including noninvasive procedures), early entry into a rehabilitation program, and GXT results aid in this stratification process. After

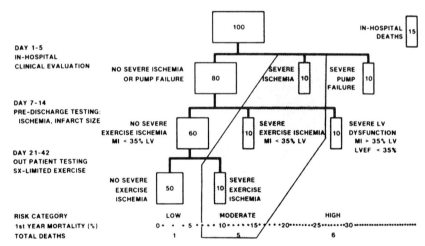

Figure 8–2. Prognostic stratification after acute myocardial infarction as proposed by DeBusk, R.F., et al.[53] The size of each patient subset (numbers in boxes) in the algorithm is approximate and will vary according to the patient population. Stratification of patients into the three main risk categories (low, moderate, and high) is based on the extent of myocardial ischemia (MI) and left ventricular (LV) dysfunction. A variety of clinical observations and tests may be used to detect these abnormalities at various times after acute myocardial infarction. LVEF = left ventricular ejection fraction, SX = symptom. (From DeBusk, et al.: Identification and treatment of the low-risk patient after acute myocardial infarction and coronary-artery bypass graft surgery. **N. Engl. J. Med.** 314:161–166, 1986. Published with permission.)

patients are classified as to their relative risk, the low-risk patients (approximately 50 percent) can be placed into a home program or, once the convalescence period is complete, can be treated like most participants entering an adult fitness program. A longer formal program is recommended for the moderate- and high-risk patients, with both groups receiving telemetric monitoring for up to 6 to 12 weeks. High-risk patients in particular may receive extended participation privileges in a formal program but may not need monitoring by telemetry every day.

The Cardiac Rehabilitation Plan

Based on the evidence and rationale for program results, safety, formal versus informal programs, risk stratification of patients, and types of monitoring, what type of program plan should be recommended for cardiac patients? First a brief review summarizes what has been recommended in the recent past.

In 1980, the American Heart Association, Wisconsin Affiliate, approved recommendations for insurance coverage of supervised cardiac exercise rehabilitation programs from its Exercise and Cardiac Rehabilitation Committee. The committee made the following recommendations for third party carriers:[95]

The response to exercise rehabilitation will vary with the severity of cardiovascular disease, clinical status of the patient, and coexisting medical problems. Components of total rehabilitation also include: patient education, risk factor modification, and individual counseling to increase adherence. The committee suggests a total of 6 to 9 months of rehabilitation as the optimum target for the majority of patients described above. The 9 months may be partitioned between three clinical phases, which are defined as follows:

Phase I Involves immediate inpatient exercise rehabilitation emphasizing patient education and risk factor modification combined with musculoskeletal range of motion, muscle tone, and activity of daily living exercise. This phase lasts approximately 12 to 21 days, and patients who are candidates for a continuing exercise rehabilitation program are referred at this point to Phase II.

Phase II Involves continuing outpatient exercise rehabilitation, usually within a medical center or clinic program. Exercise training includes progressive light to moderate endurance activities with approximately three supervised and monitored exercise sessions per week. Phase II generally extends 2 to 3 months, depending on patient progress. Occasionally, patients may require 4 to 6 months in Phase II. After satisfactory completion of Phase II, patients are

referred to Phase III. The transition to Phase III is based on clinical and physiological responses to exercise.

Phase III Is conducted within community level supervised exercise programs. . . . In Phase III there is continuing emphasis on patient education and risk factor modification combined with participation and prescribed endurance exercise. The objective of this phase is to achieve a state of self-regulated physical activity. A total of 6 months should be available for optimum results.

The committee also described the minimal criteria for a supervised phase-III program.

Cardiovascular exercise programs require the direction of a qualified physician who will assume medical responsibility for the program. For the purposes of rendering emergency medical care, in the absence of a physician, a qualified nurse with the appropriate cardiovascular training must be present. It is recommended that ideally, exercise sessions be directed by physical therapists, occupational therapists, nurses, or allied health personnel with certification in exercise rehabilitation, as specified by the American College of Sports Medicine.[67]

In smaller programs a nurse with cardiovascular training who is also trained in cardiac exercise and rehabilitation would be acceptable. In addition, all persons involved in the supervision of patient exercise must be certified in basic life support according to standards for cardiopulmonary resuscitation and emergency cardiac care.[96–98]

The physical setting for supervised exercise programs may be outside the immediate domain of a medical center. In most instances, a YMCA, a high school or university gymnasium, or Jewish Community Center may be the best available setting. Programs must have emergency equipment and supplies available for potential medical problems.

Patient exercise should be monitored by frequent determination of pulse rate, blood pressure, and work intensity. These data should be maintained in a patient record and reviewed periodically to determine progress in the program.

The elaborately organized cardiac rehabilitation plan developed by North Carolina has been accepted by both professionals and third-party carriers and is recommended for one year.[99] Although the North Carolina Plan is a one-year program, it appears to be administered at a low cost per patient-day in the program. Cost effectiveness has been evident as a result of careful planning to use existing facilities (e.g. university gymnasiums) and to keep telemetric monitoring to a minimum. For example, the Wake Forest University Program accepts phase-II patients into their gymnasium type program immediately after hospital discharge. Only periodic telemetric monitoring is used based on patient status-risk profile.

Fox[100] has suggested a one-year graduated step-down program. The patient attends a supervised program 3 days per week for 6 months, followed by 2 days per week for 3 months and one day per week the final 3 months. The latter approach allows a transitional period in which the patient begins to make the adjustment to a less supervised home or community noncardiac program. The program suggested by Fox also de-emphasizes the need for continuous long-term telemetric monitoring for all patients.

Oldridge proposed the scheme shown in Figure 8–3.* This scheme follows the premise that all patients should receive six ECG-monitored sessions. At that time, patients would be classified as to low, moderate, or high risk and triaged into the program with the proper monitoring and supervision. He then proposes another six sessions whereby moderate-risk patients remain in a supervised setting and are ECG monitored periodically, whereas the low-risk patient can graduate to an unsupervised program with periodic supervision. The high-risk patient would remain in the ECG-monitored, supervised program.

The American College of Sports Medicine (ACSM),[67] the American Association for Cardiovascular and Pulmonary Rehabilitation,[71] the American Heart Association,[101] and the American College of Cardiology[70] do not recommend a definitive plan for cardiac rehabilitation programs. They all favor comprehensive rehabilitation including behavioral and risk factor education programs and not just exercise treatment. They all support outpatient phase-II

---

*(Presented at the Indiana Heart Institute's Symposium on Cardiac Rehabilitation, September 15, 1988, Indianapolis, IN.)

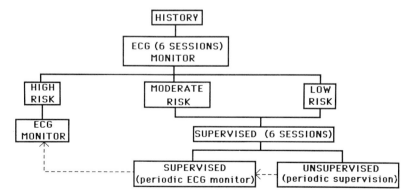

Figure 8–3. Scheme for triaging patients into monitored (telemetry), supervised, or unsupervised cardiac rehabilitation programs. (From Oldridge, N.: Presented at the Indiana Heart Institute's Cardiac Rehabilitation Symposium, September 15, 1988, Indianapolis, IN. Published with permission.)

programs of 6 to 12 weeks in length, with patients being triaged as to their level of risk and need for specific educational programs. It seems reasonable that these professional organizations should work with insurance companies as well as program directors to implement programs that better meet the needs of the patient and that are safe but cost effective.

A note should be made here in regard to the final report of the OHTA on cardiac rehabilitation services.[101a] The OHTA evaluates the safety and effectiveness of new and unestablished medical technologies that are being considered for coverage under Medicare. Their extensive report states, "Data suggest that three weekly one-hour exercise sessions for 12 weeks yield physiological benefits. A consensus opinion suggests that these programs improve the function and symptomatic status of selected patients and are associated with little risk of adverse events." The report generally supports the need of cardiac rehabilitation services as a multi-interventional program but emphasizes that routine ECG monitoring is unnecessary for most patients.

In summary, it appears that most experts recommend medically supervised cardiac rehabilitation programs but have varying opinions on how long and how much monitoring is necessary. The authors feel that a patient stratification plan as described by DeBusk and associates[53] should be encouraged and implemented. If possible, the stratification should include a cardiac rehabilitation scheme as described by Oldridge (see Fig. 8–3). In addition, the authors propose that all patients receive a symptom-limited GXT (SL-GXT) within 3 to 6 weeks of occurrence of their event or surgery to help fine tune the stratification and the exercise prescription. The second stratification period suggested by Oldridge (after 12 sessions) should be coordinated to coincide with the scheduling of the patient's SL-GXT (at 3 to 6 weeks). This provides the physician with more complete information to make a decision on stratification.

The cardiac rehabilitation staff should be aware of escalating health care costs and should listen to the concerns of their professional organizations and insurance carriers. Patients should not be monitored indiscriminately with expensive monitoring devices. The goal should be for patients to progress to nontelemetry and less expensive community types of programs as rapidly as possible. In phase II, the transition could take place for many patients as early as 3 to 6 weeks. High-risk patients may have to be monitored with telemetry for periods longer than 3 months, and supervision may be required indefinitely for some. For patients who start home programs, a plan using periodic telephone calls or revisits to the physician, rehabilitation center, or both seems warranted. Research needs to better define this plan, but adherence to exercise and behavior modification are significantly related to reinforcement.

The concern of many is whether cardiac patients should ever be allowed to train on their own. Again, this is not known, and because coronary disease continues to progress, one can never be certain. As mentioned earlier, many cardiac arrests occur after patients have been participating in the program for more than a year. Thus, supervised programs, whether denoted as cardiac or noncardiac, seem advisable for many patients. If this is not practical, it would be advisable to train with someone who knows cardiopulmonary resuscitation (CPR).

EMERGENCY CARE AND PROCEDURES

Cardiac arrests and other major cardiovascular events are not common in cardiac rehabilitation programs.[37] Even so, an adequate emergency plan is necessary for all programs. In a hospital program in which emergency medical teams are available, the situation is less complex than for the out-of-hospital community setting.

A list of drugs, equipment, and supplies that are recommended for use in cardiac rehabilitation programs can be found in Appendix B, Tables B–1 and B–2. All staff members involved in the conduct of the cardiac rehabilitation program should have current certification in CPR. If possible, someone should be trained in advanced cardiac life support. A plan should be established for handling emergencies. For programs outside a hospital, the following should be taken into account: telephone communications with local physicians, hospitals, paramedics, and emergency medical technicians; physician and nurse coverage; CPR; in the absence of a physician, standing orders for nurses (for example, see Appendix B, Figure B–1); and crowd control and the handling of other patients. The emergency plan should be reviewed and rehearsed on a regular basis.

To handle emergency situations, a minimum of one physician and one nurse or a team of two nurses who are trained in acute cardiac care is preferable. For non–hospital-based programs, telephone monitoring systems would be advantageous for emergency situations. For outdoor programs conducted away from the main headquarters, golf carts equipped with a walkie-talkie or short-wave radio may be necessary for adequate communications. For in-hospital programs, emergency "stat" buttons placed on the walls in the exercise area, classroom, restroom, and locker and shower room take the place of a telephone and can hasten communications to emergency teams.

Other safety features for programs include a minimal 15-minute recovery and surveillance period after completion of the program. As mentioned earlier, 40 to 50 percent of cardiac arrests that occur in cardiac rehabilitation programs occur in the warm-up or cool-down periods.[34, 37] In addition, it is wise not to allow patients to train alone or to leave the exercise area by themselves during class sessions. The causes of exercise-related cardiovascular emergencies, their signs and symptoms, and recommended emergency procedures, as well as precise information on CPR and emergency cardiac care (ECC), are found in American Heart Association publications.[96–98]

A COMPREHENSIVE CARDIAC REHABILITATION PROGRAM

Cardiac rehabilitation programs should incorporate a multidimensional approach. Exercise should be a major part of the program, but the program should also include proper education and counseling regarding the control of risk factors associated with the development of CAD.[67, 70, 71, 101] In addition, particularly in the earlier stages of rehabilitation, many questions and concerns arise and should be answered about medical status, incision care instructions (for surgery, percutaneous transluminal coronary angioplasty [PTCA], and pacemaker patients), medications, dietary restrictions and recommendations, activities of daily living, return to work, individualized exercise prescription, guidelines for sex during convalescence, pulse-taking techniques, realistic expectations of the recovery process, and when to call the doctor. Thus, to best cope with the many needs of the patient, a variety of staff expertise is recommended. Staff members may include a physician (medical director), one or more nurses (educators and cardiac rehabilitation specialists), an exercise physiologist, physical and occupational therapists, a clinical psychologist, an exercise specialist-physical educator, a social worker, a vocational rehabilitation counselor, a dietician, and a pharmacologist.[10, 12, 14, 16, 100, 102] The cardiac rehabilitation nurse should be trained and have experience in a critical coronary care unit. Obviously, small programs are not able to provide many full-time staff members dealing only with cardiac rehabilitation, but a variety of staff members from other departments of the hospital and community could be available for patient or staff consultation and education. More details concerning organization and administration of cardiac rehabilitation programs and staff responsibilities can be found elsewhere.[14, 16, 103–107]

Even though many types of staff members are recommended for a comprehensive cardiac rehabilitation program, their role is only to assist the primary physician in the management of his or her patient. The primary physician can use the information attained through the cardiac rehabilitation staff to help assess patient status and make decisions about management. A strong patient education program further assists the primary physician in reinforcing important health habits and goals.

Exercise Prescription for the Cardiac Patient

Many of the principles of exercise prescription outlined for noncardiac patients in Chapter 7 are appropriate for use with the cardiac patient. The major differences in programs are related to the application of these principles to the patient and how they affect the regulation of frequency, intensity, and duration of training; the rate of progression; and the selection of mode of training. In addition, because of potential medical and hemodynamic problems associated with the diseased heart and the time required for MI and postsurgical patients to heal properly, program modifications and avoidance of certain activities are generally necessary.

Basic Components of a Training Session for the Cardiac Patient

The basic components of a training session for cardiac patients are shown in Table 8–3. In contrast to the healthy adult (see Table 7–1), the cardiac patient may need a longer warm-up period and may require modifications of the endurance (aerobic) phase of the session, depending on medical status and phase of training.

Table 8–3. Components of a Training Session for Cardiac Patients

Component	Duration (min)	Phase
Warm-up	15–20	I
	10–15	II, III
Muscular conditioning	10–20	II, III
Aerobic exercise	5–20	I
	20–60	II
	30–60	III
Cool-down	10	I, II, III

As a result of the low state of fitness and the adverse effects of bed rest and surgery on the musculoskeletal systems of the cardiac patient, the need for special stretching and joint readiness is apparent. Thus, warm-up usually takes longer during phases I and II. During phase III, the warm-up period for the cardiac patient may be similar to that of the normal adult.

Once patients enter the phase-II program, they are generally ready for low-level muscle-conditioning activities (3 to 4 weeks after MI or surgery). Emphasis is placed on dynamic and rhythmical exercise that does not impede normal breathing. Activities could include light calisthenics, light weight training (initially 1- to 5-pound weights), and various other low-resistance apparatus. More specific recommendations for weight training and progression in training are discussed under phase-II programs.

The aerobic phase of training starts with a short ambulation period, which is performed two to three times daily. The phase-I patient is generally weak and cannot tolerate long bouts of physical activity. Thus, a program of shorter bouts with greater frequency is the best initial approach. A second daily training period would also be recommended to the patient after discharge and before returning to work. More specific details about suggested duration of activity and rate of progression are discussed under the various phases of the program. The 300 kcal minimum daily dosage (1,000 kcal/week) prescribed for normal adults is also recommended for the patient. Because cardiac patients generally train at lower intensities, they require training of longer duration, greater frequency, or both to reach this goal. In addition, it usually takes the cardiac patient 3 to 6 months longer than the healthy adult to reach this goal.[65, 72] Because of the lower intensity factor (kcal/min), the minimal duration of a training session during phases II and III may be 10 to 15 minutes longer for the cardiac patient than for the normal adult.

Rate of Progression in Training

The initial training load is lower and the rate of progression slower in the cardiac patient than in the healthy adult. Figure 8–4 shows the general progression of cardiac and noncardiac groups. The figure shows average estimates of progression for each group, progression being dependent on the participant's age, level of fitness, and health status. As discussed in Chapter 7 (see Fig. 7–4), normal participants generally start at 150 to 200 kcal per exercise session and progress to the 300 kcal level by 8 to 12 weeks.

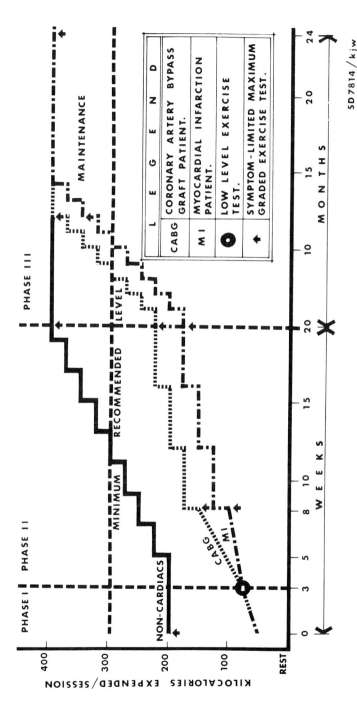

Figure 8–4. Comparison of progression of training among normal healthy adults, coronary artery bypass graft (CABG) surgery patients, and myocardial infarction (MI) patients. (From Pollock, M.L., et al.: Exercise prescription for rehabilitation of the cardiac patient. In Pollock, M.L., and Schmidt, D.H. (eds.): **Heart Disease and Rehabilitation**, 2nd Ed. New York, Churchill Livingstone, Inc., 1986, pp. 477–516. Reprinted with permission.)

In contrast, the cardiac patient begins (phase I) at a level below 50 kcal per session[108] and requires several weeks to months longer to reach the 300 kcal level.[65] The slightly slower rate of progression for the MI patient, as compared with the CABG patient, results from a reluctance to have the patient progress very rapidly until 4 to 6 weeks after the MI. Generally, by 4 to 6 weeks, depending on the size of infarct, scar tissue has adequately developed on the heart, and the healing process is nearly complete.[109] After this time, training intensity can increase more rapidly, and the patient progresses at a faster rate. During the first 4 to 6 weeks of recovery, or if the risk status is determined earlier and the patient is put in a low-risk category, the MI patient is exercised more conservatively than the CABG patient. Surgical patients with perioperative infarcts are progressed like MI patients. It also takes approximately 6 weeks for the sternum to heal fully after surgery; thus, a 20- to 25-pound lifting restriction is recommended (only 10 pounds over the head). In addition, during this healing period, activities that place undue pressure on the sternum should be avoided. During the inpatient phase, activities are of a low intensity and a short to moderate duration and are designed to offset problems associated with bed rest.

The suggested rates and levels of progression for cardiac and noncardiac groups shown in Figure 8–4 are realistic estimates. Whether or not patients can progress faster without added risk of an event is not known at this time. Research by DeBusk and colleagues[74] and Ehsani and colleagues[59] suggests that during the first 12 weeks of rehabilitation, low-risk patients can progress at a rate faster than that shown in Figure 8–4, but more research is necessary to clarify this question. Experts agree that until patients are clearly determined to be at low risk and have completed their convalescence period, the slower, conservative approach seems appropriate.

The progression in Figure 8–4 stops at the 300 to 400 kcal level per exercise session and does not take into account further increases (additional kilocaloric expenditure) in training or changes in intensity. For example, noncardiac participants entering a jogging program usually begin with short periods of jogging interspersed with equal distances of walking. As they progress, they will walk less and jog more. As they adapt, their total time and distance may also increase. An important point here is that the participant can reach the 300 kcal level fairly rapidly and before reaching the maintenance phase of a training program.

As with noncardiac participants, the exercise prescription for cardiac patients involves three stages of progression: starter, slow to moderate progression, and maintenance. The starter phase is conducted at a low intensity and includes joint readiness, stretching and light calisthenics, and low-level aerobic activities.The purpose of this stage of the program is to introduce the participant to exercise at a low level and to allow the patient the time to adapt properly to the initial rigors of training. During this phase, the patient progresses by increasing frequency and duration of training first, then intensity. If this phase is properly introduced, the participant experiences a minimum of muscle soreness and avoids debilitating injuries or discomfort.

The slow progression phase differs from the starter phase in that the participant progresses at a more rapid rate. During this stage of training, the duration or intensity of training, or both, are increased consistently every one to four weeks. How well the exerciser adapts to the present level of training dictates the frequency and magnitude of progression. As a general rule, older more fragile and less fit participants require longer to adapt and to progress in a training regimen.[110–114]

A healthy adult usually reaches the maintenance stage of training after 6 to 12 months. At this stage, the participant has attained a satisfactory level of fitness and may no longer be interested in increasing the training load; further development is minimal, and the emphasis of the program becomes that of maintaining fitness rather than of seeking further development. Progression for the cardiac patient is slower and may take from 6 to 18 months longer than for noncardiac subjects. Kavanagh and associates[72] have shown that younger cardiac patients improve their aerobic capacity for up to 2 years.

Table 8–4 lists guidelines for exercise prescription for cardiac patients. Phases I and II of these guidelines show the slower progression and intensity levels for cardiac patients in their earlier stages of training and coincide with the kilocaloric progression shown in Figure 8–4. As the patient reaches phase III, the program begins to be comparable with the general guidelines recommended for noncardiac participants. The big difference in the exercise prescription guidelines for the phase-III cardiac patient versus the noncardiac participant would be the greater frequency (4 to 5 days per week) and duration (30 to 60 minutes) of training for cardiac patients needed to compensate for their lower training intensity. Further, many cardiac patients will never be capable of moderate-to high-intensity training; thus, their program would always include a greater frequency and duration of training. A phase-IV program is referred to as a long-term maintenance program and is often unsupervised. Low-risk patients could graduate directly to an

Table 8-4. Guidelines for Exercise Prescription for Cardiac Patients as Compared with Healthy Adults

Prescription	Phase I (Inpatient Program)	Phase II (Discharge to 3 Months)	Phase III, IV* (After 3 Months)	Healthy Adults
Frequency	2–3 times/day	1–2 times/day	3–5 times/wk	3–5 times/wk
Intensity	MI: RHR + 20 CABG: RHR + 20	MI: RHR + 20*†, RPE 13 CABG: RHR + 20*†, RPE 13	60–85% HRmax reserve	60–85% HRmax reserve
Duration	MI: 5–20 min CABG: 10–20 min	MI: 20–60 min CABG: 20–60 min	30–60 min	20–60 min
Mode–activity	ROM, TDM, bike, 1 flight of stairs	ROM, TDM (walk, walk-jog), bike, arm erg, cal, Wt Tr	Walk, bike, jog, swim, cal, Wt Tr, endurance sports	Walk, jog, run, bike, swim, endurance sports, cal, Wt Tr

MI = myocardial infarction patient; CABG = coronary artery bypass graft surgery patient; HR = heart rate (beats/min); RHR = standing resting HR; ROM = range of motion exercise; TDM = treadmill; arm erg = arm ergometer; cal = calisthenics; Wt Tr = weight training; RPE = rating of perceived exertion.

*Sometimes the term Phase IV is used to denote long-term maintenance programs for cardiac patients and can be unsupervised.

†3 to 6 weeks after surgery or MI, a symptom-limited exercise test is recommended. Heart rate intensity is then based on 60 to 70 percent of maximal heart rate reserve.

(From Pollock, M. L., et al.: Exercise prescription for rehabilitation. In Pollock, M. L., and Schmidt, D. H. (eds.): **Heart Disease and Rehabilitation,** 2nd Ed. New York, Churchill Livingstone, 1986, pp. 477–516.)

adult fitness program as soon as they are through the convalescence period (after approximately 6 weeks). More specific aspects of exercise prescription for cardiac patients are described under the various phases of rehabilitation.

The starter program has a similar purpose for both cardiac and noncardiac participants. The starter program for the cardiac patient involves the first 4 to 6 weeks of training and encompasses phase I and the first part of phase II. As mentioned previously for MI patients, the scar tissue has developed and other aspects of the healing process are completed by this time. For the surgery patient, it takes about 6 to 8 weeks for the sternum to heal, for hemoglobin to approach normal, and for other aspects related to surgery to normalize. For example, data collected 2 weeks after CABG showed hemoglobin and hematocrit values to be 11 g and 33 percent, respectively. These values were normalized by 8 weeks after surgery.[76]

At 3 to 6 weeks after MI or CABG surgery, an SL-GXT is recommended. The purpose of the test is to evaluate medical status (risk stratification) and improvement (or regression) resulting from the cardiac rehabilitation program and to refine the exercise prescription. If the test results are unremarkable, then a faster rate of progression in training may begin.

INPATIENT CARDIAC REHABILITATION—PHASE I

The MI and postoperative CABG patients present with unique sets of physiological, medical, and psychological characteristics that affect their readiness to begin the exercise portion of the rehabilitation program safely. Thorough medical, nursing, and physical therapy assessments, along with review of medical records (admission, operative, and progress notes and reports from diagnostic studies such as cardiac catheterization, electrophysiology, echocardiography, and nuclear tests), form the basis for appropriate exercise prescription.

For the surgical inpatient, an important aspect of the physical assessment is the condition of the sternum and the incisions. Sternal instability, as evidenced by clicking, grating, or movement on careful palpation, should be promptly reported to the physician. When this occurs (in approximately 4 to 5 percent of surgery patients),[66] upper extremity and trunk ROM exercise should be avoided. Suspected wound infection should be thoroughly evaluated, and the appropriate treatment and isolation precautions should be instituted. Vital signs should be carefully monitored. The use of elastic stockings may be indicated to treat edema at the site of the saphenous vein incision.

The accurate differentiation of normal postoperative chest discomfort from angina pectoris or other signs and symptoms of impending complications is critical to safe exercise prescription. Chest discomfort, whether incisional or chest wall, must be clearly distinguished from angina, since unstable angina is a contraindication to exercise.

Patients who have undergone surgery may exhibit alterations of the blood, including hypovolemia and decreased hemoglobin concentration.[76] These are caused by blood loss during the surgical procedure and may help to explain in part the postoperative tachycardia and fatigue commonly experienced by surgery patients.

Pulmonary function is diminished after surgery as a result of the combined effects of anesthesia, bed rest, and a reluctance to breathe deeply because of sternal discomfort. For the patient with associated pulmonary disease and a previously compromised oxygen exchange system, a decrease in pulmonary ventilation could be significant. The program of progressive activity and early ambulation serves to minimize pulmonary complications in both the MI and postoperative patient.

The medication regimen of patients often includes a variety of agents, which may or may not directly affect exercise performance or prescription. The administration of drugs should be timed to coincide with planned activity periods if they protect or can enhance the exercise tolerance of that patient.

Mental status is an important factor to consider in patient care and can affect the patient's readiness to participate in the progressive activity program. The cardiac rehabilitation team must be sensitive to the patient's psychological adjustment to the surgical experience or MI event itself, to a changed body image, and to his or her attitude of hopefulness or helplessness. Coping skills are uniquely challenged through this life-threatening event. If time permits, the patient and his or her family should receive preoperative teaching to assist them in developing realistic expectations of the postoperative course, including ROM exercise and the progressive activity regimen.

The inpatient cardiac rehabilitation program is intended to help alleviate problems associated with bed rest, reduce anxiety and depression, develop the patient's confidence, provide education regarding modification of risk factors, increase the chance of earlier hospital discharge and return to work, provide surveillance for optimal patient management, and provide the basis for a home program.[65, 67, 101, 115]

Patients enter the cardiac rehabilitation program on referral of their cardiac surgeon or primary physician and then are assessed by the program medical director and rehabilitation team. In general, the postoperative patient who is clinically stable and infection free may safely begin the progressive activity portion of the inpatient cardiac rehabilitation program.

The inpatient cardiac rehabilitation program should begin as soon as the patient is considered stable. Depending on the type of patient, it is usually within 2 to 4 days for an uncomplicated MI patient and one to two days for a postsurgical patient.[65] The following contraindications to exercise have been used as guidelines for the inpatient program.[65, 116] The suggested contraindications to exercise have been modified for inpatients from recommendations of the ACSM:[67]

A. Absolute Contraindications
 1. Patients on bed rest with motion restrictions
 2. Prolonged or unstable angina pectoris
 3. Recent acute MI and unstable condition
 4. Resting diastolic BP over 110 mmHg (ACSM prefers a 100 mmHg limit) or resting systolic BP over 200 mmHg
 5. Inappropriate BP response: orthostatic or exercise-induced and patient symptomatic. ACSM adds a 20 mmHg or more drop in systolic BP from the patient's average level, which cannot be explained by medications
 6. Severe atrial or ventricular dysrhythmias
 7. Second- or third-degree heart block
 8. Recent embolism, either systemic or pulmonary
 9. Thrombophlebitis
 10. Dissecting aneurysm
 11. Fever greater than 100°F; for the patient in the critical care area, 102°F
 12. Excessive sternal movement—contraindication for upper extremity and trunk ROM exercises
 13. Uncompensated heart failure
 14. Active pericarditis (primary) or myocarditis
 15. Severe aortic stenosis (> 50 mmHg gradient) and idiopathic hypertrophic subaortic stenosis
 16. Acute systemic illness
B. Relative Contraindications
 1. Resting diastolic BP over 100 mmHg or resting systolic BP over 180 mmHg
 2. Inappropriate increase in BP with exercise
 3. Hypotension (see subsequent comments)
 4. Moderate aortic stenosis (25 to 50 mmHg gradient)

5. Compensated heart failure
6. Significant emotional stress
7. Pericarditis associated with myocardial revascularization surgery
8. Resting S-T–segment depression (> 3 mm)
9. Uncontrolled diabetes
10. Neuromuscular, musculoskeletal, or arthritic disorders that would prevent activity
11. Excessive incisional drainage
12. Sinus tachycardia greater than 120 beats/min at rest
13. New ECG changes after surgery or MI that are indicative or suggestive of fresh infarct
14. Ventricular aneurysm
15. Symptomatic anemia (hematocrit < 30 percent)

C. Conditions Requiring Special Consideration and/or Precautions
    1. Conduction disturbances
       a. Left bundle-branch block
       b. Wolff-Parkinson-White syndrome
       c. Lown-Ganong-Levine syndrome
       d. Bifascicular block
    2. Controlled dysrhythmias
    3. Fixed-rate pacemaker
    4. Mitral valve prolapse
    5. Angina pectoris and other manifestations of coronary insufficiency
    6. Electrolyte disturbance
    7. Cyanotic heart disease
    8. Marked obesity (20 percent above desirable body weight)
    9. Renal, hepatic, and other metabolic insufficiency
    10. Moderate to severe pulmonary disease
    11. Intermittent claudication

Some of the previous contraindications may seem somewhat vague and arbitrary. The reason for this is that it is difficult to get a consensus on many of the conditions considered. In most cases, clinical judgment takes precedence, and this may vary greatly among physicians. For example, a resting S-T–segment depression of 3 mm or greater is the consensus of experts, but who is to say that 2 or 4 mm may be a better criterion? Another vague issue is what constitutes dangerous dysrhythmias. Clinical judgment about what individual medical directors and referring physicians are comfortable with is important. In addition, the competence of the staff and the extent of supervision, as well as whether the patient is being monitored for ECG rhythm, would make a difference. In many institutions, the monitored inpatient program is used in conjunction with other methods to evaluate drug therapy for dys-rhythmias. In this situation, even ventricular tachycardia (VT) may not be an absolute contraindication to exercise. In addition, patient records, including physical and mental status and medications, are reviewed by the medical director of the cardiac rehabilitation program and by the attending physician before acceptance into the program. An example of an inpatient medical evaluation form can be found in Appendix B, Figure B–2.

Once the patient is accepted into the program, the physical activity and education program schedule guidelines listed in Table 8–5 for MI patients and in Table 8–6 for open heart surgery patients are initiated. The various exercises and stages of progression for the MI patient have been modified from the program outlined by Wenger.[115] The guidelines are designed in three parts: (1) the activity program when the cardiac rehabilitation staff is supervising the patient; (2) the ward activity when the primary nurse or patient supervises the program; and (3) patient education. These guidelines were designed so that at step 6 of the MI protocol and step 5 of the surgery protocol, the patient goes to an inpatient exercise center once a day for the activity part of the program.[117] This is discussed further later, but if treadmills and stationary cycles are not available, the program would be continued in the patient's room and adjacent ward.

Generally, the patient progresses one step each day. The rate of progression is individualized and depends on how successfully the patient adapts to each stage of the program. The following guidelines are used either to modify (reduce) or to terminate the exercise routine.[65, 67]

1. Fatigue
2. Failure of the monitoring equipment
3. Lightheadedness, confusion, ataxia, pallor, cyanosis, dyspnea, nausea, or any peripheral circulatory insufficiency
4. Onset of angina with exercise
5. Symptomatic supraventricular tachycardia
6. S-T–segment displacement ($\geq$ 3 mm horizontal or down-sloping from rest)
7. Ventricular tachycardia (3 or more consecutive premature ventricular contractions [PVCs])
8. Exercise-induced left or right bundle-branch block
9. Onset of second- and third-degree heart block
10. R on T (PVC)
11. Frequent unifocal PVCs (> 10/min, ACSM states > 30 percent of complexes)
12. Frequent multifocal PVCs (> 4/min, ACSM states 30 percent of complexes)

Table 8–5. Inpatient Physical Activity and Education Program Schedule and Guidelines for Myocardial Infarction Patients

Cardiac Rehabilitation/Physical Therapy	Ward Activity*	Patient Education
Step 1, 1.5 METs *Ward TX:* Passive ROM to major joints, active ankle exercises, 5 repetitions; deep breathing (supine) twice a day.	Bed rest May feed self	Orient to CCU. Orient to exercise component of rehabilitation program
Step 2, 1.5 METs *Ward TX:* Active-assistive ROM to major muscle groups, active ankle exercises, 5 repetitions; deep breathing (supine/sitting) twice a day.	Feed self Partial morning care (washing hands and face, brushing teeth in bed) Bedside commode	Answer patient and family questions regarding progress, procedures, reason for activity limitation Explain RPE scale
Step 3, 1.5 METs *Ward TX:* Active ROM to major muscle groups, active ankle exercises, 5 repetitions; deep breathing (sitting) twice a day.	Begin sitting in chair for short periods as tolerated 2 times a day Bathe self Bedside commode	
Step 4, 1.5 METs *Ward TX:* Active exercises: shoulder flexion and abduction; elbow flexion; hip flexion; knee extension; toe raises; ankle exercises; 5 repetitions; deep breathing (standing) twice a day.	Bathroom privileges Sit in chair 3 times a day Up in chair for meals Bathe self, dress, comb hair (sitting)	
Step 5, 1.5–2 METs *Ward TX:* Active exercises: shoulder flexion, abduction, and circumduction; elbow flexion; trunk lateral flexion; hip flexion and abduction; knee extension; toe raises; ankle exercises; 5 repetitions (standing); twice a day. Monitored ambulation of 100–200 ft, twice a day, with physician approval.	Bathroom privileges Up as tolerated in room Stand at sink to shave and comb hair Bathe self and dress Up in chair as tolerated	Answer patient and family questions Orient to ICCU phase of recovery Present discharge booklet and other printed material (AHA) Encourage patient and family to attend group classes or do 1:1 sessions

Step 6, 1.5–2 METs
Ward TX: Standing; Exercises outlined in step 5, 5–10 repetitions; once daily. Monitored ambulation for 5 min (440 ft).
Exercise Center: Transport to IEC for monitored ROM/strengthening exercises from step 5, 5–10 repetitions; leg stretching (posterior thigh muscles, gastrocnemius), 10 repetitions; treadmill and/or bicycle 5 min; and stair climbing (2–4 stairs) with physician approval.

Continue ward activity from step 5
Increase ambulation up to 1 lap† (440 ft) with assistance if appropriate, two times per day
Walk short distance in hall (room and quad areas) as tolerated

Instruction in pulse taking and rationale
Explain value of exercise
Present T-shirt and activity log
Begin discharge instructions with patient and family when appropriate
Encourage group class attendance or offer 1:1 as needed

Step 7, 1.5–2.5 METs
Ward TX: Standing; Exercises from step 5 with 1 lb weight each extremity, 5–10 repetitions; once daily. Monitored ambulation for 5–10 min (440–1,000 ft)
Exercise Center: Transport to IEC for monitored ROM/strengthening exercises from step 6 with 1 lb weight each extremity, 5–10 repetitions; leg stretching, 10 repetitions; treadmill and/or bicycle 5–10 min; and stair climbing (4–8 stairs).

Continue ward activity from step 6
Sit up in chair most of the day
Increase ambulation up to 3 laps† (up to 1,100 ft) daily

Step 8, 1.5–2.5 METs
Ward TX: Standing; Exercises from step 5 with 1 lb weight each extremity, 10 repetitions; once daily. Monitored ambulation for 10 min (up to 1,980 ft) if appropriate.
Exercise Center: Ambulate to IEC for monitored ROM/strengthening exercises from step 6 with 1 lb weight each extremity, 10 repetitions; leg stretching, 10 repetitions; treadmill and/or bicycle 10–20 min; and stair climbing (10–12 stairs).

Continue ward activity from step 7
Increase ambulation up to 5 laps† (up to 1,980 ft) daily

Give instruction in home exercise program
Initiate referral to phase II if appropriate
Explain PDGXT and upper-limit heart rate

Table continued on following page

Table 8–5. Inpatient Physical Activity and Education Program Schedule and Guidelines for Myocardial Infarction Patients *Continued*

Cardiac Rehabilitation/Physical Therapy	Ward Activity*	Patient Education
Step 9, 1.5–2.5 METs *Ward TX:* Standing: Exercises from step 5 with 2 lb weight each extremity, 10 repetitions; once daily. Monitored ambulation if appropriate. *Exercise Center:* Ambulate to IEC for monitored ROM/strengthening exercises from step 6 with 2 lb weight each extremity, 10 repetitions; leg stretching, 10 repetitions; treadmill and/or bicycle 20–25 min; and stair climbing (12–14 stairs).	Up as tolerated in room and quad area Increase ambulation to 6 laps† (up to 2,640 ft) daily	
Step 10, 1.5–3 METs *Ward TX:* Exercises from step 5 with 2 lb weight each extremity, 10 repetitions; once daily. Monitored ambulation if appropriate. *Exercise Center:* Ambulate to IEC for monitored ROM/strengthening exercises from step 6 with 2 lb weight each extremity, 10 repetitions; leg stretching, 10 repetitions; treadmill and/or bicycle 25–30 min; and stair climbing (14–15 stairs).	Up as tolerated in room and quad area Increase ambulation up to 8 laps† (up to 3,300 ft) daily	

Heart rates, blood pressures, and comments are recorded on the Inpatient Data Record or Exercise Log.
ROM = range of motion; RPE = rating of perceived exertion; CCU = cardiac care unit; AHA = American Heart Association; IEC = inpatient exercise center; ICCU = intensive cardiac care unit; PDGXT = predischarge graded exercise test.
*Activities performed alone, with family, or with primary nurse.
†Lap around ICCU at Mount Sinai Medical Center, Milwaukee = distance of approximately 424 feet.
(From the Cardiac Rehabilitation Program, Cardiovascular Disease Section, Mount Sinai Medical Center, Milwaukee, WI. Published with permission.)

13. Couplets ($>$ 2 /min)

14. Increase in HR over 20 beats/min above standing resting HR for both MI and CABG surgery patients

15. Inappropriate drop in resting (orthostatic) and exercise (no more than 10 mmHg drop) systolic BP. See comments that follow

16. Excessive BP rise (systolic $\geq$ 220 or diastolic $\geq$ 110 mmHg)

17. Inappropriate bradycardia (drop in heart rate $\geq$ 10 beats/min) with increase or no change in work load

Early Phase-I Program

The early part of the phase-I program is conducted in the critical care units and the intermediate critical care areas. As mentioned earlier, the program begins in the critical care unit as soon as the patient is considered stable. Although the guidelines listed in Tables 8–5 and 8–6 are geared for the MI and CABG surgery patients, they can be adapted for use with patients having varied diagnoses and symptoms. Patients who appear to be at a higher risk or who are symptomatic with exercise are treated more conservatively. For example, patients who develop angina or severe dysrhythmia with exercise usually train at an HR below the level at which signs or symptoms occur. Special precautions or management techniques used for patients with intermittent claudication, severe dysrhythmia, angina pectoris, arthritis, hypertension, excess fat, pacemakers, pulmonary disease, other surgical procedures (valve, septum, or aneurysm repair), perioperative MIs, and PTCA are discussed later.

The programs for MI and CABG surgery patients differ in the following ways:

1. Surgical patients begin the program sooner and usually ambulate on the first treatment day.

2. Surgical patients progress at a slightly higher intensity (approximately 0.5 mph, 0.5 to 1 MET), and duration of ambulation is more accelerated.

3. Upper extremity ROM exercise is emphasized more with the surgical patient.

Although cardiac rehabilitation programs have similar components, they often differ in their execution. Most inpatient programs include ROM exercise, ambulation, stationary cycling, and stair-climbing activities. One exception is the reluctance of some surgeons to allow surgical patients to do upper extremity ROM activities. Since 1977, Mount Sinai Medical Center in Milwaukee, Wisconsin, has used active ROM exercise with surgical patients.

Table 8-6. Inpatient Physical Activity and Education Program Schedule and Guidelines for Open Heart Surgery Patients

Cardiac Rehabilitation/Physical Therapy	Ward Activity*	Patient Education
Step 1, 1.5 METs		
am Ward TX: Sitting with feet supported: Active-assistive to active ROM to major muscle groups, active ankle scapular elevation/depression, retraction/protraction, 3–5 repetitions; deep breathing. Monitored ambulation of 100 ft as tolerated.	Begin sitting in chair (when stable) several times a day for 10–30 min May ambulate 100–200 ft with assistance, 1–2 times daily	Orient to CVICU Reinforce purpose of physical therapy and deep breathing exercises Orient to exercise component of rehabilitation program Answer patient and family questions regarding progress
pm Ward TX: Sitting with feet supported: Active ROM to major muscle groups, 5 repetitions; deep breathing. Monitored ambulation of 100–200 ft with assistance as tolerated.		
Step 2, 1.5 METs		
Ward TX: Sitting: Repeat exercises from step 1 and increase repetitions to 5–10; deep breathing twice a day. Monitored ambulation of 200 ft with assistance as tolerated (stress correct posture) twice a day.	Continue activities from step 1	Continue above
Step 3, 1.5–2 METs		
Ward TX: Standing: Begin active upper-extremity and trunk exercise bilaterally without resistance (shoulder flexion, abduction, internal/external rotation, hyperextension, circumduction backward; elbow flexion; trunk lateral flexion and rotation; knee extension (if appropriate); ankle exercises; 5–10 repetitions; twice a day. Monitored ambulation of 300 ft twice a day.	Increase ambulation to 300 ft or approximately 3 corridor lengths at slow pace with assistance twice a day	Begin pulse-taking instruction when appropriate and explain RPE scale Answer questions of patient and family Reorient patient and family to ICUU Encourage family attendance at group classes
Step 4, 1.5–2 METs		
Ward TX: Standing: Active exercises from step 3, 10–15 repetitions; twice a day. Monitored ambulation of 424 ft twice a day.	Increase ambulation to 1 lap at slow pace with assistance twice a day	
Step 5, 1.2–2.5 METs		
Ward TX: Standing: Active exercises from step 3, 15 repetitions; once daily. Monitored ambulation for 5–10 min (424–848 ft) as tolerated. *Exercise Center:* Walk to IEC for monitored ROM/strengthening exercises from step 3, 15 repetitions; leg stretching (posterior thigh muscles, gastrocnemius), 10 repetitions; treadmill or bicycle 5–10 min (refer to treadmill/bicycle protocol) with physician approval.	Increase ambulation up to 3 laps (up to 1,320 ft) daily as tolerated Begin participating in daily ADL and personal care as tolerated Encourage chair sitting with legs crossed	Orient to IEC Continue instruction in pulse taking and use of RPE scale Explain value of exercise Present T-shirt and activity log

Step 6, 1.5–2.5 METs

Ward TX: Standing: Active exercises from step 3 with 1 lb weight each upper extremity, 15 repetitions; once daily. Monitored ambulation for 10–15 min (up to 1,980 ft) if appropriate.

Exercise Center: Walk to IEC for monitored ROM/strengthening exercises from step 5 with 1 lb weight each upper extremity, 15 repetitions; leg stretching, 10 repetitions; treadmill and/or bicycle 15–20 min; and stair climbing (6–12 stairs) with assistance.

Increase ambulation up to 5 laps (up to 1,980 ft) daily
Encourage independence in ADL
Encourage chair sitting with legs elevated

Give discharge booklet and general discharge instructions to patient and family
Encourage group class attendance
Individual instruction by physical therapist, nutritionist, pharmacist

Step 7, 2–3 METs

Ward TX: Standing: Active exercises from step 3 with 1 lb weight each upper extremity, 15 repetitions; once daily. Monitored ambulation for 15–20 min (up to 3,300 ft) if appropriate.

Exercise Center: Walk to IEC for monitored ROM/strengthening exercises from step 5 with 1 lb weight each upper extremity, 15 repetitions; leg stretching, 10 repetitions; treadmill and/or bicycle 20–30 min; and stair climbing (up to 14 stairs) with assistance.

Continue activities from step 6
Increase ambulation up to 8 laps (up to 3,300 ft) daily

Discuss and initiate referral to phase II program if appropriate
Reinforce prior teaching
Give instruction in home exercise program
Explain PDGXT and upper-limit heart rate

Step 8, 2–3 METs

Ward TX: Standing: Exercises from step 3 with 2 lb weight each upper extremity, 15 repetitions; once daily. Monitored ambulation if appropriate.

Exercise Center: Walk to IEC for monitored ROM/strengthening exercise from step 5 with 2 lb weight each upper extremity; 15 repetitions; leg stretching, 10 repetitions; treadmill and/or bicycle 20–30 min; and stair climbing (up to 16 stairs).

Continue activities from step 7
Increase ambulation up to 9 laps (up to 3,746 ft) daily

Reinforce prior teaching

Table continued on following page

Table 8–6. Inpatient Physical Activity and Education Program Schedule and Guidelines for Open Heart Surgery Patients *Continued*

Cardiac Rehabilitation/Physical Therapy	Ward Activity*	Patient Education

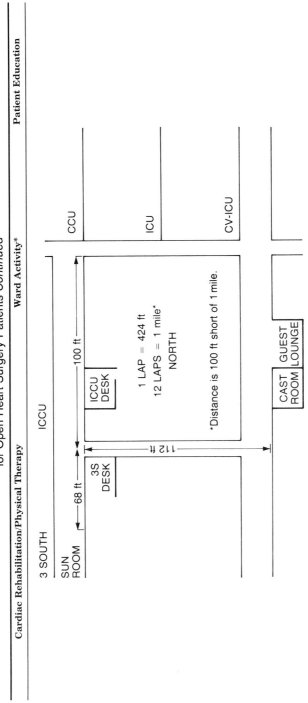

Heart rates, blood pressures, and comments are recorded on the Inpatient Data Record or Exercise log.
TX = treatment; ROM = range of motion; CVICU = cardiovascular intensive care unit; RPE = rating of perceived exertion; ICCU = intensive coronary care unit; IEC = Inpatient Exercise Center; ADL = activities of daily living; PDGXT = predischarge graded exercise test.
*Activities performed alone, with family, or with primary nurse.
†Lap around ICCU at Mount Sinai Medical Center, Milwaukee = distance of approximately 424 feet.
(From the Cardiac Rehabilitation Program, Cardiovascular Disease Section, Mount Sinai Medical Center, Milwaukee, WI. Published with permission.)

Their experience shows that approximately 95 percent of surgical patients can do upper extremity ROM exercises with no overt problems.[65, 66, 108] As mentioned earlier, patients who experience sternal movement or who have postsurgical sternal wound complications do not perform these exercises.

Why is upper extremity ROM exercise important in the early recovery from open heart surgery? Significant soft tissue and bone damage of the chest wall and of the anterior and superior regions of the arms and shoulders occurs during surgery. If these areas (joints, muscles, and other supporting tissues) are not taken through a full ROM, adhesions develop, and musculature becomes weaker and may foreshorten. Patients also favor these areas, which accentuates later problems of poor posture and difficulties in attaining their previous strength and full ROM. In addition, exercise increases blood flow to the damaged area and thus should accelerate tissue repair. Therefore, it appears that the longer the delay in receiving upper-extremity ROM exercise, the more difficult it is for the open heart surgery patient to reach full recovery.

Tables 8–5 and 8–6 outline the exercise prescription (ROM exercises, aerobic phase, and stair climbing) and patient education program for inpatient cardiac rehabilitation. The guidelines listed under the column entitled "Cardiac Rehabilitation/Physical Therapy" are performed by the cardiac rehabilitation staff. Ideally, the formal program takes place twice a day. Most treatments are performed in the patient's room or ward, but in the program outlined in Tables 8–5 and 8–6, patients begin receiving treatments once a day in an inpatient exercise center (step 6 for MI and step 5 for CABG surgery patients). The diagram shown as a part of Table 8–6 illustrates how the cardiac ward can be measured for distance and used to provide a more precise progression in training.

Activities listed under "Ward Activity" are generally carried out by the patient under the supervision of the primary care nurse. As the patient becomes stronger and is considered a low risk, much of the ambulation part of the program can be carried out by the patient with minimal supervision. The patient education program can be conducted by specialized educators, the primary nurse, or some combination thereof.[118]

The education program usually involves both individual and group sessions. For the CABG patient, it can include presurgery assessment and instructions. The presurgery instructions contain an evaluation of ROM and strength. Knowing patient limitations and weaknesses before surgery often helps in the postsurgical assessment and recommendation of the exercise routine. If possible, the spouse is included in the education process. The main educational topics that can be covered include anatomy and physiology, risk factors and the importance of intervention, diet, pharmacology, stress reduction, return to sexual activity, exercise, getting ready to go home, and a general question and answer period. Special education booklets, films, and filmstrips have been developed for the MI and CABG patients and are available through several sources.[119–126]

The ROM exercises used in the cardiovascular intensive care unit for surgical patients typically include shoulder flexion, abduction, and internal and external rotation; elbow flexion; hip flexion, abduction, and internal and external rotation; and ankle plantar and dorsal flexion, inversion, and eversion.[108] The protocol for MI patients in the critical care unit involves most of the same exercises as for surgical patients, excluding hip abduction and lower extremity internal and external rotation.

Before initiating the ROM exercises, each patient is evaluated by a physical therapist (exercise specialist). Patient position (lying, sitting, or standing) and type of exercise vary, depending upon the results of the evaluation. Tables 8–5 and 8–6 provide guidelines for the patients during this stage of their rehabilitation. Note the differences in patient position and progression of MI and surgical patients. Once patients leave the critical care areas, the ROM exercises described later in this chapter for surgical patients and for medical patients are used. Upper extremity ROM exercise with sticks or canes has been helpful with surgical patients. Initially, five repetitions of each exercise are performed with a progression to ten to 15 repetitions. When patients can comfortably execute ten to 15 repetitions, 1- to 3-pound wrist weights can be added progressively.

Ambulatory activity and progression are described in Tables 8–5 and 8–6. Because hypotension is one of the major medical problems associated with the early treatment of patients,[66] the following guidelines are recommended for use in patients first starting a cardiac rehabilitation program:

All patients will have orthostatic BP measurements before beginning exercise. After the patient's BP is obtained in the sitting position, a second reading will be taken after the patient has been in a standing position for 30 seconds. Patients should be reminded to stand slowly from a sitting position to avoid lightheadedness. The systolic BP should be at least 90 mmHg before patients are allowed to exercise. Typically, systolic BP and HR rise with exercise. However, patients may be anxious initially, and resting BP and HR may be higher than usual.[127] During low-level exercise, systolic BP and HR may not increase over resting levels in this case.

The following procedure will be utilized to check for orthostatic and exercise-induced hypotension on the ward or later in the inpatient and outpatient exercise programs.

1. Symptomatic patients will not exercise.
2. If the standing systolic BP is below 90 mmHg (without symptoms), the attending physician will be notified, and the patient will not be allowed to exercise until consulting with the medical director or attending physician.
3. If the patient exhibits a 10 to 20 mmHg orthostatic drop in the systolic BP (without symptoms), the medical director will be consulted before the patient exercises.
4. If the patient exhibits more than a 20 mmHg orthostatic drop in the systolic BP (without symptoms), the attending physician will be notified. If the attending physician wishes his or her patient to continue, the medical director will be consulted before the exercise session is begun.
5. Before the medical director or the attending physician is consulted regarding hypotension, BP measurements will be taken in both arms by two staff members.

Range-of-Motion Exercises for the Surgical Patient*

UPPER EXTREMITY EXERCISES

The purpose of these exercises is to stretch and strengthen muscles of the chest and shoulder girdle.

Text continued on page 543

---

*(Photographs from the cardiac rehabilitation program, Mount Sinai Medical Center, Milwaukee, WI. Published with permission.)

1. BEHIND HEAD PRESS

Starting Position: Stand erect with feet shoulder-width apart, and hold stick in front of body, with arms extended. Note that wrist weights are used only when patient can satisfactorily complete 15 repetitions without weights.

Movement: Raise stick straight out and up over head. Lower stick behind head and then raise up over head. Keeping arms straight, return stick to starting position.

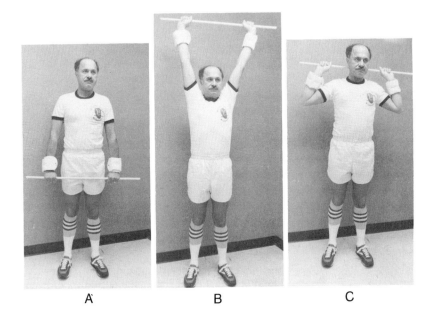

A   B   C

2. SWINGING STICK

Starting Position: Stand with feet shoulder-width apart and hold stick in front of body, with arms extended.

Movement: Using stick, move both arms laterally to side and with one arm pushed up to ear level. Repeat to other side.

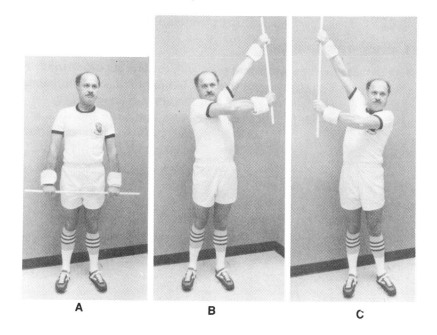

A   B   C

3. STICK BEHIND BACK

Starting Position: Stand erect with feet shoulder-width apart and hold stick behind back, with hands shoulder-distance apart, arms extended.

Movement: Move stick backward, keeping arms straight. All movement should come from shoulders. Do not lean forward. Return to starting position.

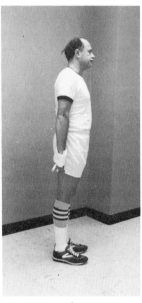 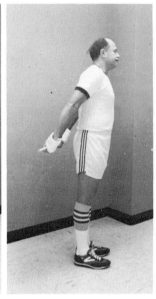

A   B

4. STICK SLIDING UP BACK

Starting Position: Stand erect with feet shoulder-width apart and stick behind back, with hands together and arms extended.

Movement: Raise elbows and slide stick up back as high as possible. Return to starting position.

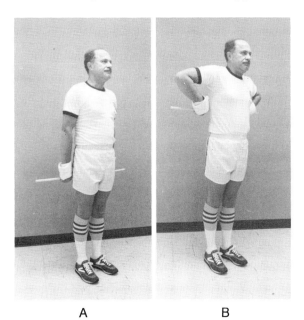

A   B

5. ARM CIRCLES

Starting Position: Stand erect with fingertips touching shoulders.

Movement: Rotate elbows in large circles backward, emphasizing upward and outward movements of shoulders.

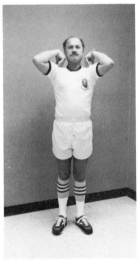
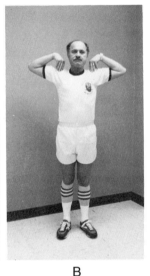

A   B

6. ADVANCED ARM CIRCLES

Starting Position: Stand erect with arms extended sideways, parallel to floor.

Movement: Rotate arms backward in large circles. One- to three-pound wrist weights are ordinarily used with this exercise.

Note: Initially, completing this exercise with one arm at a time may be advisable with many patients.

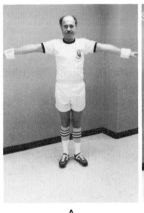
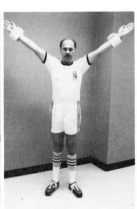
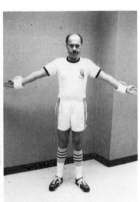

A   B   C

TRUNK EXERCISES

The purpose of these exercises is to stretch the muscles of the trunk area.

7. SIDE BENDS

Starting Position: Stand erect with feet shoulder-width apart and hands on hips.

Movement: Without twisting trunk or bending knees, lean trunk to left as far as possible, pause and return to starting position. Repeat to right side. Keep feet flat on ground.

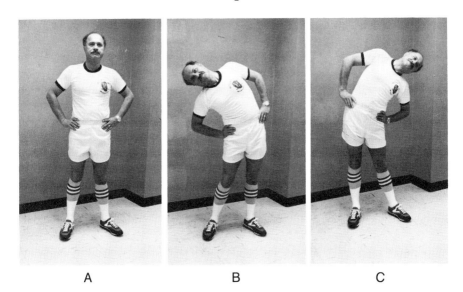

A   B   C

8. TRUNK ROTATION

Starting Position: Stand with feet shoulder-width apart and hands on hips.

Movement: Twist trunk to right, pause and return to starting position. Repeat to left. Head should be kept to front.

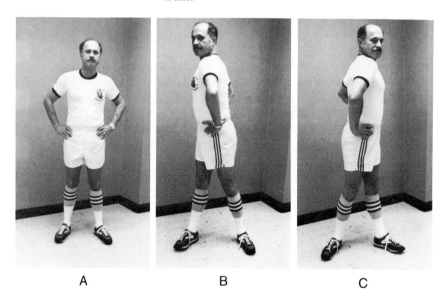

A   B   C

LOWER EXTREMITY EXERCISES

The purpose of these exercises is to stretch the calf muscles and posterior thigh muscles.

9. CALF STRETCH

Starting Position:	Stand arm's length away from wall with feet less than shoulder-width apart and toes turned slightly inward. Lean against wall, with head resting on forearms. Relax upper body.
Movement:	Slowly move hips forward, keeping back straight, until stretch is felt in back of lower legs (calves). Hold for 30 to 60 seconds. Keep heels on floor.

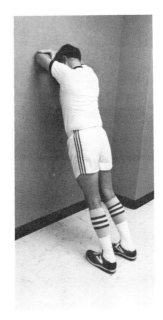

10. HAMSTRING STRETCHES

Starting Position: Sit on floor with legs extended in front.

Movement: Keeping back of knees against floor, slowly reach hands toward feet and hold for 5 seconds. Do not bounce or hold breath. Repeat 2 to 5 times.

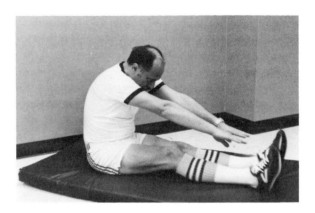

Range-of-Motion Exercises for Medical Patients*

UPPER EXTREMITY EXERCISES

1. ARM RAISES

Starting Position: Stand erect with feet shoulder-width apart and arms at side. Note that wrist weights are used only when patient can satisfactorily complete ten repetitions without weights.

Movement: Raise both arms out straight and over head. Return to starting position.

---

*(Photographs from the cardiac rehabilitation program, Mount Sinai Medical Center, Milwaukee, WI. Published with permission.)

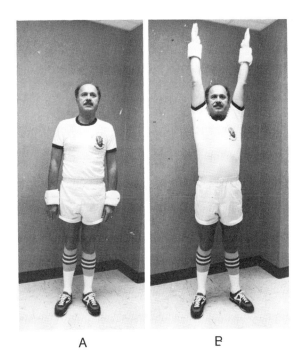

A   B

2. ARM RAISES TO SIDE

Starting Position: Same as arm raises.

Movement: Simultaneously raise arms to side laterally and up over head. Return to starting position.

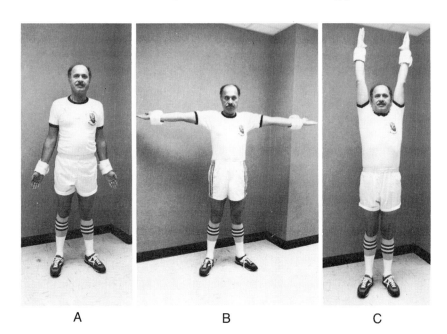

A   B   C

3. ARM CIRCLES

Same as exercise number 5 for surgical patients.

4. ADVANCED ARM CIRCLES

Same as exercise number 6 for surgical patients. Exercise both forward and backward.

5. ELBOW FLEXION

Starting Position: Stand erect with feet shoulder-width apart and with arms at side.

Movement: Flex elbows and bring fingertips to shoulders.

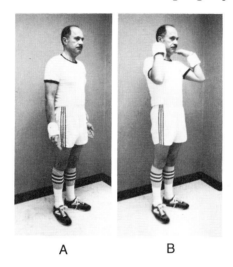

A   B

6. SIDE BENDS

Same as exercise number 7 for surgical patients.

LOWER EXTREMITY EXERCISES

7. MARCHING IN PLACE

Starting Position: Stand erect (use wall for balance purposes only) with feet placed comfortably apart.

Movement: March in place, raising leg to comfortable height.

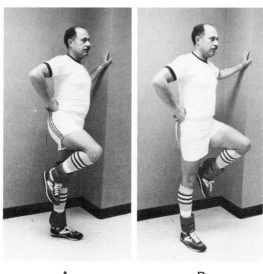

A   B

8. KNEE LIFT (may be substituted for exercise number 7)

Starting position: Sit in chair with feet flat on floor.

Movement: Flex hip and raise one knee upward. Return to starting position. Repeat with other leg.

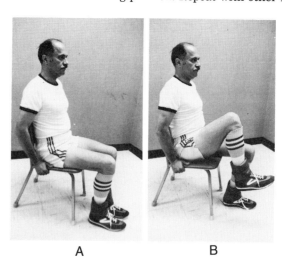

A   B

9. SIDE LEG LIFTS

Starting Position: Stand flat-footed, holding onto support.

Movement: Raise right leg out to side and return to starting position. Repeat movement with left leg.

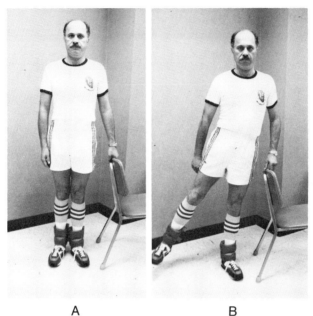

A   B

10. TOE RAISE

Starting Position: Stand next to table (for balance) with feet 6 inches apart.

Movement: Raise up on toes, bringing heels off floor. Return to starting position.

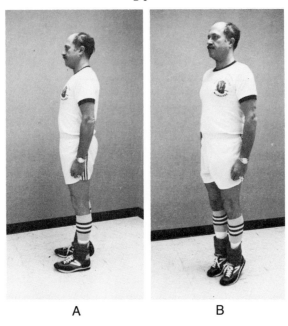

A   B

11. KNEE EXTENSION

Starting Position: Sit in chair with feet flat on floor.

Movement: Fully extend right leg. Return leg to initial position. Repeat with left leg.

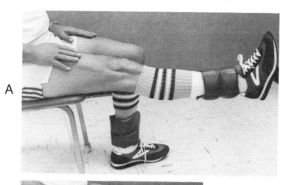

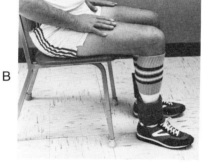

12. CALF STRETCH

        Same as exercise number 9 for surgical patients.

13. ANKLE EXERCISE (may be substituted for number 12)

Starting Position: Sit in chair with feet flat on floor.

Movement: Extend one leg and point toes, first up and then down. Follow by rotating foot in circle, with motion occurring at ankle. Repeat with other ankle.

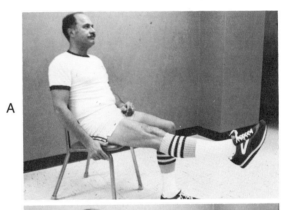

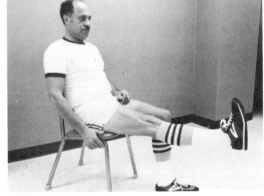

14. HAMSTRING STRETCH

        Same as exercise number 10 for surgical patients.

Early inpatient exercise is usually performed within a 2 to 3 MET level. Exercise HRs usually increase no more than 5 to 10 beats/min above resting levels for either ROM exercise or ambulation.[66, 108] Systolic BP usually rises no more than 5 mmHg for ROM exercise and 10 mmHg for ambulation.[66, 108] Because of comprehension problems resulting from fatigue and medications associated with an MI or surgery, the RPE concept is not presented to the patient until the third or fourth treatment day (see Chapter 6 for more details on RPE). The latter part of the early treatment phase is usually rated between 10 and 12 (fairly light) for both ROM and ambulation exercise.[66, 108]

Two other important points to consider during the early rehabilitation phase are breathing exercises and how the patient sits on the side of the bed. When the patient begins to sit on the edge of the bed, the feet should be supported. Leg dangling is no longer permitted in most hospitals because the pressure of the mattress edge under the thighs tends to impede venous blood return to the heart. This pressure promotes the same clotting tendency in blood that the sitting up was intended to avoid. Therefore, a stool should be placed under the feet to lift the knees and thighs off the edge of the bed when the patient is sitting up on the side of the bed. Diaphragmatic or "belly" breathing helps avoid atelectasis of the lower lobes of the lung near the diaphragm, i.e., the collapse of some air spaces of the lung that makes gas exchange impossible in the involved segments. A respiratory therapist, trained nurse, or exercise specialist should initially provide instruction in these maneuvers. Some patients have great difficulty in belly breathing when lying on their backs, since they are used to elevating the ribs and chest. The maneuver is often easier for these patients if they try it when lying on their side.

In the early phase-I cardiac rehabilitation program, some monitoring of the ECG during the rehabilitation program may be helpful in evaluating patient status (direct wire or telemetered ECG units). A portable monitor can be used in the critical care areas, where direct monitors may be detached when the patient ambulates. Early ambulation in the critical care unit for surgery patients is supervised by a cardiac rehabilitation staff member (therapist member of the team) with the assistance of the primary nurse. In the intermediate coronary care area, patients receive instructions on how to count HR. The palpation technique as described in Chapter 7 is used.

Figure 8–5 shows an example of a cardiac rehabilitation inpatient data record form. A special section entitled "Cardiac Rehabilitation" is recommended in the patient's chart. The availability of the inpatient daily record form, as well as the appropriate

Inpatient Data Record

Date of MI/Surgery ______________________ Name ______________________

					Heart Rate		Blood Pressures			
Date	Time (0–2400)	Weight lb/kg	Step No.	Feet Amb	*Rest*	*Immed. Post Ex.*	*Rest*	*Immed. Post Ex.*	RPE*	Comments/Signature
/ /							/	/		
/ /							/	/		
/ /							/	/		
/ /							/	/		
/ /							/	/		
/ /							/	/		
/ /							/	/		
/ /							/	/		
/ /							/	/		
/ /							/	/		
/ /							/	/		
/ /							/	/		
/ /							/	/		
/ /							/	/		
/ /							/	/		

* Rating of Perceived Exertion.

Figure 8–5. The inpatient data record form is used to record vital information obtained during the inpatient cardiac rehabilitation. It is recommended that this record be included in the patient's chart. (Courtesy of the Cardiac Rehabilitation Program, Cardiovascular Disease Section, Mount Sinai Medical Center, Milwaukee, WI.)

MI or surgical protocol inserted in the patient's chart, can be helpful to the attending or primary physician in patient assessment and in understanding at what level his or her patient is in the rehabilitation program.

Later Inpatient Phase-I Program

At this stage of rehabilitation, patients generally feel stronger; CABG surgery patients are able to ambulate approximately 400 feet (usually the fifth or sixth postoperative day) and MI patients, 200 feet (usually the seventh or eighth day after the MI). In addition, they can complete ten repetitions of the ROM exercises. At this stage, patients progress more rapidly in their ambulation program, and stair climbing can be introduced. Electrocardiographic monitoring during training can become less frequent, and patients may become more independent in their ambulation program; i.e., during their regularly scheduled exercise sessions, the cardiac rehabilitation staff may not find it necessary to spend the full time with the patient. As patients feel stronger, they should be encouraged to ambulate on their own in addition to the precribed formal program.

As mentioned earlier and as outlined in Tables 8–5 and 8–6, much of the later inpatient phase-I program can be conducted in a specially designed exercise room (step 5 of the CABG protocol and step 6 of the MI protocol). If an exercise room is used, it may be feasible for a patient to exercise there only once a day. The second session would then be conducted in the ward. An example of an inpatient exercise center is shown in Figure 8–6.[117] In this example, the inpatient exercise center is located adjacent to the cardiology ward. It contains four treadmills, a cycle ergometer, a special set of stairs with a handrail for stair climbing, and a mat for ROM exercises. In the inpatient center, four patients can be monitored by telemetry at one time. A special inpatient exercise record has been developed for use in the inpatient exercise center (see example in Appendix B, Fig. B–3). This additional record makes it easier to evaluate different activities separately.

In order to keep track of patient activity outside the formal program and to help reinforce certain monitoring techniques, activity logs may be used (see Appendix B, Fig. B–4). The log reminds patients of the need for keeping track of time and the distance ambulated or the resistance used for stationary cycling and for taking periodic determinations of HR and RPE. The back of the log has an RPE scale and a table for converting HR to beats per minute.

Because most patients live in homes or visit facilities that

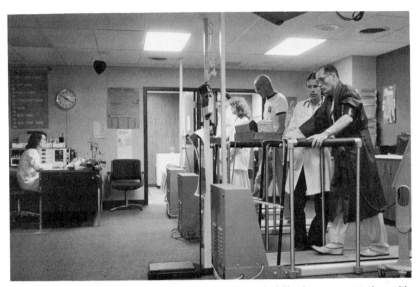

Figure 8–6. Inpatient Exercise Center. Cardiac rehabilitation nurse station with 4-channel ECG monitor at left and inpatient education classroom entrance in center background. A physical therapist is supervising a patient during treadmill walking (right foot). (Courtesy of the Cardiac Rehabilitation Program, Mount Sinai Medical Center, Milwaukee, WI.)

require stair climbing, practice on stairs is recommended before hospital discharge. The practice of proper pacing gives the patient confidence in using stairs after discharge. Initially, all patients should be monitored for BP before and immediately after stair climbing. Patients should climb stairs at a slow, comfortable pace, as tolerated. When taking the BP reading after stair climbing, have the patient alternately shift weight from one leg to the other (step in place) to help prevent venous pooling and hypotension. A BP reading should be taken before and immediately after climbing approximately six stairs. If there is less than a 10 to 20 mmHg drop in the systolic BP (without symptoms), the patient may climb six additional stairs, and a final BP reading is taken. If the systolic BP drops more than 20 mmHg (without symptoms), no further stair climbing should be done that day, and the attending physician should be notified.

Does the sequence of activity make a difference in the patient's response to training? Usually not. Traditionally, patients begin their program with ROM exercise followed by either stair climbing or ambulation (stationary cycling). For asymptomatic patients who tend to develop hypotension during stair climbing, ambulating before stair climbing sometimes improves their response to subsequent stair climbing.

Because of the cost differences between treadmills and cycles and the ease of moving and storing cycles as compared with treadmills, many centers prefer the use of stationary cycles. This is fine and has worked satisfactorily in programs for years. Keep in mind, though, that when patients go home, their main mode of transportation will be walking; thus it is recommended that 50 percent of their aerobic phase of training include walking. As mentioned earlier, treadmills are not a necessity for an inpatient program, but a convenience.

Patient Discharge

A recent major problem that must be dealt with in the inpatient program is the earlier hospital discharges. In the late 1970's and early 1980's, the average hospital stay for MI patients was 12 to 14 days and for the CABG surgery patient 10 to 12 days. Since 1983 and 1984 and the advent of imposed regulations such as diagnosis-related groups (DRGs), hospital stays have become significantly shorter. In many cases, low-risk patients without complications are leaving the hospital at 6 to 8 days. This requires that the cardiac rehabilitation staff and primary nurse initiate the patient discharge plan as early as possible.

During the final couple of days in the hospital, patients should be primed in regard to continuing their program after discharge. If available, an organized outpatient program can be recommended. An organized program at this stage would be most important if patients are confused or apprehensive, if patients are considered at moderate to high risk, and if medical management is in transition— i.e., new medications are being used, or medications are being adjusted. For the latter reason, this type of surveillance can be important to the physician for patient management.

The predischarge plan includes strategy for risk factor modifications, dietary counseling, education on medications, and a home discharge consultation on exercise prescription. In addition, educational booklets designed to aid the patients in understanding their disease and how to cope with it are available and recommended.[120–126] The American Heart Association* and the National Heart, Lung, Blood Institute† have many excellent educational materials. These booklets often include a glossary of terms and a

---

*7320 Greenville Avenue, Dallas, TX 75231
†Kit '89, Ideas and Materials for Preventing Heart Disease, Lung Disease, and Stroke, U.S. Department of Health and Human Services, Public Health Service, National Institutes of Health, Building 31, Room 4A21, Bethesda, MD 20892

question and answer section on important issues. The advent and availability of videos for program and home use should prove important for reinforcement of educational and program goals. It is advisable to have the spouse and/or significant others be a part of the discharge planning.

Redman[121] has an excellent text for the health professional concerning principles of education and applies them to health-related learning situations. The author gives insight into learning theory and is a proponent of the philosophy that all patients are ready to learn something. The key is that the educator must learn what and when. The book contains many practical suggestions and illustrations of patient education that can be applied to the cardiac rehabilitation setting.

The exercise plan for home use should include a list and description of the ROM exercise, information on a walking or stationary cycling program, and recommendations for stair climbing and other potential activities. Basic guidelines on exercise prescription should be re-emphasized (warm-up, cool-down, progression, frequency, intensity, duration, modes of activity, taking HR, and RPE). To help regulate intensity, patients should be given an upper limit target (training) HR. A list of unfavorable symptoms to watch for should help make their program safer. If necessary, special instructions for exercising in a hot or cold environment should be included (see Chapter 9).

For inclement weather (hot, cold, or rain) indoor shopping malls are often available for walking. Maps of malls may be developed and given to patients for home use.

An important part of the discharge plan should include a summary progress report sent to the referring physician. The report may include information on progress in the various stages and activities of the inpatient program (including HR and BP responses); medical problems associated with or observed during the program; ECG strips, if available; patient limitations; and recommended home program. An example of an inpatient progress report can be found in Appendix B, Figure B–5.

Determination of the Discharge Upper Limit Target (Training) Heart Rate

There is no set answer as to the best manner in which to determine the target or training HR. A survey of experts in the field of cardiac rehabilitation from 18 inpatient centers showed that training intensity was kept low in all programs and below the patient's level of symptoms, but the means of determining an upper limit HR was quite varied.[65] There were 11 different ways in which the upper limit target (training) HR was established. The two most common guidelines were (1) the use of a fixed low-level HR (12 of 18) and (2) a certain HR above standing resting HR (five of eighteen). In the former method, the upper limit HRs were usually between 110 and 120 beats/min. In the latter method, 10 to 20 beats/min above resting was most commonly used. One program used an HR of 140 beats/min as its upper limit of intensity. It must be noted that the ultimate determination should be signs, symptoms, and perception of effort (RPE).

As mentioned earlier, the authors feel that in lieu of significant signs or symptoms, the upper limit target (training) exercise HR for both medical and surgical patients should be approximately 20 beats/min above the standing resting HR for the inpatient. The ACSM[67] recommends 20 to 30 beats/min above standing resting HR, but 30 beats/min above standing resting HR may be too high. The rationale for this follows. Unless a predischarge GXT is performed, this same standard is generally used until an SL-GXT is performed at 3 to 6 weeks after the MI or surgery.

Why use 20 beats/min above standing resting HR and why not use a fixed low-level HR? Most inpatient activities are performed at an HR of 5 to 15 beats/min above standing resting HR (RPE is approximately 11 to 12).[66, 108] In addition, because of the generally wide range of resting HRs in cardiac patients, that is, 50 to 120 beats/min, a fixed HR seems inappropriate. For example, if a fixed HR of 110 or 120 beats/min were used, patients at one extreme would be allowed to double their resting HR, while those at the other extreme would not be allowed to exercise because the resting HR was already at the fixed HR. Surgical patients are generally tachycardic, and many have resting HRs of 110 to 120 beats/min. In addition, SL-GXT data at hospital discharge have shown that 30 to 40 beats/min above standing resting HR is nearly maximum for many patients, and 13 on the RPE scale is approximately 20 beats/min above standing resting HR.[128]

What about the patient on beta-adrenergic–blocking drugs? When these drugs are administered, the patient's HR is significantly depressed.[129, 130] A dose-response relationship also exists between the quantity of the drug administered and HR reduction.[131, 132] Even so, because the relationship between the percentage of HRmax and percentage of $\dot{V}O_2$max is still similar during submaximal exercise, the prescription of target HR and method for doing so would be similar for patients on or off beta blockade.[131, 134–138] It should also be noted that the relationship between percentage of HRmax (or $\dot{V}O_2$max) and RPE does not differ during submaximal exercise.[137–140] See Wilmore's review on exercise and beta-adrenergic blockers.[140a]

A study conducted on patients early after CABG surgery showed the average HR increment per MET increase in exercise intensity was 6 beats/min for patients not on propranolol therapy and 4 beats/min for patients using propranolol.[128] Thus, a chronotropic response is apparent after CABG surgery, whether the patient is on propranolol therapy or not. The same chronotropic response has been shown with MI patients.[141, 142] This response seems to persist approximately 8 to 12 weeks after the MI or surgery.

Figure 8–7 shows the HR and RPE response to submaximal exercise using a modified Naughton protocol (2-minute stages) with patients who were administered propranolol and with ones who were not.[146] These data reveal that even though HR is significantly depressed at each work load with the propranolol group, RPE is the same. This is in agreement with similar studies conducted with cardiac and noncardiac subjects.[137–140a, 143–147] These findings, along with the data from figure 7–3, are significant and give important information for exercise prescription. The data show that the

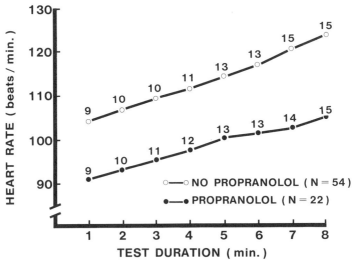

Figure 8–7. Increase in heart rate and rating of perceived exertion (RPE) during graded exercise testing in patients taking and not taking propranolol. Numbers above circles represent RPE. (Reprinted with permission from Squires, R.W., Rod, J.L., Pollock, M.L., and Foster, C.: Effect of propranolol on perceived exertion soon after myocardial revascularization surgery. **Med. Sci. Sports Exerc.** 14:276–280, 1982.)

guidelines used for determining target (training) HR for patients not taking beta-adrenergic–blocking drugs can also be used for patients taking these drugs.[133, 137–140a, 143–147]

Thus, as a result of the previously mentioned information, the following guidelines can be used for determining an upper limit target (training) HR at hospital discharge:

1. Patients who *do* complete a GXT before hospital discharge
   a. Medical status (signs and symptoms)
   b. Evaluation of patients' performance on the predischarge GXT and participation in the inpatient program
   c. Heart rate that corresponds to an RPE of 13 (somewhat hard) on the predischarge GXT
   d. Clinical judgment
2. Patients who *do not* complete a GXT before hospital discharge. In lieu of medical problems, an HR of 20 beats/min above standing rest should be used.
3. If significant signs or symptoms can be identified, an HR of 5 to 10 beats/min below that HR at which these signs and symptoms occur is often used.

Tables 8–7 and 8–8 give examples of the results from a predischarge GXT and subsequent determination of upper limit target (training) HR of two patients without complications. The patients had no significant signs or symptoms and had normal HR, BP, and RPE responses to exercise. The recommended upper limit HR of patient number one was set at 143 beats/min. This was higher than the 133 beats/min HR achieved during his last training session in the cardiac rehabilitation program. Since his medical course was unremarkable and an HR of 143 was rated 13 on the RPE scale, 143 beats/min was recommended. Patient number 2 was taking a beta-adrenergic–blocking drug. Because the patient had ambulated for 30 minutes (2 mph) at an HR of 90 beats/min the previous day with no apparent difficulty, an HR of 92 beats/min (RPE 14) was advised. As shown in both examples, clinical judgment based on the factors listed under guideline 1, a to c, was used in making the final HR designation.

It is important to note that because of the earlier hospital discharge now occurring with cardiac patients, fewer predischarge GXTs are being performed. Although there are no data to support this, it appears that more programs are waiting until one to two weeks after discharge (approximately 3 weeks after the event or surgery) to do their first GXT. The exercise prescription based on a GXT administered as an outpatient and usually 3 to 6 weeks after the event or surgery is discussed later in this chapter under outpatient programs.

Table 8–7. Results from a Predischarge Graded Exercise Test and Determination of Upper Limit Target and Training Heart Rate: Patient Number One*

Patient #1	Age 44	Ht 6'2"	Wt 193 lb	
Sex M	Previous MI Yes		Surgery 3 Grafts 7-23-80	
Medication Warfarin				
Type of test Predischarge 8-7-80			Protocol Modified Naughton	

Time	METs	HR	BP	RPE
Rest	—	110	116/70	—
1		111		6
2	2	108	124/60	7
3		115		8
4	3	112	132/60	8
5		119		8
6	4	127	140/60	9
7		132		11
8	5	136	154/60	12
9		143		13
10	6	147	160/60	15
11		152		16
12	7	157	160/60	17

Recovery Normal   Reason for stopping Fatigue

Recommended upper limit HR 143

Highest training HR inpatient center 133, Work load 2.5–3 mph, 30 min

*Patient was recovering from CABG surgery and had an above-average MET capacity.

Table 8–8. Results from a Predischarge Graded Exercise Test and Determination of Upper Limit Target and Training Heart Rate: Patient Number Two*

Patient #2	Age 51	Ht 5'10"	Wt 210 lb
Sex M	Previous MI Yes	Surgery 5 Grafts 9-30-80	
Medication Warfarin, isosorbide dinitrate, propranolol			
Type of test Predischarge 9-12-80		Protocol Modified Naughton	

Time	METs	HR	BP	RPE
Rest	—	75	120/60	—
1		82		7
2	2	85	126/60	8
3		86		11
4	3	87	136/60	13
5		92		14
6	4	95	160/60	16
7	4.5	101	170/60	18

Recovery Normal   Reason for stopping Leg fatigue—Dyspnea

Recommended upper limit HR 92

Highest training HR inpatient center 90, Work load 2 mph, 30 min

*Patient was recovering from CABG and had an average MET capacity.

Should patients attend cardiac rehabilitation sessions the same day they receive a predischarge GXT? To prevent undue fatigue, the patient is advised to keep ambulation to a minimum on the day of the GXT. Undue fatigue before taking the test affects the results. Other guidelines include the following:

1. Patients undergoing an exercise test (predischarge GXT or rest and exercise nuclear dynamic studies) in the afternoon may receive rehabilitation in the morning for ROM exercises.

2. Patients undergoing an exercise test in the morning may receive rehabilitation in the afternoon for ROM exercises. Depending on patient fatigue, ambulatory activity may have to be modified.

Resumption of Sexual Activity

One of the chief objectives of the predischarge exercise evaluation is to assess the risks of beginning sexual activity and to help compose a convincing presentation of the facts to both the patient and the spouse. Studies show that sexual intercourse with one's spouse approximates a 4 to 5 MET level of work and, in most cases, is associated with an HR lower than 130 beats/min.[148–150] Extra-marital sexual relations are likely to cause a higher HR response.[151] Larson and associates[152] developed a two-flight stair-climbing test for patients and found it to be comparable with the energy require-ment for sexual activity. The test had patients climb 20 steps in 10 seconds. Their results showed that the patients' HR increased to 127 beats/min and BP rose to 145/72 mmHg. Thus, it appears that a low-level GXT to a minimum of 5 METs or the two-flight stair-climbing test could be used as a guide to determine the readiness for resumption of customary sexual activity.

Data suggest that there is a frequent reduction in sexual activity after an MI or CABG surgery.[148, 150] Much of this reduction can be attributed to anxiety in the patient or spouse, or both, and apprehension of a recurring cardiac event. Thus, it is important that the cardiac rehabilitation team instruct the patient and spouse on how to achieve a healthy sex life through modifying the intensity and orchestrating the encounter with a light touch of low energy demand.[150, 153] Patient education materials that discuss the problem of resuming sexual activity and offer suggestions for coping with this situation are available.[119] If the evaluation suggests that sex can be undertaken at acceptably low risks, the patient needs to be reassured that he or she can resume sex and be an adequate partner. It is crucial, although not easy, to provide counseling in this area, even with the help of an early discharge evaluation. It is also important that the physician or other designated members of the rehabilitation staff initiate a discussion with and solicit questions from partners on this sometimes embarrassing topic. Usually, if the patient is medically stable and asymptomatic and has a functional capacity of at least 5 METs, sexual activity can be recommended as soon after hospital discharge as the patient desires, usually within 3 to 6 weeks for low-risk patients.

OUTPATIENT CARDIAC REHABILITATION—PHASE II

Organized, supervised outpatient and unsupervised home pro-grams have become an important part of the rehabilitation process. The earlier strategy was to send patients home to rest for a few weeks and then encourage them to participate in an organized phase-III community program, some 2 to 3 months after discharge. A survey of experts in the field showed a lack of organized and supervised outpatient cardiac rehabilitation programs.[65] A review of exercise training in patients with CAD published by the Amer-ican Heart Association emphasized the need in the early stages of rehabilitation for formal supervised classes with personnel trained in exercise prescription and CPR.[154] Although most of the experts surveyed agreed with this concept, only six of 17 institutions had organized and supervised programs that commenced within a week of discharge. Of these six programs, two were not hospital based, and two were research programs.

Including home programs, ten of 17 centers had varied times in which they initiated their programs after the patient had been discharged from the hospital: four of 17, within 2 to 4 weeks, and three of 17, within 6 to 12 weeks. Most experts agree that the first 2 to 6 weeks of rehabilitation are often the most critical for the patient. Because of the many anxieties and apprehensions that are apparent when the healing process is still incomplete and because medication dosage is often being altered to find the proper balance, it seems contradictory not to have well-planned and administered outpatient programs available for patients soon, if not immediately, after hospital discharge. Therefore, to start patients early after hospital discharge and give them more definitive guidelines and instructions before going home is important.

The outpatient program can begin when the patient is discharged from the hospital and is generally organized as a hospital-based or free-standing program, as a recommended home program, or as a program based in a community gymnasium facility. The outpatient phase of cardiac rehabilitation is the intermediate phase during which the patient progresses from a restricted low-level training program and a condition of unknown stability to a less restricted moderate-level training program and more stability. Programs conducted in hospitals and clinics usually include more telemetry monitoring of HR and ECG than those in the community setting. Details on the organization, administration, and facilities of various outpatient programs are available elsewhere.[14, 16, 102, 104–106] Of particular interest is the October 1982 issue of the *Journal of Cardiac Rehabilitation* (name changed to *Journal of Cardiopulmonary Rehabilitation* in 1985).[102] This issue includes the description (of programs and facilities) of 17 different well-established cardiac rehabilitation programs. An example of facilities used for outpatient cardiac rehabilitation hospital-based programs is shown in Figures 8–8 to 8–11. Free-standing clinics may look similar. A new hospital trend is to establish a wellness or fitness center and have a portion of the facility dedicated to cardiac and pulmonary rehabilitation. The larger facility often allows for the sharing of staff and facility space, thus potentially making programs more cost effective. With the advent of risk stratification, the wellness or fitness-rehabilitation type facility could accommodate the low-

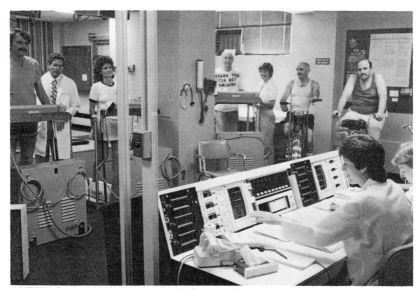

Figure 8–8. The figure shows a hospital-based outpatient exercise center. The nurses' station is shown in the foreground (8 ECG telemetry monitoring units). The patient range-of-motion (ROM) and strengthening exercise area is in the background. Overhead monitors (upper left) can be rotated for observation in the ROM and strength training area. Exercise leaders are supervising patients on treadmills and cycle ergometers. Not shown are men's and women's locker rooms, education classroom, and lounge. (Courtesy of the Cardiac Rehabilitation Program, Mount Sinai Medical Center, Milwaukee, WI.)

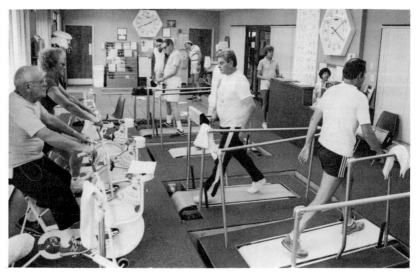

Figure 8–9. The figure shows an outpatient exercise center. The nurse's station is shown at the right (8 ECG telemetry units are available), and the range-of-motion (ROM) strength training area is in the background. (Courtesy of the Cardiac Rehabilitation Program, Arizona Heart Institute, Phoenix, AZ. From **J. Cardiac Rehabil.** 2:453–456, 1982.)

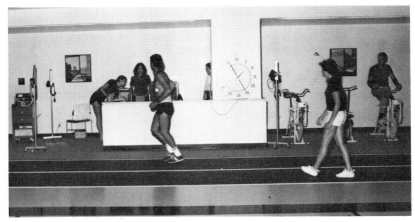

Figure 8–10. An outpatient exercise center with small indoor track and exercise facilities. The facility is used for both phase II and III programs. The nurse monitoring station is in the center. (Courtesy of the Cardiac Rehabilitation Program, Sid W. Richardson Institute for Preventive Medicine, the Methodist Hospital, Houston, TX. From **J. Cardiac Rehabil.** 2:453–456, 1982.)

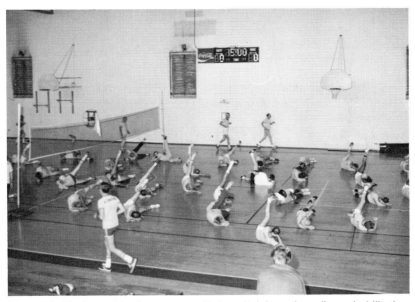

Figure 8–11. A combination community-hospital–based cardiac rehabilitation program facility. The gymnasium is connected to the Georgia Baptist Medical Center and houses a phase II and III program. (Courtesy of Cardiac Rehabilitation Program, Georgia Baptist Medical Center, Atlanta, GA. From **J. Cardiac Rehabil.** 2:453–456, 1982.)

as well as the high-risk patient. The various levels of monitoring (e.g., telemetry) and supervision would be available under one roof, thus providing an excellent avenue for the early triage of patients and placing them in the type of program that best meets their needs. Community programs such as those shown in Figures 8–12 to 8–14 also accommodate high- and low-risk patients in a phase-II program. Thus, depending upon available space, equipment, size of program, and so forth, the cardiac outpatient facility varies.

As mentioned previously, patients should begin their home program as soon as possible. Keeping records of the home program on a log, as shown in Figure B–4 (Appendix B), is important. The information can be helpful to the patient's physician (or designate) on subsequent visits. Progress and improvement (or nonimprovement or regression) can be noted and problems resolved or modifications made.

Although more research is necessary to determine the optimal amount of supervision that is necessary or cost effective for patient compliance with cardiac rehabilitation programs, most experts feel that 6 to 12 weeks may be a minimum. As discussed earlier under "Supervision and Monitoring of Cardiac Rehabilitation Programs," it was mentioned that home-based exercise programs have proved to be safe and realistic as far as improvement in $\dot{V}O_2max$ is concerned for the low-risk patient. It was also mentioned that some type of reinforcement is necessary for the best program compliance. Periodic visits to their physician or outpatient center, telephonic

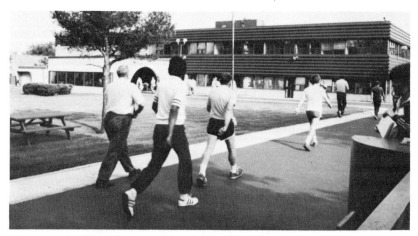

Figure 8–12. The outdoor walk-run track of the Toronto Rehabilitation Centre. The nurse's and exercise leader's station is at the right. The Centre's indoor facilities are shown in the background. (Courtesy of the Toronto Rehabilitation Centre, Toronto, Ontario, Canada. From **J. Cardiac Rehabil.** 2:453–456, 1982.)

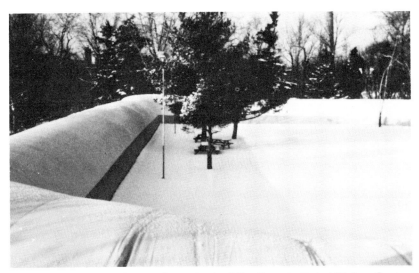

Figure 8–13. The outdoor walk-run track of the Toronto Rehabilitation Centre has a plastic bubble cover for the winter months. (Courtesy of the Toronto Rehabilitation Centre, Toronto, Ontario, Canada. From **J. Cardiac Rehabil.** 2:453–456, 1982.)

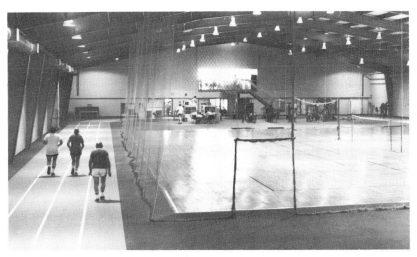

Figure 8–14. The Reh-Fit Program. A community-based program for healthy adults and cardiac patients. Graded exercise testing and sports medicine rehabilitation equipment and facilities and the program observation deck are located at the far end of the track. (Courtesy of the Reh-Fit Program, Winnepeg, Manitoba, Canada. From **J. Cardiac Rehabil.** 2:453–456, 1982.)

monitoring or a telephone call from a staff member, and keeping daily records on a log seem to increase compliance.

In programs in which patients live too far away from or do not have transportation to an outpatient facility, other methods of monitoring the home program are being used. For example, the Gunderson Clinic, La Crosse, Wisconsin, rents stationary cycle ergometers to their patients for home use and requires periodic but systematic visits to their center for progress checks. Patients who are at higher risk have telemetry by a telephonic system. In this way, an HR and ECG rhythm strip can be transmitted from the patient's home to the physician's office.

The formal outpatient program can begin as soon after discharge as the patient is referred. Having the referral forms signed before patient discharge can prevent unnecessary delays in program entrance. An example of an outpatient referral form is shown in Appendix B, Figure B–6. Upon entrance into the program, the program director or designate should explain the various aspects of the program to the patient. Realistic goals and expectations of the program should be covered. Patients should then be asked to read and sign an informed consent form. An example of an outpatient consent form is shown in Appendix B, Figure B–7.

The contraindications and guidelines used to modify or terminate the exercise routine listed for the inpatient program are also appropriate for the outpatient program. Exceptions to this should be mentioned in regard to S-T–segment displacement and the systolic BP rise during exercise. There is no exact standard of how much S-T–segment displacement should be allowed during an exercise program. Most experts agree that 1 mm of horizontal or downsloping displacement 0.08 sec from the J-point as compared with rest is significant, but depending on other medical factors concerning the patient's clinical status, opinions are varied with regard to the proper standard. The same variance of opinion exists with the upper limit for exercise systolic BP. Many experts feel that after the acute stage of recovery for CABG surgery or MI, the upper limit for systolic BP should be approximately 250 mmHg.[67] The upper limit target and training HR is calculated differently in the outpatient program and is discussed in the following section.

Determination of Intensity of Training in the Outpatient Program

The upper limit target (training) HR standard used can vary significantly, depending on medical status, number of weeks in the program, RPE, symptomatology, method of calculation, personal preference, and whether the patient had a GXT.[65, 67, 155, 156] Table 8–4, under phase-II program, describes the standards recommended for use in outpatient programs. The method of estimating the target (training) HR described earlier for hospital discharge is used for the first 3 to 6 weeks of the outpatient program or until the SL-GXT is administered.

As in phase I, the philosophy is to keep the intensity low and to raise the work load first by increasing duration of training. Table 8–9 shows a 12-step walking program that can be used in an outpatient program. The patients progress from step to step, as tolerated. Usually a patient should be stable at a step for a

Table 8–9. Twelve-Step Walking Program for Outpatients

Functional Capacity (METs)	Step	Speed (mph)	Elevation (%)	Duration (min)	METs	Calories (kcal/ min)
5	1	1.5	0	20–30	2.0	2.0
	2	2.0	0	20–30	2.0	2.5
5–8	3	2.0	0	5	2.0	2.5
		2.5		40–60	2.5	3.0
	4	2.5	0	5	2.5	3.0
		3.0	0	40–60	3.0	3.7
8 or more	5	3.0	0	5	3.0	3.7
		3.5	0	40–60	3.5	4.2
	6	3.0	0	5	3.0	3.7
		3.5	0 (1 min)*	40–60	3.5	4.2
		3.5	2.5 (min)		4.2	5.9
	7	3.0	0	5	3.0	3.7
		3.5	0 (1 min)*	40–60	3.5	4.2
		3.5	2.5 (6 min)		4.2	5.9
	8	3.0	0	5	3.0	3.7
		3.5	0 (1 min)*	40–60	3.5	4.2
		3.5	2.5 (10 min)		4.2	5.9
	9	3.0	0	5	3.0	3.7
		3.5	0 (1 min)*	40–60	3.5	4.2
		3.5	2.5 (14 min)		4.2	5.9
	10	3.0	0	5	3.0	3.7
		3.5	2.5	40–60	4.2	5.9
	11	3.0	0	5	3.0	3.7
		3.5	0 (1 min)*	40–60	3.5	4.2
		3.5	5.0 (2 min)		6.9	7.5
	12	3.0	0	5	3.0	3.7
		3.5	0 (1 min)*	40–60	3.5	4.2
		3.5	5.0 (2 min)		6.9	7.5

*Two lines denote interval training; for example, in step six, the patient will alternate one minute at 0-percent grade with 4 minutes at 2.5 percent. If a treadmill is not available, the higher intensity segment can include a faster walk and/or use of hand weights (see Chapter 7 for use of hand weights).

(Reprinted with permission from Pollock, M.L., Pels, A.E., Foster, C., and Ward, A.: Exercise prescription for rehabilitation of the cardiac patient. In Pollock, M.L., and Schmidt, D.H. (eds.): **Heart Disease and Rehabilitation,** 2nd Ed. New York, Churchill Livingstone, 1986, pp. 477–515.)

minimum of one to two weeks before progressing to a higher level. The duration of training varies and depends on the patient's level of tolerance and available time. As mentioned earlier, the ultimate goal is to have the patient progress in such a way that a minimum of 300 kcal per session, or 1,000 kcal per week, are expended. Therefore, at a slow to moderate walking speed, patients must eventually walk 45 to 60 minutes per session or increase the training frequency, or both. Although patients are not necessarily expected to reach these kilocaloric levels during the outpatient program (many do), those patients who have a lower exercise tolerance or who are limited in time when visiting the outpatient exercise center may be encouraged to train twice a day, once at the center and once at home.

As shown in Table 8–4, 3 to 6 weeks after surgery or MI, an SL-GXT is recommended. Then the HR intensity is based on 60 to 70 percent of HRmax reserve. This usually increases the target and training HR by approximately 10 beats/min.[157] An example of an SL-GXT 6 weeks after surgery and the determination of upper limit target (training) HR is shown in Table 8–10. Compare Table 8–7, predischarge GXT results, with Table 8–10 for differences in MET capacity and target (training) HR. It should be noted that the target (training) HR as described here (all phases) refers to an upper limit HR. Many programs use a lower HR limit as well as the upper limit. This approach has been suggested by the ACSM[67] as one alternative to the exercise prescription. For example, the target (training) HR could range from 50 to 75 percent of HRmax reserve. The idea would be to train the patient within that HR training zone.

As patients improve, higher levels of intensity may be prescribed, depending on medical and risk status. How soon can this higher intensity limit occur, and how does this relate to the initiation of a jogging program? Although not generally recommended, a few programs allow patients to begin jogging in the early part of phase II. These patients have had an SL-GXT 3 to 4 weeks after MI or surgery, have had no medical complications (low-risk classification), and have an above-average fitness level. Philosophically, it does not seem necessary to accelerate the rehabilitation process until after the estimated 6- to 8-week healing period. Thus, after approximately 6 weeks and assuming they had an SL-GXT, patients without complications who are above average in fitness may safely initiate a walk-jog program. These patients are usually younger than average (less than 50 years of age) or have an MET capacity of 8 and above. The authors' experience has shown that once a patient can walk at 3.5 mph, 5-percent grade, he or she

Table 8–10. Results from 8-Week Symptom-Limited Graded Exercise Test*

Patient #1	Age 44	Ht 6'2"		Wt 193 lb
Sex M	Previous MI Yes		Surgery 3 Grafts 7-23-89	
Medication Procainamide		Protocol Modified Naughton		

Time	METs	HR	BP	RPE
Rest	—	100	116/70	—
1		99		6
2	2	100	134/70	6
3		103		6
4	3	104	134/70	7
5		109		8
6	4	112	136/70	10
7		120		10
8	5	126	146/70	11
9		133		12
10	6	138	160/70	12
11		142		13
12	7	145	166/70	14
13		152		14
14	8	158	170/70	15
15		163		16
16	9	167	172/70	16
17	9.5	173		17

Recovery Normal   Reason for stopping Fatigue

Based on 70% of maximum (Karvonen)

Recommended upper limit HR 151

*Data show improvement from the predischarge test (Table 8–8). New upper limit target and training heart rate is based on 70 percent of the maximum heart rate reserve.

can jog on a level surface. A five-step walk-jog program is shown in Table 8–11. The starting jogging speed may vary from 4.75 to 5.5 mph and walking from 3.0 to 4 mph. The speed of walking and jogging should be regulated to keep the HR at a level within the training zone. Thus, the walking HR should not be allowed to go below 50 to 60 percent of HRmax reserve. Initially, the jogging HR may reach 75 to 85 percent of HRmax reserve. Of those patients who receive an SL-GXT at 6 weeks post MI or surgery and continue in an outpatient program, approximately 30 percent have been capable of initiating a jogging program. After several weeks of a

Table 8–11. Five-Step Walk-Jog Program for Outpatients

Step	Speed (mph)	Elevation (%)	Duration (min)	METs	METs (avg/workout)	Energy Cost* (kcal/min)
1	3.0	0	5			3.7
	3.0 (1 min)†	0		3.0		3.7
	5.5 (1 min)	0	30–40	8.3	6.5	12.0
2	3.0	0	5			3.7
	3.0 (1 min)†	0		3.0		3.7
	5.5 (2 min)	0	30–40	8.3	7.24	12.0
3	3.0	0	5			3.7
	3.0 (1 min)†	0		3.0		3.7
	5.5 (4 min)	0	30–40	8.3	7.5	12.0
4	3.0	0	5			3.7
	3.0 (1 min)†	0		3.0		3.7
	5.5 (7 min)	0	30–40	8.3	7.7	12.0
5	3.0	0	5			3.7
	3.0 (1 min)†	0		3.0		3.7
	5.5 (10 min)	0	30–40	8.3	7.8	12.0

*Energy cost of kcal is based on an individual of 154 pounds of body weight (70 kg) walking 3.0 mph, expending approximately 3.7 kcal/min, and jogging 5.5 mph, expending about 12.0 kcal/min. To calculate the number of calories expended during a workout, multiply the number of the calories expended per minute for each work load by the number of minutes at that work load.

†Two lines represent interval training program. For example, in step 1, after a 5-minute warm-up, the patient will alternate walking for 1 minute with jogging for 1 minute.

(Reprinted with permission from Pollock, M.L., Pels, A.E., Foster, C., and Ward, A.: Exercise prescription for rehabilitation of the cardiac patient. In Pollock, M.L., and Schmidt, D.H. (eds.): **Heart Disease and Rehabilitation,** 2nd Ed. New York, Churchill Livingstone, 1986, pp. 477–515.)

walk-jog program or on reaching step 8 (Table 8–10) of walking, a patient is encouraged to progress to a community-based program. Some patients who are considered stable and who do not wish to progress to step 8 of walking also are encouraged to graduate to a community-based program.

It should be noted that the 3- to 6-week SL-GXT results could be used to classify patients into a fitness category, as shown in Table 6–3. Then the suggested starter programs and 20-week walk or walk-jog programs listed in Chapter 7 may be used.

What did the survey of experts mentioned earlier have to say about regulating intensity of training in a phase-II program? The results show that as in the inpatient program, training intensity was kept at a low level in all programs and maintained below the patient's level of symptoms.[65] The standard used for determining the upper limit of training intensity varied. The diversity in program organization and philosophy (structured versus unstructured, supervised versus unsupervised, monitored with telemetry versus unmonitored, and different policies regarding GXT determination) added to the variety of methods used in prescribing training intensity for the outpatient. In general, exercise intensity was more conservative in the unsupervised programs.

With regard to intensity of training, the survey dichotomized the phase-II program into early and late stages. The early stage was one to six weeks after discharge and generally culminated with an SL-GXT. In many programs, the later stage (after the SL-GXT) marked the beginning of entrance into a phase-III program. This was generally true with programs that had no organized phase-II program.

In the early stage, the most common guidelines for estimating the upper limit of training intensity were 20 to 30 beats/min above standing resting HR, an HR of 120 to 130 beats/min, and 5 to 10 beats/min below symptoms or endpoint on discharge GXT. Five programs had no set HR standard and instructed their patients to train at low work levels and to slow down or stop if symptoms occurred.

In the later stage of phase II, the guidelines for intensity used were 5 to 10 beats/min below achieved HR on SL-GXT, 60 to 85 percent of HR calculated as a percentage from zero to peak, or 70 to 75 percent HRmax reserve on an SL-GXT. One medical director had established different guidelines according to whether the patient was in a supervised or an unsupervised program; i.e., in the later stage of phase II, the patient would train at either 80 to 85 percent (supervised) or 70 to 75 percent of HRmax (unsupervised). Before making a decision on what technique should be used to calculate target (training) HR, refer to the section on estimation of exercise intensity in Chapter 7 and refer to information in this chapter about patient risk and risk stratification. As mentioned earlier, the conservative approach to exercise prescription is best; however, once the patient has completed an SL-GXT, is beyond the convalescence period of rehabilitation (4 to 6 weeks), and is classified as low risk, then he or she can be treated much like a participant entering an adult fitness program.

Frequency and Duration of Training

The recommended frequency and duration of training during phase II is shown in Table 8–4. A daily program is recommended. If a patient is active in an organized outpatient program, this would usually represent 3 days per week in the organized program and 4 days per week in a home program. For patients who are not stable, whose medications are still being adjusted, whose status of risk has not been determined, or who are at high risk, the home program (unsupervised) would not be recommended. This may necessitate the patient attending the outpatient center 5 days per week. In the early stages of rehabilitation when the kilocaloric expenditure of a program is low, and before the patient goes back to work, an extra session per day at home may be recommended.

Table 8–4 shows the duration of aerobic training starting at where it left off in the inpatient program. This varies greatly, depending on whether a patient is involved in an inpatient program, medical status, length of hospital stay, and time of entry into the outpatient program. The goal is to increase the time of aerobic training to 45 minutes as rapidly as the patient can adjust. For most patients this may take 4 to 6 weeks after surgery or MI.

Mode of Training

WALKING, JOGGING, AND STATIONARY CYCLING

The modes of training recommended for phase II are listed in Table 8–4. Steps for a walking and jogging program have been outlined in Tables 8–9 and 8–11 (also see Chapter 7). Stationary cycling is of equal value, and the time components and progressive stages used for walking and walking-jogging in Tables 8–9 and 8–11 can be used by substituting resistance for speed. Usually, stationary cycling can be initially tolerated at 100 to 300 kpm/min (17 to 50 watts). If one's power output cannot be tolerated for the required time span, then the interval training method should be used. For patients with low fitness, this may include some zero-resistance pedaling.

Often patients have uncalibrated stationary cycles for home use, thus making it more difficult to regulate their home program. In this case, more trial and error is involved. The patients should use the same time components as they would with the calibrated cycle, but intensity is estimated solely by HR and RPE. In essence, the program conducted on a calibrated cycle is regulated in a manner similar to that used with the uncalibrated cycle, but because of the known power output settings adjustments can be made more quickly and accurately with the calibrated cycle. A new cycle ergometer has been developed for home (clinic) use that regulates the power output (resistance) by using the patient's monitored HR.[158] The cycle can be programmed to be used in a continuous or interval training mode.

SWIMMING

Although swimming can be introduced in the phase-II program, it is not recommended until after an SL-GXT has been administered and completion of 6 to 8 weeks of rehabilitation. Before commencing with a swimming program, the patient should be able to comfortably complete the ROM exercises mentioned earlier. This period allows sufficient time for healing of the sternum and leg incisions in the surgery patient and heart tissue in the MI patient. In addition, patient stability is particularly important before entering a swimming program. The advantages of a swimming program are many: it is an aerobic activity involving both arms and legs; it puts the patient in a nongravity type of situation, thus helping venous return; it keeps the HR lower (may allow symptomatic patients to do more exercise); it causes fewer musculoskeletal injuries; and it can be therapeutic for patients with arthritis, intermittent claudication, limb amputations, or paralysis.[159–162] Swimming or other water activities, such as walking or jogging in water (using arms to paddle in combination with legs), can be the best alternative aerobic mode of training for the aforementioned patients. If done vigorously, they can become high–energy-cost activities.[161a]

The wide variations in skill level and energy cost of swimming among patients are major problems in regulating such programs.[159–164] For nonswimmers and those with poor skills, swimming would most likely be an anaerobic activity and is not recommended. Walking in waist- or chest-deep water while paddling backward with the arms and the use of flotation devices around the waist for swimming on the back are two excellent ways of introducing water activities to patients and are of particular help for the nonswimmer and swimmer with poor skills.[161a] Ekelund[161a] has outlined a set of less vigorous and vigorous water exercise routines that can be adapted to most populations. Use of old tennis or walking shoes while walking and exercising in the water is helpful when the pool surface is slippery.

Initially, it is recommended that nonswimmers begin their program on their side or back, using the side or elementary back strokes. Frequent stops at the side of the pool should be made to count the pulse. It is also important to have the patient avoid either entering too cold water or getting uncomfortably cold in a pool in which the temperature is too cold.[162] Usually, having patients remain active counteracts the latter cooling effect.

After patients have had a sufficient amount of time to adjust to their water activities, their program can be regulated in much the same way as with other aerobic activities; i.e., pacing is regulated by HR and RPE, with total time of the exercise period being increased to 45 minutes. In regard to regulating intensity of training by HR, it has been shown that the HR in the water (prone position) is lower for a given work load as measured on the treadmill[160, 163] or cycle ergometer.[161, 164] Therefore, if the target (training) HR for water activity is estimated by a treadmill or cycle GXT, then the calculated prone or supine swimming HR should be reduced 5 to 10 beats/min. For exercising upright in the water, the same HR values that are recommended for use out of the water are appropriate.

RESISTANCE/STRENGTH TRAINING

Along with the ROM exercises previously mentioned, resistance/strength training can also be emphasized at this stage of recovery. These activities are integrated as part of a total fitness program and as a result of the need a patient may have in preparation for return to work or leisure activities.

What is the safety of strength training types of exercise? Before this question is answered, certain physiological responses to static and dynamic exercise must be discussed. Traditionally, MI and CABG patients were told to avoid moderate to heavy static exercise as well as dynamic strength training. Dynamic endurance exercise is associated with an increased volume overload on the heart, which is proportional to the cardiac output or percentage of $\dot{V}O_2$max.[166–170] The normal response to dynamic endurance exercise is associated with an increase in HR, systolic BP, end-diastolic volume (EDV), myocardial contractility and a decrease in diastolic BP, end-systolic volume (ESV), and peripheral resistance. Mean arterial pressure (MAP) usually goes up moderately. Static exercise is associated with an increased pressure load on the heart.[166, 169, 171] This would include an increase in HR, systolic BP, diastolic BP, and MAP, with peripheral resistance remaining unchanged. In static exercise, EDV remains generally unchanged, thus ruling out the Starling mechanism as a means of adaptation to the needs of exercise, and ESV is decreased with static exercise. The increased pressure load found in isometric exercise can be of some benefit in that it causes an increase in perfusion pressure, thus facilitating blood flow to the myocardium. On the other hand, one of the main differences between static and dynamic exercise is the reduced ability in static exercise of increasing (accelerating) the venous return because of the absence of an active muscle pump.[166] Static exercise conducted with the Valsalva maneuver results in an even greater increase in BP than that found when the Valsalva maneuver is not used.[172] Both dynamic and isometric exercise can cause left ventricular dysfunction (reduced ejection fraction, regional wall motion abnormalities, and, sometimes, increased ectopy) in patients with CAD and, in particular, patients with an already compromised ventricle.[169, 171, 173] Patients with left ventricular dysfunction have a reduced capacity to increase cardiac output with static (and dynamic) exercise, thus showing a reduced ability of increasing HR with a concomitant decrease in stroke volume.[169, 171, 174] Reddy and associates[174] also found that patients with chronic heart failure showed a greater degree of lactate production in the exercising forearm with light isometric exercise as compared with that of normal subjects. This condition persisted into recovery and was associated with a limited cardiovascular capacity and resulted in perceived breathlessness.

The classic study of Lind and McNicol,[175] comparing isometric versus dynamic endurance exercise responses to HR and BP, is often shown to illustrate why isometric exercise is potentially dangerous to patients (Fig. 8–15). Although these data have been replicated, their interpretation may be misleading. There is an abundance of data now that supports the premise that the pressure response to exercise is mostly related to the size of the active muscle mass being exercised and its absolute $\dot{V}O_2$.[165, 167–170] Thus, in contrast to what some have interpreted about arm exercise, the HR, $\dot{V}O_2$, and BP response is greater for leg exercise than for arm exercise. These findings are consistent with those of Lewis and associates[168] (Table 8–12), when comparing handgrip and double-legged knee extension exercise; MacDougall and associates[176] (Fig. 8–16), when comparing the single-arm curl, single-leg press, and double-leg press; and Haslam and associates[177] (Fig. 8–17), when comparing single-arm curl, single-leg press, and double-leg press exercises at 20, 40, 60, and 80 percent of maximum.

Lewis and associates[168] have also shown that there is not that much difference in BP response betwen isometric and dynamic exercise when similar activities are compared. For example, when comparing static and dynamic exercise performed by handgrip and double-legged knee extension with local muscular fatigue (approximately 6 minutes of exercise), the authors found increases in MAP to be similar for each mode of exercise, but greater for knee extension than for handgrip (see Table 8–12). Based on the previously mentioned research, the rehabilitation specialist should keep the following points in mind when recommending strength training exercises:

1. Moderate to heavy static and dynamic exercise both increase systolic and diastolic BP, and MAP.

2. The increase in BP is related to the size of the muscle mass

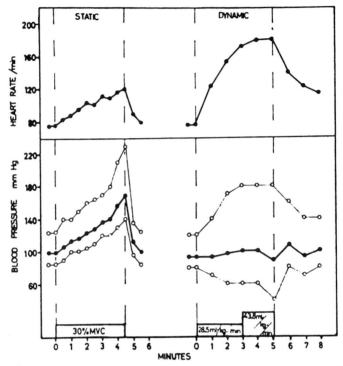

Figure 8–15. Comparison of heart rate and blood pressure (systolic, diastolic, and estimated mean pressures) in response to a fatiguing, sustained handgrip contraction at 30% of maximal volitional contraction (MVC), and to an exhaustive treadmill walking test. (From Lind, A.R., and McNicol, G.W.: Muscular factors which determine the cardiovascular responses to sustained and rhythmic exercise. **Canad. Med. Assoc. J.** 96:706–713, 1967. Published with permission.)

being exercised and at the relative percentage of maximum at which it is stimulated.

The reason for the differences in BP response between static and dynamic exercise as shown in Figure 8–15 is the way the stimulus was applied to the muscle. In the handgrip, the stimulus is applied to a smaller muscle mass, but the relative load (percentage) is greater than for walking and running exercise. If the handgrip is held for more than a short time, the 30 percent of maximum volitional contraction (MVC) can eventually become 100 percent. In an activity like running or walking, even though the cardiorespiratory system may be working to maximum, the percentage of muscle mass being used is small in relation to the total size of the muscle mass involved. The latter type of activity also allows for a significant vasodilation effect, thus keeping diastolic

BP (MAP) down. The more specific the exercise (isolation of muscle groups), such as shown in Figures 8–16 and 8–17 and Table 8–12, the greater is the potential for a pressor response. This is why the more traditional aerobic exercises have generally been recommended for the cardiac patient.

Now back to the question "Is strength/resistance training safe for use with cardiac patients?" The answer is an unequivocal yes for low-risk cardiac patients who have normal left ventricular function. Patients with normal left ventricular function have the same cardiovascular and hemodynamic response to resistance exercise (both isometric and dynamic) as do normal subjects.[169, 171, 178] It also appears that S-T–segment depression, angina pectoris, left ventricular wall motion abnormalities, and arrhythmias are not precipitated more with arm exercise than with leg exercise in cardiac patients.[178–182] Patients with left ventricular dysfunction and a low functional capacity are generally symptomatic or show signs of exercise intolerance with strength training. One study showed that patients with a resting left ventricular ejection fraction of less than 35 percent tolerated weight carrying of up to 50 pounds as well as patients with a normal left ventricle.[183] It appears that even though diastolic BP increases during strength training, its

Table 8–12. Cardiovascular and Hemodynamic Responses to Static and Dynamic Exercise

Variable	Rest	Type Contraction	Handgrip	Double-Legged Knee Extension
Cardiac output (l/min)	5.5	S	6.8	10.1*
		D	7.4	13.1*†
Stroke volume (ml)	72	S	76	77
		D	76	101*†
DBP (mmHg)	67	S	94	114*
		D	95	101†
SBP (mmHg)	118	S	150	193*
		D	151	193*
HR (beats/min)	76	S	91	134*
		D	99	128*
MAP (mmHg)	84	S	113	140*
		D	114	132*

DBP = diastolic blood pressure; SBP = systolic blood pressure; MAP = mean arterial blood pressure; S = static exercise; D = dynamic exercise.
*$p < 0.05$, values different from those of handgrip.
†$p < 0.05$, values different from those for S.
(Data from Lewis, S.F., et al.: Role of muscle mass and mode of contraction in circulatory responses to exercise. **J. Appl. Physiol.** 58:146–151, 1985.)

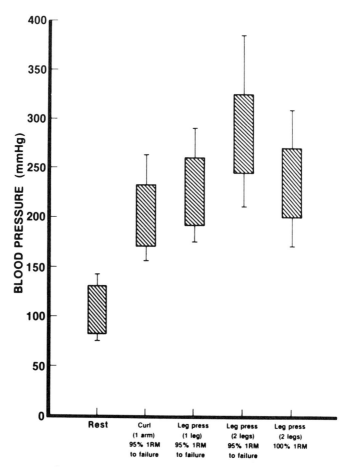

Peak systolic and diastolic blood pressures reached during
various exercises. X̄ and SD, N = 5

Figure 8–16. Mean ± SD peak blood pressures for all subjects during various exercises at 95% and 100% of their single maximum lift (1 RM). (From MacDougall, J.D., et al.: Arterial blood pressure response to heavy resistance exercise. **J. Appl. Physiol.** 58:785–790, 1985. Published with permission.)

greater perfusion effect on blood to the myocardium may offset some of the adverse effects of the BP increase.

The chronic effects of resistance/strength training have been shown to yield similar benefits in patients and in normals.[184–187] As shown in Chapter 7, the main effect is associated with increased muscular strength and endurance. These programs, which most often have included only low-risk patients, have been shown to be safe, with no added incidence of ischemia or dysrhythmia with training.[184–188] One program observed and followed patients for up to 3 years.[188] Another important point concerning strength training is its effect on submaximal BP. Most patients need and must do some form of lifting, carrying, or pushing activity in their daily routine. Lewis and associates[189] found that the pressor response was less at an absolute submaximal workload after training. Thus, including strength training as part of the patients' normal exercise program will better prepare them to perform other strength tasks safely and more efficiently.

How should patients be screened for doing resistance training? DeBusk and associates[180–182] in a series of three experiments comparing arm work with leg work, static with dynamic exercise (using 25 and 50 percent of an MVC), and handgrip with forearm lifting, found the SL-GXT to be an appropriate test for screening. Although

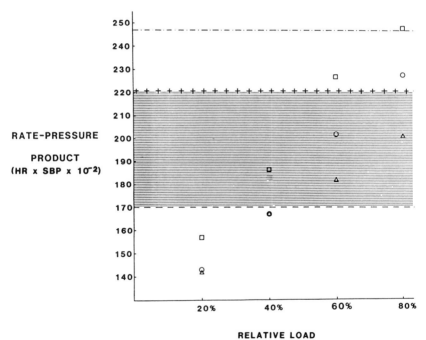

RELATIVE LOAD

Figure 8–17. The mean maximum rate-pressure product (mean maximum peak heart rate × mean maximum peak systolic pressure × 10^{-2}) responses to single-arm curl (△), single-leg press (○), and double-leg press (□) exercises are shown as functions of relative work intensity (plotted as a percentage of single maximum lift). Also shown are the mean rate-pressure product values in progressive incremental cycle ergometer testing at 60% (----), 85% (+ + + +), and 100% (— · —·) of the maximum achieved work. Data are shown as mean ± SEM; n = 8. (From Haslam, D.R.S., et al.: Direct measurement of arterial blood pressure during formal weightlifting in cardiac patients. **J. Cardiopul. Rehabil.** 8:213–225, 1988. Published with permission.)

static, handgrip, and arm exercise significantly increased systolic BP and HR, dynamic leg exercise such as walking or running elicited the highest maximal rate-pressure product (RPP = HR × Systolic BP) on the SL-GXT. Also, any combination of static (handgrip, forearm lifting) or dynamic-static exercise did not produce any greater incidence of abnormal responses (angina, S-T–segment depression, or dysrhythmia) to exercise. DeBusk and associates[181, 182] suggest that because the SL-GXT elicits a higher RPP than handgrip or arm exercise or other lifting-type tasks, it can be used satisfactorily for screening patients for returning to work and resuming lifting tasks or training. An addition of a graded weight-carrying task test as described by Sheldahl and associates[183] and Knapp and associates[190] may also be appropriate for patients returning to work who will be doing heavy lifting tasks.

Whether strength training is appropriate for patients who are at moderate to high risk should be evaluated on an individual basis. Since patients with depressed left ventricular function and a history of chronic heart failure have greater potential for a cardiac event, moderate to heavy lifting should not be recommended.

For the most part, the authors are in agreement with DeBusk and associates[181, 182] and their statement on the SL-GXT being the test of choice for screening patients for returning to work and clearing them for doing heavy lifting tasks. Patients who are screened in this manner and are considered at low risk have an MET capacity of 8 and above and have not been shown to have added complications doing lifting tasks or training. Even so, the reader should be aware of the data of MacDougall and colleagues[176] from young healthy participants doing heavy resistance training exercises. As shown in Figure 8–16, highly motivated individuals can drive BPs to alarmingly high levels. Thus, under these severe conditions, the SL-GXT may have limited value. On the other hand, Haslam and colleagues,[177] from the same group of investigators, have shown that cardiac patients performing light- to moderate-intensity strength training of up to 60 percent of MVC kept their RPP at or below that 85 percent of maximum RPP that was found during an SL-GXT (Fig. 8–17). These studies did not elicit any adverse responses to resistance training. Thus, light- to moderate-intensity resistance training can be recommended for most cardiac patients who have an 8 + MET capacity and who are considered at low risk.

Another point to emphasize here concerns the manner in which BP is assessed during strength training. MacDougall and colleagues[176] have shown that BP returns to within normal limits 10 to 15 seconds after stopping heavy resistance training. Thus, if BP is assessed after a patient stops exercise, which is usually the case with arm training and other types of weight training exercise, then the values measured are not representative of the actual BP that occurred during exercise.

What strength/resistance training exercise should be included in a cardiac rehabilitation program? In general, strength training of a light intensity can be started early in the outpatient program. Usually dynamic exercise, using the larger muscle groups of the body (arms-shoulders, back-trunk, and legs), should be included as part of a well-rounded program. Avoid heavy dynamic or static lifting, breath-holding, and activities that put undue pressure on the sternum (for surgery patients).

Because strength development is specific to how the muscle is trained, a more specific strength training routine is recommended for the surgery patient. Therefore, a combination of calisthenic and weight-lifting exercises can be used. For example, Figure 8–18 outlines an upper body strength routine that can be used by patients without complications beginning the second week of an outpatient phase-II program. Most patients begin the strength training program with 3-pound weights and progress to 5- to 7-pound weights before the 6-week SL-GXT. Depending on test results and patient needs, they may increase their weight up to 12 to 15 pounds before completing the phase-II program. French curls are not recommended for use with the surgical patient until the sternum is adequately healed.

Additional leg exercises are not included (except for ROM) because most patients are already getting leg strengthening with their aerobic activities. For the abdominal muscles, a modified bent-legged sit-up is used. In this modification, most patients will rest their arms across the chest and sit up through just the first one third of the ROM. Patients should be taught not to hold their breath during any exercise and to take at least one full inspiration and expiration with each repetition. Most of the exercises recommended for home use (see Chapter 7) are recommended for use in the outpatient program.

Some programs use a circuit method of training.[65, 104] This method incorporates a combination of leg stations (stationary cycling, treadmill walking, and bench stepping) and arm stations (rowing, arm cranking and wheeling, wall pulleys, and light weights). This method produces improvement in both aerobic fitness and upper body strength.

For patients without complications after the 6-week SL-GXT, many of the general restrictions on lifting or pushing weight with the arms and shoulders can be eliminated. This may include the

WARM-UP

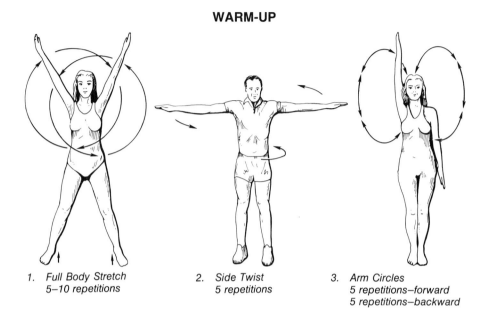

1. *Full Body Stretch*
   5–10 repetitions

2. *Side Twist*
   5 repetitions

3. *Arm Circles*
   5 repetitions–forward
   5 repetitions–backward

WEIGHT TRAINING

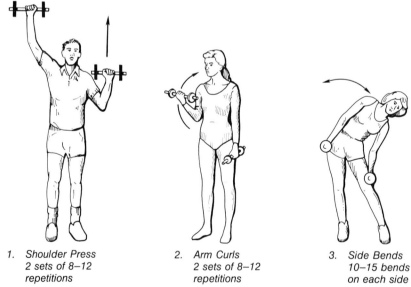

1. *Shoulder Press*
   2 sets of 8–12
   repetitions

2. *Arm Curls*
   2 sets of 8–12
   repetitions

3. *Side Bends*
   10–15 bends
   on each side

Figure 8–18. The upper body warm-up and weight training routine is introduced as early as 2 weeks after hospital discharge. This routine is used in the outpatient cardiac rehabilitation program of Mount Sinai Medical Center, Milwaukee, Wisconsin.

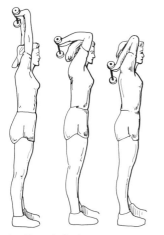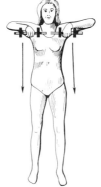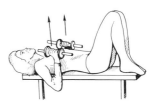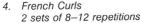

4. *French Curls*
   2 sets of 8–12 repetitions

5. *Upright Rowing*
   2 sets of 8–12
   repetitions

6. *Bench Press*
   2 sets of 8–12 repetitions

addition of arm and shoulder ergometer activities, i.e., a combination arm-leg cycle ergometer (Air Dyne, produced by Excelsior Fitness Corporation, Chicago, Illinois), rowing machine, and so on. The Air Dyne ergometer (see Fig. 8–8) allows a participant to train with a combination of arms and legs, legs only, and arms only. The arm-shoulder action is a push-pull movement that develops the muscles that will be used in many commonly performed work and recreation types of activities.

Strength training with weight training machines can also be introduced at this time. As shown in Chapter 7, these machines are designed to exercise the major muscle groups. They are ideal for use in cardiac rehabilitation because each machine's weight stack starts at a very low resistance and is graduated at acceptably small increments. Many of these machines are designed to protect the lower back and to avoid hand gripping. Also, balance- and skill-related problems that are associated with lifting barbells are not a factor in the new machine-type equipment.

In initiating a strength training program, start with the lightest weight on the weight stack. Have patients perform ten to 12 repetitions or exercise to an RPE of no greater than 13 (somewhat hard). Progress them to the next higher weight increment (5 or 10 pounds) every one to two weeks. Once the patients are thoroughly indoctrinated into the program, they can be progressed in training much as was suggested for the poorly fit healthy adult (Chapter 7).

More research is needed to determine further the safe limits of strength training using heavier weights. At this time, it seems probable that many patients without complications can train with heavier weights in much the same fashion as recommended for healthy adults. Possibly, weight training without the hand gripping component allows patients to do more, safely. Patients who have a low left ventricular function but a good functional capacity (8+ METs and asymptomatic) should be capable of doing strength training activities safely, although more research is needed in this area before making a more definitive statement.

Patient Education, Additional Forms, and Program Progress Report

As mentioned with the inpatient program, patient education should be a continuing process and an integral part of all phases of cardiac rehabilitation. For the formal outpatient program, examples of a physician referral form and an informed consent form were described earlier and are shown in Appendix B, Figures B–6 and B–7. Other forms that may be helpful include a daily exercise record, a data record of pertinent information, and an outpatient progress report (see Appendix B, Figures B–8 to B–10). The daily exercise record is used to keep accurate records of the patient's program. Pertinent information is kept on the various phases of the program, such as warm-up, weight training, treadmill or cycle ergometer activity, and cool-down. In addition, ECG strips (when appropriate) are taken each day (rest, peak exercise, and recovery) and are mounted separately.

The data record form summarizes important medical, physiological, and psychological information on each patient. Much of the information on this form should be self-explanatory. Line three lists risk factors and any special diet the patient may be on. Patient education (listed under V) includes initial assessment, introduction, risk factor education, and follow-up sessions. The body composition data are based on the sum of three skinfold fat measures (refer to the section on body composition measurement in Chapter 6).

Upon completion or termination of the outpatient program, patients are given a summary of their results (progress, potential problems, precautions, and so on) in the outpatient program. They are also given recommendations for a home program as well as a phase-III community-based program. The outpatient progress report is mailed to the patient's referring physician.

Community-Based Cardiac Rehabilitation Program— Phase III

As mentioned earlier, the phase-III program can be described in an organized and supervised community-based setting or in an unsupervised home or community program. The discussion in this section is directed toward the organized and supervised program, but many of the guidelines and suggestions can be applied to the unsupervised program.

A supervised phase-III program is generally conducted at a YMCA, Jewish Community Center, community or private rehabilitation-prevention center, or university campus. Figures 8–10 to 8–14 show examples of indoor and combination indoor-outdoor facilities used for phase-III cardiac rehabilitation programs. Both the Toronto Rehabilitation Centre and the Reh-Fit program do service some phase-II patients. Although described under phase-II programs, Figures 8–10 and 8–11 show facilities used for both phase-II and phase-III programs. Further descriptions of these programs are published elsewhere.[102]

A patient is admitted to the phase-III program after receiving a physical examination and an SL-GXT and after completing a medical history questionnaire. A physician referral form should also be required. Information related to medical status and the risk of further development of CAD is usually obtained during the physical examination, SL-GXT, and other tests. This information should be documented on the physician referral form. A current SL-GXT is important and should not be more than 3 months old. Phase-III programs usually accept the same type of patient as described for phase-II programs. Phase-III patients have had more time to recover from their MI or surgical procedure and are generally more stable medically and stronger physically. The same contraindications to exercise and guidelines for modifying the training program described for the phase-II program are also recommended for the phase-III program. As a result of studies showing that the distance traveled to and from an exercise facility correlates well with program adherence,[191] patients should be advised to attend the programs that are most convenient to their office or home.

The phase-III facility is generally not attached or necessarily close to a hospital; thus a portable defibrillator with ECG recorder and monitoring scope, sphygmomanometer, and emergency drugs, equipment, and supplies should be on site for all training sessions.[14, 16, 101, 192]

Table 8–4 shows the guidelines for exercise prescription used in the community-based phase-III programs. At this phase of training, the exercise prescription is similar for both MI and CABG patients. In addition, the exercise prescription becomes more similar to that recommended for the healthy adult. The intensity of the training is based on the patient's medical and physical status (risk classification) and on the results of the entry SL-GXT. The initial intensity prescribed is usually 60 to 70 percent of the HRmax reserve. As a patient progresses in the program (one to six months), the intensity can be adjusted upward, and some participants may reach 85 percent of maximum. When patients enter the program 6 to 12 months after the MI or surgery and have already been quite active, they can progress at a faster rate. If such a patient is asymptomatic and has a high functional capacity, he or she could progress to a higher intensity HR after just a couple of orientation sessions. Usually a functional capacity of 8 to 10 METs is sufficient to place a patient into a jogging regimen. Once patients are placed into a jogging type of program, it will be difficult for them to stay at the 70 percent intensity level. If the patient has not been observed previously in a supervised program, however, waiting approximately a week to a month before increasing the intensity is recommended. As in the case of other phases of the program, the level of intensity is individualized, and the patient progresses only if it is considered safe and the patient so desires.

The duration of training is between 30 and 60 minutes and depends on available time and intensity of training. Table 8–13 shows a 16-step walk, walk-jog program for patients in a phase-III program. The duration of training shown does not reflect the time needed for a warm-up, muscular conditioning, and cool-down (see Table 8–3). The guidelines for progression in Table 8–13 are the same as those described for the outpatients; i.e., a patient should be considered stable for at least one to two weeks before advancing to a higher step. Initially, the patient is placed at the step that corresponds to his or her functional capacity and proven experience in another phase of the program. If there is any question regarding the proper step, take the conservative approach and place the patient in a lower step.

It should be noted that the starter programs and 20-week walking or walking-jogging programs listed in chapter 7 may also be appropriate for use with cardiac patients. See Table 6–3 for assignment to the proper fitness category.

Patients with low functional capacities or those limited as a result of impaired coronary and ventricular function are not as likely to progress to a jogging program. Although many of these

Table 8–13. Sixteen-Step Walk, Walk-Jog Program for Cardiac Patients in Phase-III (Community-based–Home) Exercise Program

Functional Capacity (METs)	Step	Speed (mph)	Duration (min)	METs	METs (avg/workout)	Energy Cost (kcal)
5	1	2.5	30–60	2.5	2.5	3.0
	2	3.0	30–60	3.0	3.0	3.7
	3	3.25	30–60	3.25	3.25	4.0
5–8	4	3.5	30–60	3.5	3.5	4.2
	5	3.75	30–60	4.0	4.0	4.9
	6	4.0	30–60	4.6	4.6	5.5
8 or more	7	3.75 (2 min)*	30–45	4.0	4.6	4.9
		5.0 (30 sec)		6.9		8.3
	8	3.75 (2 min)*	30–45	4.0	5.0	4.9
		5.0 (1 min)		6.9		8.3
	9	3.75 (2 min)*	30–45	4.0	5.5	4.9
		5.0 (2 min)		6.9		8.3
	10	3.75 (1 min)*	30–45	4.0	6.0	4.9
		5.0 (2 min)		6.9		8.3
	11	3.75 (1 min)*	30–45	4.0	6.3	4.9
		5.0 (4 min)		6.9		8.3
	12	3.75 (1 min)*	30–45	4.0	6.5	4.9
		5.0 (6 min)		6.9		8.3
	13	3.75 (1 min)*	30–45	4.0	6.6	4.9
		5.0 (8 min)		6.9		8.3
	14	3.75 (1 min)*	30–45	4.0	6.6	4.9
		5.0 (10 min)		6.9		8.3
	15	3.75 (1 min)*	30–45	4.0	7.9	4.9
		5.5 (10 min)		8.3		10.1
	16	3.75 (1 min)*	30–45	4.0	8.0	4.9
		5.5 (12 min)		8.3		10.1

*Two lines denote interval training; for example, in step seven, the patient will alternate 2 minutes of walking at 3.75 mph with 30 seconds of jogging at 5.0 mph.

(Reprinted with permission from Pollock, M.L., Pels, A.E., Foster, C., and Ward, A.: Exercise prescription for rehabilitation of the cardiac patient. In Pollock, M.L., and Schmidt, D.H. (eds.): **Heart Disease and Rehabilitation,** 2nd Ed. New York, Churchill Livingstone, 1986, pp. 477–515.)

patients cannot tolerate higher intensity work, they generally adapt well to activity of lower intensity and longer duration.[193–198] In this situation, the patient progresses by duration of training and in increments of 5 minutes. This situation should not be confused with the patient who has a low ejection fraction (less than 40 percent) but has a moderate to normal functional capacity (8+ METs). These patients have a limited ventricular function but can often tolerate jog or walk-jog programs.[194] The suggested progression shown in Table 8–13 and subsequent remarks are only guidelines; patient stability and perception of effort should override any predetermined plan.

The duration of training shown in steps 1 to 6 is longer than that of steps 7 to 16 because steps 1 to 6 are of lower intensity. The attempt is to fit the program to the patient's daily schedule or time frame and to increase the kilocaloric level (total work) of the program toward a 300-kcal level.

Community-based programs usually require patients to attend class 3 days per week. Minimal acceptable attendance is usually 75 percent. It is strongly recommended that the patients train 3 to 5 days per week. As previously mentioned in Chapter 3, 300 kcal expenditure per training session and 1,000 kcal per week seem to be important thresholds for developing and maintaining fitness. Concerning the latter, Sidney, Shephard, and Harrison[199] showed that older participants who trained at approximately 200 to 250 kcal for a minimum of 4 days per week showed adequate improvement in cardiorespiratory function. The important point is that if the patient is training at a lower intensity, either the duration or frequency of training or both should be increased. Because of busy schedules, it is often difficult for patients to complete any more than a 30-minute aerobic program per session; thus, an increase in frequency (4 to 6 days per week) may be preferable. To maintain the necessary frequency of training, a home program is often needed. In this regard, a home program should follow the same guidelines as those described for the phase-II outpatient program.

Table 8–4 shows that a wider variety of activities are available for the patient in a phase-III program. The activity still depends on medical status, functional capacity, needs and desires, time, and available facilities. Games and various endurance sport activities may not be recommended at this time. For example, unless a patient has successfully participated in a walk-jog, jog regimen for several weeks to 3 months, sport activities that include a jog-run component would not be recommended. In addition, activities such as golf and tennis may require the patient to have special preparation (strength and flexibility training) before starting. Once a patient has participated satisfactorily in the phase-III program and can easily attain the MET requirement to take part in a specific activity (see Table 7–6), other activities can be encouraged. Highly competitive games and situations are not recommended for the high-risk patient. In certain situations, before a patient resumes normal work or lesiure activities, he or she can perform the required or desired activity while being monitored by telemetry or a Holter monitor. In addition, it may be important to evaluate BP. This type of monitoring may be useful in assessing the heart rhythm, BP, and HR responses under conditions that simulate those of the unsupervised setting. Although this technique of evaluating patient activity has some limitations, the results tend to eliminate certain apprehensions and thus help the patient toward a full recovery.

Monitoring of the patient during the phase-III program is accomplished through systematic checks of HR, BP, rhythm, and RPE. Heart rate and rhythm strips are determined before, approximately halfway through, and at the end of the training session, and before the patient leaves the exercise area (approximately 10 to 15 minutes). The rhythm monitoring may be accomplished with a defibrillator or quickly applied electrodes that are attached to a recorder. Blood pressure is checked before the training session and before the patient leaves the exercise area. If patients are symptomatic or have a questionable BP response to exercise, then more frequent readings (during exercises and recovery) should be taken. Heart rate is usually checked by the patient, using the palpation technique. Both HR and RPE are checked at the middle and end of the muscular conditioning and aerobic exercise periods. In general, no routine continuous monitoring of patients with telemetry is usually done at this stage of training.

If local patients prefer to train at home rather than as part of a supervised program, they are encouraged to have periodic evaluations of their training routines. These evaluations may occur once every 2 weeks to several months, depending on their medical status and stage of training. These sessions can be conducted in the doctor's office or in either the community-based or the phase-II outpatient setting. If desirable, patients can be monitored in their training program to simulate exercise conditions at home. These specially monitored sessions are encouraged when the patient is making a major change in training intensity or duration, is having modifications in medications, and if there is any question concerning his or her medical status. As mentioned earlier under "Supervision and Monitoring of Cardiac Rehabilitation Programs," this periodic visit is important in reviewing the patient's records and reinforcing any education goals important for risk reduction.

As mentioned earlier, strength training and flexibility exercises should be an integral part of a well-rounded program. For patients with normal left ventricular function and average to above-average MET capacities, more strenuous exercise can be recommended. Other patients who are medically stable may also be encouraged to perform more strenuous activity, but they should initiate these activities under supervision. All patients should continue to avoid heavy static holds and other activities that include a moderate but steady static component, such as water skiing.

Survey of Experts

In the survey of experts in the field, 17 phase-III programs were examined.[65] Of the 17 programs, eight accepted patients at 8 weeks and five at 12 weeks after MI or surgery. The others accepted patients earlier, and these programs coincided with ongoing out-patient programs. All but one required an SL-GXT before entry into the program. The one program required a GXT to 90 percent of age-predicted HRmax.

The frequency of training for the community-based programs was 3 days per week (± 0.7). Several programs used a combination of supervised (community-based) and unsupervised (home) training sessions. Two of 17 programs had patients train 3 days per week in a supervised program for the first 3 months, then 2 days supervised and 1 day unsupervised for the next 3 months, and finally 1 day supervised and 2 days unsupervised for the next 3 months. The idea was to have the patients gradually become independent, so that they would not always have to rely on a supervised program. About 50 percent of the programs encouraged their patients to walk at home on days they did not have to report to the formal program.

Duration of training (aerobic phase) averaged 31.3 minutes (± 7.2) per exercise session. Although the duration of training ranged from 20 to 60 minutes, few programs increased the duration of aerobic work beyond 40 minutes (six of 17). Two of 17 programs had durations of 20 to 25 minutes for aerobic training.

Intensity of training for phase-III programs centered mainly on the following two methods: 60 to 85 percent of HRmax and 60 to 85 percent of HRmax reserve. Heart rate monitoring was accomplished by telemetry or hard wire hook-ups, using either quick hook-up electrodes from an ECG or paddles from a defibrillator, and by palpating the pulse. In five of 17 programs, patients were routinely monitored by telemetry or hard wire hook-ups at least once a week for the first 2 to 4 weeks of training. Another three programs monitored exercise sessions by telemetry on a few patients, when deemed necessary. Most programs required the patients to check their HRs when they entered the exercise area, at the middle and end of their aerobic workouts, and before leaving the exercise area. Initially, BP was determined before and after each training session in 13 of 17 programs. Less attention was paid to BP monitoring and the number of times that HR was counted as the patients progressed in the program.

The community-based programs used a single mode of aerobic training (12 of 17), a single mode plus recreational game activities (four of 17), or circuit training (one of 17). Walking, walking-jogging, jogging, and stationary cycling were the activities most used.

Seven of 17 programs required a physician and eight of 17 required a nurse to be present at all training sessions. Three other programs always had a physician present in the building or adjacent area, and four programs had a physician present at least once a week. The physician generally used this time to review cases, to modify exercise prescriptions, and to speak with patients.

PROGRAMS FOR CARDIAC PATIENTS WITH SPECIAL MEDICAL PROBLEMS

There are specific problems or program modifications that are associated with exercise prescription for cardiac patients with angina pectoris, diabetes mellitus, pacemaker implants, peripheral vascular disease (intermittent claudication), arthritis, amputations, paralysis, and pulmonary disease. Also, cardiac transplantation and PTCA have become popular procedures and present the rehabilitation specialist with additional challenges.[200, 201]

Angina Pectoris

Angina is the squeeze or strangling in the chest first and best described by Heberden in 1772.[202] Although actual pain is present in moderately severe cases, angina is more frequently experienced as a severe discomfort or sense of constriction behind the breast bone.[203] Radiation of the discomfort up to the neck, jaw, individual teeth, or arms is typical. Since the appearance of anginal symptoms can be quite varied, upper abdominal discomfort without the chest component must be taken seriously. Palpation of the discomfort area may help to differentiate musculoskeletal pain from that of true angina.

The symptoms of angina can provide a warning to the individual approximately proportional to the ECG evidence of ischemia. Thus, the discomfort can be interpreted as a signal to ease up on either exertional intensity or psychological involvement. When the patient does recognize the chest discomfort, it can be a useful guide to making the appropriate adjustments for such influences as cold, heat, humidity, previous meals, or continued psychological burden after a tense situation.

Because the perception of pain differs widely, attempts to grade the degree of discomfort on some simple scale have been extremely difficult. A rating from grade 1 to 4 has been useful, although more precise assessment would be preferable. A 1-to-4 grading system is advised by the American Heart Association, the Canadian Cardiovascular Society, and the ACSM.[67, 203, 204] The following descriptive comments listed by each grade are recommended for use by Samuel Fox, M.D., past president of the American College of Cardiology.[205]

Grade-1 (light) is the discomfort that is established—but just established. Some patients speak of grade-½ discomfort as that premonitory sensation that precedes the grade-1 level as they walk, have sex, or get emotionally upset.

Grade-2 (light-moderate) discomfort is that from which one can be distracted by a noncataclysmic event. It can be "pain" but usually is not.

Grade-3 (moderate-severe) discomfort or pain prevents distraction by a beautiful woman, handsome man, TV show, or other consuming interest. Only a tornado, earthquake, or explosion can distract one from grade-3 discomfort or pain. During exercise testing, it should rarely be permitted for long, even when no other evidence of danger exists. In an unsupervised situation, it should definitely be avoided.

Grade-4 (severe) discomfort is the most excruciating pain experienced or imaginable. It should be avoided completely.

Borg and coworkers[206] have used a 9-point scale to rate angina pectoris. The scale is as follows: 1, no discomfort; 2, extremely light; 3, very light; 4, rather light; 5, not so light, rather strong; 6, strong; 7, very strong; 8, extremely strong; and 9, maximum, unbearable.

Nitroglycerin tablets should be available at all exercise classes. The anginal patient should carry nitroglycerin tablets in a light-resistant container. To ensure freshness, they should be replaced at least every 6 months. Storage in the refrigerator may help preserve effectiveness. The nitroglycerin is sufficiently strong if it has a sharp, "bitey" taste and gives a pounding in the head, if not a brief (10- to 20-minute) headache.

The effective action of nitroglycerin should occur in one to three minutes and last for 10 to 30 minutes. If relief does not occur, one or two repeat tablets can be taken at 5-minute intervals. Pain or discomfort for more than 15 minutes that persists after three rounds of active nitroglycerin tablets is usually considered sufficient cause to seek emergency medical treatment.

Two common ways of determining the upper limit training (target) HR for anginal patients are (1) having patients exercise at an HR that is 5 to 10 beats/min below the onset of angina, and (2) calculating an HR that is 70 to 85 percent of the anginal threshold. Some experimentation can be helpful. For example, sometimes a longer, slower warm-up period of 10 to 15 minutes may prevent or relieve symptoms or shift the anginal threshold upward. Although there is some controversy about allowing more stable patients to train with some anginal discomfort, it is generally not recommended to have patients attempt to walk through their angina when the discomfort level reaches 2 (on a 4-point scale). If patients become proficient in detecting and rating their anginal discomfort, then they can be counseled to train at a level just below their threshold of discomfort. The trial-and-error process should be accomplished in a supervised setting.

Taking nitroglycerin to help alleviate angina during training is an accepted practice. It is particularly useful for patients with a low angina threshold. Some institutions premedicate their angina patients before beginning their exercise routine.

Silent Myocardial Ischemia

Silent myocardial ischemia has been defined as "objective evidence for myocardial ischemia in the absence of angina or equivalent symptoms."[207] Its prevalence is estimated at 2 to 4 percent of the total asymptomatic middle-aged male population (USA: 1 to 2 million persons), 20 to 30 percent of asymptomatic post-MI patients (USA: 50,000 to 100,000 persons per year), and 80 to 90 percent of patients with angina (USA: 3 million persons).[207] Weiner and coworkers[208] reported on 2,982 patients from the coronary artery surgery study. Seven-year follow-up data showed survival rates to be similar for patients with exercise-induced S-T–segment depression and no angina (76 percent), exercise-induced angina with no S-T–segment depression (77 percent), and both exercise-induced angina and S-T–segment depression (78 percent) and were significantly better for the group with no angina or S-T–segment depression during exercise (88 percent). Thus, it is important for the rehabilitation specialist to know that many patients have silent ischemia and that it is significantly related to both the severity of disease and long-term survival. When these patients are identified, they should be treated as angina patients.

Diabetes Mellitus

Researchers are beginning to understand the complexities of glucose metabolism and how it is regulated for the diabetic patient. The potential hazards of acute exercise and chronic benefits of exercise training, as well as patient management during rehabilitation and exercise training are discussed. It has been estimated that approximately 11 million people have diabetes, with roughly 10 to 15 percent of them having type-I insulin-dependent diabetes mellitus (IDDM).[209] Diabetes is ranked sixth among leading causes of death in the U.S. Diabetes is a risk factor for cardiovascular diseases and thus is prevalent among the CAD and stroke patients found in cardiac rehabilitation programs.

Type-I IDDM is also called juvenile diabetes because it generally occurs in young people. In IDDM, the pancreas lacks the ability to produce enough insulin. Type-II diabetes is often called non–insulin-dependent diabetes mellitus (NIDDM) and is usually found in adults over the age of 40 years. Type-II NIDDM is usually slow in onset and is a result of the pancreas producing less insulin or the beta receptor cells becoming less sensitive to insulin. Type-I IDDM is of rapid onset, more difficult to control, and is treated with insulin injections. Type-II NIDDM is first treated by diet and exercise, oral medications, and finally, for some, insulin injections.

Hanson, Ward, and Painter[210] made the following comments in a review on exercise training in the diabetic patient:

METABOLIC RESPONSES TO ACUTE EXERCISE. During exercise, skeletal muscle substrate uptake varies according to intensity (%$\dot{V}O_2$max) and duration of work. At rest, free fatty acids (FFA) are the primary energy source. Glucose and FFA are both used during the initial phase of submaximal exercise, whereas FFA becomes the dominant substrate during prolonged submaximal (50% to 60% $\dot{V}O_2$max) exercise. Small amounts of glucose from skeletal muscle glycogen stores are required for prolonged exercise, however, and the depletion of these stores results in prompt muscle fatigue.[211]

The control of hepatic glucose and adipose-tissue FFA release is mediated by a characteristic pattern of neurohormonal and hormonal response (Table 8–14). Insulin levels are pivotal in maintaining the balance between hepatic glucose production and increased muscle

Table 8–14. Metabolic Effect of Submaximal Exercise in Normal and Diabetic Subjects

	Regulatory Hormone				Circulating Substrates		
	IN	*GL*	*E*	*NE*	*Glucose*	*FFA*	*Ketone*
Normal	↓	↑	↑	↑	↑ early → or ↓ late	↑	→
IDDM							
In (−)	0	↑↑	↑↑	↑↑	↑↑	↑↑	↑
In (+)	→ or ↑	↑	↑	↑	→ early ↓ late	↑	→ or ↑
NIDDM	↑ or ↓	↑	↑	↑	↑ early → or ↓ late	↑	→

↑ = increased; ↓ = decreased; → = no change; IDDM = insulin-dependent diabetes; NIDDM = non–insulin-dependent diabetes; In = insulin; E = epinephrine; NE = norepinephrine; GL = glucagon; FFA = free fatty acids.
(From Hanson, P., Ward, A., and Painter, P.: Exercise training in special patient populations. **J. Cardiopul. Rehabil.** 6:104–112, 1986. Published with permission.)

glucose use during exercise. In normal subjects pancreatic insulin release is inhibited by increased catecholamine levels, and hepatic glycogenolysis and gluconeogenesis are stimulated by increased levels of glucagon, epinephrine, and possibly growth hormone and cortisol. Plasma FFA also increases because of norepinephrine-mediated lipolysis. Skeletal muscle uptake of glucose is simultaneously increased through insulin-independent transport mechanisms. Circulating glucose levels remain stable or decline only slightly, although with prolonged exercise, hypoglycemia may occur in normal subjects.[212]

Type-I Diabetes Mellitus. Insulin-dependent diabetics who have absent or insufficient insulin levels are hyperglycemic at rest and respond to exercise with marked increases in glucose, FFA, and ketone production stimulated by excessive catecholamine, glucagon, and growth hormone release.[213]

With exogenous insulin therapy, type-I diabetics exhibit near normal patterns of glucose and FFA response to exercise. The relatively high circulating levels of insulin combined with additional insulin released from subcutaneous injection sites may inhibit hepatic glucose release, however, so that hypoglycemia ensues.[214] This effect is more pronounced when exercise is attempted during the time of peak insulin rise.

When exercise is performed in the immediate postprandial period, the usually high circulating levels of glucose are attenuated, presumably because of non–insulin-dependent uptake of glucose by exercising muscle.[215] Accordingly, this pattern of daily exercise may be most useful for controlling postprandial hyperglycemia.

Type-II Diabetes Mellitus. Non–insulin-dependent diabetics exhibit a variable spectrum of peripheral insulin resistance and show hyperglycemia and impaired glucose tolerance and either increased or reduced insulin levels.[216] During exercise, glucose levels usually decrease gradually because of enhanced use by skeletal muscle. Hepatic glucose production may be inhibited in the presence of high insulin levels; however, hypoglycemia is unlikely during short-term exercise.[216]

CARDIOVASCULAR AND AUTONOMIC RESPONSES. Hemodynamic responses to exercise are frequently abnormal in type-I diabetic patients who have evidence of autonomic neuropathy. Heart rate, blood pressure, cardiac output, and peripheral blood-flow responses to dynamic and static exercise are typically attenuated, presumably because of combined effects of impaired sympathetic drive and diabetic cardiomyopathy. Postural hypotension and postexertional orthostatic hypotension are also common in diabetics with autonomic neuropathy.[217]

Exercise Training in Type-I Diabetes. Most training studies have shown that significant increases in $\dot{V}O_2$max are achieved in subjects with uncomplicated type-I diabetes. These responses are accompanied by evidence of increased peripheral insulin sensitivity and variable improvement in glucose regulation, measured by fasting glucose (FG), 24-hour glucose excretion, oral glucose tolerance (OGT), intravenous glucose tolerance (IVGT), and hemoglobin Alc(HbAlc).

An initial training study by Soman and associates[218] showed increased insulin sensitivity (euglycemic clamp method) but no change in FG. Peterson and coworkers[219] subsequently showed significant decreases in mean glucose and HbAlc levels and reduction in muscle capillary basement membrane thickness. Wallberg-Henricksson and associates[220] found increased insulin sensitivity and muscle oxidative enzyme activity but no change in 24-hour urinary glucose excretion or HbAlc. In contrast, Champaigne and collagues[221] recently showed reduction in FG and HbAlc in younger type-I diabetics after vigorous exercise for 12 weeks.

These findings probably reflect the marked heterogeneity of this population and emphasize the necessity for individual evaluation and follow-up monitoring to determine the effects of exercise on glucose control.

Exercise Training in Type-II Diabetes. Type-II diabetics are usually obese and unfit. Most exercise-training studies show increased peripheral insulin sensitivity and improved glycemic control. The degree of improvement, however, may vary with the intensity of exercise training, diet, and simultaneous weight loss.

Barnard and coworkers[222] reported significant decreases in FG and use of oral hypoglycemic agents and insulin therapy after a 26-day rigid diet and exercise program. Reitman and colleagues[223] found decreased FG and improved OGT, and Trovati and associates[224] also found decreased FG, IVGT, and HbAlc after 6 to 10 weeks of training. Leon and colleagues[225] recently reported no change in FG, OGT, or insulin levels in type-II diabetics who trained for 12 weeks without weight loss.

These findings indicate a generally predictable trend toward improved glucose levels in type-II diabetics who follow prescribed exercise. Simultaneous weight loss, however, may be a major factor in this response.

Recommendations and Precautions. Exercise training appears to be useful as an adjunct to traditional dietary and insulin or oral hypoglycemia treatment of uncomplicated diabetes. Its objective with respect to diabetic patients is to optimize functional capacity, control body weight, modulate glucose levels, and reduce other metabolic risk factors for CHD.

Exercise testing is recommended to determine baseline functional capacity and to identify potential abnormal responses such as hypertension, hypotension, asymptomatic myocardial ischemia, or impaired heart-rate response. Patients with diabetic complications of retinal microangiopathy, peripheral or autonomic dysfunction, peripheral vascular disease, or asymptomatic coronary disease are not appropriate candidates for exercise training and may be at increased risk during imposed exercise.[213, 217]

Exercise should be prescribed according to accepted guidelines used for cardiac rehabilitation, with emphasis on aerobic training at 60% to 75% $\dot{V}O_2$max for 30 to 40 minutes daily or at least four times weekly. Initially, exercise training is best performed in intervals of 5 to 10 minutes with several minutes of recovery between intervals. As exercise tolerance increases, the duration of steady-state training is gradually extended to achieve a total of 30 to 40 minutes. High-intensity or prolonged (more than 60 minutes) exercise should be avoided. In addition, warm-weather exercise may be poorly tolerated in type I or obese type-II patients.

Signs or symptoms of exercise or postexercise hypoglycemia should be anticipated in type-I diabetics. Appropriate adjustments in insulin dose, injection site, caloric intake, and the timing of exercise may be used to correct the hypoglycemic response. Insulin dosage may be reduced in small (2 unit) increments and insulin injections placed in subcutaneous sites over nonexercising muscle. Carbohydrate intake should be increased before exercise, using one bread exchange (15 g carbohydrate) for each 30 minutes of anticipated exercise. The need for increased caloric intake may be alleviated by exercising during the early postprandial period.[215] Blood glucose levels should be routinely monitored to verify the outcome of these changes.

Sports Participation. Many individual and team sports are appropriate for well-controlled young diabetic patients. Indeed, diabetic athletes have competed successfully in national and international endurance sports events such as swimming, track, tennis, and soccer. In addition, some diabetic patients play traditional contact sports such as football, basketball, wrestling, and hockey.

Medical clearance for participation in endurance or contact sports should be based on individual clinical status and the following important factors:

1. Stable diabetic control as judged by history and self-monitoring of blood glucose. A diabetic patient should not exercise when the blood glucose is lower than 60 mg/dl or higher than 300 mg/dl or when ketotic.

2. The absence of diabetic complications such as microangiopathic retinal changes, autonomic neuropathy (heart rate, blood pressure), altered renal function, hypertension, ischemic heart disease, and cardiomyopathy.

3. A thorough understanding of the prevention and treatment of hypoglycemia. Alterations in insulin treatment and caloric intake will be similar to those previously outlined for aerobic exercise training. Patients should also wear a tag identifying themselves as being diabetic.

Unfortunately, there are no completely satisfactory guidelines for participation in a specific sport. In the majority of uncomplicated insulin-dependent diabetic patients, a cautious trial of training or competition is the best way of determining an exercise regimen for a given individual.

The ACSM recommends that the diabetic patient exercise 5 to 7 days per week.[67] For the type-I diabetic, daily training aids in keeping the pattern of diet-insulin dosage regulated. For the type-II diabetic, greater frequency of training (moderate intensity, low impact) aids in weight control and diabetes management.

Just as recommended for the cardiac patient, the diabetic patient should have an exercise partner. Within this framework of exercise, all persons involved in the training regimen (patient, exercise partner, program director) should be aware of the common symptoms of diabetes and its treatment. Leon[226] lists the common symptoms and signs of diabetes as fatigue, weakness, weight loss, hunger (polyphagia), thirst (polydipsia), frequent urination (polyuria), elevated blood sugar level (hyperglycemia), sugar in the urine (glycosuria), and acetone in the blood and urine (ketosis). Common symptoms of hypoglycemia include excessive sweating, trembling, drowsiness, dizziness, dilated pupils, blurred vision, nervousness, and irritability.

Since a hypoglycemic reaction can occur 24 to 48 hours after completion of an exercise training session, the patients must be educated to this potentially dangerous problem. Most problems with hypoglycemia occur in patients who exercise at a high intensity or for a prolonged period of time.[67, 227] Also, exercising immediately after an insulin injection when the patient's blood insulin level is at its peak or injecting insulin at the site of the exercising muscle (usually within 45 minutes) can precipitate a hypoglycemic response. Thus, the patient should be instructed to carry nourishment such as simple sugar (candy), fruit juice, or other easily digestible carbohydrates.[227, 228] These same nourishments should be available at the rehabilitation center. Many experts suggest the abdominal area as being a good neutral site for insulin injection.[226, 228]

Because of the long-term effect that elevated blood glucose has on the peripheral circulation and sweating mechanism, diabetic patients should be particularly careful in selecting the proper footwear and pay close attention to foot hygiene.[67, 226, 229] They should also be cautious in exercising in the heat.[67] Patients with foot problems should be guided to low-impact activities that do not cause further aggravation.

The ACSM guidelines emphasize the importance of the exercise program director knowing patients who are taking both insulin and beta-blocking drugs, because the hypoglycemic symptoms can be masked by the beta blocker.[67] For more detailed information on diabetes risk factors, complications, and management see Leon[226] and Goldberg and Coon (for the elderly patient).[230]

Pacemakers

Exercise testing of and prescription for the patient with a pacemaker is common in cardiac rehabilitation programs. Pacemaker technology is becoming more and more complex; thus constant interaction with an electrophysiologist is helpful. The two most common reasons for pacemaker implantation are sick sinus syndrome (mainly episodes of bradycardia, episodic atrial tachyarrhythmias, and chronotropic insufficiency) and high-degree atrial-ventricular node block (mainly associated with complete heart block).

The pacing system consists of a small generator and one or two leads. Most pacemakers are implanted in the subclavicular area, with lead wires placed in the right ventricle (apex, single-chamber pacer), or right atrium and right ventricle (dual-chamber pacer). The signals that come in from the lead wires allow the generator to sense intrinsic cardiac activity. Fearnot, Smith, and Gedders[231] describe the various pacemaker algorithms that are available for generator control. Most of these can be programmed to best meet the needs of the patient.

A once commonly used pacemaker, the VVI paces the ventricle, senses the ventricle, but paces at a preset rate (usually around 75 beats/min) and is inhibited when the preset ventricular rate is exceeded. A dual-chamber pacemaker can pace or sense either chamber at programmable rates. It is widely used now and offers potential hemodynamic advantages for use during exercise. Other exciting and promising new rate-responsive pacemakers are being clinically examined and include sensing of pH, Q-T interval, respiration rate, body motion, and central venous temperature.[231] The recent work of denDulk and associates[232] shows promising results for an activity-sensing detector and circuitry. As summarized by Fearnot, Smith, and Gedders,[231] more advanced sensors will allow for more optimal detection of physiological needs.

In general, exercise prescription can be based on an SL-GXT as described for other cardiac patients, but careful attention should be placed on BP response and symptoms of exercise intolerance. For demand-type (rate-response) pacemakers, training HR can be calculated as described for MI and CABG surgery patients. Patients on fixed HR response–type pacemakers for episodes of bradycardia, but who otherwise have a normal HR response, can also calculate their training HRs in a conventional manner. Patients who are pacemaker dependent have no target HR and usually exercise at a more moderate intensity and emphasize more gradual build-up (warm-up) and cool-down periods. The ACSM[67] recommends that pacemaker-dependent patients should have their BP checked at least three times during the training session and until the exercise leader is assured of a satisfactory exercise response.

The intensity of exercise for fixed HRs can be developed by use of a modified Karvonen equation, substituting BP for HR. This technique was first mentioned by Superko[233] and later recommended by the ACSM.[67] The equation is as follows:

$$\text{TSBP} = (\text{SBP}_{max} - \text{SBP}_{rest})\,(0.6 \text{ to } 0.8) + \text{SBP}_{rest}$$
$$\text{TSBP} = \text{training systolic BP}$$

Thus, the patient would train at a level that would not exceed the percent of specified systolic BP, based on data from an SL-GXT.

Use of the RPE is particularly helpful in monitoring the exercise prescription of pacemaker patients. Other factors important to the management of the pacemaker patient include a regular check of battery and pacemaker function.

For patients with new subclavicular permanent pacemaker implantation, no upper extremity movement with the affected arm is recommended for the initial 24 to 48 hours. After 48 hours, upper extremity exercise is limited to that associated with normal daily activity. To prevent the pacemaker wire from dislodging, no additional ROM exercise should be performed for approximately the first 2 weeks. After this, upper extremity ROM exercises may commence. Patients with new abdominal permanent pacemaker implantation should not perform hamstring or gastrocnemius stretching for 2 weeks. The ACSM states that even though electrodes tend to become relatively fixed with time, caution is still advised regarding excessive stretching and body manipulation.[67]

Intermittent Claudication

Patients with intermittent claudication are often limited in their ambulation (cycling) program by their peripheral vascular disease rather than their heart condition. In this case, patients use an interval training method of exercise.[67, 234] This includes one- to five-minute bouts of low-level aerobic exercise followed by 2 to 10 minutes of rest. This procedure may be repeated four to six times. As patients progress, longer periods of aerobic exercise should be introduced. Others have recommended the use of more continuous training at low levels just below the onset of significant pain symptoms (grade 2, moderate).[235, 236] Some have recommended that this training procedure be repeated twice daily.[67, 237] Because both techniques appear to give similar results, the authors recommend one training session per day.

Depending on where their blockage is located, some patients tolerate stationary cycling better than walking. In this case, at least 50 percent of their aerobic program should be completed on the stationary cycle. Because walking is a patient's major mode of transportation and walking training significantly improves walking performance,[234-238] some walking training is always recommended. Alternative exercises—e.g., swimming and rowing—can be considered as part of the training program for phases II and III.

In addition to using the RPE scale for monitoring one's general perception of effort during the aerobic phase of training, it is also useful in rating peripheral discomfort (pain). Usually when leg discomfort reaches 13 to 15 (somewhat hard to hard), the rest period should commence. Once the discomfort reaches the hard level, patients must usually terminate their exercise program for that day, because recovery is often quite slow and painful. Boyd and colleagues[236] found excellent improvements in performance in intermittent claudication patients who were trained relatively pain free for 12 weeks. Thus, using 13 on the RPE scale or grade 2, moderate, discomfort (grade 1 to 4 scale recommended by the ACSM[67]) as a means of monitoring training allows the patient to accomplish repeated bouts of exercise training.

Arthritis and Amputees

Arthritic or paralyzed patients or amputees exercise in the activities that they can perform without undue symptoms. Alternate aerobic activities may be substituted. For example, if lower extremity activities such as walking and stationary cycling cannot be performed or tolerated, arm ergometry with little or no resistance may be used. Patients with wheelchairs may be allowed to propel themselves slowly during the early stage of their training program. Crutch walking is too strenuous at the earlier phases of recovery and is not recommended. Caution should be taken with surgery patients that little pressure is placed on the sternum. If sternal movement or clicking occurs, the arm cycle activity should be discontinued.

For phases II and III, other alternative activities—e.g., swimming, walking, or jogging in water—may be substituted. Generally, for arthritic patients, high-impact activities should be avoided. Also, during periods of high joint inflammation or pain, a reduction in intensity and duration of training is often necessary. Most often, high-intensity exercise should be avoided, but low- to moderate-intensity exercise through a full ROM is desirable. As mentioned earlier under strength/resistance training, many of the new weight-lifting machines can be pinned to limit the ROM of the exercise. This would be applicable to the arthritic patient who is often having pain in only part of the ROM.

Ekblom and Nordemar[239] review the many clinical and treatment aspects of the rheumatoid arthritis patient. They also show that light to moderate exercise is beneficial to the arthritic patient. Panush and Brown[240] are in agreement with Ekblom and Nordemar and further state that sensible exercise is generally safe for the arthritic patient.

Chronic Obstructive Pulmonary Disease (COPD)

Patients with COPD are quite varied in physical and medical impairment and their ability to perform exercise and activities of daily living (ADL).[241–244] It is also well known that although pulmonary rehabilitation improves most patients' functional capacity, it does not appear to improve the underlying disease.[241, 243, 245–247] In a more recent review, Hodgkin[243] reported that most studies evaluating the effects of pulmonary rehabilitation showed patients to report fewer respiratory symptoms, less anxiety and depression, increased ability to perform ADLs, a better quality of life, and improved exercise tolerance. The data on survival and return to work were mixed but promising. Programs that showed better survival used multi-interventional approaches including exercise, hygiene, and supplemental oxygen therapy, as well as good follow-up.

Most COPD patients stop during an SL-GXT because of dyspnea. Patients with COPD who have mild symptoms (FEV_1 is approximately 80 percent of predicted maximum) can usually do quite well with an exercise prescription as described for cardiac patients. Usually high-intensity exercise is not recommended, but moderate exercise with increased frequency and duration is. Hodgkin[243] recommends the normally used target HR techniques for these patients but adds that RPE and signs of dyspnea are sometimes better indicators for monitoring intensity.

With more moderate (FEV_1 is 60 to 80 percent of predicted maximum) and severe (FEV_1 is less than 60 percent of predicted maximum) COPD patients, the use of dyspnea and the use of RPE are the recommended monitoring techniques. For patients with more severe disease and for those whose partial pressure of oxygen drops to 55 mmHg or whose oxygen saturation drops to 88 percent or lower, supplemental oxygen is recommended.[243] Patients with significant limitations are often trained similarly to what was described for intermittent claudication patients—low-level interval training. This type of program can be easily monitored by walking or with the use of a stationary cycle. Hodgkin[243] recommends the use of a 12-minute walk test at the beginning and periodically throughout the program. This test has been shown to be safe and easy to administer and can aid in determining the patient's progress in the program.

Connors and coworkers[248] emphasize the importance of a good evaluation. Their experience has shown that many COPD patients have multiple medical problems other than their pulmonary condition. These problems include hypertension, arrhythmias, CAD, nasal and sinus abnormalities, and similar conditions. Hodgkin[243] feels that an SL-GXT is most important for COPD patients in helping to quantify their medical status and is particularly useful in the following situations: "(1) to select a target HR to use during the exercise training period; (2) to determine whether there is any reason, other than pulmonary impairment, for dyspnea or exercise limitations, e.g., coronary artery disease, cardiac valve disease, or peripheral vascular disease; and (3) to determine if a patient's level of impairment precludes them from certain types of work."

For many patients, special respiratory muscle training is recommended.[249] COPD patients should have special training (educational programs) on pulmonary hygiene and breathing exercises.[241, 249] Lastly, for information on drugs most used by COPD patients and other aspects of pulmonary rehabilitation, other references should be consulted.[241, 242, 250–253]

Percutaneous Transluminal Coronary Angioplasty (PTCA)

The PTCA procedure has become an accepted alternative for many patients needing revascularization. The procedure was performed in more than 133,000 patients in the U.S. in 1986.[254] King,[255] in a more recent review, stated that in the more than 8,000 procedures performed at Emory University Hospital, the overall mortality rate was 0.2 percent for all cases and under 0.1 percent in single-vessel disease.

The major problem in the management and rehabilitation of the PTCA patient is restenosis.[201, 255] The restenosis rate most often quoted is 25 percent,[255] but it can range up to 30 to 35 percent.[201] The restenosis process is usually complete by 4 to 6 months[255] and is rare after 6 to 8 months.[201, 255] Repeat PTCA has shown success similar to that found with the original procedure, with no increased rate of restenosis. The advent of multiple-vessel PTCA and emergency PTCA in acute MI[256] creates a greater challenge for patient management.

The factors related to restenosis include male gender, unstable angina, a short history of angina, total occlusion of the dilated vessel, and location of the stenosis (proximal anterior descending artery, ostium of the right coronary artery, or body of a vein graft.)[255] Like many CAD or CABG surgery patients, PTCA patients are on multiple drugs including calcium antagonists and antiplatelet agents.

What type of program is given to patients who have had PTCA? Because the patients are discharged within 2 to 3 days after the procedure, there is little time to provide them with an inpatient program. Patients can begin slow ambulation and ROM exercise approximately 24 hours after PTCA. The incision used for the procedure should be stable by this time. Education concerning risk factors, primary and secondary prevention, home exercise, and similar topics that is given to CAD patients is also desirable for the PTCA patient. Of particular importance is their knowledge concerning the possibility of restenosis and ensuing signs and symptoms.

Most hospitals that perform PTCA routinely give SL-GXTs and other diagnostic tests before and after the procedure. This would leave possibly a day for an evaluation from the cardiac rehabilitation staff. The exercise session should include the various components of a training program. The ROM exercises for MI patients are recommended. Usually, patients can complete the entire ten repetitions of exercise, climb and descend one flight of stairs, and ambulate or stationary cycle for 20 to 30 minutes. If the patients have had their SL-GXT before their training session, the test results should be used as a guide for exercise prescription. A patient with a 5+ MET capacity should be able to complete the program as outlined for the CABG surgery patient (Table 8–6), with ambulation being conducted at 2 to 3.0 mph for 30 minutes. After completion of the training session and SL-GXT, a review of the principles of exercise and some instruction on counting HR and the use of the

RPE scale would be helpful. Then, a 12-week home exercise program is designed and recommended for the patient. The program is individually designed, and PTCA patients usually can progress at a faster rate than can MI and CABG surgery patients.[257,*] Progression in training and determination of whether patients need to be exercised in a supervised program depend on their estimated risk. High-risk patients and ones who are at high risk of restenosis should be recommended to exercise in an organized, supervised program for up to 6 months. If they choose to train at home, exercising with a partner and in populated areas where emergency help is available is recommended.

At 2 weeks after discharge, PTCA patients usually return for a consultation with their cardiologist. If these patients are not involved in an organized outpatient program, it may be advisable to have them meet with someone from the cardiac rehabilitation staff for an exercise prescription update. Depending on time and facilities, the consultation can be simply a review and discussion of how the patients have progressed in their home programs. If time and facilities are available, the home program can be actually simulated in the outpatient clinic. The consultation would help clear up any questions and confusion that patients may have concerning their program, and if necessary, their existing program can be modified.

Cardiac Transplantation

The first cardiac transplant procedure was performed in 1967.[258] Even so, its popularity had not greatly increased until the recent advances in immunosuppression drugs.[259] In particular, cyclosporine and other pharmacological agents (azathioprine and low-dose prednisone on a long-term basis and the use of rabbit antithymocyte globulin (RATG) or OKT3 for resistant rejection episodes) have increased survival immensely.[200, 259] Within this framework, one-year survival rates average 80 percent, and 5-year survival rates are 60 percent, up dramatically from reports before 1981.[200] Other technical factors such as controlling infections and better patient selection have helped increase survival. Better survival rates have resulted in an exponential growth in the number of transplants performed each year in the U.S., with more than 1,000 being performed in 1987. With the projected need of 15,000 available

*(Unpublished data, Ben-Ari, E., and Rothbaum, D., Indiana Heart Institute, 1989.)

patients annually, the donor supply appears to be a major problem for increasing the numbers of yearly transplantations.[200]

General indications for cardiac transplantation include the patient having end-stage heart disease, being unlikely to benefit from standard therapy, and having a poor prognosis for survival.[200, 260] Patients are generally under the age of 55 years, healthy other than having end-stage cardiac disease, medically compliant, and emotionally stable, with a realistic attitude toward their illness.[200, 260] The most common reason for cardiac transplantation is a result of end-stage CAD (43 percent), cardiomyopathy (49 percent), and advanced valvular disease (5 percent).[200] These diagnoses are important for the rehabilitation team to know because not all of these patients have CAD and, thus, may not need much education in regard to risk reduction for CAD. It is also evident that some of these patients have had severe disease for a number of months or years and thus, as a whole, tend to be weaker (low functional capacity) than most patients and normal individuals without heart disease. Table 8–15 shows data on 36 cardiac transplant patients compared with 45 age-matched normals.[261] The data show that the patients were significantly lighter in body weight, which was mainly a result of less fat-free weight. The data also

Table 8–15. Comparison of Physiological Variables of Cardiac Transplant Patients Before and After Endurance Training and in a Comparison with an Aged-Matched Normal Group

Variable	Normals (n = 45)	Cardiac Transplant Patients Before (n = 36)	After (n = 36)
Age (yr)	45.4	47.3	48.9†
Weight (kg)	80.7*	69.9	73. 9†
Fat (%)	22.1	19.1	20.2
Fat-free wt, (kg)	62.6*	56.2	58.2†
HRrest (beats/min)	76.8*	103.9	100.3†
HRmax (beats/min)	176.2*	135.5	148.2‡
BPrest (mmHg)	127*/84*	138/95	125‡/86‡
BPmax (mmHg)	214*/96*	178/100	174/92‡
$\dot{V}O_2$max (ml · kg^{-1} · min^{-1})	34.0*	21.7	25.8‡
Peak power (W)	219*	101	150‡
RPEmax	19.4*	18.3	19.1†
$\dot{V}_E$max (l/min)	101.4*	70.5	90.9‡
$\dot{V}_E/\dot{V}O_2$	37.3*	48.1	48.1
R	1.18	1.14	1.16

(Data from Kavanagh, T., et al.: Cardiorespiratory responses to exercise training after orthotopic cardiac transplantation. **Circulation** 77:162–171, 1988.)

*p < 0.01, normals compared with transplants (before).

†p < 0.05, transplants after training as compared with before.

‡p < 0.01, transplants after training as compared with before.

showed that the transplant recipients had a limited functional capacity. These factors as well as the threat of rejection and infection make the early stages of recovery and rehabilitation more complex with the cardiac transplant patient than with most MI or CABG surgery patients.

With the cardiac transplant patient, preoperative rehabilitation is often necessary because many patients have to be hospitalized several days to 2 weeks before the transplant procedure.[262, *] Oftentimes, patients at this stage are bedridden, have a limited functional capacity (New York Heart Association Class IV) or both. Their low capacity is associated with weeks of debilitation, severe cardiac dysfunction, or both. The cardiac rehabilitation team can be helpful to patients by giving them energy conservation training, which can help them with their daily ADLs.[262] The patients may also need assistance in learning diversional activities and relaxation techniques. Low-level exercise in both ROM and slow ambulation or stationary cycling without resistance may be helpful in maintaining the patient's function capacity before surgery. This time period also gives the rehabilitation team the opportunity to evaluate the patient for other potential medical problems such as orthopedic limitations.

The inpatient stay for the cardiac transplant patient varies but, most often, is a minimum of 21 to 28 days. The first 3 to 7 days are in the intensive care unit. Rehabilitation can begin as soon as the surgeon gives approval. Progress in the program is individualized and is quite varied from patient to patient. In general, the same program that has been recommended for a CABG surgery patient can be adapted to the cardiac transplant patient. The big difference is in its application. The program for the cardiac transplant patient begins 3 to 7 days after surgery, and the patient is usually weaker than an average CABG surgery patient. Thus the progression in training is much slower, with the speed of ambulation or resistance on a stationary cycle and repetitions in the ROM exercise being less initially. Once patients get to the step-down units or ward, the rehabilitation program continues in the patients' room. As they get stronger, they can be allowed to ambulate in the wards. Usually during this period of rehabilitation, it is recommended that ambulation take place during the low-traffic hours of the day. More specific step programs for inpatient and outpatient rehabilitation for the cardiac transplant patient are available through other sources (Mayo Clinic, Rochester, MN;

---

*(Personal communication, Ray Squires, Ph.D., Mayo Clinic, Rochester, MN, January, 1988.)

Stanford University, Palo Alto, CA; and Shands Hospital–University of Florida, College of Medicine, Gainesville, FL).

Serious infections, acute rejection, and rapid-onset atherosclerosis are the most serious problems confronting the cardiac transplant patient.[200, 259] Endomyocardial biopsies are taken frequently and are performed on a step-down basis. Severe rejection is most prevalent the first 3 months after transplant.[259] It is important to time the rehabilitation program so that it does not take place immediately after a biopsy procedure. It is also important to know the various responses to the immunosuppression drugs and signs of rejection or infections.[259, 262] Cyclosporine has many side effects, but the most important for the rehabilitation team is its effect on BP. Hypertension is a common problem with cyclosporine treatment.[200, 263, 269] This hypertensive response tends to be less with time.[263, 269] Also, exercise training has been associated with a decrease in BP in cardiac transplant patients.[261, 264] Sources are available that give specific actions and side effects of the various drugs.[259, 262] Antithymocyte globulin, which is given in the very early stages of the postoperative course and during episodes of severe rejection, is usually injected in the quadriceps muscle. A side effect from this drug is swelling around the injection site and, sometimes, leg pain and cramps. Light ROM exercise during this time may be helpful in relieving some of these symptoms.

The exercise response to the denervated heart is different from that found for the normal heart.[261, 264–270] Although there is a significantly altered HR-hemodynamic and cardiorespiratory effect on the denervated heart, its contractile characteristic and reserve appear to be intact and unaffected.[271] Data from Savin and associates[267] (Figs. 8–19 and 8–20) and Kavanagh and associates[261] (see Table 8–15) show values at rest and the acute response to exercise of cardiac transplant patients as compared with age-matched normals. Values for HR, BP, and cardiorespiratory function during rest and exercise are shown. The resting HR response of a denervated heart is higher than normal because of the lack of vagal tone. The HR approximates the inherent rate of the sinoatrial node. Resting HR usually averages 100 to 110 beats/min initially and is often paced at that rate during the early recovery period. The denervated heart adjusts more gradually to the exercise load being mediated by circulating catecholamine levels. The HRmax for the denervated heart is also significantly less than that predicted for its age. As shown in Figure 8–20, the HR during recovery from exercise for the transplanted heart is much slower and more gradual than the normal response. As mentioned earlier, the increased resting BP is related to the use of cyclosporine.[200, 263, 269] As shown

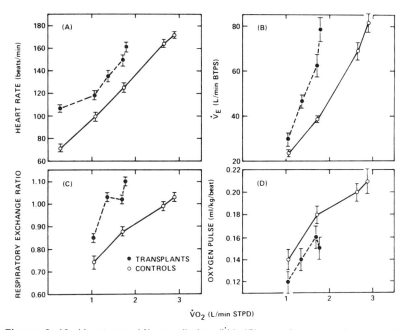

Figure 8–19. Heart rate (A), ventilation ($\dot{V}_E$) (B), respiratory exchange ratio (C), and oxygen pulse (D), plotted against $\dot{V}O_2$ at 30%, 60%, 90%, and 100% of peak workload for patients after cardiac transplantation and for normal men. Values are mean ± SEM. (Data from Savin, W., et al.: Cardiorespiratory responses of cardiac transplant patients to graded, symptom-limited exercise. **Circulation** 62:55–60, 1980. Published with permission.)

in Table 8–15, there is a dramatic difference between cardiac transplant patients and normals in regard to peak HR and systolic BP, $\dot{V}O_2$max, peak power output, and pulmonary ventilation. At the onset of exercise, increases in cardiac output of the denervated heart are primarily a result of increase in stroke volume. The increase in stroke volume is a function of increased preload and associated Frank-Starling mechanism.[265–267, 270] Later increases in cardiac output are related to a combination of chronotropic and inotropic responses associated with increased levels of circulating catecholamines.[265–267, 270] Because of the lag in the neurosympathetic response to exercise, there is a steeper increase in HR, respiratory exchange ratio, pulmonary ventilation, and blood lactate level for any given level of $\dot{V}O_2$ (see Fig. 8–19).[267]

Thus, in prescribing exercise for the cardiac transplant patient, a longer warm-up period and a more gradual increase in workload are necessary during the aerobic training period. This longer adaptation period allows the catecholamine response to augment the increase in cardiac output during work. Although the upper

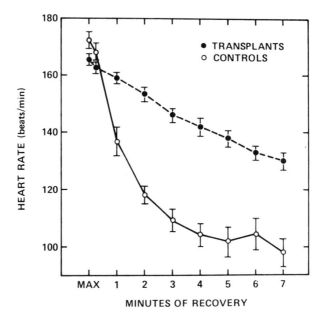

Figure 8–20. Mean heart rate (± SEM) is shown at peak exercise and during 7 minutes of recovery for patients after cardiac transplant and for normal controls. (Data from Savin, W., et al.: Cardiorespiratory responses of cardiac transplant patients to graded, symptom-limited exercise. **Circulation** 62:55–60, 1980. Published with permission.)

limit exercise guidelines that are recommended for the CABG surgery patient (see Table 8–4) can also be used for the cardiac transplant patient, many think the use of RPE and general symptoms of fatigue to be more appropriate.[261, 264]

When monitoring the cardiac transplant patient, the ECG characteristically shows two P-waves. One is produced by the rate of the native sinoatrial node. This tissue is left intact from the original heart but does not cross the suture line and has no effect on the QRS complex. The second P-wave is produced by the donor's sinoatrial node and is associated with the QRS complex. This ECG complex is associated only with orthotopic transplanted heart (native heart removed). With the heterotopic heart transplant, the patient has two hearts, the donor's plus the native heart, still intact. This procedure is rarely used in the U.S.

The effects of endurance exercise training in the transplant patient have been studied by Squires and associates[264] and Kavanagh and associates.[261, 272] Kavanagh (Toronto Rehabilitation Centre) and Yacoub (Harefield Hospital) have had the most experience in studying the long-term effects of endurance training on cardiac transplant patients. Their report on 36 patients who were endurance trained for 16 months is shown in Table 8–15. Patients were 21 to 57 years of age, were 2 to 23 months after transplant (average 7.4 months), and were New York Heart Association Class IV before transplant. Exercise training initially included 20 minutes of stretching followed by walking one mile 5 times per week. The initial pace ranged from 17.5 to 22.5 minutes/mile. An RPE of 14 (between somewhat hard and hard) was used as a guide (upper limit) for training. Patients increased their distance by one mile every 2 weeks until they could walk 3 miles in 45 minutes. Most patients could accomplish this by the end of 4 months of training. Many who accomplished this training goal began to walk-jog (200 to 800 meters initially) until they could attain 3 miles in 36 minutes. At the end of 16 months training, many could jog-walk 4 miles in 48 minutes (average of the total group was 15 miles/week at approximately a 13.5 minutes/mile pace). One highly motivated patient ran and satisfactorily completed the Boston Marathon in 1985. The results show many favorable improvements in body composition and in resting and exercise HR-hemodynamics and cardiorespiratory fitness.*

SUMMARY

This chapter has described in detail the manner in which exercise is prescribed to cardiac patients in an inpatient (phase-I), outpatient (phase-II), and community-based (phase-III) program setting. The risks and medical problems associated with cardiac rehabilitation programs were discussed. The risks of fatal or non-fatal coronary events were shown to be low and significantly reduced in more recent years. Guidelines for staffing, medical safety, and monitoring patients were discussed. Although medical problems exist, it was shown that initiating programs early after MI or CABG surgery is safe and beneficial to the patient.

Inpatient programs for patients without complications usually begin 3 days after MI or one to two days after open-heart surgery. Programs are conducted at a low intensity and emphasize ROM exercise, ambulation, and stair climbing. Outpatient programs are recommended for at least 8 to 12 weeks after hospital discharge, followed by 3 to 6 months in a community-based program. The

*The authors would like to express their thanks to Ray Squires, Ph.D., Cardiovascular Health Clinic, Mayo Clinic; Susan Quan, P.T., Department of Physical and Occupational Therapy, Stanford University Hospital; and Alice Joslin, P.T., Department of Physical Therapy, University of Florida Medical Center, for their help in providing information concerning the cardiac transplant program at their respective institutions.

importance of classifying patients as to low, medium, and high risk for future events was emphasized. Low-risk patients need little or no telemetric ECG monitoring and can safely conduct their exercise program at home or in a low-cost supervised setting.

The standards for exercise prescription were outlined, and the common features of training programs for normal healthy adults and cardiac patients were discussed. Because of the physical limitations of the cardiac patient, progression of exercise is slower, intensity is lower, frequency is greater, and duration is longer than in healthy individuals.

The need for a well-rounded training program for patients was discussed. It was recommended that strength training be included early in the recovery process (phase-II) so that patients may be better prepared to carry out work and leisure activities. In addition, the importance and need for ROM exercise in surgical patients as early as one to two days after surgery was stressed.

Monitoring of exercise sessions was accomplished in a variety of ways. Early ambulation was usually monitored by direct wire or telemetry systems for HR and ECG rhythm. Although there were diverse opinions regarding how long and to what extent sophisticated monitoring should take place, most experts believed that 8 to 12 weeks of continuous or periodic monitoring was ideal for moderate-risk patients. Longer periods of monitoring were recommended for patients at high risk and with dangerous rhythm disturbances. Guidelines for BP monitoring and the use of the RPE scale for exercise prescription were discussed. Most directors administered an SL-GXT 3 to 6 weeks after surgery or MI. The predischarge GXT or SL-GXT is a standard procedure for diagnosis, exercise prescription, and risk stratification. In general, exercise prescription for the cardiac patient should start early but progress slowly, include rhythmical activity of low intensity, emphasize greater frequency and longer duration, be individualized, and help the patient become independent and return to a normal life.

The later part of this chapter reviews exercise prescription and management procedures recommended for use in special patient populations. The special groups include those with the following conditions: angina pectoris, silent myocardial ischemia, diabetes mellitus, pacemaker implant, intermittent claudication, arthritis, COPD, PTCA, and cardiac transplant.

References

1. Lewis, T.: **Diseases of the Heart**. New York, Macmillan, 1933, pp. 41–49.
2. Levine, S. A., and Lown, B.: The chair treatment of acute coronary thrombosis. **Trans. Assoc. Am. Physicians** 64:316–327, 1951.

3. Cain, H. D., Frasher, W. G., and Stivelman, R.: Graded activity program for safe return to self-care after myocardial infarction. **JAMA** 177:111–115, 1961.
4. Hellerstein, H. K., and Ford, A. B.: Rehabilitation of the cardiac patient. **JAMA** 164:225–231, 1957.
5. Wenger, N. K. The use of exercise in the rehabilitation of patients after myocardial infarction. **J SC Med. Assoc.** 65:(Suppl. 1–12) 66–68, 1969.
6. Naughton, J., Bruhn, J. G., and Lategola, M. T.: Effects of physical training on physiologic and behavioral characteristics of cardiac patients. **Arch. Phys. Med. Rehabil.** 49:131–137, 1968.
7. Zohman, L. R.: Early ambulation of post-myocardial infarction patients: Montefiore Hospital. In Naughton, J. P., Hellerstein, H. K., and Mohler, L. C. (eds.): **Exercise Testing and Exercise Training in Coronary Heart Disease.** New York, Academic Press, 1973, pp. 329–336.
8. Karvonen, M. J., and Barry, A. J. (eds.): **Physical Activity and the Heart.** Springfield, IL, Charles C Thomas, 1967.
9. Fox, S. M., Naughton, J. P., and Haskell, W. L.: Physical activity and the preventions of coronary heart disease. **Ann. Clin. Res.** 3:404–432, 1971.
10. Naughton, J. P., Hellerstein, H. K., and Mohler, L. C. (eds.): **Exercise Testing and Exercise Training in Coronary Heart Disease.** New York, Academic Press, 1973.
11. Amsterdam, E. A., Wilmore, J. H., and DeMaria, A. N. (eds.): **Exercise in Cardiovascular Health and Disease.** New York, Yorke Medical Books, 1977.
12. Wenger, N. K., and Hellerstein, H. K. (eds.): **Rehabilitation of the Coronary Patient,** 2nd Ed. New York, John Wiley and Sons, 1984.
13. Leon, A. S., and Blackburn, H.: Exercise rehabilitation of the coronary heart disease patient. **Geriatrics** 32:66–76, 1977.
14. Pollock, M. L., and Schmidt, D. H. (eds.): **Heart Disease and Rehabilitation,** 2nd Ed. New York, Churchill Livingstone, 1986.
15. Kellerman, J. J. (ed.): **Comprehensive Cardiac Rehabilitation.** Basel, S. Karger, 1982.
16. Fardy, P. S., Yankowitz, F. G., and Wilson, P. K.: **Cardiac Rehabilitation, Adult Fitness, and Exercise Testing,** 2nd Ed. Philadelphia, Lea & Febiger, 1988.
17. Kallio, V., Hamalainen, H., Hakkila, J., and Luurila, O. J.: Reduction in sudden deaths by a multifactorial intervention programme after acute myocardial infarction. **Lancet** 2:1091–1094, 1979.
18. Hjermann, I., Velve Dyre, K., and Holme, I.: Effect of diet and smoking interventions on the incidence of a randomized trial in healthy men. **Lancet** 2:1303–1310, 1981.
19. Oldridge, N. B., Guyatt, G. H., Fischer, M. E., and Rimm, A. A.: Cardiac rehabilitation after myocardial infarction. **JAMA** 260:945–950, 1988.
20. Taylor, H. L., Henschel, A., Brozek, J., and Keys, A.: Effects of bed rest on cardiovascular function and work performance. **J. Appl. Physiol.** 2:233–239, 1949.
21. Saltin, B., Blomqvist, G., Mitchell, J., Johnson, R. L., Widenthal, K., and Chapman, C. B.: Response to exercise after bed rest and after training. **Circulation** 37 and 38(Suppl. 7):1–78, 1968.
22. Convertino, V., Hung, J., Goldwater, D., and DeBusk, R. F.: Cardiovascular responses to exercise in middle-aged men after 10 days of bed rest. **Circulation** 65:134–140, 1982.
23. Cassem, N. H., and Hackett, T. P.: Psychological rehabilitation of myocardial infarction patients in the acute phase. **Heart Lung** 2:382–388, 1973.
24. Morgan, W. P., and Pollock, M. L.: Physical activity and cardiovascular health: psychological aspects. In Landry, F., and Orban, W. A. R. (eds.): **Physical Activity and Human Wellbeing.** Miami, Symposium Specialists, 1978, pp. 163–181.
25. Blumenthal, J. A.: Psychologic assessment in cardiac rehabilitation. **J. Cardiopul. Rehabil.** 5:208–215, 1985.

26. Taylor, C. B., Houston-Miller, N., Ahn, D. K., Haskell, W., and DeBusk, R. F.: The effects of exercise training programs on psychosocial improvement in uncomplicated postmyocardial infarction patients. **J. Psychosom. Res.** 30:581–587, 1986.

27. Burgess, A. W., Lerner, D. J., D'Agostino, R. B., Vokonas, P. S., Hartman, C. R., and Gaccione, P.: A randomized control trial of cardiac rehabilitation. **Soc. Sci. Med.** 24:359–370, 1987.

28. Krantz, D. S., and Blumenthal, J. A. (eds.): **Behavioral Assessment and Management of Cardiovascular Disorders.** Sarasota, FL, Professional Resource Exchange, 1987.

29. MacDougall, J. M., Dembroski, T. M., Dimsdale, J. E., and Hackett, T. P.: Components of type A, hostility, and anger: further relationships to angiographic findings. **Health Psych.** 4:137–152, 1985.

30. Froelicher, V. F.: **Exercise and the Heart: Clinical Concepts,** 2nd Ed. Chicago, Year Book Medical Publishers, 1987.

31. Shephard, R. J.: Do risks of exercise justify costly caution? **Phys. Sportsmed.** 5:58–65, 1977.

32. Mead, W. F., Pyfer, H. R., Trombold, J. C.: Successful resuscitation of two near simultaneous cases of cardiac arrest with a review of 15 cases occurring during supervised exercise. **Circulation** 53:187–189, 1972.

33. Fletcher, G. F., and Cantwell, J. D.: Ventricular fibrillation in a medically supervised cardiac exercise program. JAMA 238:2627–2629, 1977.

34. Haskell, W. L.: Cardiovascular complications during training of cardiac patients. **Circulation** 57:920–924, 1974.

35. Hossack, K. F., and Hartwig, R.: Cardiac arrest associated with supervised cardiac rehabilitation. **J. Cardiac Rehabil.** 2:402–408, 1982.

36. Shephard, R. J., Kavanagh, T., Tuck, J.: Marathon jogging in post-myocardial infarction patients. **J. Cardiac Rehabil.** 3:321–329, 1983.

37. Van Camp, S. P., and Peterson, R. A.: Cardiovascular complications of outpatient cardiac rehabilitation programs. JAMA 256:1160–1163, 1986.

38. Gibbons, L. W., Cooper, K. H., Meyer, B. M., and Ellison, R. C.: The acute cardiac risk of strenuous exercise. JAMA 244:1799–1801, 1980.

39. Vander, L., Franklin, B., and Rubenfire, M.: Cardiovascular complications of recreational activity. **Phys. Sportsmed.** 10:89–97, 1982.

40. Thompson, P. D., Funk, E. J., Carleton, R. A., and Sturner, W. Q.: Incidence of death during jogging in Rhode Island from 1975 through 1980. JAMA 247:2535–2538, 1982.

41. Siscovick, D. S., Weiss, N. S., Fletcher, R. H., and Lasky, T.: The incidence of primary cardiac arrest during vigorous exercise. **N. Engl. J. Med.** 311:874–877, 1984.

42. Rogsta, M., Crabtree, J., Sturner, W., and Thompson, P. D.: Death during recreational exercise in the state of Rhode Island. **Med. Sci. Sports Exerc.** 16:339–342, 1984.

43. Thompson, P. D., Stern, M. P., Williams, P., Duncan, K., Haskell, W. L., and Wood, P. D.: Death during jogging and running. A study of 18 cases. JAMA 242:1265–1267, 1979.

44. Marion, B. J., Epstein, S. E., and Roberts, W. C.: Causes of sudden death in competitive athletes. **J. Am. Coll. Cardiol.** 7:204–214, 1986.

45. Van Camp, S. P., and Choi, J. H.: Exercise and sudden death. **Phys. Sportsmed.** 16:49–52, 1988.

45a. Thompson, P.: Cardiovascular hazards of physical activity. In Terjung, R. (ed.): **Exercise and Sport Sciences Reviews.** New York, MacMillan, 1982, pp. 208–235.

46. Cooper, K. H.: **Running Without Fear.** New York, M. Evans and Co., 1985.

46a. Sandaniantz, A., Clayton, M. A., Sturner, W. W., and Thompson, P. D.: Sudden death immediately after a record-setting athletic performance. **Am. J. Cardiol.** 63:375, 1989.

47. Granath, A., Sodermark, T., Winge, T., Volpe, U., and Zetterquist, S.: Early

work load tests for evaluation of long-term prognosis of acute myocardial infarction **Br. Heart J.** 39:758–763, 1977.

48. Theroux, P., Waters, D. D., Halphen, C., Debaisieux, J. D., and Mizgala, H. F.: Prognostic value of exercise testing soon after myocardial infarction. **N. Engl. J. Med.** 301:342–345, 1979.

49. Dillahunt, P. H., and Miller, A. B.: Early treadmill testing after myocardial infarction. **Chest** 76:150–155, 1979.

50. Davidson, D. M., and DeBusk, R. F.: Prognostic value of a single exercise test 3 weeks after uncomplicated myocardial infarction. **Circulation** 61:236–242, 1980.

51. Starling, M. R., Crawford, M. H., Kennedy, G. T., and O'Rourke, R. A.: Exercise testing early after myocardial infarction: predictive value for subsequent unstable angina and death. **Am. J. Cardiol.** 46:909–914, 1980.

52. Koppes, G. M., Kruyer, W., Beckmann, C. H., and Jones, F. G.: Response to exercise early after uncomplicated acute myocardial infarction in patients receiving no medication: long-term follow-up. **Am. J. Cardiol.** 46:764–769, 1980.

53. DeBusk, R. F., Blomqvist, C. G., Kouchoukos, N. T., Luepker, R. W., Miller, H. S., Moss, A. J., Pollock, M. L., Reeves, T. J., Selvester, R. H., Stason, W. B., Wagner, G. S., and Willman, V. L.: Identification and treatment of low-risk patients after acute myocardial infarction and coronary-artery bypass graft surgery. **N. Engl. J. Med.** 314:161–166, 1986.

54. Corne, R. A.: Risk stratification in stable angina pectoris. **Am. J. Cardiol.** 59:695–697, 1987.

55. Cheitlin, M. D.: Finding the high risk patient with coronary heart disease. **JAMA** 259:2271–2277, 1988.

55a. Haskell, W. L.: Safety of outpatient cardiac exercise programs—issues regarding medical supervision. In Franklin, B. A., and Rubenfire M. (eds.): **Clinics in Sports Medicine—Cardiac Rehabilitation.** Philadelphia, W.B. Saunders Co., 1984, pp. 455–470.

56. McNeer, J. F., Margolis, J. R., Lee, K. L., Kisslo, J. A., Peter, R. H., Kong, Y., Behar, V. S., Wallace, A. G., McCants, C. B., and Rosati, R. A.: The role of the exercise test in the evaluation of patients for ischemic heart disease. **Circulation** 57:64–70, 1978.

57. Epstein, S. E.: Implications of probability analysis on the strategy used for noninvasive detection of coronary artery disease. **Am. J. Cardiol.** 46:492–499, 1982.

58. Akhtar, M., Wolf, F., and Denker, S.: Sudden cardiac death. In Pollock, M. L., and Schmidt, D. H. (eds.): **Heart Disease and Rehabilitation,** 2nd Ed. New York, Churchill Livingstone, 1986, pp. 115–130.

59. Ehsani, A. A., Heath, G. W., Hagberg, J. M., Sobel, B. E., and Holloszy, J. O.: Effects of 12 months of intense exercise training on ischemic ST-segment depression in patients with coronary heart disease. **Circulation** 64:1116–1124, 1981.

60. Ehsani, A. A., Biello, D. R., Shultz, J., Sobel, B. E., and Holloszy, J. O.: Improvement of left ventricular contractile function by exercise training in patients with coronary artery disease. **Circulation** 74:350–358, 1986.

61. Martin, W. H., and Ehsani, A. A.: Reversal of exertional hypotension by prolonged exercise training in selected patients with ischemic heart disease. **Circulation** 76:548–555, 1987.

62. Hellerstein, H. K., and Franklin, B. A.: Exercise testing and prescription. In Wenger, N. K., and Hellerstein, H. K. (eds.): **Rehabilitation of the Coronary Patient,** 2nd Ed. New York, Churchill Livingstone, 1984, pp. 197–284.

63. Shephard, R. J.: Cardiac rehabilitation in prospect. In Pollock, M. L., and Schmidt, D. H. (eds.): **Heart Disease and Rehabilitation,** 2nd Ed. New York, Churchill Livingstone, 1986, pp. 713–740.

64. Shephard, R. J.: Recurrence of myocardial infarction in an exercising population. **Br. Heart J.** 42:133–138, 1979.

65. Pollock, M. L., Pels, A. E., Foster, C., and Ward, A.: Exercise prescription for rehabilitation of the cardiac patient. In Pollock, M. L., and Schmidt, D. H. (eds.): **Heart Disease and Rehabilitation,** 2nd Ed. New York, Churchill Livingstone, 1986, pp. 477–515.
66. Dion Faraher, W., Grevenow, P., Pollock, M. L., Squires, R. W., Foster, C., Johnson, W. D., and Schmidt, D. H.: Medical problems and physiologic responses during supervised inpatient cardiac rehabilitation: the patient after coronary bypass grafting. **Heart Lung** 11:248–255, 1982.
67. American College of Sports Medicine: Guidelines for Graded **Exercise Testing and Exercise Prescription,** 3rd Ed. Philadelphia, Lea & Febiger, 1986.
68. Sennett, S. M., Pollock, M. L., Pels, A. E., Foster, C., Dolatowski, R., Laughlin, J., Patel, S., and Schmidt, D. H.: Medical problems of patients in an outpatient cardiac rehabilitation program. **J. Cardiopul. Rehabil.** 7:458–465, 1987.
69. Fletcher, B., Thiel, J., and Fletcher, G. F.: Phase II intensive monitored cardiac rehabilitation for coronary artery disease and coronary risk factors—a six session protocol. **Am. J. Cardiol.** 57:751–756, 1986.
70. American College of Cardiology: Recommendations of the American College of Cardiology on cardiovascular rehabilitation. **J. Am. Coll. Cardiol.** 7:451–453, 1986.
71. American Association for Cardiovascular and Pulmonary Rehabilitation: Cardiac rehabilitation services: a scientific evaluation. **J. Cardiopul. Rehabil.** in press.
71a. Public Health Service: Medical technology: scientific evaluation; cardiac rehabilitation services. **Fed. Register** 50:32911–32912, 1985.
71b. Greenland, P. G., and Chu, J. S.: Efficacy of cardiac rehabilitation services with emphasis on patients after myocardial infarction. **Ann. Intern. Med.** 109:650–663, 1988.
72. Kavanagh, T., Shephard, R. J., Doney, H., and Pandit, V.: Intensive exercise in coronary rehabilitation. **Med. Sci. Sports** 5:34–39, 1973.
73. Franklin, B. A., Besseghini, I., and Golden, L. H.: Low intensity physical conditioning: effects on patients with coronary heart disease. **Arch. Phys. Med. Rehabil.** 59:276–280, 1978.
74. DeBusk, R. F., Houston, N., Haskell, W., Fry, G., and Parker, M.: Exercise training soon after myocardial infarction. **Am. J. Cardiol.** 44:1223–1229, 1979.
75. Savin, W. M., Haskell, W. L., Houston-Miller, N., and DeBusk, R. F.: Improvement in aerobic capacity soon after myocardial infarction. **J. Cardiac Rehabil.** 1:337–342, 1981.
76. Foster, C., Pollock, M. L., Anholm, J. D., Squires, R. W., Ward, A., Dymond, D. S., Rod, J. L., Saichek, R. P., and Schmidt, D. H.: Work capacity and left ventricular function during rehabilitation after myocardial revascularization surgery. **Circulation** 69:748–755, 1984.
77. Marten, P. F., Simons, L., Zwiers, G., Boardman, T., Brower, R. W., Kazemir, M., and Hugenholtz, P. G.: Value of predischarge data for the prediction of exercise capacity after cardiac rehabilitation in patients with recent myocardial infarction. **Eur. Heart J.** 8:33–38, 1987.
78. Blumenthal, J. A., Rejeski, W. J., Wash-Riddle, M., Emery, C. F., Miller, H., Roark, S., Ribisl, P. M., Morris, P. B., Brubaker P., and Williams, S.: Comparison of high- and low-intensity exercise training early after acute myocardial infarction. **Am. J. Cardiol.** 61:26–30, 1988.
79. Simons, M., Lap, C., and Pool, J.: Heart rate levels and ventricular ectopic activity during cardiac rehabilitation. **Am. Heart J.** 100:9–14, 1980.
80. Williams, M. A., and Fardy, P. S.: Limitations in prescribing exercise. **Cardiovasc. Pulmon. Technique** 8:33–36, 1980.
81. Fardy, P. S., Doll, N., Taylor, J., and Williams, M.: Monitoring cardiac patients: how much is enough? **Phys. Sportsmed.** 10:146–152, 1982.
82. Dolatowski, R. P., Squires, R. W., Pollock, M. L., Foster C., and Schmidt, D. H.: Dysrhythmia detection in myocardial revascularization surgery patients. **Med. Sci. Sports Exerc.** 15:281–286, 1983.

83. Mitchell, M., Franklin, B., Johnson, S., and Rubinfire, M.: Cardiac exercise programs: role of continuous electrocardiographic monitoring. **Arch. Phys. Med. Rehabil.** 65:463–466, 1984.
84. Fagan, E. T., Wayne, V. S., and McConachy, D. L.: Serious ventricular arrhythmias in a cardiac rehabilitation programme. **Med. J. Australia** 141:421–424, 1984.
85. Rubin, D. A., Nieminski, K. E., Manteferrante, J. C., Magee, T., Reed, G. A., and Herman, M. V.: Ventricular arrhythmias after coronary artery bypass graft surgery: incidence, risk factors, and long-term prognosis. **J. Am. Coll. Cardiol.** 6:307–310, 1985.
86. Greenland, P., and Pomilla, P. V.: Electrocardiographic monitoring in cardiac rehabilitation: an assessment. **Phys. Sportsmed.** 17:75–82, 1989.
87. Stevens, R., and Hansen, P.: Comparison of supervised and unsupervised exercise training after coronary artery bypass surgery. **Am. J. Cardiol.** 53:1524–1528, 1984.
88. Houston-Miller, N. H., Haskell, W. L., Berra, K., and DeBusk, R. F.: Home versus group exercise training for increasing functional capacity after myocardial infarction. **Circulation** 70:645–649, 1984.
89. Heath, G. W., Maloney, P. M., and Fure, C. W.: Group exercise versus home exercise in coronary artery bypass graft patients: effects on physical activity habits. **J. Cardiopul. Rehabil.** 7:190–195, 1987.
90. Hands, M. E., Briffa, T., Henderson, K., Antico, V., Thompson, P., and Hung, J.: Functional capacity and left ventricular function: the effect of supervised and unsupervised exercise rehabilitation soon after coronary artery bypass graft surgery. **J. Cardiopul. Rehabil.** 7:578–584, 1987.
91. Massie, J. F., and Shephard, R. J.: Physiological and psychological effects of training: a comparison of individual and gymnasium programs with a characterization of the exercise "dropout." **Med. Sci. Sports** 3:110–117, 1971.
92. Gettman, L. R., Pollock, M. L., and Ward, A.: Adherence to unsupervised exercise. **Phys. Sportsmed.** 11:56–66, 1983.
93. Juneau, M., Rogers, F., De Santos, V., Yee, M., Evans, A., Bohn, A., Haskell, W. L., Taylor, C. B., and DeBusk, R. F.: Effectiveness of self-monitored, home-based, moderate-intensity exercise training in middle-aged men and women. **Am. J. Cardiol.** 60:66–70, 1987.
94. King, A. C., Taylor, C. B., Haskell, W. L., and DeBusk, R. F.: Strategies for increasing early adherence to and long-term maintenance of home-based exercise training in healthy middle-aged men and women. **Am. J. Cardiol.** 61:628–632, 1988.
95. American Heart Association/Wisconsin Affiliate: **Recommendations for Insurance Coverage of Supervised Cardiac Exercise Rehabilitation Programs.** Milwaukee, American Heart Association/Wisconsin Affiliate, 1980.
96. American Heart Association: Standards and guidelines for cardiopulmonary resuscitation (CPR) and emergency cardiac care (ECC). **JAMA** 255:2905–2989, 1986.
97. American Heart Association: **Heartsavers Manual: A Student Handbook for Cardiopulmonary Resuscitation and First Aid for Choking.** Dallas, American Heart Association, 1987.
98. American Heart Association: **Textbook of Advanced Cardiac Life Support.** Dallas, American Heart Association, 1987.
99. North Carolina Cardiac Rehabilitation Association: **North Carolina Cardiac Rehabilitation Plan.** Raleigh, North Carolina Division of Vocational Rehabilitation Services, 1983.
100. Fox, S. M.: Heart disease and rehabilitation: scope of the problem. In Pollock, M. L., and Schmidt, D. H. (eds.): **Heart Disease and Rehabilitation.** New York, John Wiley and Sons, 1979, pp. 3–14.
101. Erb, B. D., Fletcher, G. F., and Scheffield, T. L.: AHA Committee report: standards for cardiovascular exercise treatment programs. **Circulation** 59:1084A–1090A, 1979.

101a. Feigenbaum, E., and Carter, E.: **Health Technology Assessment Report, No. 6.** Rockville, M.D., Cardiac Rehabilitation Services, U.S. Department of Health and Human Services, 1987.

102. Froelicher, V. F., and Pollock, M. L. (eds.): **J. Cardiac Rehabil.** 2:429–514, 1982.

103. Brammel, H. L., Robertson, D. R., Darnell, R., McDaniel, J. W., and Niccoli, S. A.: **Cardiac Rehabilitation Handbook for Vocational Rehabilitation Counselors.** Denver, Webb-Waring Lung Institute, 1979.

104. Fardy, F. S., Bennett, J. L., Reitz, N. L., and Williams, M.D. (eds.): **Cardiac Rehabilitation Implications for the Nurse and Other Health Professionals.** St. Louis, C. V. Mosby, 1980.

105. Fry, G., and Berra, K.: **YMCAardiac Therapy.** Chicago, National Council of the YMCA, 1981.

106. Howley, E. T., and Franks, B. D.: **Health/Fitness Instructor's Handbook.** Champaign, IL, Human Kinetics, 1986.

107. American College of Sports Medicine: **Resource Manual for Guidelines for Exercise Testing and Prescription.** Philadelphia, Lea & Febiger, 1988.

108. Silvidi, G. E., Squires, R. W., Pollock, M. L., and Foster, C.: Hemodynamic responses and medical problems associated with early exercise and ambulation in coronary artery bypass graft surgery patients. **J. Cardiac Rehabil.** 2:355–362, 1982.

109. Wenger, N. K.: The physiological basis for early ambulation after myocardial infarction. In Wenger, N. K. (ed.): **Exercise and the Heart.** Philadelphia, F. A. Davis, 1978, pp. 107–116.

110. DeVries, H. A.: Physiological effects of an exercise training regimen upon men aged 52 to 88. **J. Gerontol.** 24:325–336, 1970.

111. Pollock, M. L., Dawson, G. A., Miller, H. S., Jr., Ward, A., Cooper, D., Headly, W., Linnerud, A. C., and Nomeir, M. M.: Physiologic responses of men 49 to 65 years of age to endurance training. **J. Am. Geriatr. Soc.** 24:97–104, 1976.

112. American College of Sports Medicine: Position statement on the recommended quantity and quality of exercise for developing and maintaining fitness in healthy adults. **Med. Sci. Sports** 10:vii–x, 1978. (Revised statement, **Med. Sci. Sports Exerc.** in press).

113. Seals, D. R., Hagberg, J. M., Hurley, B. F., Ehsani, A. A., and Holloszy, J. O.: Endurance training in older men and women. I. Cardiovascular responses to exercise. **J. Appl. Physiol.** 57:1024–1029, 1984.

114. Hagberg, J. M., Graves, J. E., Limacher, M., Woods, D. R., Leggett, S., Cononie, C., Gruber, J., and Pollock, M. L.: Cardiovascular responses of 70–79 year old men and women to exercise training. **J. Appl. Physiol.** 66:2589–2594, 1989.

115. Wenger, N. K.: Rehabilitation of the patient with acute myocardial infarction: early ambulation and patient education. In Pollock, M. L., and Schmidt, D. H. (eds.): **Heart Disease and Rehabilitation,** 2nd Ed. New York, Churchill Livingstone, 1986, pp. 405–422.

116. Metier, C. P., Pollock, M. L., and Graves, J. E.: Exercise prescription for the coronary artery bypass graft surgery patient. **J. Cardiopul. Rehabil.** 6:85–103, 1986.

117. Pollock, M. L., Foster, C., Knapp, D., and Schmidt, D. H.: Cardiac rehabilitation program at Mount Sinai Medical Center, Milwaukee. **J. Cardiac Rehabil.** 2:458–463, 1982.

118. Knapp, D., Hansen, M., Rogowski, B., and Pollock, M. L.: A comparison of effectiveness of education of cardiac surgery patients: nurse educators and primary nurses. **J. Cardiopul. Rehabil.** 5:429–434, 1985.

119. American Heart Association: **Professional Catalog for Physicians, Nurses, and Allied Health Professionals.** Dallas, American Heart Association, 1982.

120. Billie, D. A. (ed.): **Practical Approaches to Patient Teaching.** Boston, Little, Brown, and Co., 1981.

121. Redman, B.: **The Process of Patient Education.** St. Louis, C.V. Mosby, 1984.

122. **Health/Patient Education Catalog.** Bowie, MD, R.J. Brady Co., 1982.

123. Fletcher-Johnston, B., Cantwell, J. D., and Fletcher, G. F.: **Exercise for Heart and Health.** Atlanta, Pritchard and Hull Associates, 1985.
124. **Patient Education Materials 1989 Catalog.** Atlanta, Pritchard and Hull Associates, 1989.
125. Hansen, M., Laughlin, J., Oldridge, N. B., Schmidt, D. H., and Pollock, M. L.: **Heart Care—After Heart Attack,** 2nd Ed. Redmond, WA, Medic Publishing Co., 1987.
126. Hansen, M., Laughlin, J., Oldridge, N. B., Schmidt, D. H., and Pollock, M. L.: **Heart Care—After Heart Surgery,** 2nd Ed. Redmond, WA, Medic Publishing Co., 1987.
127. Taylor, H. L., Wang, Y., Rowell, L., and Blomqvist, G.: The standardization and interpretation of submaximal and maximal tests of working capacity. **Pediatrics** 32:703–722, 1963.
128. Rod, J. L., Squires, R. W., Pollock, M. L., Foster, C., and Schmidt, D. H.: Symptom-limited graded exercise testing soon after myocardial revascularization surgery. **J. Cardiac Rehabil.** 2:199–205, 1982.
129. Epstein, S. E., Robinson, B. E., Kahler, R. L., and Braunwald, E.: Effects of beta-adrenergic blockade on the cardiac response to maximal and submaximal exercise in man. **J. Clin. Invest.** 44:1745–1753, 1965.
130. Tesch, P. A., and Kaiser, P.: Effects of beta-adrenergic blockage on O_2 uptake during submaximal and maximal exercise. **J. Appl. Physiol.** 54:901–905, 1983.
131. Pollock, M., Foster, C., Rod, J., Stoiber, J., Hare, J., and Schmidt, D.: Effect of propranolol dosage on the response to submaximal and maximal exercise. (Abstr.) **Am. J. Cardiol.** 49:1000, 1982.
132. Hughson, R. L.: Dose-response study of maximal exercise with propranolol, metoprolol, and oxprenolol in normal subjects. **J. Cardiac Rehabil.** 4:50–54, 1984.
133. Kaiser, P., Tesch, P. A., Frisk-Holmberg, M., Juhlin-Dannfelt, A., and Kaijer, L.: Effect of beta-selective and non-selective beta-blockade on work capacity and muscle metabolism. **Clin. Physiol.** 6:197–207, 1986.
134. Hossack, K. F., Bruce, R. A., and Clark, L. J.: Influence of propranolol on exercise prescription training heart rates. **Cardiology** 65:47–48, 1980.
135. Gordon, N. F., Van Rensburg, J. P., Russell, H. M. S., Kalwasky, D. L., Celliers, C. P., Cilliers, J. F., and Myburgh, D. P.: Effect of beta-selective adrenoceptor blockade on physiological response to exercise. **Br. Heart J.** 54:96–99, 1985.
136. Areskog, N. H., and Wilmore, J.: Workshop I: developing the exercise prescription for patients on chronic beta-blockade. **Am. J. Cardiol.** 55:167D–168D, 1985.
137. Pollock, M. L., and Foster, C.: Exercise prescription for participants on propranolol. (Abstr.) J. Am. Coll. Cardiol. 2:624, 1983.
138. Pollock, M. L., Jackson, A. S., and Foster, C.: The use of the perception scale for exercise prescription. In Borg, G., and Ottoson, D. (eds.): **The Perception of Exertion in Physical Work.** London, MacMillan Press, 1986, pp. 161–175.
139. Davies, C. T. M., and Sargeant, A. J.: The effects of atropine and practolol on the perception of exertion during treadmill exercise. **Ergonomics** 22:1141–1146, 1979.
140. Onodera, K., and Miyashita, M.: Rating of perceived exertion: a study on Japanese scale for rating of perceived exertion in endurance exercise. **Jpn. J. Phys. Educ.** 21:191–203, 1976.
140a. Wilmore, J. H.: Exercise testing, training, and beta-adrenergic blockade. **Phys. Sportsmed.** 16:45–51, 1988.
141. Powles, A. C. P., Sutton, J. R., Wicks, J. R., Oldridge, N. B., and Jones, N. L.: Reduced heart rate response to exercise in ischemic heart disease: the fallacy of the target heart rate in exercise testing. **Med. Sci. Sports** 11:227–233, 1979.
142. Haskell, W. L., and DeBusk, R.: Cardiovascular responses to repeated treadmill exercise testing soon after myocardial infarction. **Circulation** 60:1247–1251, 1979.

143. Demello, J. J., Cureton, K. J., Boineau, R. E., and Singh, M. M.: Ratings of perceived exertion at lactate threshold in trained and untrained men and women. **Med. Sci. Sports Exerc.** 19:354–362, 1987.

144. Borg, G., Hassmen, P., and Lagerstrom, M.: Perceived exertion related to heart rate and blood lactate during arm and leg exercise. **Eur. J. Appl. Physiol.** 65:679–685, 1987.

145. Borg, G., Van Den Burg, M., Hassmen, P., Kaijser, L., and Tanaka, S.: Relationships between perceived exertion, HR and HLa in cycling, running and walking. **Scand. J. Sports Sci.** 9:69–77, 1987.

146. Squires, R. W., Rod, J. L., Pollock, M. L., and Foster, C.: Effects of propranolol on perceived exertion soon after myocardial revascularization surgery. **Med. Sci. Sports Exerc.** 14:276–280, 1982.

147. Hartzell, A. A., Freund, B. J., Jilka, S. M., Joyner, M. J., Anderson, R. L., Ewy, G. A., and Wilmore, J. H.: The effect of beta-adrenergic blockade on ratings of perceived exertion during submaximal exercise before and following endurance training. **J. Cardiopul. Rehabil.** 6:444–456, 1986.

148. Hellerstein, H. K., and Friedman, F. H.: Sexual activity and the post-coronary patient. **Arch. Intern. Med.** 125:987–999, 1970.

149. Nemec, E. D., Mansfield, L., and Kennedy, J. W.: Heart rate and blood pressure responses during sexual activity. **Am. Heart J.** 92:274–277, 1976.

150. Skinner, J. S.: Sexual relations and the cardiac patient. In Pollock, M. L., and Schmidt, D. H. (eds.): **Heart Disease and Rehabilitation,** 2nd Ed. New York, Churchill Livingstone, 1986, pp. 587–596.

151. Ueno, M.: The so-called coition death. **Jpn. J. Leg. Med.** 17:333–340, 1963.

152. Larson, J. L., Naughton, M. W., Kennedy, J. W., and Mansfield, L. W.: Heart rate and blood pressure responses to sexual activity and a stair-climbing test. **Heart Lung** 9:1025–1030, 1980.

153. Scalzi, C., and Dracup, K.: Sexual counseling of coronary patients. **Heart Lung** 7:840–845, 1978.

154. Scheuer, J., Greenberg, M. A., and Zohman, L. R.: Exercise training in patients with coronary artery disease. **Mod. Concepts Cardiovasc. Dis.** 47:85–90, 1978.

155. Pollock, M. L., Foster, C., Rod, J. L., and Wible, G.: Comparison of methods for determining exercise training intensity for cardiac patients and healthy adults. In Kellerman, J. J. (ed.): **Comprehensive Cardiac Rehabilitation.** Basel, S. Karger, 1982, pp. 129–133.

156. Franklin, B. A., Hellerstein, H. K., Gordon, S., and Timmis, G. C.: Exercise prescription for the myocardial infarction patient. **J. Cardiopul. Rehabil.** 6:62–79, 1986.

157. Gutman, M. C., Squires, R. W., Pollock, M. L., Foster, C., and Anholm, J.: Perceived exertion–heart rate relationship during exercise testing and training in cardiac patients. **J. Cardiac Rehabil.** 1:52–59, 1981.

158. Tennant, K. L., Allen, R. E., Pollock, M. L., Graves, J. E., Conti, C. R., and Carmichael, M.: The evaluation of a heart rate controlled cycle ergometer for use in cardiac rehabilitation. **J. Cardiopul. Rehabil.** 9:195–201, 1989.

159. Magder, S., Linnarsson, D., and Gullstrand, L.: The effect of swimming on patients with ischemic heart disease. **Circulation** 63:979–986, 1981.

160. Thompson, D. L., Boone, T. W., and Miller, H. S.: Comparison of treadmill exercise and tethered swimming to determine validity of exercise prescription. **J. Cardiac Rehabil.** 2:363–370, 1982.

161. McMurray, R. G., Fieselman, C. C., Avery, K. E., and Shops, D. S.: Exercise hemodynamics in water and on land in patients with coronary artery disease. **J. Cardiopul. Rehabil.** 8:69–75, 1988.

161a. Ekelund, C.: **Exercise in Water: A Scientific Approach.** Durham, NC, Duke University, 1985.

162. Fletcher, G. F., Cantwell, J. D., and Watt, E. W.: Oxygen consumption and hemodynamic response of exercises used in training of patients with recent myocardial infarction. **Circulation** 60:140–144, 1979.

163. Holmer, I., Stein, E. M., Saltin, B., Ekblom, B., and Åstrand, P.O.: Hemody-

namic and respiratory responses compared in swimming and running. **J. Appl. Physiol.** 37:49–54, 1974.

164. Heigenhauser, G. F., Boulet, D., Miller, B., and Faulkner, J. A.: Cardiac outputs of post-myocardial infarction patients during swimming and cycling. **Med. Sci. Sports** 9:143–147, 1977.

165. Blomqvist, C. G., Lewis, S. F., Taylor, W. F., and Graham, R. M.: Similarity of the hemodynamic responses to static and dynamic exercise of small muscle groups. **Circ. Res.** (Suppl. I) 48:87–92, 1981.

166. Asmussen, E.: Similarities and dissimilarities between static and dynamic exercise. **Circ. Res.** (Suppl. I) 48:3–10, 1981.

167. Lewis, S. F., Taylor, W. F., Graham, R. M., Pettinger, W. A., Schutte, J. E., and Blomqvist, C. G.: Cardiovascular responses to exercise as functions of absolute and relative workload. **J. Appl. Physiol.** 54:1314–1323, 1983.

168. Lewis, S. F., Snell, P. G., Taylor, W. F., Hamra, M., Graham, R. M., Pettinger, W. A., and Blomqvist, C. G.: Role of muscle mass and mode of contraction in circulatory responses to exercise. **J. Appl. Physiol.** 58:146–151, 1985.

169. Mitchell, J. H., and Blomqvist, C. G.: Response of patients with heart disease to dynamic and static exercise. In Pollock, M. L., and Schmidt, D. H. (eds.): **Heart Disease and Rehabilitation,** 2nd Ed. New York, Churchill Livingstone, 1986, pp. 85–95.

170. Bezucha, G. R., Lenser, M. C., Hanson, P. G., and Nagle, F. J.: Comparison of hemodynamic responses to static and dynamic exercise. **J. Appl. Physiol.** 53:1589–1593, 1982.

171. Painter, P., and Hanson, P.: Isometric exercise: implications for the cardiac patient. **Cardiovasc. Rev. Reports** 5:261–279, 1984.

172. Ewing, D. J., Kerr, F., Leggett, R.: Interaction between cardiovascular responses to sustained handgrip and Valsalva manoeuvre. **Br. Heart J.** 38:483–490, 1976.

173. Atkins, J. M., Matthews, O. A., Blomqvist, C. G., and Mullins, C. B.: Incidence of arrhythmias induced by isometric and dynamic exercise. **Br. Heart J.** 38:465–471, 1976.

174. Reddy, H. K., Weber, K. T., Janick, J. S., and McElroy, P. A.: Hemodynamic, ventilatory and metabolic effects of light isometric exercise in patients with chronic heart failure. **J. Am. Coll. Cardiol.** 12:353–358, 1988.

175. Lind, A. R., and McNicol, G. W.: Muscular factors which determine the cardiovascular responses to sustained and rhythmic exercise. **Can. Med. Assoc. J.** 96:706–713, 1967.

176. MacDougall, J. D., Tuxen, D., Sale, D. G., Moroz, J. R., and Sutton, J. R.: Arterial blood pressure response to heavy resistance exercise. **J. Appl. Physiol.** 58:785–790, 1985.

177. Haslam, D. R. S., McCartney, N., McKelvie, R. S., and MacDougall, J. D.: Direct measurements of arterial blood pressure during formal weightlifting in cardiac patients. **J. Cardiopul. Rehabil.** 8:213–225, 1988.

178. Sagiv, M., Hanson, P., Goldhammer, E., Ben-Sira, D., and Rudoy, J.: Left ventricular and hemodynamic responses during upright isometric exercise in normal young and elderly men. **Gerontology** 34:165–170, 1988.

179. Ben-Ari, E., and Kellermann, J. J.: Comparison of cardiocirculatory responses to intensive arm and leg training in patients with angina pectoris. **Heart Lung** 12:337–340, 1983.

180. Markiewicz, W., Houston, N., and DeBusk, R.: A comparison of static and dynamic exercise soon after myocardial infarction. **Isr. J. Med. Sci.** 15:894–897, 1979.

181. DeBusk, R. F., Valdez, R., Houston, N., and Haskell, W.: Cardiovascular responses to dynamic and static effort soon after myocardial infarction. Application to occupational work assessment. **Circulation** 58:368–375, 1978.

182. DeBusk, R., Pitts, W., Haskell, W., and Houston, N.: Comparison of cardiovascular responses to static-dynamic effort and dynamic effort alone in patients with chronic ischemic heart disease. **Circulation** 59:977–983, 1979.

183. Sheldahl, L. M., Wilkie, N. A., Tristani, F. E., and Kalbfleisch, J. H.: Responses

of patients after myocardial infarction to carrying a graded series of weight loads. **Am. J. Cardiol.** 52:698–703, 1983.

184. Vander, L. B., Franklin, B. A., Wrisley, D., and Rubenfire, M.: Acute cardiovascular responses to Nautilus exercise in cardiac patients: implications for exercise training. **Ann. Sports Med.** 2:165–169, 1986.

185. Kelemen, M. H., Stewart, K. J., Gillilan, R. E., Ewart, C. K., Valenti, S. A., Manley, J. D., and Kelemen, M. D.: Circuit weight training in cardiac patients. **J. Am. Coll. Cardiol.** 7:38–42, 1986.

186. Butler, R. M., Beierwaltes, W. H., and Rodgers, F. J.: The cardiovascular response to circuit weight training in patients with cardiac diseases. **J. Cardiopul. Rehabil.** 7:402–409, 1987.

187. Harris, K. A., and Holly, R. G.: Physiological response to circuit weight training in borderline hypertensive subjects. **Med. Sci. Sports Exerc.** 19:246–252, 1987.

188. Stewart, K. J., Mason, M., and Kelemen, M. H.: Three year participation in circuit weight training improves muscular strength and self-efficacy in cardiac patients. **J. Cardiopul. Rehabil.** 8:292–296, 1988.

189. Lewis, S. F., Nygaard, E., Sanchez, J., Egeblad, H., and Saltin, B.: Static contraction of the quadriceps muscle in man. Cardiovascular control and responses to one-legged strength training. **Acta Physiol. Scand.** 122:341–353, 1984.

190. Knapp, D., Gutmann, M. C., Tristani, F., Sheldahl, L., and Wilke, N.: Returning the patient to work. In Pollock, M. L., and Schmidt, D. H. (eds.): **Heart Disease and Rehabilitation,** 2nd Ed. New York, Churchill Livingstone, 1986, pp. 647–678.

191. Oldridge, N. B., Wicks, J. R., Hanley, C., Sutton, J. R., and Jones, N. L.: Noncompliance in an exercise rehabilitation program for men who have suffered a myocardial infarction. **Can. Med. Assoc. J.** 118:361–364, 1978.

192. Strauss, W. E., Scaramuzzi, M. S., Panton-Lapsley, D., and McIntryre, K. M.: Emergency plans and procedures for an exercise facility. In Blair, S. N., Painter, P., Pate, R. R., Smith, L. K., and Taylor, C. B. (eds.): **Resource Manual for Guidelines for Exercise Testing and Prescription.** Philadelphia, Lea & Febiger, 1988, pp. 278–284.

193. Lee, A. P., Ice, R., Blessey, R., and Sanmarco, M. E.: Long-term effects of physical training on coronary patients with impaired ventricular function. **Am. J. Cardiol.** 49:296–300, 1982.

194. Cohn, E. H., Sanders, R. S., and Wallace, A. G.: Exercise responses before and after physical conditioning in patients with severely depressed left ventricular function. **Am. J. Cardiol.** 49:296–300, 1982.

195. Musch, T. I., Moore, R. L., Leathers, D. J., Bruno, A., and Zelis, R.: Endurance training in rats with chronic heart failure induced by myocardial infarction. **Circulation** 74:431–441, 1986.

196. Smith, L. K., Layton, K., Newmark, J. L., and Diethrich, E. B.: An intensive cardiovascular rehabilitation program for patients with disabling angina and diffuse coronary artery disease. **J. Cardiopul. Rehabil.** 7:425–429, 1987.

197. Kellermann, J. J.: The role of exercise therapy in patients with impaired ventricular function and chronic heart failure. **J. Cardiovasc. Pharmacol.** (Suppl. 6) 10:S172–S177, 1987.

198. Sullivan, M. J., Higginbotham, M. B., and Cobb, F. R.: Exercise training in patients with severe left ventricular dysfunction: hemodynamic and metabolic effects. **Circulation** 78:506–515, 1988.

199. Sidney, K. H., Shephard, R. J., and Harrison, H.: Endurance training and body composition of the elderly. **Am. J. Clin. Nutr.** 30:326–333, 1977.

200. Schroeder, J. S., and Hunt, S.: Cardiac transplantation update 1987. **JAMA** 258:3142–3145, 1987.

201. American College of Cardiology/American Heart Association: Guidelines for percutaneous transluminal coronary angioplasty. **Circulation** 78:486–502, 1988.

202. Willius, F. A., and Keys, J. E.: **Cardiac Classics.** St. Louis, C.V. Mosby, 1941.
203. Hurst, W. J.: **The Heart,** 6th Ed. New York, McGraw-Hill, 1986.
204. Champeau, L.: Grading of angina pectoris. **Circulation** 54:522–523, 1976.
205. Pollock, M. L., Wilmore, J. H., and Fox, S. M.: **Health and Fitness through Physical Activity.** New York, John Wiley and Sons, 1978.
206. Borg, G., Holmgren, A., and Lindblad, I.: Quantitative evaluation of chest pain. **Acta Med. Scand.** (Suppl.) 644:43–45, 1981.
207. Pepine, C. J.: Silent ischemia: etiology, prevalence and prognosis. **Heart House Learning Center Highlights** 2:14–18, 1986.
208. Weiner, D. A., Ryan, T. J., McCabe, C. H., Luk, S., Chaitman, B. R., Sheffield, L. T., Trisani, F., and Fisher, L. D.: Significance of silent myocardial ischemia during exercise testing in patients with coronary artery disease. **Am. J. Cardiol.** 59:725–729, 1987.
209. National Institutes of Health, U.S. Department of Health and Human Service, Bethesda, MD, 1985.
210. Hanson, P., Ward, A., and Painter, P.: Exercise training in special populations. **J. Cardiopul. Rehabil.** 6:104–112, 1986.
211. Wahren, J.: Glucose turnover during exercise in man. **Ann NY Acad. Sci.** 301:45–55, 1977.
212. Felig, P., Cherif, A., Minagawe, A., and Wahren, J.: Hypoglycemia during prolonged exercise in normal man. **N. Engl. J. Med.** 306:895–900, 1982.
213. Richter, E. A., Ruderman, N. B., and Schneider, S. H.: Diabetes and exercise. **Am. J. Med.** 70:201–209, 1981.
214. Koivisto, V. A., and Felig, P.: Effects of leg exercise on insulin absorption in diabetic patients. **N. Engl. J. Med.** 298:78–83, 1978.
215. Caron, D., Poussier, P., and Marliss, E. B.: The effect of postprandial exercise on meal-related glucose tolerance in insulin-dependent diabetic individuals. **Diabetes Care** 5:364–369, 1982.
216. Zinman, B., Minuk, H. L., Hanna, A. K., Leibel, B. S., Albisser, A. M., and Marliss, E. B.: The metabolic response to exercise in obese diabetic men treated with sulfonylureas. (Abstr.) 10th Congress of the International Diabetes Federation. **Excerpta Medica International Congress Series** 481:264, 1979.
217. Hilsted, J.: Pathophysiology in diabetic autonomic neuropathy. Cardiovascular hormonal and metabolic studies. **Diabetes** 31:730–737, 1982.
218. Soman, V. R., Koivisto, V. A., Deibert, D., Felig, P., and DeFronzo, R. A.: Increased insulin sensitivity and insulin binding to monocytes after physical training. **N. Engl. J. Med.** 301:1200–1204, 1979.
219. Peterson, C. M., Jones, R. L., Easterly, J. A., Wantz, G. E., and Jackson, R. L.: Changes in basement membrane thickening and pulse volume concomitant with improved glucose control in patients with insulin-dependent diabetes. **Diabetes Care** 3:586–589, 1980.
220. Wallberg-Henricksson, H., Gunnerson, R., DeFronzo, R., Felig, P., Ostman, J., and Wahren, J.: Increased peripheral insulin sensitivity and muscle mitochondrial enzymes but unchanged blood glucose control in type I diabetics after physical training. **Diabetes** 31:1044–1050, 1982.
221. Campaigne, B., Gilliam, T. B., Spencer, M. L., Lampman, R. M., and Schork, M. A.: Effects of physical activity program on metabolic control and cardiovascular fitness in children with insulin-dependent diabetes mellitus. **Diabetes Care** 7:57–62, 1984.
222. Barnard, R. J., Lattimore, L., Holly, R. G., Cherny, S., and Pritikin, N.: Response of noninsulin-dependent diabetic patients to an intensive program of diet and exercise. **Diabetes Care** 5:370–374, 1982.
223. Reitman, J. S., Vasquez, B., Klimes, I., and Nagulesparan, M.: Improvement in glucose hemostasis after exercise training in noninsulin-dependent diabetes. **Diabetes Care** 7:434–441, 1984.
224. Trovati, M., Carta, Q., Cavalot, F., Vitali, S., Banaudi, C., Luccina, P. G., Fioccli, F., Emanuelli, G., and Lenti, G.: Influence of physical training on blood glucose, glucose tolerance, insulin secretion, and insulin action in noninsulin-dependent diabetic patients. **Diabetes Care** 7:416–420, 1984.

225. Leon, A. S., Conrad, J. C., Casal, D. C., Serfass, R., Bonnard, R. A., Goetz, F. C., and Blackburn, H.: Exercise for diabetics: effects of conditioning at constant body weight. **J. Cardiac Rehabil.** 4:278–286, 1984.
226. Leon, A. S.: Diabetes. In Skinner, J. S. (ed.): **Exercise Testing and Exercise Prescription for Special Cases.** Philadelphia, Lea & Febiger, 1987, pp. 115–133.
227. Richter, E. A., Ruderman, N. B., and Schneider, S. H.: Diabetes and exercise. **Am. J. Med.** 70:201–209, 1981.
228. Costill, D. L., Miller, J. M., and Fink, W. J.: Energy metabolism in diabetic distance runners. **Phys. Sportsmed** 8:64–71, 1980.
229. Cantu, R. C.: **A Practical Positive Way to Control Diabetes, Diabetes and Exercise.** New York, E. P. Dutton, 1982.
230. Goldberg, A. P., and Coon, P. J.: Non–insulin-dependent diabetes mellitus in the elderly. **Endocrin. Metabol. Clin.** 16:843–865, 1987.
231. Fearnot, N. E., Smith, H. J., and Geddes, L. A.: A review of pacemakers that physiologically increase rate: the DDD and rate responsive pacemakers. **Prog. Cardiovasc. Dis.** 29:145–164, 1986.
232. denDulk, K., Bouwels, L., Lindemans, F., Rankin, I., Brugada, P., and Wellens, H. J. J.: The Activitrax rate response pacemaker system. **Am. J. Cardiol.** 61:107–112, 1988.
233. Superko, H. R.: The effects of cardiac rehabilitation in permanently paced patients with third degree heart block. **J. Cardiac Rehabil.** 3:561–568, 1983.
234. Skinner, J. S., and Strandness, P. E.: Exercise and intermittent claudication. II. Effect of physical training. **Circulation** 36:23–29, 1967.
235. Hall, J. A., and Barnard, R. J.: The effects of an intensive 26-day program of diet and exercise on patients with peripheral vascular disease. **J. Cardiac Rehabil.** 2:569–574, 1982.
236. Boyd, C. E., Bird, P. J., Charles, C. D., Wellons, H. A., MacDougall, M. A., and Wolfe, L. A.: Pain free physical training in intermittent claudication. **J. Sports Med.** 24:112–122, 1984.
237. Ernst, E. E., and Matrai, A.: Intermittent claudication, exercise and blood rheology. **Circulation** 76:1110–1114, 1987.
238. Ernst, E.: Physical exercise for peripheral vascular disease—a review. **VASA** 16:227–231, 1987.
239. Ekblom, B., and Nordemar, R.: Rheumatoid arthritis. In Skinner, J. S. (ed.): **Exercise Testing and Exercise Prescription for Special Cases.** Philadelphia, Lea & Febiger, 1987, pp. 101–114.
240. Panush, R. S., and Brown, D. G.: Exercise, the musculoskeletal system, and arthritis. **Postgrad. Adv. Rheumat.** 2–4:1–20, 1987.
241. Moser, K. M., Archibald, C., Hansen, P., Ellis, B., and Whelan, D.: **Better Living and Breathing. A Manual for Patients.** St. Louis, C.V. Mosby, 1980.
242. Unger, K. M., Moser, K. M., and Hansen, P.: Selection of an exercise program for patients with chronic obstructive pulmonary disease. **Heart Lung** 9:68–76, 1980.
243. Hodgkin, J. E.: Pulmonary rehabilitation: structure, components and benefits. **J. Cardiopul. Rehabil.** 8:423–434, 1988.
244. Ries, A. L., and Archibald, C. J.: Endurance exercise training at maximal targets in patients with chronic obstructive pulmonary disease. **J. Cardiopul. Rehabil.** 7:594–601, 1987.
245. Corriveau, M. L., Harris, C. M., Chun, D. S., Keller, C., and Dolan, G. F.: Relationship between multiple physiologic variables and change in exercise capacity after a pulmonary rehabilitation program. **J. Cardiopul. Rehabil.** 8:303–308, 1988.
246. Carter, R., Nicotra, B., Clark, L., Zinkgraf, S., Williams, J., Deavler, M., Fields, S., and Berry, J.: Exercise conditioning in the rehabilitation of patients with chronic obstructive pulmonary disease. **Arch. Phys. Med. Rehabil.** 69:118–122, 1988.
247. Hass, A., and Cardon, H.: Rehabilitation in chronic obstructive pulmonary disease: a 5-year study of 252 male patients. **Med. Clin. North Am.** 53:593–606, 1969.

248. Connors, G. A., Hodgkin, J. E., and Asmus, R. M.: A careful assessment is crucial to successful pulmonary rehabilitation. **J. Cardiopul. Rehabil.** 8:435–438, 1988.
249. Pardy, R. L., Reed, W. D., and Belman, M. J.: Respiratory muscle training. In Belman, M. J. (ed.): **Clinics in Chest Medicine,** Vol. 9. Philadelphia, W.B. Saunders Co., 1988, pp. 287–296.
250. Hodgkin, J. E. (ed.): Pulmonary rehabilitation. **J. Cardiopul. Rehabil.** 8:423–497, 1988.
251. Andrews, J. L.: Pulmonary disease: improving the prognosis. **Mod. Med.** 55:88–94, 105, 106, 1987.
252. Wasserman, K., Hansen, J. E., Sue, D. Y., Whipp, B. J.: **Principles of Exercise Testing and Interpretation.** Philadelphia, Lea & Febiger, 1987.
253. Jones, N. L., Berman, L. B., Bartkiewicz, P. D., and Oldridge, N. B.: Chronic obstructive respiratory disorders. In Skinner, J. S. (ed.): **Exercise Testing and Exercise Prescription for Special Cases.** Philadelphia, Lea & Febiger, 1987, pp. 175–188.
254. National Center for Health Statistics: **1986 Summary: National Hospital Discharge Survey.** Advance data from vital and health statistics. No. 145, DHHS Pub. No. (PHS) 87-1250. Hyattsville, MD, Public Health Service, 1987.
255. King, S. B.: Current status of percutaneous transluminal coronary angioplasty. **Cardiovasc. Rev. Reports** 9:27–32, 1988.
256. Rothbaum, D. A., Linnemeier, T. L., Landin, R. J., Steinmetz, E. F., Hillis, J. S., Hallam, C. C., Noble, R. J., and See, M. R.: Emergency percutaneous transluminal angioplasty: a 3 year experience. **J. Am. Coll. Cardiol.** 10:264–268, 1987.
257. Maresh, C. M., Harbrecht, J. J., Flick, B. L., Hartzler, G. O.: Comparison of rehabilitation benefits after percutaneous transluminal coronary angioplasty and coronary artery bypass graft surgery. **J. Cardiac Rehabil.** 5:124–130, 1985.
258. Barnard, C. N.: The operation: a human cardiac transplant: an interim report of a successful operation performed at Groote Schuur Hospital, Cape Town. **S. Afr. Med. J.** 41:1271–1274, 1967.
259. Murdock, D., Collins, E., Lawless, C., Molnar, Z., Scanlon, P., and Pifarre, R.: Rejection of the transplanted heart. **Heart Lung** 16:237–245, 1987.
260. Carmichael, M., Salomon, D., and Sadler, L.: Cardiac transplantation: the first year's experience at the University of Florida–Shands Hospital. **J. Florida Med. Assoc.** 73:849–854, 1986.
261. Kavanagh, T., Yacoub, M., Mertens, D., Kennedy, J., Campbell, R., and Sawyer, P.: Cardiorespiratory responses to exercise training after orthotopic cardiac transplantation. **Circulation** 77:162–171, 1987.
262. Sadowsky, H., Rohrkemper, K., and Quon, S.: **Rehabilitation of Cardiac and Cardiopulmonary Recipients. An Introduction for Physical & Occupational Therapists.** Unpublished manual. Palo Alto, CA, Stanford University Hospital, 1986.
263. Greenburg, M., Uretsky, B., Reddy, P., Bernstein, R., Griffith, B., Hardesty, R., Thompson, M., and Bahnson, H.: Long-term hemodynamic follow-up of cardiac transplant patients treated with cyclosporine and prednisone. **Circulation** 71:487–494, 1985.
264. Spuires, R., Arthur, P., Gau, G., Muri, A., and Lambert, W.: Exercise after cardiac transplantation: a report of two cases. **J. Cardiac Rehabil.** 3:570–574, 1983.
265. Schroeder, J.: Hemodynamic performance of the human transplanted heart. **Transplant. Proc.** 11:304–308, 1979.
266. Pope, S., Stinson, E., Daughters, G., Schroeder, J., Ingels, N., and Alderman, E.: Exercise response of the denervated heart in long-term cardiac transplant recipients. **Am. J. Cardiol.** 46:213–218, 1980.
267. Savin, W., Haskell, W., Schroeder, J., and Stinson, E.: Cardiorespiratory responses of cardiac transplant patients to graded, symptom-limited exercise. **Circulation** 62:55–60, 1980.

268. Degre, S., Niset, G., DeSmet, J., Ibrahim, T., Stoupel, E., LeClerc, J., and Primo, G.: Cardiorespiratory response to early exercise testing after orthotopic cardiac transplantation. **Am. J. Cardiol.** 60:926–928, 1987.
269. Corcos, T., Tamburino, C., Leger, P., Vaissier, E., Rossant, P., Mattei, M., Daudon P., Gandjbakhch, I., Pavie, A., Cabrol, A., and Cabrol, C.: Early and late hemodynamic evaluation after cardiac transplantation: a study of 28 cases. **J. Am. Coll. Cardiol.** 11:264–269, 1988.
270. Pflugfelder, P., Purves, P., McKenzie, F., and Kostuk, W.: Cardiac dynamics during supine exercise in cyclosporine-treated orthotopic heart transplant recipients: assessment by radionuclide angiography. **J. Am. Coll. Cardiol.** 10:336–341, 1987.
271. Borow, K., Neumann, A., Arensman, F., and Yacoub, M.: Left ventricular contractility and contractile reserve in humans after cardiac transplantation. **Circulation** 71:866–872, 1985.
272. Kavanagh, T., Yacoub, M., Campbell, R., and Mertens, D.: Marathon running after cardiac transplantation: a case history. **J. Cardiopul. Rehabil.** 6:16–20, 1986.

9

SPECIAL CONSIDERATIONS IN PRESCRIBING EXERCISE

INTRODUCTION

Once the commitment has been made to begin an exercise program, whether for its health benefits or for rehabilitation from disease, attention must be given to a number of factors that can directly influence the program's success or failure. What type of clothing should be worn when exercising, and how important is proper footwear? What steps can be followed to minimize the possibility of serious orthopedic injury? Is warm-up necessary, and what is the proper way in which to cool down after a bout of vigorous exercise? How does altitude or extreme variations in temperature and humidity influence the daily workout? Do age and gender become factors in modifying the exercise prescription or limit the degree of improvement that might be expected to result from the exercise program? How can the exercise prescription be followed when traveling or when forced inside during inclement weather? How does one stay motivated to continue his or her exercise program from day to day or year to year? These and many other practical questions of a similar nature are discussed in this chapter.

CLOTHING, SHOES, AND SPECIAL EQUIPMENT

The selection of improper or inappropriate clothing, shoes, or related equipment can create many problems for participants just beginning an exercise program. Overdressing or underdressing, wearing the wrong size or type of shoe, or using the wrong piece of

621

equipment can lead to serious problems of heat or cold stress, disability, injury, overstress, or unnecessary expense. Appropriate care must be taken when making decisions in each of the following areas.

Clothing

The choice of clothing is totally dependent on the specific activity selected and the environmental conditions under which the activity is performed. With swimming, the conditions are relatively stable throughout the year, and as a result, special considerations are not required when selecting a swimming suit. For hiking, walking, jogging, running, bicycling, or any other sporting activity that is performed outdoors, the attire should be comfortable, reasonably loose fitting, and of the proper weight to ensure protection from the sun, heat, cold, and wind. As a general rule, it is better to underdress than overdress, since the exercise itself will have a considerable warming effect on the body. Avoid restrictive support garments or clothing that would impede movement or blood flow. Bras may or may not be worn, depending on the size of the breasts. "Athletic bras" are now available to provide additional support for large breasts.[1] Although men should wear supporters when participating in vigorous or contact sports, supporters are not essential during an activity such as jogging and may lead to skin irritations during long periods of activity.

The clothing material or fabric is also an important consideration. The fabric should be nonabrasive and nonirritating. Many new synthetic materials are being used that provide features that are of importance to both the safety and performance of the athlete and the noncompetitive exerciser. Materials are available that are water repellent, light in weight, aerodynamically advanced to reduce friction with air, and designed to either release body heat or retain body heat during hot or cold weather. The wicking characteristics of clothing are also important, as wicking allows the removal of moisture from perspiration without saturating the fabric. A good wicking fabric will help prevent heat-stress injury.[1]

Although there is a great deal of individual variation when exercising at different temperatures, the following suggestions should prove helpful. When a person is exercising at temperatures between 60°F and 80°F, a light T-shirt or blouse and shorts should be adequate; between 40°F and 60°F, the addition of a lightweight jacket or sweat shirt is advisable; and below 40°F, sweat pants, thermal underwear, or both may be required. Gloves and stocking caps are also desirable when the temperature drops below 40°F. Kaufman[2] provides a good summary of his work on short-term and long-term exposure to cold relative to clothing needs. At temperatures above 80°F, men may wish to exercise without a shirt, and women may elect to wear a halter top. These recommendations are made on the assumption that there are low to moderate levels of humidity and wind. With higher humidities, the extremely high and low temperatures are considerably more stressful. Direct radiation from the sun is also an important consideration at the higher temperatures, and hats can be worn to reduce the radiant load.

Under no circumstances should one exercise while wearing rubberized or plastic clothing. This is common practice among individuals trying to use exercise as a means of losing weight. Athletes such as jockeys and wrestlers frequently use this technique to get down to their prescribed weight limit. The increased sweat loss does not result in a permanent loss of body weight, and this practice can be very dangerous.[3] Rubberized or plastic clothing does not allow the body sweat to evaporate. Since the heat loss through the evaporation of sweat is the principal manner in which the body regulates its temperature during exercise, a reduction in sweating or reduced evaporation of sweat can lead to a dramatic increase in body temperature and possible heat stroke or heat exhaustion.[3] For additional, more detailed information on the physiological and biophysical effects of clothing for exercise under a variety of environmental conditions, the reader is referred to the excellent review by Gonzalez published in 1987.[4]

Shoes and Socks

The type of shoe selected and the proper fit of the shoe are important considerations for any activity program. For most activities, a well-fitting tennis, basketball, or general gym shoe of good quality is perfectly adequate. For walking, jogging, or running activities, however, a special and carefully fitted walking or running shoe designed specifically for these activities is highly recommended. The foot strikes the ground many times during a single workout. This places considerable stress on the foot and its associated structures. Thus, a shoe that gives good support and protection and has good shock-absorbing qualities is highly desirable.

Most walking and running shoes have a strong, highly supportive heel counter, a heel wedge and midsole, a good arch support, a comfortable innersole, a relatively pliable outer sole, and a comfortable toe box.[5] The heel counter, which provides support and stabilization of the heel, should be firm, should fit snugly, and should come at least 4 inches forward from the rear point of the heel.[5] The heel wedge and midsole combine to form the heel lift, which helps to reduce pressure on the Achilles tendon and serves as the primary shock absorber. The outer sole should be durable and tough, to prevent rapid wear, but must be pliable. The toe box is often overlooked but is extremely important for total foot comfort. Black toenails result from blood blisters that form under the toenail, which are caused by a toe box that has insufficient clearance between the toes and the underside of the toe box. The sockliner and the insole provide additional protection from shock and from blister formation and should feel comfortable, with no seams to cause irritation.

Shoes should be selected on the basis of one's individual needs. Factors to be considered include the need for rear foot stabilization and pronation control, shock-absorbing characteristics, and the wear characteristics of the outer sole and the upper. Prices vary between 30 and 125 dollars or more for a good pair of shoes. Several running magazines publish annual ratings of the various running shoes on the market. These publications should be consulted when selecting a running shoe for the first time or when changing from one shoe to another. Despite the ratings, however, the most important factor is proper shoe fit and comfort. Some brands come in different widths, and this is important for the individual with an extremely narrow or wide foot. Figure 9–1 illustrates the "anatomy" of a running shoe.

Socks are also important items for the beginning exerciser. Wool or cotton socks are appropriate, provided they fit properly after washing. Tube socks have become quite popular, for they fit a variety of sizes, do not shrink appreciably, and tend to stay fixed to the foot. This last point is important, since creeping socks tend to bunch up and cause painful blisters.

Special Equipment

An activity such as swimming or jogging requires no special equipment other than that described previously. If, however, the exercise prescription specifies games like tennis or racketball, or an indoor exercise device such as a stationary cycle, proper knowledge of the equipment under consideration is important. It would be impossible to discuss here all possible items of equipment likely to be used in an exercise program designed to promote cardiores-

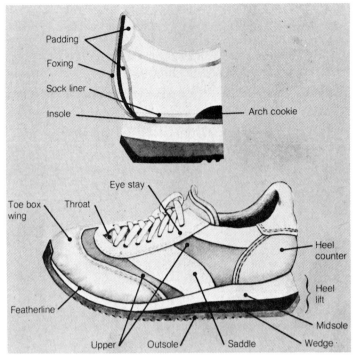

Figure 9–1. The anatomy of a running shoe. (Reprinted with permission from Bates, W.T.: Selecting a running shoe. **Physician Sportsmed.** 10:154–155, 1982.)

piratory fitness. However, there are certain guidelines that can be applied in the purchase of most specialized exercise equipment, including the following:

- Deal with reputable businesses that stand behind their products. If possible, make sure the product can be serviced locally, or conveniently and within a reasonable period of time if local service is not available.
- Consult experts in the field or various consumer reports if there is any question about a company or its product. Most YMCAs, colleges, or universities have experts in this area who are willing to provide valuable information.
- Avoid devices that claim to do all of the work. Active participation is essential to obtain the desired benefits of exercise.
- Do not be misled into thinking that the more expensive the item, the better job it does. Many items of equipment are greatly overpriced.
- Do not buy something that will not be used. Many expensive

pieces of exercise equipment end up being stored in the garage, basement, or attic.

- Do not buy on impulse after receiving a high-powered sales pitch. Wait at least 3 days before making the final decision.
- Understand completely the purpose of the exercise device and its principle of operation.

WARM-UP, COOL-DOWN, AND INJURY PREVENTION

Warm-Up Period

It is particularly important to incorporate a brief, but basic, warm-up routine into any training program. This was discussed in Chapter 7, and appropriate stretching exercises were illustrated. Stretching exercises develop and maintain flexibility as well as prepare the muscles, joints, and ligaments for the added stress of the strength or cardiorespiratory endurance training session.[3] Barnard and associates[6] demonstrated serious electrocardiogram abnormalities in middle-aged adults when sudden exercise was undertaken without proper warm-up. Strength and muscular endurance exercises can be performed as a part of the initial warm-up period, but they should be preceded by the stretching exercises. If jogging or running, bicycling, hiking, or similar activities are the participant's main endurance activity, then strength and muscular endurance exercises should concentrate more on the upper body, because the lower body is the primary focus of these cardiorespiratory endurance programs. Proper warm-up may help alleviate many potential injuries such as muscle pulls, strains, sprains, and low-back discomfort, in addition to reducing the extent of muscle soreness. However, several epidemiological studies have failed to identify stretching and increased flexibility as critical in reducing the risk of running injuries.[7, 8]

Cool-Down Period

The cool-down period is equal to the warm-up period in importance. This is the period immediately after the cardiorespiratory endurance portion of each exercise session. The major purpose of the cool-down period is to keep the primary muscle groups, which were involved in the endurance exercise, continuously active. Since most cardiorespiratory endurance exercises involve the legs and are typically performed in an upright position, blood will pool in the lower half of the body if the individual does not perform light activity such as walking or slow jogging during the recovery period. Postexercise hypotension, resulting in dizziness and fainting, is particularly evident after stationary cycling. Thus, easy pedaling against light or no resistance should be continued during the cool-down period. This light activity allows the leg muscles to assist the return of the pooled blood to the heart. As the muscles in the legs contract, they create pressure against the veins, which in turn pushes the blood toward the heart, with the venous valves permitting blood to flow in only one direction—back to the heart. Without this light activity, blood will continue to pool in the lower body, and the participant may experience dizziness and can even pass out because of inadequate blood flow to the brain (vasovagal response). Plasma catecholamine levels are also greatly elevated during the immediate postexercise recovery period, which increases the risk of cardiac arrhythmias, ischemia, and hypotension.[9] An active recovery period greatly reduces this risk.

Light activity during the cool-down period also helps to prevent extreme muscle soreness. This is particularly true if the cool-down period includes a few selected stretching exercises that concentrate on the legs and lower back. The length of the cool-down period need not exceed 5 to 10 minutes. After the workout, the participant should take a warm, *not hot*, shower, since hot showers after endurance exercise can create serious cardiovascular complications, i.e., peripheral dilation, increasing blood pooling in the periphery.

Injury Prevention

The potential for serious injury exists in almost any exercise program if the proper precautions are not followed. As discussed earlier, sudden vigorous exercise has been shown to place a potentially lethal strain on the heart.[6] A proper warm-up period decreases the likelihood of this occurring. The participant must be aware of the various warning signs that may result from vigorous endurance exercise. Zohman, in her booklet *Beyond Diet . . . Exercise Your Way to Fitness and Heart Health*,[10] has listed a number of potential warning signs and symptoms that could occur either during or immediately after exercise. These may be grouped into the following categories:

A. *Stop exercising*. See a physician before resuming if the following occur:

    1. Abnormal heart activity, including arrhythmias, fluttering, jumping, or palpitations in the chest or throat; sudden burst of rapid heartbeats; or a sudden slowing of a rapid pulse rate.

2. Pain or pressure in the center of the chest, the arm, or the throat during or immediately after exercise.
3. Dizziness, lightheadedness, sudden lack of coordination, confusion, cold sweating, glassy stare, pallor, cyanosis, or fainting.
4. Illness, particularly viral infections, can lead to myocarditis, that is, viral infection of the heart muscle. Avoid exercise during and immediately after an illness, particularly when fever is present.

B. *Attempt self-correction.*
1. Persistent rapid pulse rate throughout 5 to 10 minutes of recovery or longer. *Self-correction technique:* reduce the intensity of the activity (use a lower training heart rate) and progress to higher levels of activity at a slower rate. Consult a physician if the condition persists.
2. Nausea or vomiting after exercise. *Self-correction technique:* reduce the intensity of the endurance exercise and prolong the cool-down period. Avoid eating for at least 2 hours before the exercise session.
3. Extreme breathlessness lasting more than 10 minutes after the cessation of exercise. *Self-correction technique:* reduce the intensity of the endurance exercise. Consult a physician if the condition persists.
4. Prolonged fatigue up to 24 hours after exercise. *Self-correction technique:* reduce the intensity of the endurance exercise and reduce the duration of the total workout session if this symptom persists. Consult a physician if these self-correcting techniques do not remedy the situation.

In addition to the preceding, there are a number of potential injuries or medical complications of an orthopedic nature that are usually minor but can also result in many participants' dropping out of their exercise programs. Sharkey has listed a number of these in his book *Fitness and Work Capacity*[11] and has suggested a sound course of action to follow in an attempt to correct the situation. The list includes the following:

Blisters. These are a common problem, particularly when one is breaking in a pair of new shoes. Prevention begins with purchasing properly fitting shoes and socks that stay in place and do not creep or bunch up. When blisters occur, puncture the edge of the blister with a sterile needle, drain the fluid, apply a topical antiseptic, and cover with gauze or an adhesive bandage. Use precaution to avoid possible infection.

Muscle Soreness. Soreness usually accompanies the start of any exercise program or results from a sudden change in exercise habits. The degree of soreness can be reduced by starting at low levels of exercise and progressing slowly through the first few weeks and by thorough warm-up and cool-down periods that include stretching exercises. Massage and warm baths help to relieve the soreness when present. Reducing the eccentric component of the exercise routine also reduces the potential for soreness.[12]

Muscle Cramps. These are involuntary muscle contractions that may be due to salt, potassium, or calcium imbalances in the muscle. Stretching and massaging the muscle usually bring immediate relief. Proper warm-up, replacement of electrolytes that were lost through sweating, and postexercise stretching should prevent most muscle cramps.

Bone Bruises. These are painful bruises, usually on the bottoms of the feet, caused by a single blow or repeated trauma to the bone. Ice and padding of the bruised area provide some relief, but proper footwear, including good midsoles, usually prevents the problem.

Low-Back Pain. Low-back pain is usually the result of poor flexibility, weak abdominal and back muscles, and poor posture. Stretching and muscle-strengthening exercises, along with a conscious effort to improve posture, remedy the problem in the majority of cases. See Chapter 7 for details on exercises for a healthy back.

Knee Problems. These can be caused or aggravated by the endurance conditioning program. This is a frequent area of complaint among joggers and runners. Wearing proper footwear and running on soft, even surfaces such as grass tend to reduce or eliminate the problem. Stay away from sharp turns or roads with high crowns. A physician or podiatrist should be consulted if the problem persists.

Shin Splints. A shin splint is manifested as a sharp pain on the front aspect of the tibia. Shin splints are probably the result of a lowered arch, irritated membranes, tearing of muscle where it attaches to bone, hairline or stress fracture of the bone, or other factors. Although rest is the only sure cure, limited exercise is possible with the leg wrapped or taped, or an alternate form of exercise—e.g., cycling or swimming—may be chosen. Prevention of shin splints can be accomplished by using proper footwear, running on soft surfaces such as grass, and strengthening the surrounding musculature.

Achilles Tendon Injuries. These injuries are a frequent source of trouble in distance runners. Improper footwear, including shoes without heel wedges and high-back shoes that rub against the Achilles tendon, are considered to be the primary cause. Reduced activity or total rest combined with applying ice packs appears to be the only remedy, and surgical repair may be necessary. Prevention through selection of proper footwear and adequate warm-up is strongly advised. The warm-up should include a heel-stretching exercise, but caution must be exerted to prevent over-stretching (see Chapter 7).

Ankle Problems. These are a frequent problem for those who play sports that require a quick change in direction. A sprained ankle should be iced immediately to prevent major swelling and to facilitate recovery. Serious sprains should be examined by a physician. Prevention is best achieved by strengthening the surrounding musculature, by wearing high-topped gym or basketball shoes, and by preventive taping or ankle wraps, although this latter recommendation is controversial.

If a jogger has an injury to the lower extremity and rest is required, he or she can use alternate activities such as cycling (stationary or free wheeling) or swimming. In this way, general fitness can be maintained while the jogging injury has a chance to heal. The reader is referred to several good textbooks on athletic injuries for a more comprehensive review of this area.[13-16]

ENVIRONMENTAL CONSIDERATIONS

In a temperature-controlled swimming pool or inside an air-conditioned or heated building, the environment remains stable from day to day and month to month, independent of changes in the outer environment. However, most individuals exercise outside these controlled conditions, and factors such as heat, cold, humidity, and quality of air become major considerations. In addition, whether exercising under controlled conditions or not, any marked change in altitude also significantly influences one's ability to exercise.

Heat

The body's temperature is maintained consistently at approximately 98.6°F under normal conditions. When confronted with variations in outside temperature, the body makes rather remarkable adjustments to preserve its temperature. In extreme cold, the body shivers, which generates metabolic heat to maintain body temperature. In extreme heat, the body relies primarily on the evaporation of sweat to keep a constant temperature. Sweating is effective only as long as the sweat can evaporate, since it is the loss of heat resulting from the evaporation of the sweat that cools the body. Wind also aids in the evaporative process. In very humid weather, since the air is nearly saturated with water, evaporation becomes limited, and thus the body has difficulty being cooled. The lethal combination of high temperature and high relative humidity has resulted in a number of deaths related to exercise, including football[17] and jogging.[18]

The ability of an individual to perform successfully in a hot environment depends on the magnitude of heat, the existing humidity, the air movement, the intensity and duration of the exercise, and the extent of his or her previous exposure to heat, i.e., acclimatization. The amount of direct radiation is also a critical factor, for direct exposure to the sun, as opposed to shade or cloud cover, is a major source of heat gain. Sources of heat gain and loss are illustrated in Figure 9–2.[19]

The higher the temperature, the greater the heat stress on the individual. With low humidity and acclimatization, the individual can tolerate air temperatures in excess of 90°F without too much trouble, since the individual can sweat at rates in excess of 2 liters per hour, and the dry air can evaporate most of the sweat.[3] As the humidity increases, the tolerable heat level reduces considerably. In a dry climate, the individual is not even aware he or she is

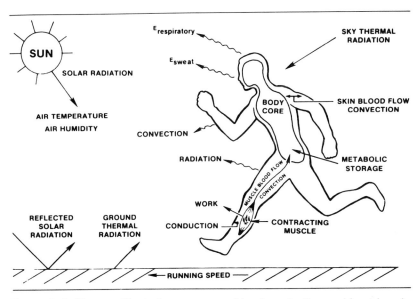

Figure 9–2. Diagram illustrating avenues of heat production and heat loss in the exercising body. (Reprinted with permission from Gisolfi, C.V., and Wenger, C.B.: Temperature regulation during exercise: old concepts, new ideas. **Exerc. Sport Sci. Rev.** 12:339–372, 1984. Copyright American College of Sports Medicine, 1984.)

sweating, since the sweat evaporates the moment it reaches the skin. Under conditions of high humidity, the individual is quite conscious of sweating since very little can be evaporated into the nearly saturated air, and the sweat seems to roll off unceasingly. Another factor that is critical to determining the total thermal stress is air movement. The greater the air movement, the greater the cooling effect. Still air stagnates and becomes saturated with water, and evaporation is reduced.

A heat-stress index has been developed that takes into account the absolute temperature (dry bulb temperature), the humidity (dry bulb and wet bulb temperature), and solar radiant energy (black globe temperature). This index is referred to as the wet bulb globe temperature (WBGT). By using the WBGT heat-stress index, it is possible to assign a relative risk for heat injury to the prevailing environmental conditions.[20] A much simpler index, using only absolute temperature and humidity, is illustrated in Figure 9–3.

The intensity and duration of the activity are also factors in determining the total heat stress experienced by the individual.[21] Since the body produces heat as it exercises, the higher the intensity of the exercise and the longer the duration, the greater will be the resulting heat load and the subsequent stress to the body. It is possible to partially adapt or acclimatize to heat through repeated exposure, but total adaptation never occurs; i.e., heat will always be a major limitation to peak performance.[21]

One of the primary concerns when exercising in the heat is

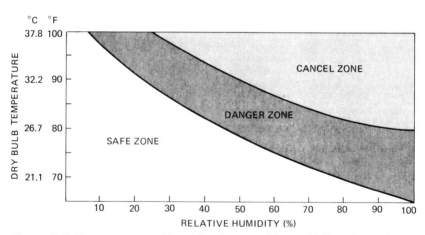

Figure 9–3. Temperature and humidity chart providing guidelines for environmental conditions under which it is safe to exercise. (Reprinted with permission from Lamb, D.R.: **Physiology of Exercise: Responses and Adaptations**, 2nd Ed. New York, Macmillan, 1984.)

dehydration. With high sweat rates, the body loses a large volume of water. Since a major portion of this water loss comes from the blood volume, a serious situation exists unless rehydration is accomplished by consuming the appropriate fluids.[21] Water and a diluted electrolyte solution appear to be the best fluids for quick rehydration. Fluids high in sugar content, i.e., over 10 percent, are not rapidly absorbed by the body.[22-24] Since a salt loss occurs with these high sweat rates, a liberal salting of food is recommended. Patients with hypertension and on salt-restricted diets or diuretics, or both, should consult their physicians before increasing their salt intake.

Since people respond quite differently to heat, the adjustments to exercising in the heat should be made on an individual basis. In the summer, it is often important to exercise during the cooler parts of the day, preferably when the sun's radiation is minimal, i.e., night, early morning or early evening. Drink fluids abundantly before, during, and after the exercise session. Avoid exercise altogether when the combination of temperature and humidity is such that severe heat stress resulting in heat exhaustion or heat stroke is unavoidable. It is most likely that both the intensity and the duration of the activity will have to be reduced to maintain the same training heart rate. In 1987, the American College of Sports Medicine published a position statement on *Prevention of Thermal Injuries During Distance Running.*[25] This is included in Appendix C.

Continued daily exposure to heat results in a gradual adaptation of the body to this stress, and the heat can be tolerated much more effectively. If a participant must play vigorous game activities or run races in the heat, then much of his or her training should be done under similar conditions. For example, many runners had a bad experience at the 1975 Boston Marathon when the temperature reached in excess of 90°F. They had not prepared themselves for the heat. One can become more than 90 percent acclimatized in approximately 14 days.[3, 21] If one becomes sporadic in exercising in the heat and chooses to train during the cool part of the day, then part of the acclimatization is lost in just a few days.[21]

Cold

Exercise in the cold presents far fewer problems. The exercise itself provides considerable body heat, and additional clothing can always be worn. Since the hands, feet, and head are particularly sensitive to extreme cold, proper gloves, extra socks, and a stocking hat with a face mask are strongly advised. As with heat, the degree of humidity and air movement is important. The more humid the air and the greater the wind velocity, the greater is the cold stress for the same absolute temperature. On the other hand, in a very dry, cold environment, care must be taken not to overdress, since sweating occurs once the individual warms up. The sweat-soaked clothing is subject to evaporation, which leads to rapid cooling and chills. If possible, easily unzipped layers of light clothing that can be ventilated (opened from the front) or even removed are often better than one or two heavy garments. Table 9–1 outlines the interaction between temperature and wind speed and should be used as a guide to plan winter exercise sessions. On a cold, windy day, it is recommended that a participant start out by running against the wind (coldest segment) and return with the wind to his or her back. Kavanagh[26] has prepared extensive guidelines for cardiac patients exercising outdoors in cold weather.

Air Pollution

Air pollution has become a major consideration over the recent years because of its effect on the exercising subject.[27-32] Although

Table 9–1. Wind-Chill–Factor Chart

Estimated Wind Speed (mph)	Actual Thermometer Reading (°F)											
	50	40	30	20	10	0	−10	−20	−30	−40	−50	−60
	Equivalent Temperature (°F)											
Calm	50	40	30	20	10	0	−10	−20	−30	−40	−50	−60
5	48	37	27	16	6	−5	−15	−26	−36	−47	−57	−68
10	40	28	16	4	−9	−24	−33	−46	−58	−70	−83	−95
15	36	22	9	−5	−18	−32	−45	−58	−72	−85	−99	−112
20	32	18	4	−10	−25	−39	−53	−67	−82	−96	−110	−124
25	30	16	0	−15	−29	−44	−59	−74	−88	−104	−118	−133
30	28	13	−2	−18	−33	−48	−63	−79	−94	−109	−125	−140
35	27	11	−4	−20	−35	−51	−67	−82	−98	−113	−129	−145
40	26	10	−6	−21	−37	−53	−69	−85	−100	−116	−132	−148

	Green	Yellow	Red
Wind speeds greater than 40 mph have little additional effect.	**Little Danger** (for properly clothed person) Maximal danger of false sense of security.	**Increasing Danger** Danger from freezing or exposed flesh.	**Great Danger**

Trenchfoot and immersion foot may occur at any point on this chart.

(Adapted from **Runner's World** 8:28 (1973). Reproduced by permission of the publisher.)

this may not be a problem in many rural communities, it is a major problem in most large metropolitan areas. Carbon monoxide has a much greater affinity or attraction to hemoglobin than oxygen. Since almost all oxygen is transported through the blood by hemoglobin, high concentrations of carbon monoxide greatly reduce one's working capacity.[31] Other air pollutants, particularly ozone, have also been shown to have a significant negative effect on exercise capacity.[27] In certain areas of the United States, smog alerts have been instituted to warn individuals to stay indoors and to restrict physical activity levels on days when smog levels exceed a certain critical level. Exercising along heavily traveled roads can also expose the exerciser to fairly high, concentrated doses of pollutants, which are also potentially dangerous. Exercising in nonpolluted areas or restricting activity when pollution levels are high is strongly suggested. Raven has published an excellent summary of the national ambient air quality standards and has recommended federal episode criteria for various pollutants (Table 9–2).[32]

Altitude

The percentage of oxygen in the atmosphere at an altitude of 10,000 feet is exactly the same as that at sea level. However, the atmospheric pressure is much less at 10,000 feet, and thus, pressure exerted by oxygen at that altitude is proportionally less than at sea level. As a result, it is more difficult to deliver oxygen to the working muscles of the body, and the absolute working capacity is reduced in direct proportion to the altitude.[3] This has little, if any, effect on short bursts of activity such as sprinting, but it greatly affects activities of an endurance nature. For the same heart rate, more work can be done at sea level than at high altitude. As a result, the intensity of the workout at high altitudes should be reduced to maintain approximately the same cardiovascular stress as experienced at sea level. Dehydration is also a significant problem or concern at altitude, which should be considered when planning workouts or competition. The body starts to adapt to the stress of a particular altitude shortly after arriving at that altitude. After several weeks at that altitude, the body partially acclimatizes, but performance is still compromised.[3] Particular caution must be exerted by postcoronary and pulmonary patients when exercising at altitude.

Table 9–2. National Ambient Air Quality Standards and Recommended Federal Episode Criteria

Pollutant (units/averaging time)	Secondary	Primary	Alert*	Warning*	Emergency*	Significant Harm†
Sulfur dioxide µg/m³ (ppm)						
1 year		80 (0.03)				
24 hours		365 (0.14)	800 (0.3)	1,600 (0.6)	2,100 (0.8)	2,620 (1.0)
3 hours	1,300 (0.5)					
Particulate matter µg/m³ (COH)						
1 year	60	75				
24 hours	150	260	375 (3.0)	625 (5.0)	875 (7.0)	1,000 (8.0)
Product of sulfur dioxide and particulate matter $[\mu g/m^3]^2$ (ppm × COH)			6.5×10^4 (0.2)	2.61×10^5 (0.8)	3.93×10^5 (1.2)	4.90×10^5 (1.5)
Carbon monoxide mg/m³ (ppm)						
8 hours	10 (9)	10 (9)	17 (15)	34 (30)	46 (40)	57.5 (50)
1 hour	40 (35)	40 (35)				144 (125)
Oxidants µg/m³ (ppm)						
1 hour	160 (0.08)	160 (0.08)	200 (0.1)	800 (0.4)	1,200 (0.6)	1,400 (0.7)
Nitrogen dioxide µg/m³ (ppm)						
1 year	100 (0.05)	100 (0.05)				
24 hours			282 (0.15)	565 (0.3)	750 (0.4)	938 (0.5)
1 hour			1,130 (0.6)	2,260 (1.2)	3,000 (1.6)	3,750 (2.0)
Hydrocarbons µg/m³ (ppm)						
3 hours (6 to 9 AM)	160 (0.24)	160 (0.24)				

*The federal episode criteria specify that meteorological conditions are such that pollutant concentrations can be expected to remain at these levels for 12 or more hours or increase; or, in case of oxidants, the situation is likely to reoccur within the next 24 hours unless control actions are taken.

†Priority I regions must have a contingency plan that shall, as a minimum, provide for taking any emission control actions necessary to prevent ambient pollutant concentration from reaching these levels at any location.

(Reprinted with permission from Raven, P.B.: Questions and answers. **J. Cardiac Rehabil.** 2:411–414, 1982.)

AGE AND GENDER CONSIDERATIONS

Do individuals adapt differently to exercise depending upon their age and gender? Are we "over the hill" by the age of 30 years? Are women genetically inferior to men when it comes to exercise capacity? These questions have been asked for many years, and the answers are just now starting to surface.

First, endurance capacity does increase with age up to the middle to late 20's.[33, 34] Strength, muscular endurance, and cardiovascular endurance follow similar patterns of development.[34] Women tend to reach their peak much earlier, that is, shortly after puberty.[3, 33, 35] Men tend to maintain their peak values until the age of 30, after which there is a gradual decline throughout their lives.[33] Women start to decline shortly after attaining their peak and continue to do so gradually throughout the rest of their lives. The earlier peak and decline for women is thought to be a result of their lack of participation at an early age.[3] Up to the point of puberty, there are essentially no differences between men and women for practically all aspects of physical performance, that is, speed, strength, power, agility, and muscular and cardiorespiratory endurance. Beyond puberty, men become faster and considerably stronger in upper body strength and have greater power and muscular and cardiorespiratory endurance.[3, 35]

Two questions arise from the preceding observations. Are the sex differences seen after puberty—i.e., the fact that women tend to discontinue or reduce participation in vigorous activity or sports after puberty—genetically determined, or are they the result of different cultural and social expectations? Are the declines in physical ability noted with aging purely biological phenomena, or are they the result of an increasingly sedentary lifestyle? To answer the first question, studies that have compared highly trained female athletes with male athletes of similar training have found few physiological differences between the sexes, with the exception of upper body strength.[36] Therefore, it appears that the large differences seen between normal men and women beyond the age of puberty result primarily from comparing moderately active men with relatively sedentary women. The implications are obvious. Women are not second-class citizens physically but can enjoy all the same benefits of exercise enjoyed by men![35]

With respect to the decline in performance with age,[37] studies have shown that individuals who have remained physically active, even to the point of international class competition for their age category, have not experienced the same rate of decline in physiological function.[38–40] There does appear to be a decrease, as would be expected, but the decrease is greatly accentuated by a decline in daily physical activity patterns. Since there are a large number of men and women who are vigorously active in their 50's, 60's, and 70's, and even older, including those who are competing in races of 26.2 miles (marathon) or longer, it does appear that age is not a barrier to an active lifestyle.[41] For example, Kasch and associates[42] studied a group of middle-aged men ranging in age from 45 to 55 years who trained for 20 years. The men maintained their level of training during this period and showed only a 3-percent reduction in $\dot{V}O_2$max by 18 years and a 12-percent reduction by 20 years. The older individual may need to start the exercise program at a much lower level and progress at a slower rate, but given time, the benefits will be the same.[38] See Chapter 3 for additional information on the effect of age on cardiorespiratory fitness.

SPECIFICITY OF TRAINING

Over the past few years, research has continued to confirm what many have suspected for years, i.e., training benefits are specific to the activity. Athletes who participate in both football and basketball are frequently shocked to find that all of the hard training that conditioned them for the sport of football did little to prepare them for a full court scrimmage on the first night of basketball practice. Playing basketball conditions players for a game of basketball but does little to prepare them for running a 5-mile race. Endurance training in a swimming pool has little or no carry-over for long-distance running. Changes that result from physical training are very specific to the actual muscles involved and to the pattern in which the muscles are used. This is an important concept to remember. Researchers are just now probing into why the training responses are so specific.[3, 43]

EXERCISE PROGRAMS FOR TRAVELING AND AT HOME

Frequently, an individual just gets started on an exercise program when the program is interrupted by a vacation, business travel, or inclement weather. This problem has been of major concern to physicians, exercise physiologists, and program staff, since this interruption frequently signals the end of the program for that particular individual. By the time he or she returns or the weather improves, the urge to exercise has passed or considerable deconditioning has occurred.[3]

To combat such a situation, several approaches have been taken to develop indoor home and travel programs in order to maintain the continuity of the exercise program. Some good indoor activities are available. The stationary cycle is probably the best home device. It can be set in front of the television or by an outside window to provide variety while exercising, thus eliminating potential boredom. Stationary cycles should have an adjustable knob to vary the resistance against which the individual pedals. The resistance should be set to provide an intensity of exercise equivalent to that used in the individual's jogging, running, or swimming program, i.e., should use the same training heart rate. Duration and frequency would also be the same as that prescribed for jogging, walking, or swimming. Because of the specificity of training, it will probably take a few workouts to get the legs sufficiently in shape for a full program.

Rope skipping and running in place are two additional exercises that can be performed indoors at home or when traveling on the road, although these may not be appropriate for some patient populations, e.g., postcoronary patients or the elderly. Both exercises are excellent when performed correctly for the same duration and frequency and at the same intensity as stationary cycling. A word of caution is necessary, however. Extreme muscle soreness in the calf muscles is very common during the first few weeks of both rope-skipping and running-in-place programs. As with all other forms of exercise, the intensity is regulated on the basis of the training heart rate. In addition, calf-stretching exercises help alleviate muscle soreness and cramping. The injury potential with rope skipping is high, since it is a high-impact activity.

Home video exercise programs have become very popular. Aerobic dance and stretching exercise tapes are available that are of professional quality and are scientifically sound. Many of the early tapes were not well designed and included unsafe exercises. This appears to be less of a problem with the more recent tapes.

When traveling, it is also possible to substitute long, brisk walks or stair climbing for the activity normally pursued. It is also becoming widely acceptable for joggers and runners to take their workout gear with them on trips. Usually there are parks or lightly traveled roads within a short distance of most hotels or motels. Once the individual overcomes the embarrassment of riding an elevator and walking through the lobby in his or her running gear, the rest is easy! Many hotels have up-to-date exercise facilities and provide maps of walking and jogging trails located in the immediate vicinity. Winson[44] provides a guide for hotels with fitness facilities, running trails, and swimming facilities in 33 North American cities.

MOTIVATION

The success or failure of any exercise program is directly related to the motivation of the individual participants. Those who are highly motivated will continue their exercise program indefinitely, even when faced with injury. Those who are poorly motivated will have great difficulty adhering to their exercise program. It has been estimated that only 50 to 60 percent of those who start an exercise program will adhere to this program for 6 months or longer, whereas the remaining 40 to 50 percent drop out.[45, 46] Studies have attempted to identify those factors that might be responsible for adherence versus dropout. Some of these include the attitude of the participant's spouse toward involvement in the program, the proximity of the participant to the testing and exercise facility, inconvenient time and conflict with work schedule, the intensity of training, being overweight, smoking, being a blue-collar worker, low self-motivation, and freedom from serious illness or injury.[46, 47] Factors such as behavior pattern, health consciousness, attitude toward physical activity, level of physical fitness, and previous athletic experiences apparently have little or no relationship to adherence rates.[47] Factors that have not been studied, but would appear to be important, include the degree of supervision and guidance provided in the exercise program and the optimization of the exercise prescription, i.e., mode, frequency, intensity, and duration. This has become a major area of interest and will be the focus of future research.[48]

Physical activity must be a lifetime pursuit, and therefore, proper motivation is critical to continued participation in the exercise program. One of the most important aspects of motivation is to have participants properly educated about why regular exercise should be an important component of their lifestyle. Films, books, booklets, lectures, seminars, workshops, and group discussions are all excellent methods to help them understand the importance of regular physical activity.

A second factor of equal importance is having participants engage in activities they enjoy or helping them to learn to enjoy activities that would be of greatest benefit and interest to them. Unfortunately, too many people have been under the false impression that jogging and running are the only activities that have any long-term benefits and value. Many people simply do not enjoy jogging or running. To insist that all people must jog or run to gain the benefits associated with physical activity is creating a situation in which a high percentage of the participants will drop out of the exercise program after a relatively short period of time. Alternative activities that have a high aerobic or cardiorespiratory endurance component should be suggested and prescribed if they are more attractive to the participant. Brisk walking, hiking, swimming, bicycling, and vigorous sports such as handball, racquetball, and tennis would all be acceptable substitutes for jogging or running. Although individuals may not improve as rapidly with these alternative modes of exercise, the important factor is that they will improve, and there is no rigid time frame within which optimal levels of fitness must be attained.

It is argued by some, with good logic, that a sport should not be used to gain physical fitness but rather to maintain fitness. In other words, as an example, rather than using tennis as an activity to get into shape, use an activity like jogging for several months to increase the basic level of fitness to a respectable level and then switch to tennis to maintain that optimal level. It is felt that the individual will be better able to enjoy participation in the sport if this approach is followed.

Other factors that have been shown to facilitate adherence include exercising at a regular time of day as a fixed part of a daily routine. Professionals who have conducted fitness programs for many years generally agree that the attrition rate is much lower for those who exercise in the early morning before going to work. First, there is the obvious advantage that there are few interruptions early in the morning—no phone calls, unscheduled meetings, early dinner, and so on. Second, when the weather is warm, this is an ideal time to exercise, since heat stress is minimized. However, it must be recognized that not everyone is a "morning person," and an early morning program would be largely unacceptable to some participants, particularly in winter months when it is dark and cold. Whatever the agreed-upon time, consistency is the critical factor.

Exercising with a partner or as a member of a formal group, as opposed to doing it alone, has been found to reduce the drop-out rate. Companionship and knowing that others are waiting is a potent motivator to show up for group exercise sessions. A word of caution must be introduced at this point, however. Group participation frequently leads to competition, and this is usually not recommended. Almost everyone is intrigued by competition, but it is unwise for the novice who is just beginning his or her exercise program. The potential for orthopedic injury is there, as well as other medical risks.

Simple tests, self-administered on a regular basis, are also motivating, since progress can be seen from week to week. Monitoring the resting pulse rate before getting up in the morning, after a good night's sleep, should show a decrease of approximately 1 beat/min every two weeks for the first 15 to 20 weeks of training. After 10 weeks, it is not unusual to see a resting pulse rate of 70 beats/min drop to 65 beats/min. This change reflects improvement in cardiorespiratory efficiency, which is a positive reinforcement to the participant and acts to encourage the individual to continue the present program. Many simple tests are available, can be self-administered, and can help to maintain a high level of participant enthusiasm and motivation.

The ultimate in motivation has been noted by Glasser, who in his book *Positive Addiction*,[49] has reported that joggers or runners who exercise 30 to 60 minutes per day for 4 days a week, or more, frequently become addicted to this routine. If illness, injury, travel, or some other interruption disrupts their exercise routine, these individuals actually go through withdrawal-like symptoms. Of course, this would be a highly desirable outcome, but unfortunately too many individuals do not have the patience, persistence, or psychological strength to get to this point of "positive addiction." Also, some carry this addiction too far to the point of injury and disrupted lives, e.g., divorce, emotional disturbances.

Most recently, attempts have been made to apply the concepts of behavioral modification to increase adherence to exercise programs. Since this is a relatively new approach, it is too early to predict whether it will be any more successful than traditional approaches. Behavior modification uses a system of rewards to promote changes in behavior. Many programs have provided rewards to their participants in the form of 100-Mile Club, 500-Mile Club, 1,000-Mile Club, and 10,000-Mile Club T-shirts. These programs have been shown to be very effective. It is somewhat ironic to watch mature men and women who are wealthy enough to buy the entire company that makes the T-shirts fight to get one of these relatively inexpensive rewards. If past experience provides any indication of the future, behavior modification techniques, applied more broadly, should have a significant impact on increasing adherence rates.

SUMMARY

Participation in any exercise program requires that attention be given to a number of factors, each of which directly influences how successful the individual participant will be in his or her exercise program. Ignoring such things as correct shoes, clothing, and special equipment; warm-up, cool-down, and injury prevention; and environmental factors such as heat, cold, humidity, air pollution, and altitude can lead the participant into an unpleasant if not hazardous situation that may have serious and sometimes tragic consequences. A knowledge of the specificity of training and how the sexes and individuals of varying ages differ in their response to an exercise program is also extremely important. Total education of the participant is important to prevent possible medical complications or injury and to promote a healthy, positive attitude toward the program. Exercise must become the reward and not the punishment.

References

1. Adrian, M.J.: Proper clothing and equipment. In Haycock, C.E. (ed.): **Sports Medicine for the Athletic Female.** Oradell, NJ, Medical Economics Co., 1980.
2. Kaufman, W.C.: Cold-weather clothing for comfort or heat conservation. **Physician Sportsmed.** 10:71–75, 1982.
3. Wilmore, J.H., and Costill, D.L.: **Training for Sport and Activity: The Physiological Basis of the Conditioning Process,** 3rd Ed. Dubuque, IA, William C. Brown, 1988.
4. Gonzalez, R.R.: Biophysical and physiological integration of proper clothing for exercise. **Exerc. Sport Sci. Rev.** 15:261–295, 1987.
5. Bates, W.T.: Selecting a running shoe. **Physician Sportsmed.** 10:154–155, 1982.
6. Barnard, R.J., Gardner, G.W., Diaco, N.V., MacAlpin, R.N., and Kattus, A.A.: Cardiovascular responses to sudden strenuous exercise—heart rate, blood pressure, and ECG. **J. Appl. Physiol.** 34:833–837, 1973.
7. Powell, K.E., Kohl, H.W., Caspersen, C.J., and Blair, S.N.: An epidemiological perspective on the causes of running injuries. **Physician Sportsmed.** 14:100–114, 1986.
8. Blair, S.M., Kohl, H.W., and Goodyear, N.N.: Rates and risks for running and exercise injuries: Studies in three populations. **Res. Q. Exerc. Sports** 58:221–228, 1987.
9. Dimsdale, J.E., Hartley, L.H., Guiney, T., Ruskin, J.N., and Greenblatt, D.: Postexercise peril: plasma catecholamines and exercise. **JAMA** 251:630–632, 1984.
10. Zohman, L.R.: **Beyond Diet . . . Exercise Your Way to Fitness and Heart Health.** Englewood Cliffs, NJ, Mazola Products, Best Foods, 1974.
11. Sharkey, B.J.: **Fitness and Work Capacity.** U.S. Department of Agriculture, Forest Service Equipment Development Center, Missoula, Montana, 1976, No. 7661-2811.
12. Evans, W.J.: Exercise-induced skeletal muscle damage. **Physician Sportsmed.** 15:89–100, 1987.
13. Klafs, C.E., and Arnheim, D.D.: **Modern Principles of Athletic Training,** 4th Ed. St. Louis, C.V. Mosby, 1977.
14. Kuprian, W. (ed.): **Physical Therapy for Sports.** Philadelphia, W.B. Saunders Co., 1982.
15. Fahey, T.D.: **What to Do About Athetic Injuries.** New York, Butterick Publishing, 1979.

16. Fahey, T.D.: **Athletic Training: Principles and Practice.** Palo Alto, CA, Mayfield Publishing Co., 1986.
17. Murphy, R., and Ashe, W: Prevention of heat illness in football players. **JAMA** 194:650–654, 1965.
18. Sutton, J.R., and Bar-Or, O.: Thermal illness in fun running. **Am. Heart J.** 100:778–781, 1980.
19. Gisolfi, C.V., and Wenger, C.B.: Temperature regulation during exercise: Old concepts, new ideas. **Exerc. Sport Sci. Rev.** 12:339–372, 1984.
20. Vogel, J.A., Jones, B.H., and Rock, P.B.: Environmental considerations in exercise testing and training. In American College of Sports Medicine: **Resource Manual for Exercise Testing and Prescription.** Philadelphia, Lea & Febiger, 1988.
21. Buskirk, E.R., and Bass, D.E.: Climate and exercise. In Johnson, W.R., and Buskirk, E.R. (eds.): **Science and Medicine of Exercise and Sport,** 2nd Ed. New York, Harper and Row, 1974, pp. 190–205.
22. Harrison, M.H.: Heat and exercise effects on blood volume. **Sports Med.** 3:214–223, 1986.
23. Murray, R.: The effects of consuming carbohydrate-electrolyte beverages on gastric emptying and fluid absorption during and following exercise. **Sports Med.** 4:322–351, 1987.
24. Costill, D.L.: **Inside Running: Basics of Sports Physiology.** Indianapolis, Benchmark Press, 1986.
25. American College of Sports Medicine: Position stand on the prevention of thermal injuries during distance running. **Med. Sci. Sports Exerc.** 19:529–533, 1987.
26. Kavanagh, T.: Guidelines for cold weather exercise. **J. Cardiac Rehabil.** 3:70–73, 1983.
27. Adams, W.C.: Effects of ozone exposure at ambient air pollution episode levels on exercise performance. **Sports Med.** 4:395–424, 1987.
28. Gliner, J.A., Raven, P.B., Horvath, S.M., Drinkwater, B.L., and Sutton, J.C.: Man's physiologic response to long-term work during thermal and pollutant stress. **J. Appl. Physiol.** 39:628–632, 1975.
29. Horvath, S.M., Raven, P.B., Dahms, T.E., and Gray, D.J.: Maximal aerobic capacity at different levels of carboxyhemoglobin. **J. Appl. Physiol.** 38:300–303, 1975.
30. Raven, P.B., Drinkwater, B.L., Ruhling, R.O., Bolduan, N., Taguchi, S., Gliner, J., and Horvath, S.M.: Effect of carbon monoxide and peroxyacetyl nitrate on man's maximal aerobic capacity. **J. Appl. Physiol.** 36:288–293, 1974.
31. Raven, P.B.: Heat and air pollution: the cardiac patient. In Pollock, M.L., and Schmidt, D.H. (eds.): **Heart Disease and Rehabilitation,** 2nd Ed. New York, John Wiley and Sons, 1986, pp. 549–574.
32. Raven, P.B.: Questions and answers. **J. Cardiac Rehabil.** 2:411–414, 1982.
33. Åstrand, I.: Aerobic work capacity—its relation to age, sex, and other factors. **Circ. Res.** (Suppl. I) 20 and 21:211–217, 1967.
34. Skinner, J.S.: Age and performance. In **Limiting Factors of Physical Performance.** Stuttgart, George Thieme, 1973, pp. 271–282.
35. Wilmore, J.H., and Thomas, E.L.: Importance of differences between men and women for exercise testing and exercise prescription. In Skinner, J.S. (ed.): **Exercise Testing and Exercise Prescription for Special Cases.** Philadelphia, Lea & Febiger, 1987.
36. Wilmore, J.H.: Inferiority of female athletes: myth or reality. **J. Sports Med.** 3:1–6, 1975.
37. Bottiger, L.E.: Regular decline in physical working capacity with age. **Br. Med. J.** 3:270–271, 1973.
38. Pollock, M.L., Dawson, G.A., Miller, H.S., Jr., Ward, A., Cooper, D., Headley, W., Linnerud, A.C., and Nomeir, M.M.: Physiologic responses of men 49 to 65 years of age to endurance training. **J. Am. Geriatr. Soc.** 24:97–104. 1976.
39. Wilmore, J.H., Miller, H.L., and Pollock, M.L.: Body composition and physiolog-

ical characteristics of active endurance athletes in their eighth decade of life. **Med. Sci. Sports** 6:44–48, 1974.

40. Pollock, M.L., Foster, C., Knapp, D., Rod, J.L., and Schmidt, D.H.: Effect of age and training on aerobic capacity and body composition of master athletes. **J. Appl. Physiol.** 62:725–731, 1987.

41. Cureton, T.K.: A physical fitness case study of Joie Ray (improving physical fitness from age 60 to 70 years). **J. Assoc. Phys. Mental Rehabil.** 18:64–72, 1964.

42. Kasch, F.W., Wallace, J.P., VanCamp, S.P., and Verity, L.: A longitudinal study of cardiovascular stability in active men aged 45 to 65 years. **Physician Sportsmed.** 16:117–126, 1988.

43. Wilmore, J.H.: Testing the elite Masters athlete. In Sutton, J.R., and Brock, R.M. (eds.) **Sports Medicine for the Mature Athlete.** Indianapolis, Benchmark Press, 1986.

44. Winson, J.: **Fitness on the Road.** Bolinas, CA, Shelter Publications, 1986.

45. Dishman, R.K.: Compliance/adherence in health-related exercise. **Health Psychology** 1:237–267, 1982.

46. Dishman, R.K.: Exercise compliance: a new view for public health. **Physician Sportsmed.** 14:127–145, 1986.

47. Morgan, W.P.: Involvement in vigorous physical activity with special reference to adherence. **Proceedings, National College of Physical Education for Men.** Orlando, FL, January 1977.

48. Dishman, R.K. (ed.): **Exercise Adherence: Its Impact on Public Health.** Champaign, IL, Human Kinetics, 1988.

49. Glasser, W.: **Positive Addiction.** New York, Harper and Row, 1976.

APPENDIX A

Medical Screening and Exercise

**MEDICAL
HISTORY
QUESTIONNAIRE**

Institute for Aerobics Research
11811 Preston Road
Dallas, Texas 75230

This is your medical history form for your visit to The Institute for Aerobics Research. All information will be kept confidential. The doctor or exercise physiologist you see at the Institute will use this information in his evaluation of your health. You will want to make it as accurate and complete as possible, yet free of meaningless details. Please fill out this form carefully and thoroughly. Then check it over to be sure you haven't left out anything.

Note: Please PRINT all responses so that your data will be compatible with computer storage and analysis.

Name _____ Exam Date _____ ,19 _____

Figure A–1. Medical history questionnaire. (Published with permission of the Institute for Aerobics Research, Dallas, TX, and John Wiley and Sons, New York, NY.)

Institute for Aerobics Research
11811 Preston Road
Dallas, Texas 75230

Patient Medical History Form

All information is private and confidential. Please Print.

DO NOT WRITE IN THIS SPACE; FOR OFFICE USE ONLY.
PATIENT NUMBER VISIT CARD FORM CLINIC
0 1 M 0 2 B

I. GENERAL INFORMATION

- ☐ Mr.
- ☐ Ms.
- ☐ Miss
- ☐ Mrs.
- ☐ Dr.

NAME

FIRST   MIDDLE   LAST

ADDRESS

NUMBER AND STREET

0.2   CITY   STATE ZIP CODE

COUNTRY (IF OUTSIDE U.S.A.)

HOME PHONE   SOCIAL SECURITY NUMBER   DATE OF BIRTH   TODAY'S DATE

( )   AREA CODE   MONTH DAY YEAR   MONTH DAY YEAR

FAMILY PHYSICIAN

Dr.   FIRST NAME, IF KNOWN   INITIAL LAST NAME

DOCTOR'S ADDRESS (if known)

NUMBER AND STREET   PHONE

04   CITY   STATE ZIP CODE   ( ) AREA CODE

May we send a copy of your consult to your physician?   Yes ☐   No ☐

MARITAL STATUS

Single ☐   Married ☐   Divorced ☐   Widowed ☐   Separated ☐

SEX

Male ☐   Female ☐   PRESENT AGE

EDUCATION (Check highest level attained)

- ☐ Grade School
- ☐ Junior High School
- ☐ High School
- ☐ Two-year College (or 4-year college; degree not completed)
- ☐ College Graduate
- ☐ Postgraduate School

OCCUPATION

FOR OFFICE USE ONLY
OCCUP CODE ☐

EMPLOYER (use abbreviations if necessary)

05

EMPLOYER'S ADDRESS

NUMBER AND STREET   BUSINESS PHONE

06   CITY   STATE ZIP CODE   ( ) AREA CODE

What is/are your purpose(s) in coming to the Institute?

- ☐ To participate in a research study.
- ☐ To determine my current level of physical fitness and to receive recommendations for an exercise program.
- ☐ Other (please explain):

07

PLEASE PRINT

Medical History

PRESENT HISTORY   1 0 M 0 2 B   2

Check the box in front of those questions to which your answer is yes. Leave others blank.

10

Has a doctor ever said that your blood pressure was too high or too low?
Do you ever have pain in your heart or chest?
Are you often bothered by a thumping of the heart?
Does your heart often race like mad?
Do you ever notice extra heart beats or skipped beats?
Are your ankles often badly swollen?
Do cold hands or feet trouble you even in hot weather?
Has a doctor ever said that you had or have heart trouble,
an abnormal electrocardiogram (ECG or EKG), heart attack, or coronary?
Do you suffer from frequent cramps in your legs?
Do you often have difficulty breathing?
Do you get out of breath long before anyone else?
Do you sometimes get out of breath when sitting still or sleeping?
Has a doctor ever told you your cholesterol level was high?

Comments: **11**

                   12

                   13

Do you now have or have you recently had:

14

A chronic, recurrent or morning cough?
Any episode of coughing up blood?
Increased anxiety or depression?
Problems with recurrent fatigue, trouble sleeping or increased
irritability?
Migraine or recurrent headaches?
Swollen or painful knees or ankles?
Swollen, stiff or painful joints?
Pain in your legs after walking short distances?
Back pain?
Kidney problems such as passing stones, burning, increased frequency,
decreased force of stream of difficulty in starting or stopping your stream?
Prostate trouble (men only)?
Any stomach or intestinal problems such as recurrent heartburn,
ulcers, constipation or diarrhea?
Any significant vision or hearing problem?
Any recent change in a wart or mole?
Glaucoma or increased pressure in the eyes?
Exposure to loud noises for long periods?

Comments: **15**

WOMEN ONLY answer the following:

16

Do you have any menstrual period problems?
Do you have problems with recurrent itching or discharge?
Did you have any significant childbirth problems?
Do you have any breast discharges or lumps?
Do you sometimes lose urine when you cough, sneeze or laugh?

Please give number of: Pregnancies |__|__| Living children |__|__| First day of last |__|__|__|__|__|__|
                                                                          menstrual period MONTH DAY YEAR
Date of last pelvic exam and/or Paps smear: month |__|__| year 19 |__|__| Results: Normal ☐ Abnormal ☐

Comments: **17**

PLEASE PRINT

Medical History

DO NOT WRITE IN THIS SPACE; FOR OFFICE USE ONLY.

PATIENT NUMBER	VISIT	CARD	FORM	CLINIC	3
	2 5	M	0	2 8	

MEN and WOMEN answer the following:

List any prescribed medications you are now taking:

[25]

List any self-prescribed medications or dietary supplements you are now taking:

[26]

Date of last complete physical examination: ____ 19 ____ never ☐ can't remember ☐ Normal ☐ Abnormal ☐
                 month year

Date of last chest x-ray: [27] ____ 19 ____ never ☐ can't remember ☐ Normal ☐ Abnormal ☐
                 month year

Date of last electrocardiogram: ____ 19 ____ never ☐ can't remember ☐ Normal ☐ Abnormal ☐
                 month year

Date of last dental check-up: ____ 19 ____ never ☐ can't remember ☐ Normal ☐ Abnormal ☐
                 month year

List any other medical or diagnostic test you have had in the past two years:

[28]

[29]

List hospitalizations including dates of and reasons for hospitalization:

[30]

[31]

[32]

List any drug allergies:

[33]

PAST HISTORY

Have you ever had:

[34]
- ☐ Heart Attack, how many years ago? _____
- ☐ Rheumatic Fever
- ☐ Heart murmur
- ☐ Diseases of the arteries
- ☐ Varicos veins
- ☐ Arthritis of legs or arms
- ☐ Diabetes or abnormal blood sugar test
- ☐ Phlebitis
- ☐ Dizziness or fainting spells
- ☐ Epilepsy or fits
- ☐ Strokes
- ☐ Diphtheria
- ☐ Scarlet fever
- ☐ Infectious mononucleosis
- ☐ Anemia

- ☐ Thyroid problems
- ☐ Pneumonia
- ☐ Bronchitis
- ☐ Asthma
- ☐ Abnormal chest x-ray
- ☐ Other lung diseases
- ☐ Injuries to back, arms, legs or joints
- ☐ Broken bones
- ☐ Jaundice or gallbladder problems
- ☐ Polio
- ☐ Urinary tract infections, kidney stones, or prostate problems.
- ☐ Any nervous or emotional problems

Comments: [35]

PLEASE PRINT

Medical History

DO NOT WRITE IN THIS SPACE; FOR OFFICE USE ONLY.

PATIENT NUMBER	VISIT	CARD	FORM	CLINIC
		4 0	M 0 2	B

FAMILY MEDICAL HISTORY

40 FATHER:
Alive ☐ Current age ☐☐☐ General health now: excellent ☐₁ good ☐₂ fair ☐₃ poor ☐₄ don't know ☐₅
Deceased ☐ Age at death ☐☐☐ Cause of death or reason for poor health now: ☐☐☐☐☐☐☐☐☐☐☐☐☐☐☐☐☐

MOTHER:
Alive ☐ Current age ☐☐☐ General health now: ₆₁ excellent ☐₁ good ☐₂ fair ☐₃ poor ☐₄ don't know ☐₅
Deceased ☐ Age at death ☐☐☐ Cause of death or reason for poor health now: ☐☐☐☐☐☐☐☐☐☐☐☐☐☐

41 SIBLINGS: No. of brothers ☐☐ No. of sisters ☐☐ Age range ☐☐☐ – ☐☐☐ Health Problems: ☐☐☐☐☐☐☐☐☐☐☐☐☐☐☐

FAMILIAL DISEASES: Have any of your blood relatives had any of the following?
Include grandparents, aunts, and uncles, but exclude cousins, relatives by marriage, and half relatives.

42
☐ Heart attacks under age 50
☐ Strokes under age 50
☐ High blood pressure
☐ Elevated cholesterol
☐ Diabetes
☐ Asthma or hay fever

☐ Congenital heart disease
☐ Heart operations
☐ Glaucoma
☐ Obesity (20 or more lbs. overweight)
☐ Leukemia or cancer under age 60

Comments: ☐☐☐☐☐☐☐☐☐☐☐☐☐☐☐☐☐☐☐☐☐☐☐☐☐☐☐☐

43
OTHER HEART DISEASES RISK FACTORS

SMOKING

44
Have you ever smoked cigarettes, cigars or a pipe? yes ☐₁ no ☐₂
If no, skip to Diet section.
Do you smoke presently? yes ☐₁ no ☐₂
If you did or do smoke cigarettes, how many per day? ☐☐ Age you started: ☐☐
If you did or do smoke cigars, how many per day? ☐☐ Age you started: ☐☐
If you did or do smoke a pipe, how many pipefuls per day? ☐☐ Age you started: ☐☐
If you have quit smoking, when was it? ☐☐ MONTH 19 ☐☐ YEAR

DIET

45
What do you consider a good weight for yourself? ☐☐☐ pounds

What is the most you have ever weighed? (including when pregnant) ☐☐☐ lbs. At what age? ☐☐ yrs.

Weight: Now ☐☐☐ lbs. One year ago ☐☐☐ lbs. At age 21 ☐☐☐ lbs.

Number of meals you usually eat per day. ☐☐

Average number of eggs you usually eat per week: ☐☐ (Do not count those in cooking and baking, cakes, casseroles, etc.)

Number of times per week you usually eat:

Beef ☐☐ Fish ☐☐ Desserts ☐☐
Pork ☐☐ Fowl ☐☐ French fried foods ☐☐

Number of servings (cups, glasses or containers) per week you usually consume of:

Homogenized (whole) milk ☐☐ Buttermilk ☐☐
Skim (non-fat) milk ☐☐ Tea (iced or hot) ☐☐
Two percent (2% fat) milk ☐☐ Coffee ☐☐

Do you ever drink alcoholic beverages? yes ☐ no ☐

If yes, what is your approximate intake of these beverages?

	None	Occasional	Often	If often, how many drinks per week?
Beer	☐	☐	☐	☐☐
Wine	☐	☐	☐	☐☐
Hard Liquor	☐	☐	☐	☐☐

At any time in the past were you a heavy drinker (consumption of 6 oz. of hard liquor per day or more)? yes ☐₁ no ☐₂

46 Comments: ☐☐☐

PLEASE PRINT

Medical History

DO NOT WRITE IN THIS SPACE; FOR OFFICE USE ONLY.

PATIENT NUMBER   VISIT   CARD   FORM   CLINIC

| | 5 | 0 | M | 0 | 2 | B |

EXERCISE

50

Are you currently involved in a regular exercise program?   yes ☐   no ☐

Do you regularly walk or run one or more miles continuously?   yes ☐   no ☐   don't know ☐

If yes, average no. of miles you cover per workout or day: ☐☐.☐ miles

What is your average time per mile? ☐☐:☐☐ minutes: seconds   don't know ☐

Do you practice weight lifting or home calisthenics?   yes ☐   no ☐

Are you now involved in the Aerobics program?   yes ☐   no ☐

If yes, your average Aerobics points per week: ☐☐☐

Have you taken in the past 6 months: ☐ 12 minute test   ☐ 1.5 mile   ☐ neither

If yes, your miles in 12 minutes: ☐.☐☐   or your time for 1.5 miles: ☐☐:☐☐ minutes : seconds

Do you frequently participate in competitive sports?   yes ☐   no ☐

If yes, which one or ones?

☐ Golf   ☐ Bowling   ☐ Tennis   ☐ Handball   ☐ Soccer

☐ Basketball   ☐ Volleyball   ☐ Football   ☐ Baseball   ☐ Track

☐ Other _____

Average number of times per month ☐☐

51

In which of the following high school or college athletics did you participate?

☐ None   ☐ Football   ☐ Basketball   ☐ Baseball   ☐ Soccer

☐ Track   ☐ Swimming   ☐ Tennis   ☐ Wrestling   ☐ Golf

☐ Other _____

In which of the following high school or college athletics did you earn a varsity letter?

☐ None   ☐ Football   ☐ Basketball   ☐ Baseball   ☐ Soccer

☐ Track   ☐ Swimming   ☐ Tennis   ☐ Wrestling   ☐ Golf

☐ Other _____

52

What activity or activities would you prefer in a regular exercise program for yourself?

☐ Walking and/or running   ☐ Bicycling (outdoors)   ☐ Swimming

☐ Stationary running   ☐ Stationary cycling   ☐ Tennis

☐ Jumping rope   ☐ Handball, basketball or squash

☐ Other _____

53 Comments: _____

Explain any other significant medical problems that you consider important for us to know:

5 5 _____

5 6 _____

5 7 _____

5 8 _____

5 9 _____

6 0 _____

6 1 _____

PLEASE PRINT

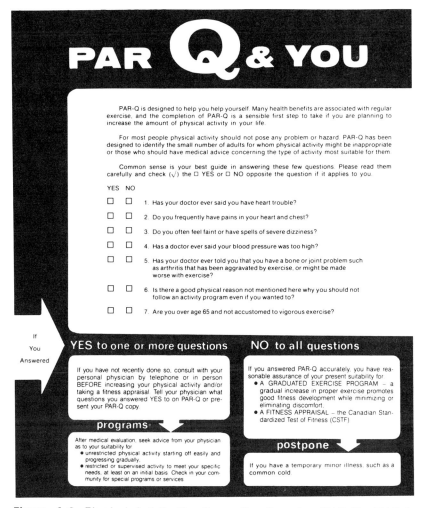

Figure A–2. Physical Activity Readiness Questionnaire (PAR-Q). (PAR-Q Validation Report. British Columbia Ministry of Health, 1978. Produced by the British Columbia Ministry of Health and the Department of National Health & Welfare. From **Canadian Standardized Test of Fitness (CSTF) Operations Manual,** 3rd Ed. With the permission of Fitness Canada, Fitness and Amateur Sport Canada, Ottawa, 1986.

MOUNT SINAI MEDICAL CENTER
Milwaukee, Wisconsin
NONINVASIVE LABORATORY
CARDIAC WORK EVALUATION LAB

I understand that this exercise test is being done to: **1.** determine the functional capacity of my heart and circulation and **2.** detect the possible presence of heart disease. *I hereby consent to voluntarily engage in an exercise test to determine the state of my heart and circulation.*

The tests which I will undergo will be performed on a treadmill, bicycle, or other methods designed to gradually increase the demands on the heart. This increase in effort will continue until symptoms such as chest discomfort or pain, excessive shortness of breath or fatigue would indicate that I should stop.

During the performance of the test, a physician and trained observer will keep under surveillance my pulse, electrocardiogram, and clinical appearance. Other tests may also be measured during or after the exercise.

There exists the possibility of certain changes occuring during the exercise tests. They include abnormal blood pressure, rapid or very slow heart beat, and very rare instances of heart attack. Every effort will be made to minimize them by the constant surveillance during testing. Emergency equipment and trained personnel are available to deal with unusual situations which may arise.

The information which is obtained will be treated as privileged and confidential and will not be released or revealed to any person other than my physician without my expressed written consent. The information obtained, however, may be used for a statistical or scientific purpose with my right of privacy retained.

I have read the foregoing, and I understand it; any questions which may have occurred to me have been answered to my satisfaction.

Signed: _____
PATIENT

_____
WITNESS

_____
PHYSICIAN SUPERVISING THE TEST

_____
DATE

Figure A–3. An example of an informed consent for graded exercise testing used mainly for diagnostic purposes. (Courtesy of Cardiac Work Evaluation Lab, Mount Sinai Medical Center, Milwaukee, WI.)

Human Performance Laboratory
Mount Sinai Medical Center
950 N. 12th Street
Milwaukee, Wisconsin 53233

CONSENT TO GRADED EXERCISE TESTING

PATIENT NAME _____

Date _____ Time _____

I authorize Drs. _____ and such assistants or designees as may be selected by them to perform a symptom-limited graded exercise test to determine maximal oxygen uptake and cardiovascular function. During the test heart rate and electrocardiogram will be intermittently monitored. This test will facilitate evaluation of cardiopulmonary function and assist the physician or exercise physiologist in prescribing or evaluating exercise programs. It is my understanding that I will be questioned and examined by a physician prior to taking the test and will be given a resting electrocardiogram to exclude contraindications to such testing.

Exercise testing will be performed on a treadmill, cycle ergometer or other device that allows workload to gradually increase until fatigue, breathlessness or when other signs or symptoms dictate cessation of the test. Blood pressure and electrocardiogram will be monitored by a physician, nurse, or exercise physiologist. In the latter cases, a physician will be readily available in case of emergency.

There exists the possibility that certain abnormal changes may occur during the progress of the test. These changes could include abnormal heart beats, abnormal blood pressure response, and in rare instances heart attack. Professional care in selection and supervision of individuals provides appropriate precaution against such problems.

The benefits of such testing are the scientific assessment of working capacity and the clinical appraisal of health hazards which will facilitate prescription of an exercise/rehabilitative program.

I have read the foregoing information and understand it. Questions concerning this procedure have been answered to my satisfaction. I have also been informed that the information derived from this test is confidential and will not be disclosed to anyone other than my physician or others that are involved in my care or exercise prescription without my permission. However, I am in agreement that information from this test not identifiable to me can be used for research purposes.

Patient/Participant Signature _____

Witness Signature _____

Test Supervisor _____

Figure A–4. An example of an informed consent for graded exercise testing used for the purpose of entering an exercise program. (Courtesy of Human Performance Laboratory, Mount Sinai Medical Center, Milwaukee, WI.)

24-HOUR HISTORY

NAME: _____ DATE: _____

TIME: _____

HOW MUCH SLEEP DID YOU GET LAST NIGHT? (Please circle one)
   1 2 3 4 5 6 7 8 9 10 (hours)

HOW MUCH SLEEP DO YOU NORMALLY GET? (Please circle one)
   1 2 3 4 5 6 7 8 9 10 (hours)

HOW LONG HAS IT BEEN SINCE YOUR LAST MEAL OR SNACK? (Please circle one)
   1 2 3 4 5 6 7 8 9 10 11 12 13 14 (hours)

LIST THE ITEMS EATEN BELOW:

_____

WHEN DID YOU LAST:

    Have a cup of coffee or tea _____

    Smoke a cigarette, cigar, or pipe _____

    Take drugs (including aspirin) _____

    Drink alcohol _____

    Give blood _____

    Have an illness _____

    Suffer from respiratory problems _____

WHAT SORT OF PHYSICAL EXERCISE DID YOU PERFORM YESTERDAY?

WHAT SORT OF PHYSICAL EXERCISE DID YOU PERFORM TODAY?

DESCRIBE YOUR GENERAL FEELINGS BY CHECKING ONE OF THE FOLLOWING:

    _____ Excellent _____ Bad

    _____ Very, Very Good _____ Very Bad

    _____ Very Good _____ Very, Very Bad

    _____ Neither Bad nor Good _____ Terrible

Figure A–5. This is an example of a 24-hour history form used to document and standardize testing conditions.

UNIVERSITY HOSPITAL
University of California
Medical Center, San Diego

REPORT OF
TREADMILL EXERCISE TEST
(Page One)

Rev. Code **750**

SEND REPORT TO		Source	Date		
				Patient Identification	
				Procedure No. 013 ☐	

TMT NO.	AGE	SEX	WT (lbs)	HT (in)	CLINICAL REASONS FOR TEST

DIAGNOSIS OF ATYPICAL SENSATION OR PAIN POSSIBLY DUE TO ASCVD (Explain) ☐

☐ INPATIENT   DATE (Mo., Day, Yr.)   24 HR. TIME
☐ OUTPATIENT

PREVIOUS TEST   >3 HRS. SINCE LAST MEAL   EVALUATION OF ANGINA
☐ No ☐ Yes, when: ☐ Yes   ☐ No   ☐ Typical   ☐ Variant   ☐ Unstable

MEDICATIONS   DYSRHYTHMIA EVALUATION
                        ☐ Calcium Antagonist   ☐
☐ Digitalis   ☐ Nitrates   ☐ PVCs   ☐ SVT   ☐ HB   ☐ Sick Sinus   ☐ Other
☐ Beta-Blocker   ☐ Quinidine/Pronestyl   OTHER HEART DISEASE   ☐ Valvular   ☐ Heart Muscle
☐ Anti-HBP   ☐ Other   ☐ Mitral Prolapse   ☐ Congenital   ☐ Other

ACTIVITY STATUS   EVALUATION   TIME SINCE LAST INFARCT
☐ Recent Bed Rest   ☐ Sedentary   ☐ Active   ☐ Athletic   POST AMI ☐   Weeks   Months   Years

PROBABILITY OF ASCVD BY HISTORY PRIOR TO TEST   SCREENING ASYMPTOMATIC   FUNCTIONAL CAPACITY
☐ Unlikely   ☐ Possible   ☐ Probable   ☐ Very Probable   INDIVIDUAL ☐   EVALUATION ☐

PHYSICAL   S3   S4   MURMUR   CORONARY BYPASS SURGERY   DATE OF SURGERY & TYPE
EXAM   ☐ Pre   ☐ Post
(PRE)   ☐ Yes ☐ No   ☐ Yes ☐ No   ☐ Yes ☐ No   OTHER ☐

STAGE	MPH/GRADE	METS	MIN/SEC IN STAGE	HR	BP (AT END OF STAGE)	P.E.	DESCRIBE: CHEST PAIN/DYSRHYTHMIA/ ST SLOPE/AMOUNT J-JCT UP OR DOWN/LEAD(S)
SUPINE							
HV FOR 30 SEC	3.5cc O_2/kg·min = 1 MET						
STAND	If 2.0 mph, 2/3 the O_2 cost						
1A	2.0/0%	2					
1B	3.3/0%	4					
2	3.3/5%	6					
3	3.3/10%	8					
4	3.3/15%	10					
5	3.3/20%	13					REASON FOR STOPPING
6	3.3/25%	15					☐ Angina ☐ Other chest pain
							☐ Claudication ☐ Other leg pain
							☐ ECG changes ☐ Dysrhythmia
							☐ Maximal effort ☐ Other
IMMED	MAX SBP (_____) x						
2 MIN	MAX HR (_____) =						
5 MIN	___ ___ . ___ x 10³						
___ MIN	Estimated Maximal O_2 Cost = _____ METS						

B248(3-83)6   WHITE - Medical Record   CANARY - Referring MD   PINK - Cardiology File   GOLD - Research File

Figure A–6. Data collection form and summary sheet for graded exercise testing. (Courtesy of Victor F. Froelicher, M.D., Chief Cardiology Section, Veterans Administration Medical Center, Long Beach, CA.)

Illustration continued on following page

UNIVERSITY HOSPITAL
University of California
Medical Center, San Diego

Rev. Code **750**

REPORT OF
TREADMILL EXERCISE TEST
(Page Two)

Source   Date

Patient Identification

Procedure No. 013 ☐

PHYSICAL EXAM (POST)	S₃ ☐ Yes ☐ No	S₄ ☐ Yes ☐ No	SIGNS/SYMPTOMS CHF	MURMUR ☐ Yes ☐ No	TYPE		

ECG RESPONSE	DYSRHYTHMIA	NO EXPLAIN	OCC PVC	FREQ PVC	VT	SVT	AF
	ST SEGMENTS	NL EXPLAIN	BORDERLINE	ABNL	ELEVATE		NORMALIZE
	CONDUCTION	NL EXPLAIN	LBBB	RBBB	BLOCK		AXIS SHIFT

PATIENT RESPONSE	MAX HR ☐ NL ☐ HI ☐ LO		MAX SYSTOLIC BP ☐ NL ☐ HI ☐ LO ☐ Drop		FUNCTIONAL CAPACITY ☐ NL ☐ HI ☐ LO	
	ANGINA ☐ Yes ☐ No	ATYPICAL CHEST PAIN ☐ Yes ☐ No	CHF ☐ Yes ☐ No	OTHER COMPLICATIONS ☐ Yes ☐ No	MAXIMAL EFFORT ☐ Yes ☐ No	

RESTING ECG ☐ Normal ☐ Abnormal	DESCRIBE

INTERPRETATION

Figure A–6. *Continued*

Figure A–7. Recording form for anthropometric measures. (Adapted with permission from the Institute for Aerobics Research, Dallas, TX.)

Table A–1. Physical Fitness and Health Standards for Men 20 to 29 Years of Age

Percentile Rankings	Resting (Sitting) Heart Rate (beats/min)	Blood Pressure Systolic (mmHg)	Blood Pressure Diastolic (mmHg)	Maximum Oxygen Uptake ($ml \cdot kg^{-1} \cdot min^{-1}$)	Maximum Heart Rate (beats/min)	Lipids CHOL (mg/dl)	HDL (mg/dl)	CHOL/HDL	TRIG (mg/dl)	Glucose (mg/dl)	Body Fat (%)
100	43	98	60	58.7	209	130	84	2.1	39	80	1.6
95	47	100	62	54.4	203	139	60	2.9	45	83	6.7
90	48	107	68	51.1	202	153	56	3.1	53	86	7.9
85	50	108	69	49.6	200	155	52	3.1	59	87	10.0
80	52	110	70	48.2	198	160	51	3.4	61	88	11.0
75	53	112	70	46.8	197	165	50	3.4	66	90	12.2
70	55	114	72	45.7	196	173	47	3.6	71	91	13.4
65	56	117	74	45.3	195	174	46	3.8	76	92	14.4
60	58	118	75	44.1	193	180	45	3.9	79	93	15.8
55	60	118	76	43.9	192	185	44	4.1	84	94	16.6
50	61	119	78	42.4	190	188	42	4.3	89	95	17.3
45	62	120	78	41.3	189	193	41	4.3	96	96	17.6
40	64	122	78	41.0	188	195	40	4.5	102	98	18.5
35	66	125	79	39.5	187	202	39	4.7	113	99	19.5
30	68	126	80	38.5	184	205	37	5.0	122	100	21.2
25	69	128	82	38.1	183	215	36	5.2	140	102	21.6
20	70	130	85	36.7	180	218	35	5.6	155	104	23.5
15	74	134	88	35.9	177	230	34	5.8	171	105	25.4
10	76	136	90	33.8	176	250	30	7.0	224	111	28.2
5	88	150	96	25.1	141	300	25	8.9	230	115	34.3
Population size	1886	1898	1898	1890	1890	1601	1037	1036	1597	1594	674
Average	61.5	120.3	77.5	43.1	190.6	189.0	44.9	4.4	116.1	96.1	17.3
Standard deviation	11.6	12.0	9.2	7.2	11.0	36.8	14.6	1.6	188.3	10.9	8.4

(Data from the Cooper Clinic Coronary Risk Factor Profile Charts, which are data collected on patients being evaluated at the Cooper Clinic and standards being established at the Institute of Aerobics Research, Dallas, Texas, 1989. Reprinted with permission. Courtesy of K. H. Cooper, M.D., S. Blair, P.Ed., and B. Barlow.)

CHOL = cholesterol; TRIG = triglycerides; CHOL/HDL = ratio of total cholesterol, divided by high-density lipoproteins.

Table A–2. Physical Fitness and Health Standards for Men 30 to 39 Years of Age

	Resting (Sitting)	Blood Pressure		Maximum		Lipids					Body Fat (%)
Percentile Rankings	Heart Rate (beats/min)	Systolic (mmHg)	Diastolic (mmHg)	Oxygen Uptake (ml·kg^{-1}·min^{-1})	Heart Rate (beats/min)	CHOL (mg/dl)	HDL (mg/dl)	CHOL/HDL	TRIG (mg/dl)	Glucose (mg/dl)	Body Fat (%)
100	44	90	64	54.0	210	143	69	2.6	46	80	6.8
95	46	100	66	52.8	200	150	63	3.1	53	85	9.8
90	48	105	68	49.6	197	165	56	3.2	56	87	10.9
85	50	108	69	48.2	195	173	53	3.4	62	89	13.0
80	52	109	70	47.0	194	175	51	3.6	70	90	13.9
75	54	110	72	46.8	192	183	50	3.9	76	91	15.2
70	56	112	75	45.3	190	187	47	4.0	82	93	16.2
65	57	115	76	43.9	189	190	46	4.2	85	94	16.9
60	58	117	77	42.4	188	195	44	4.4	90	95	17.2
55	59	118	78	41.4	187	200	43	4.5	100	96	18.6
50	60	118	78	41.0	186	202	42	4.7	104	98	19.2
45	62	119	79	40.3	184	210	41	4.9	111	99	20.2
40	64	120	80	38.5	183	215	39	5.2	118	100	20.8
35	65	122	81	38.1	180	220	38	5.3	132	101	21.3
30	66	124	83	37.4	179	223	36	5.7	141	103	22.1
25	68	128	84	36.7	178	230	35	5.9	168	105	22.9
20	70	129	86	35.2	176	235	34	6.3	182	106	24.4
15	74	130	88	33.8	174	244	32	6.6	197	109	25.4
10	75	138	94	32.3	170	260	30	7.2	251	110	28.3
5	80	140	110	29.4	165	290	24	10.8	520	121	33.5
Population size	9073	9126	9125	9122	9122	7751	4944	4943	7729	7707	3291
Average	61.4	119.4	79.1	41.6	185.5	206.0	44.3	4.9	132.0	98.5	19.0
Standard deviation	11.0	12.3	9.2	7.0	11.4	44.9	11.7	2.2	146.7	14.8	7.0

(Data from the Cooper Clinic Coronary Risk Factor Profile Charts, which are data collected on patients being evaluated at the Cooper Clinic and standards being established at the Institute of Aerobics Research, Dallas, Texas, 1989. Reprinted with permission. Courtesy of K. H. Cooper, M.D., S. Blair, P.Ed., and B. Barlow.)

CHOL = cholesterol; TRIG = triglycerides; CHOL/HDL = ratio of total cholesterol, divided by high-density lipoproteins.

Table A-3. Physical Fitness and Health Standards for Men 40 to 49 Years of Age

Percentile Rankings	Resting (Sitting)			Maximum		Lipids					Body Fat (%)
	Heart Rate (beats/min)	Systolic (mmHg)	Diastolic (mmHg)	Oxygen Uptake (ml·kg⁻¹·min⁻¹)	Heart Rate (beats/min)	CHOL (mg/dl)	HDL (mg/dl)	CHOL/HDL	TRIG (mg/dl)	Glucose (mg/dl)	
100	37	96	60	55.4	198	125	95	2.6	34	80	9.0
95	46	100	68	51.1	195	160	64	3.3	54	85	11.9
90	50	107	69	49.6	191	175	59	3.4	64	88	13.6
85	52	108	70	46.8	189	180	53	3.7	69	90	14.8
80	53	110	72	45.3	188	187	52	3.9	78	92	15.6
75	54	112	75	43.9	186	192	50	4.1	88	94	17.5
70	56	114	76	42.9	185	195	47	4.4	92	95	17.9
65	57	115	76	42.4	182	200	46	4.4	99	96	18.3
60	58	116	78	41.0	181	205	44	4.7	107	97	19.5
55	60	118	78	39.5	180	210	43	4.8	112	99	19.8
50	61	119	79	38.7	179	215	42	5.1	123	100	20.7
45	62	120	80	38.1	178	220	40	5.3	131	101	21.9
40	64	122	83	36.7	175	227	39	5.5	140	102	22.7
35	65	124	84	35.9	174	230	37	6.1	151	104	23.5
30	67	126	85	35.2	172	235	36	6.1	172	105	24.2
25	69	128	88	33.8	170	245	34	6.2	192	108	25.1
20	72	132	89	33.0	169	253	33	6.9	200	110	26.0
15	75	135	90	31.6	164	265	30	7.0	241	113	27.9
10	80	140	98	29.4	160	285	29	7.7	286	115	30.5
5	98	150	110	22.2	150	292	27	8.6	695	125	39.1
Population size	9583	9611	9611	9607	9607	8055	4906	4906	8026	8005	3568
Average	62.0	120.8	81.0	39.9	178.6	218.2	43.9	5.3	149.6	101.4	20.9
Standard deviation	11.1	13.3	9.7	7.2	13.4	43.3	11.5	2.0	128.9	16.2	7.2

(Data from the Cooper Clinic Coronary Risk Factor Profile Charts, which are data collected on patients being evaluated at the Cooper Clinic and standards being established at the Institute of Aerobics Research, Dallas, Texas, 1989. Reprinted with permission. Courtesy of K. H. Cooper, M.D., S. Blair, P.Ed., and B. Barlow.)

CHOL = cholesterol; TRIG = triglycerides; CHOL/HDL = ratio of total cholesterol, divided by high-density lipoproteins.

Table A–4. Physical Fitness and Health Standards for Men 50 to 59 Years of Age

Percentile Rankings	Resting (Sitting)			Maximum		Lipids					Body Fat (%)
	Heart Rate (beats/min)	Blood Pressure		Oxygen Uptake (ml·kg⁻¹·min⁻¹)	Heart Rate (beats/min)	CHOL (mg/dl)	HDL (mg/dl)	CHOL/HDL	TRIG (mg/dl)	Glucose (mg/dl)	
		Systolic (mmHg)	Diastolic (mmHg)								
100	45	102	60	54.0	200	162	66	2.7	46	80	4.2
95	47	104	65	46.8	189	170	64	3.4	62	85	13.3
90	50	108	70	45.3	185	180	56	3.7	73	90	14.9
85	53	110	74	42.4	181	188	54	3.8	75	92	16.6
80	54	112	75	41.0	186	195	51	4.2	82	94	17.6
75	55	116	76	39.5	179	200	48	4.4	92	95	19.3
70	56	118	78	38.1	175	205	47	4.5	95	97	20.2
65	58	119	78	37.3	174	210	45	4.8	102	98	20.5
60	59	120	79	36.7	172	215	44	4.9	109	99	21.7
55	60	122	80	35.9	171	220	43	5.2	116	100	22.4
50	62	124	82	35.2	169	225	41	5.3	127	102	22.7
45	63	125	83	33.8	168	230	39	5.5	138	104	23.6
40	64	128	85	33.0	167	236	38	5.8	146	105	24.2
35	66	130	86	32.3	164	242	37	6.0	156	106	24.7
30	68	132	88	31.6	162	245	36	6.3	169	108	26.2
25	70	134	89	30.9	158	255	34	6.7	186	110	26.8
20	72	138	90	29.4	155	262	32	6.9	204	113	27.5
15	76	142	92	28.2	152	265	30	7.3	253	115	29.8
10	79	144	98	25.1	143	280	27	8.1	320	120	30.8
5	84	154	100	22.4	130	297	26	11.4	669	160	34.1
Population size	4978	4999	4999	4975	4975	4510	2730	2729	4485	4488	1988
Average	62.5	125.4	83.2	35.8	168.1	226.6	43.8	5.6	158.1	107.2	22.6
Standard deviation	11.2	15.7	9.9	7.1	16.6	55.8	13.8	5.4	142.7	137.7	6.5

(Data from the Cooper Clinic Coronary Risk Factor Profile Charts, which are data collected on patients being evaluated at the Cooper Clinic and standards being established at the Institute of Aerobics Research, Dallas, Texas, 1989. Reprinted with permission. Courtesy of K. H. Cooper, M.D., S. Blair, P.Ed, and B. Barlow.)

CHOL = cholesterol; TRIG = triglycerides; CHOL/HDL = ratio of total cholesterol, divided by high-density lipoproteins.

Table A–5. Physical Fitness and Health Standards for Men 60 to 69 Years of Age

Percentile Rankings	Resting (Sitting) Heart Rate (beats/min)	Blood Pressure Systolic (mmHg)	Blood Pressure Diastolic (mmHg)	Maximum Oxygen Uptake ($ml \cdot kg^{-1} \cdot min^{-1}$)	Maximum Heart Rate (beats/min)	Lipids CHOL (mg/dl)	HDL (mg/dl)	CHOL/HDL	TRIG (mg/dl)	Glucose (mg/dl)	Body Fat (%)
100	44	100	60	46.8	189	138	70	2.5	48	83	7.2
95	46	106	68	43.9	178	170	63	3.1	63	86	14.0
90	50	110	70	41.0	177	176	59	3.6	70	90	15.1
85	52	112	72	40.3	173	185	54	3.7	74	92	16.1
80	53	116	74	37.3	170	190	51	4.0	78	94	17.3
75	54	118	76	36.7	168	200	50	4.2	86	95	18.5
70	56	120	78	35.2	166	205	47	4.3	91	98	19.9
65	57	122	78	33.8	165	207	46	4.6	100	99	20.5
60	59	127	79	33.0	161	210	44	4.6	106	100	22.1
55	60	128	80	32.3	160	215	43	5.1	112	102	22.4
50	61	130	82	31.1	157	220	41	5.1	124	104	23.5
45	63	132	83	30.9	156	225	39	5.4	138	105	24.6
40	64	133	84	29.4	153	230	38	5.8	142	107	25.6
35	66	138	86	28.7	150	236	37	6.0	150	109	26.4
30	68	140	88	28.0	145	243	36	6.1	166	110	26.9
25	70	142	89	27.3	144	250	34	6.5	185	114	27.5
20	73	148	90	25.1	136	260	33	6.6	200	116	29.5
15	75	150	96	23.7	134	265	32	7.2	240	122	30.3
10	84	157	98	22.4	126	290	28	7.4	254	137	31.9
5	90	168	110	20.0	95	320	27	10.3	380	145	34.7
Population size	1413	1415	1415	1402	1402	1251	796	796	1246	1242	489
Average	62.8	130.9	83.1	32.5	156.1	222.5	44.3	5.3	145.8	107.0	23.2
Standard deviation	12.6	17.8	10.5	7.3	19.9	40.7	11.8	1.8	97.2	23.1	8.0

(Data from the Cooper Clinic Coronary Risk Factor Profile Charts, which are data collected on patients being evaluated at the Cooper Clinic and standards being established at the Institute of Aerobics Research, Dallas, Texas, 1989. Reprinted with permission. Courtesy of K. H. Cooper, M.D., S. Blair, P.Ed., and B. Barlow.)

CHOL = cholesterol; TRIG = triglycerides; CHOL/HDL = ratio of total cholesterol, divided by high-density lipoproteins.

Table A–6. Physical Fitness and Health Standards for Men 70 to 79 Years of Age

Percentile Rankings	Resting (Sitting) Heart Rate (beats/min)	Blood Pressure Systolic (mmHg)	Diastolic (mmHg)	Maximum Oxygen Uptake (ml·kg⁻¹·min⁻¹)	Heart Rate (beats/min)	Lipids CHOL (mg/dl)	HDL (mg/dl)	CHOL/HDL	TRIG (mg/dl)	Glucose (mg/dl)	Body Fat (%)
100	40	60	64	42.4	194	151	72	3.0	44	80	7.4
95	49	112	66	39.5	170	167	63	3.3	56	84	12.1
90	50	118	70	38.1	165	178	60	3.6	63	89	14.5
85	52	119	71	36.7	162	180	54	3.8	66	92	16.1
80	54	120	72	35.2	160	185	51	3.9	76	93	19.3
75	56	124	74	33.8	156	193	50	4.1	84	95	19.4
70	57	126	76	32.3	155	197	48	4.3	85	97	19.7
65	58	128	78	30.9	150	200	47	4.4	98	99	21.1
60	59	130	78	29.4	149	209	44	4.6	100	100	21.5
55	60	132	79	28.3	145	210	43	4.6	104	103	22.0
50	62	138	79	28.0	142	215	42	5.0	118	104	23.1
45	63	139	80	27.3	140	220	40	5.1	124	105	24.1
40	65	140	84	26.5	138	223	39	5.3	133	107	26.8
35	66	144	86	25.1	136	230	39	5.6	137	108	28.2
30	69	148	88	23.9	133	240	38	5.8	150	110	28.9
25	69	149	89	22.6	130	250	36	6.1	167	115	29.0
20	70	150	90	21.1	120	255	34	6.4	172	117	31.1
15	72	162	94	20.8	117	273	33	6.8	210	125	32.0
10	78	168	100	19.3	110	275	30	7.1	227	132	35.4
5	105	182	105	18.1	101	309	25	8.4	309	307	37.7
Population size	207	208	208	203	203	171	120	120	171	170	51
Average	62.8	137.5	82.0	28.8	144.5	217.5	45.0	5.0	128.7	108.4	23.4
Standard deviation	11.7	20.1	10.8	7.3	22.1	39.9	11.4	1.4	71.6	29.4	7.4

(Data from the Cooper Clinic Coronary Risk Factor Profile Charts, which are data collected on patients being evaluated at the Cooper Clinic and standards being established at the Institute of Aerobics Research, Dallas, Texas, 1989. Reprinted with permission. Courtesy of K. H. Cooper, M.D., S. Blair, P.Ed., and B. Barlow.)

CHOL = cholesterol; TRIG = triglycerides; CHOL/HDL = ratio of total cholesterol, divided by high-density lipoproteins.

Table A-7. Physical Fitness and Health Standards for Women 20 to 29 Years of Age

Percentile Rankings	Resting (Sitting)			Maximum		Lipids					Body Fat (%)
	Heart Rate (beats/min)	Systolic (mmHg)	Diastolic (mmHg)	Oxygen Uptake (ml·kg⁻¹·min⁻¹)	Heart Rate (beats/min)	CHOL (mg/dl)	HDL (mg/dl)	CHOL/HDL	TRIG (mg/dl)	Glucose (mg/dl)	
100	44	89	54	54.0	205	133	83	2.1	30	72	8.8
95	46	90	57	45.3	200	138	74	2.2	37	77	8.9
90	52	94	60	44.3	198	145	69	2.4	43	80	12.3
85	54	96	62	42.4	197	150	66	2.6	45	81	13.0
80	56	98	64	41.0	195	155	62	2.7	48	83	15.5
75	57	99	67	40.0	193	160	61	2.8	50	84	16.3
70	58	100	67	39.5	192	165	59	2.9	55	85	17.0
65	60	102	68	38.1	190	166	57	3.0	58	86	18.3
60	62	104	68	36.7	190	170	56	3.1	64	88	19.0
55	63	106	69	36.0	189	175	55	3.2	65	89	20.0
50	64	108	69	35.2	188	180	53	3.3	70	90	20.2
45	66	108	70	34.4	186	182	52	3.4	75	91	21.2
40	67	109	72	33.8	185	190	50	3.5	78	92	21.6
35	68	110	74	33.0	184	191	49	3.6	82	93	22.7
30	72	112	77	31.6	182	196	48	3.7	92	94	24.1
25	73	115	78	30.9	180	200	46	3.8	100	95	25.0
20	74	118	78	29.9	178	210	43	4.1	109	98	25.6
15	17	119	79	28.2	177	218	41	4.2	112	100	30.6
10	82	120	80	28.0	173	233	38	4.7	155	101	32.4
5	88	132	90	23.7	160	245	35	5.7	182	105	35.6
Population size	864	863	863	869	868	715	499	499	713	709	263
Average	64.8	107.6	71.2	36.0	187.7	180.6	55.0	3.4	80.5	90.7	20.5
Standard deviation	11.7	11.0	8.4	6.9	10.6	32.8	11.6	0.9	50.4	15.6	7.7

(Data from the Cooper Clinic Coronary Risk Factor Profile Charts, which are data collected on patients being evaluated at the Cooper Clinic and standards being established at the Institute of Aerobics Research, Dallas, Texas, 1989. Reprinted with permission. Courtesy of K. H. Cooper, M.D., S. Blair, P.Ed., and B. Barlow.)

CHOL = cholesterol; TRIG = triglycerides; CHOL/HDL = ratio of total cholesterol, divided by high-density lipoproteins.

Table A–8. Physical Fitness and Health Standards for Women 30 to 39 Years of Age

| Percentile Rankings | Resting (Sitting) | | | Maximum | | Lipids | | | | | Body Fat (%) |
| | Heart Rate (beats/min) | Blood Pressure | | Oxygen Uptake (ml·kg⁻¹·min⁻¹) | Heart Rate (beats/min) | CHOL (mg/dl) | HDL (mg/dl) | CHOL/HDL | TRIG (mg/dl) | Glucose (mg/dl) | |
		Systolic (mmHg)	Diastolic (mmHg)								
100	45	89	56	46.8	200	135	88	2.1	34	60	7.6
95	50	90	60	43.9	197	149	77	2.3	37	80	10.5
90	53	94	62	41.0	193	150	73	2.5	42	82	14.1
85	55	96	65	40.3	192	160	70	2.5	43	84	14.8
80	56	98	66	39.5	190	165	66	2.7	48	85	16.0
75	58	99	68	38.1	189	168	65	2.8	50	86	17.5
70	60	100	68	36.7	188	170	63	2.8	54	87	18.6
65	61	102	69	35.9	186	173	61	2.9	58	88	19.4
60	62	104	69	35.2	184	178	60	3.0	60	89	20.0
55	64	106	70	34.5	183	180	57	3.1	65	90	21.2
50	65	108	72	33.8	182	185	56	3.1	67	92	22.4
45	66	108	73	33.0	180	190	55	3.2	70	93	23.4
40	68	109	74	32.0	179	195	53	3.3	76	94	23.6
35	70	110	76	30.9	178	200	52	3.5	80	95	25.5
30	71	112	78	30.2	176	205	51	3.7	86	96	26.1
25	74	116	78	29.4	175	208	48	3.8	88	98	27.6
20	76	118	79	28.7	173	215	46	4.0	100	100	30.0
15	79	120	80	28.0	170	220	44	4.2	115	102	31.0
10	80	126	85	25.1	167	230	42	4.4	140	105	34.4
5	88	150	90	24.3	160	280	37	5.5	191	140	42.9
Population size	2794	2813	2813	2845	2845	1986	1387	1384	1976	1969	696
Average	65.8	108.1	73.1	34.3	182.4	188.1	58.9	3.3	76.2	97.2	22.4
Standard deviation	11.7	11.9	8.8	6.2	11.2	45.4	21.1	0.9	107.5	205.7	8.2

(Data from the Cooper Clinic Coronary Risk Factor Profile Charts, which are data collected on patients being evaluated at the Cooper Clinic and standards being established at the Institute of Aerobics Research, Dallas, Texas, 1989. Reprinted with permission. Courtesy of K. H. Cooper, M.D., S. Blair, P.Ed., and B. Barlow.)

CHOL = cholesterol; TRIG = triglycerides; CHOL/HDL = ratio of total cholesterol, divided by high-density lipoproteins.

Table A–9. Physical Fitness and Health Standards for Women 40 to 49 Years of Age

Percentile Rankings	Resting (Sitting) Heart Rate (beats/min)	Blood Pressure Systolic (mmHg)	Blood Pressure Diastolic (mmHg)	Maximum Oxygen Uptake (ml·kg^{-1}·min^{-1})	Maximum Heart Rate (beats/min)	Lipids CHOL (mg/dl)	HDL (mg/dl)	CHOL/HDL	TRIG (mg/dl)	Glucose (mg/dl)	Body Fat (%)
100	43	90	50	45.3	205	150	84	2.3	36	70	11.8
95	52	94	60	42.4	190	160	80	2.5	42	80	16.5
90	53	98	65	38.5	188	165	73	2.6	46	83	18.1
85	56	99	68	38.1	186	170	71	2.7	48	85	18.7
80	57	100	68	36.7	185	179	70	2.8	54	87	20.7
75	58	102	69	35.2	183	180	68	2.9	58	88	21.1
70	60	104	70	33.8	180	185	65	2.9	60	89	22.9
65	61	106	71	33.0	180	191	64	3.1	64	90	23.9
60	63	108	72	32.3	179	195	62	3.2	69	92	24.0
55	64	109	74	31.6	177	198	61	3.3	72	93	25.3
50	66	110	76	30.9	175	204	59	3.4	74	94	25.6
45	67	112	77	30.2	173	209	57	3.5	80	95	26.3
40	68	115	78	29.4	172	210	55	3.6	85	97	27.6
35	70	116	78	28.7	170	214	53	3.7	90	98	28.7
30	72	118	79	28.0	169	218	52	3.9	98	99	29.7
25	74	120	80	27.3	166	225	50	4.1	104	100	31.4
20	75	124	82	25.7	163	235	47	4.3	113	102	32.1
15	78	128	85	25.1	160	245	44	4.5	141	105	34.3
10	82	130	88	23.7	156	264	38	5.2	152	110	36.9
5	86	160	120	22.2	113	380	35	7.0	233	115	48.3
Population size	2414	2438	2438	2468	2468	1881	1280	1280	1871	1860	564
Average	66.2	112.2	75.9	31.6	175.2	204.5	59.9	3.5	88.5	94.8	26.1
Standard deviation	11.2	13.6	9.4	6.2	13.3	36.5	13.1	1.0	68.7	12.1	8.4

(Data from the Cooper Clinic Coronary Risk Factor Profile Charts, which are data collected on patients being evaluated at the Cooper Clinic and standards being established at the Institute of Aerobics Research, Dallas, Texas, 1989. Reprinted with permission. Courtesy of K. H. Cooper, M.D., S. Blair, P.Ed., and B. Barlow.)

CHOL = cholesterol; TRIG = triglycerides; CHOL/HDL = ratio of total cholesterol, divided by high-density lipoproteins.

Table A-10. Physical Fitness and Health Standards for Women 50 to 59 Years of Age

Percentile Rankings	Resting (Sitting) Heart Rate (beats/min)	Blood Pressure Systolic (mmHg)	Blood Pressure Diastolic (mmHg)	Maximum Oxygen Uptake (ml·kg⁻¹·min⁻¹)	Maximum Heart Rate (beats/min)	Lipids CHOL (mg/dl)	HDL (mg/dl)	CHOL/HDL	TRIG (mg/dl)	Glucose (mg/dl)	Body Fat (%)
100	48	80	60	43.9	193	150	84	2.3	33	79	14.4
95	53	98	66	36.7	186	175	81	2.6	53	84	19.6
90	54	100	68	35.2	180	185	75	2.7	55	85	21.1
85	56	104	69	33.8	178	192	74	2.9	63	88	23.3
80	58	108	70	32.3	176	194	70	3.0	67	90	24.0
75	59	109	72	31.6	175	203	68	3.2	71	91	25.3
70	60	110	75	30.9	174	205	66	3.3	77	93	25.9
65	62	112	76	30.2	171	212	64	3.4	84	94	26.9
60	63	114	77	29.4	170	217	62	3.4	86	95	27.8
55	64	118	78	28.7	168	220	60	3.5	96	96	28.7
50	66	119	78	28.0	167	225	59	3.7	100	98	29.7
45	67	120	79	27.1	166	232	57	3.8	108	99	30.7
40	68	122	80	26.5	164	235	55	3.9	110	100	32.1
35	70	124	82	25.8	162	240	54	4.1	123	102	32.4
30	72	128	85	25.1	160	245	52	4.3	130	104	33.9
25	73	130	86	24.4	159	256	51	4.5	138	105	34.1
20	77	134	88	23.7	154	265	48	4.9	160	107	35.7
15	80	140	90	22.9	151	270	44	5.0	166	110	37.7
10	86	150	96	22.2	148	290	43	6.0	189	115	40.1
5	88	152	130	18.3	125	317	33	6.9	242	121	48.7
Population size	1464	1467	1467	1480	1479	1217	788	788	1213	1205	347
Average	66.6	120.5	79.7	28.7	166.5	226.8	61.3	3.9	112.6	99.5	29.7
Standard deviation	11.5	17.9	10.4	5.4	14.9	40.2	13.9	1.3	69.1	18.9	8.7

(Data from the Cooper Clinic Coronary Risk Factor Profile Charts, which are data collected on patients being evaluated at the Cooper Clinic and standards being established at the Institute of Aerobics Research, Dallas, Texas, 1989. Reprinted with permission. Courtesy of K. H. Cooper, M.D., S. Blair, P.Ed., and B. Barlow.)

CHOL = cholesterol; TRIG = triglycerides; CHOL/HDL = ratio of total cholesterol, divided by high-density lipoproteins.

Table A–11. Physical Fitness and Health Standards for Women 60 to 69 Years of Age

Percentile Rankings	Resting (Sitting) Heart Rate (beats/min)	Blood Pressure Systolic (mmHg)	Diastolic (mmHg)	Maximum Oxygen Uptake (ml·kg⁻¹·min⁻¹)	Heart Rate (beats/min)	Lipids CHOL (mg/dl)	HDL (mg/dl)	CHOL/HDL	TRIG (mg/dl)	Glucose (mg/dl)	Body Fat (%)
100	50	90	60	38.1	186	165	88	2.0	41	82	6.1
95	52	100	68	35.2	177	182	77	2.7	52	84	10.6
90	55	108	69	32.3	171	185	73	2.8	57	87	21.5
85	56	110	70	30.9	170	195	70	3.0	67	88	22.2
80	58	115	72	30.2	166	197	69	3.1	73	90	24.9
75	59	117	75	29.4	165	208	67	3.4	80	92	26.8
70	60	118	75	28.2	163	213	64	3.4	84	93	27.0
65	62	120	76	28.0	160	216	62	3.5	88	94	27.7
60	63	122	78	27.3	158	220	61	3.8	93	95	29.4
55	64	124	78	26.5	157	230	59	3.8	103	96	30.1
50	65	126	79	25.8	155	234	57	4.1	107	99	31.5
45	66	128	80	25.1	153	235	54	4.2	118	100	32.7
40	68	130	81	24.4	150	245	53	4.5	124	102	32.9
35	70	132	82	23.8	149	249	52	4.7	129	103	33.0
30	72	136	84	23.7	146	257	50	4.8	140	105	36.0
25	74	138	88	22.6	142	265	48	5.0	147	107	37.3
20	75	140	89	22.2	140	268	45	5.2	169	110	38.7
15	78	150	90	20.8	135	275	43	5.5	183	113	40.4
10	85	158	95	19.5	130	299	37	6.1	214	120	41.7
5	96	160	100	18.3	117	314	35	7.4	250	140	52.9
Population size	514	515	515	514	514	444	316	316	443	439	74
Average	66.8	127.8	80.4	26.7	154.5	232.5	58.9	4.3	119.0	101.6	29.9
Standard deviation	11.9	18.1	9.9	4.7	17.5	42.3	14.5	3.0	63.3	22.2	10.0

(Data from the Cooper Clinic Coronary Risk Factor Profile Charts, which are data collected on patients being evaluated at the Cooper Clinic and standards being established at the Institute of Aerobics Research, Dallas, Texas, 1989. Reprinted with permission. Courtesy of K. H. Cooper, M.D., S. Blair, P.Ed., and B. Barlow.)

CHOL = cholesterol; TRIG = triglycerides; CHOL/HDL = ratio of total cholesterol, divided by high-density lipoproteins.

Table A-12. Physical Fitness and Health Standards for Women 70 to 79 Years of Age

Percentile Rankings	Resting (Sitting)			Maximum		Lipids				Glucose (mg/dl)	Body Fat (%)
	Heart Rate (beats/min)	Blood Pressure		Oxygen Uptake (ml·kg⁻¹·min⁻¹)	Heart Rate (beats/min)	CHOL (mg/dl)	HDL (mg/dl)	CHOL/HDL	TRIG (mg/dl)		
		Systolic (mmHg)	Diastolic (mmHg)								
100	48	100	58	38.5	177	144	102	2.1	50	75	—
95	53	108	60	35.4	173	170	80	2.6	51	79	—
90	57	114	68	32.5	168	193	75	3.2	69	86	4.7
85	58	116	69	32.3	163	199	72	3.4	70	88	—
80	59	118	70	31.0	160	212	66	3.4	80	91	—
75	60	120	72	29.8	158	217	65	3.4	90	92	29.2
70	62	125	74	29.4	154	223	63	3.9	93	94	—
65	63	128	76	27.2	153	226	59	4.0	100	95	—
60	64	129	78	26.8	150	228	56	4.0	108	96	29.9
55	65	130	78	26.5	148	234	55	4.2	113	97	—
50	66	134	79	25.3	145	242	54	4.3	114	99	—
45	68	136	80	25.1	144	245	53	4.5	120	100	32.6
40	70	138	82	23.7	141	248	51	4.6	122	101	—
35	71	140	84	22.6	138	250	50	4.6	138	103	33.9
30	73	142	86	22.2	135	264	48	4.8	145	105	—
25	75	148	88	21.3	132	272	47	5.0	146	109	—
20	76	152	90	20.8	128	281	45	5.3	175	110	42.0
15	78	156	92	20.0	120	295	44	5.4	190	115	—
10	80	172	94	19.3	106	330	39	6.2	237	122	—
5	90	180	104	18.3	97	355	32	8.5	417	128	—
Population size	88	85	85	84	84	77	53	53	77	77	6
Average	67.7	134.9	80.1	26.6	145.7	241.0	58.0	4.4	128.0	101.1	28.7
Standard deviation	9.8	20.0	10.7	5.8	20.3	46.5	14.6	1.4	69.3	18.5	12.6

(Data from the Cooper Clinic Coronary Risk Factor Profile Charts, which are data collected on patients being evaluated at the Cooper Clinic and standards being established at the Institute of Aerobics Research, Dallas, Texas, 1989. Reprinted with permission. Courtesy of K. H. Cooper, M.D., S. Blair, P.Ed., and B. Barlow.)

CHOL = cholesterol; TRIG = triglycerides; CHOL/HDL = ratio of total cholesterol, divided by high-density lipoproteins.

Table A–13. Y's Way to Physical Fitness Evaluation Profile: Norms for Men 18 to 25 Years of Age

Rating	% Ranking	Resting HR	% Fat	3-Min Step Test	PWC max (kgm)	VO₂max (ml/kg)	Flexibility	Bench Press	Sit-ups
Excellent	100	49	4	70	2350	80	26	45	60
	95	52	6	72	2275	71	22	42	54
	90	55	6	78	2065	63	20	38	50
Good	85	57	8	82	1905	59	20	34	48
	80	60	10	85	1795	55	19	32	46
	75	61	10	88	1705	53	18	30	45
Above average	70	63	12	91	1630	51	18	28	42
	65	64	12	94	1570	49	17	26	41
	60	65	13	97	1515	47	17	25	40
Average	55	67	14	101	1455	46	16	22	38
	50	68	15	102	1400	45	16	22	37
	45	69	16	104	1350	43	15	21	36
Below average	40	71	17	107	1305	41	14	20	34
	35	72	18	110	1260	39	14	17	33
	30	73	20	114	1195	38	13	16	32
Poor	25	76	20	118	1135	35	12	13	30
	20	79	22	121	1090	33	12	12	28
	15	81	24	126	1050	31	10	9	26
Very poor	10	84	26	131	975	29	9	8	24
	5	89	28	137	885	26	7	2	17
	0	95	36	164	850	20	2	0	12

(Reprinted with permission from Golding, L. A., Myers, C. R., and Sinning, W. E. (eds.): **Y's Way to Physical Fitness: The Complete Guide to Fitness Testing and Instruction,** 3rd Ed. Champaign, IL, Human Kinetics, 1989.)

Table A–14. Y's Way to Physical Fitness Evaluation Profile: Norms for Men 26 to 35 Years of Age

Rating	% Ranking	Resting HR	% Fat	3-Min Step Test	PWC max (kgm)	V̇O₂max (ml/kg)	Flexibility	Bench Press	Sit-ups
Excellent	100	49	8	73	2300	70	25	43	55
	95	52	9	76	2180	64	22	40	50
	90	54	11	79	1950	58	20	34	46
Good	85	57	12	83	1820	54	19	30	45
	80	60	14	85	1740	52	18	29	42
	75	61	15	88	1665	50	18	26	41
Above average	70	62	16	91	1600	47	17	25	38
	65	64	17	94	1545	46	17	24	37
	60	65	18	97	1485	44	16	22	36
Average	55	66	18	101	1430	42	16	21	34
	50	68	20	103	1375	41	15	20	33
	45	70	20	106	1325	40	15	18	32
Below average	40	72	22	109	1270	39	14	17	30
	35	73	22	113	1225	38	13	14	30
	30	74	24	116	1180	35	12	13	29
Poor	25	77	24	119	1135	34	12	12	28
	20	78	26	122	1080	33	11	10	25
	15	81	27	126	1020	31	10	9	24
Very Poor	10	84	28	130	960	28	9	5	21
	5	88	30	140	840	26	7	2	12
	0	94	36	164	780	20	2	0	6

(Reprinted with permission from Golding, L. A., Myers, C. R., and Sinning, W. E. (eds.): **Y's Way to Physical Fitness: The Complete Guide to Fitness Testing and Instruction,** 3rd Ed. Champaign, IL, Human Kinetics, 1989.)

Table A–15. *Y's Way to Physical Fitness* Evaluation Profile: Norms for Men 36 to 45 Years of Age

Rating	% Ranking	Resting HR	% Fat	3-Min Step Test	PWC max (kgm)	V̇O₂max (ml/kg)	Flexibility	Bench Press	Sit-ups
Excellent	100	50	10	72	2250	77	24	40	50
	95	53	12	74	2055	60	21	34	46
	90	56	14	81	1815	53	19	30	42
Good	85	60	16	86	1725	49	19	28	40
	80	61	17	90	1640	46	17	25	37
	75	62	18	94	1565	44	17	24	36
Above average	70	64	19	98	1500	42	17	22	34
	65	65	20	100	1440	41	15	21	32
	60	66	21	102	1375	40	15	20	30
Average	55	68	21	105	1325	38	15	18	29
	50	69	23	108	1280	37	14	17	29
	45	70	23	111	1235	35	13	16	28
Below average	40	73	24	113	1190	34	13	14	26
	35	74	25	116	1140	33	11	13	25
	30	76	25	118	1090	32	11	12	24
Poor	25	77	27	120	1045	30	11	10	22
	20	80	28	124	995	28	9	9	20
	15	82	29	128	945	27	9	8	18
Very poor	10	86	30	132	860	25	7	5	16
	5	90	32	142	745	21	5	2	9
	0	96	39	168	700	19	1	0	4

(Reprinted with permission from Golding, L. A., Myers, C. R., and Sinning, W. E. (eds.): **Y's Way to Physical Fitness: The Complete Guide to Fitness Testing and Instruction**, 3rd Ed. Champaign, IL, Human Kinetics, 1989.)

Table A-16. *Y's Way to Physical Fitness* Evaluation Profile: Norms for Men 46 to 55 Years of Age

Rating	% Ranking	Resting HR	% Fat	3-Min Step Test	PWC max (kgm)	V̇O₂max (ml/kg)	Flexibility	Bench Press	Sit-ups
Excellent	100	50	12	78	2150	60	23	35	50
	95	53	14	81	1940	54	20	28	41
	90	57	16	84	1645	47	19	24	36
Good	85	59	18	89	1520	43	17	22	33
	80	60	19	93	1450	42	17	21	30
	75	63	20	96	1385	40	16	20	29
Above average	70	64	21	99	1335	38	15	17	28
	65	65	22	101	1285	36	15	16	26
	60	67	23	103	1240	35	14	14	25
Average	55	68	24	109	1205	35	13	13	24
	50	69	24	113	1165	34	12	12	22
	45	71	25	115	1130	32	12	10	22
Below average	40	73	26	118	1090	31	11	10	21
	35	75	26	120	1055	30	10	9	20
	30	76	27	121	1020	29	10	8	18
Poor	25	79	28	124	950	28	9	6	17
	20	80	29	126	935	27	8	5	16
	15	83	30	130	885	26	7	4	13
Very poor	10	85	32	135	830	23	6	2	12
	5	91	34	145	750	22	4	1	8
	0	97	38	158	700	18	1	0	4

(Reprinted with permission from Golding, L. A., Myers, C. R., and Sinning, W. E. (eds.): **Y's Way to Physical Fitness: The Complete Guide to Fitness Testing and Instruction**, 3rd Ed. Champaign, IL, Human Kinetics, 1989.)

Table A–17. *Y's Way to Physical Fitness* Evaluation Profile: Norms for Men 56 to 65 Years of Age

Rating	% Ranking	Resting HR	% Fat	3-Min Step Test	PWC max (kgm)	$\dot{V}O_2$max (ml/kg)	Flexibility	Bench Press	Sit-ups
Excellent	100	51	13	72	2100	58	21	32	42
	95	52	16	74	1665	49	19	24	37
	90	56	18	82	1485	43	17	22	32
Good	85	59	20	89	1400	39	17	20	29
	80	60	20	93	1315	38	15	18	28
	75	61	21	97	1240	37	15	14	26
Above average	70	64	22	98	1195	35	13	14	24
	65	65	22	100	1150	34	13	12	22
	60	67	23	101	1100	33	13	10	21
Average	55	68	24	105	1055	31	11	10	20
	50	69	24	109	1005	31	11	8	18
	45	71	25	111	965	30	11	8	17
Below average	40	72	26	113	925	29	9	6	16
	35	73	26	116	890	27	9	6	14
	30	75	27	118	860	26	9	4	13
Poor	25	76	28	122	830	25	7	4	12
	20	79	29	125	795	23	7	2	10
	15	81	30	128	740	22	5	2	9
Very poor	10	84	32	131	680	21	5	0	8
	5	88	34	136	597	18	3	0	4
	0	94	38	150	590	16	1	0	2

(Reprinted with permission from Golding, L. A., Myers, C. R., and Sinning, W. E. (eds.): **Y's Way to Physical Fitness. The Complete Guide to Fitness Testing and Instruction,** 3rd Ed. Champaign, IL, Human Kinetics, 1989.)

Table A–18. Y's Way to Physical Fitness Evaluation Profile: Norms for Men over 65 Years of Age

Rating	% Ranking	Resting HR	% Fat	3-Min Step Test	PWC max (kgm)	VO₂max (ml/kg)	Flexibility	Bench Press	Sit-ups
Excellent	100	50	14	72	1940	50	20	30	40
	95	53	16	74	1405	42	18	20	33
	90	55	18	86	1235	38	17	18	29
Good	85	58	19	89	1175	36	15	14	26
	80	59	20	92	1110	34	14	12	25
	75	61	21	95	1045	33	13	10	22
Above average	70	62	22	97	1015	32	13	10	21
	65	63	22	100	990	30	12	10	21
	60	65	23	102	945	29	11	8	20
Average	55	66	23	104	900	28	11	8	18
	50	69	24	109	870	26	10	6	17
	45	69	24	113	840	25	9	6	16
Below average	40	70	25	114	805	25	9	4	14
	35	71	26	116	765	24	8	4	13
	30	73	26	119	725	22	8	4	12
Poor	25	75	27	122	695	21	7	2	10
	20	77	28	126	665	21	6	2	9
	15	79	29	128	610	20	5	2	8
Very poor	10	83	31	133	555	18	4	0	6
	5	89	32	140	510	17	3	0	4
	0	98	38	152	490	15	0	0	2

(Reprinted with permission from Golding, L. A., Myers, C. R., and Sinning, W. E. (eds.): **Y's Way to Physical Fitness: The Complete Guide to Fitness Testing and Instruction**, 3rd Ed. Champaign, IL, Human Kinetics, 1989.)

Table A–19. *Y's Way to Physical Fitness* Evaluation Profile: Norms for Women 18 to 25 Years of Age

Rating	% Ranking	Resting HR	% Fat	3-Min Step Test	PWC max (kgm)	$\dot{V}O_2$max (ml/kg)	Flexibility	Bench Press	Sit-ups
Excellent	100	54	13	72	1830	71	27	50	55
	95	56	15	79	1640	67	25	42	48
	90	60	16	83	1440	58	24	36	44
Good	85	61	17	88	1320	54	23	32	41
	80	64	18	93	1235	50	22	29	38
	75	65	19	97	1175	48	21	28	37
Above average	70	66	20	100	1120	46	21	25	36
	65	68	21	103	1075	43	20	24	34
	60	69	22	106	1030	42	20	22	33
Average	55	70	23	110	990	41	19	21	32
	50	72	24	112	950	40	19	20	30
	45	73	25	116	915	39	18	18	29
Below average	40	74	26	118	880	37	18	16	28
	35	76	27	122	845	35	17	14	26
	30	78	28	124	810	34	17	13	25
Poor	25	80	29	128	775	32	16	12	24
	20	82	30	133	740	31	15	9	22
	15	84	31	137	705	29	14	8	20
Very poor	10	86	33	142	640	26	13	5	17
	5	90	37	149	555	22	12	2	10
	0	100	43	155	500	18	8	1	4

(Reprinted with permission from Golding, L. A., Myers, C. R., and Sinning, W. E. (eds.): **Y's Way to Physical Fitness: The Complete Guide to Fitness Testing and Instruction,** 3rd Ed. Champaign, IL, Human Kinetics, 1989.)

Table A–20. *Y's Way to Physical Fitness* Evaluation Profile: Norms for Women 26 to 35 Years of Age

Rating	% Ranking	Resting HR	% Fat	3-Min Step Test	PWC max (kgm)	$\dot{V}O_2$max (ml/kg)	Flexibility	Bench Press	Sit-ups
Excellent	100	54	14	72	1800	69	26	48	54
	95	55	15	80	1440	59	24	40	42
	90	59	16	86	1330	54	23	33	40
Good	85	60	18	91	1245	51	22	29	37
	80	63	19	93	1180	48	21	26	34
	75	64	20	97	1115	46	20	25	33
Above average	70	66	21	103	1065	43	20	22	32
	65	67	22	106	1020	42	19	21	30
	60	68	23	110	985	40	19	20	29
Average	55	69	24	112	955	38	18	18	28
	50	70	24	116	925	37	18	17	26
	45	71	25	118	885	35	18	16	25
Below average	40	72	27	121	840	34	17	14	24
	35	74	28	124	805	33	16	13	23
	30	76	29	127	765	31	16	12	21
Poor	25	78	31	129	730	30	15	9	20
	20	80	32	131	695	28	14	8	18
	15	82	33	135	655	26	14	5	16
Very poor	10	84	36	141	600	25	13	2	12
	5	88	39	148	530	22	11	1	2
	0	94	49	154	490	20	8	0	1

Table A–21. *Y's Way to Physical Fitness Evaluation Profile:* Norms for Women 36 to 45 Years of Age

Rating	% Ranking	Resting HR	% Fat	3-Min Step Test	PWC max (kgm)	V̇O₂max (ml/kg)	Flexibility	Bench Press	Sit-ups
Excellent	100	54	16	74	1780	66	25	46	50
	95	56	17	80	1360	53	23	32	38
	90	59	19	87	1215	46	22	28	34
Good	85	62	20	93	1135	44	21	25	30
	80	63	21	97	1085	41	20	22	29
	75	64	23	101	1035	39	19	21	27
Above average	70	66	24	104	980	37	19	20	26
	65	68	25	106	925	36	18	18	25
	60	69	26	109	880	34	17	17	24
Average	55	70	27	111	835	33	17	14	22
	50	71	28	114	800	32	16	13	21
	45	72	29	117	765	31	16	12	20
Below average	40	74	30	120	745	30	15	11	18
	35	76	31	122	720	29	15	10	17
	30	78	32	127	695	28	14	9	16
Poor	25	79	33	130	670	26	13	8	14
	20	80	35	135	625	25	12	6	12
	15	82	36	138	575	23	11	4	10
Very poor	10	84	38	143	530	21	10	2	6
	5	88	41	146	470	19	9	1	2
	0	92	48	152	490	18	6	0	1

(Reprinted with permission from Golding, L. A., Myers, C. R., and Sinning, W. E. (eds.): **Y's Way to Physical Fitness: The Complete Guide to Fitness Testing and Instruction,** 3rd Ed. Champaign, IL, Human Kinetics, 1989.)

Table A-22. *Y's Way to Physical Fitness* Evaluation Profile: Norms for Women 46 to 55 Years of Age

Rating	% Ranking	Resting HR	% Fat	3-Min Step Test	PWC max (kgm)	V̇O₂max (ml/kg)	Flexibility	Bench Press	Sit-ups
Excellent	100	54	17	76	1700	64	24	42	42
	95	56	19	88	1245	48	22	30	30
	90	60	21	93	1130	42	21	26	28
Good	85	61	23	96	1045	39	20	22	25
	80	64	24	100	980	36	19	21	24
	75	65	25	102	930	35	18	20	22
Above average	70	66	26	106	885	33	18	17	21
	65	68	27	111	850	32	17	14	20
	60	69	28	113	815	31	17	13	18
Average	55	70	29	117	790	30	16	12	17
	50	72	30	118	760	29	16	11	16
	45	73	31	120	730	28	15	10	14
Below average	40	74	32	121	700	27	15	9	13
	35	76	33	124	670	26	14	8	12
	30	77	34	126	640	25	14	6	10
Poor	25	78	35	127	610	24	13	5	9
	20	81	36	131	585	23	12	4	8
	15	84	38	133	545	21	11	2	6
Very poor	10	85	39	138	495	19	10	1	4
	5	90	42	147	430	18	8	0	1
	0	96	50	152	400	16	4	0	0

(Reprinted with permission from Golding, L. A., Myers, C. R., and Sinning, W. E. (eds.): **Y's Way to Physical Fitness: The Complete Guide to Fitness Testing and Instruction,** 3rd Ed. Champaign, IL, Human Kinetics, 1989.)

Table A–23. *Y's Way to Physical Fitness* Evaluation Profile: Norms for Women 56 to 65 Years of Age

Rating	% Ranking	Resting HR	% Fat	3-Min Step Test	PWC max (kgm)	V̇O₂max (ml/kg)	Flexibility	Bench Press	Sit-ups
Excellent	100	54	18	74	1650	57	23	34	38
	95	56	20	83	1165	43	21	30	29
	90	59	22	92	1015	38	20	22	25
Good	85	61	24	97	970	36	19	20	21
	80	63	25	99	895	34	18	18	20
	75	64	26	103	840	32	18	16	18
Above average	70	67	27	106	790	31	17	15	17
	65	68	28	109	750	30	17	14	14
	60	69	29	111	720	28	16	12	13
Average	55	71	30	113	690	27	15	10	12
	50	72	31	116	660	26	15	9	11
	45	73	32	117	635	25	15	8	10
Below average	40	75	33	119	605	24	14	7	9
	35	76	34	123	575	23	13	6	8
	30	77	35	127	550	22	13	4	7
Poor	25	79	36	129	530	21	12	3	6
	20	80	37	132	510	20	11	2	5
	15	81	38	136	475	19	10	1	4
Very poor	10	85	39	142	420	17	9	0	2
	5	89	41	148	355	15	7	0	1
	0	96	49	151	340	14	3	0	0

(Reprinted with permission from Golding, L. A., Myers, C. R., and Sinning, W. E. (eds.): **Y's Way to Physical Fitness: The Complete Guide to Fitness Testing and Instruction,** 3rd Ed. Champaign, IL, Human Kinetics, 1989.)

Table A–24. *Y's Way to Physical Fitness Evaluation Profile:* Norm for Women over 65 Years of Age

Rating	% Ranking	Resting HR	% Fat	3-Min Step Test	PWC max (kgm)	$\dot{V}O_2$max (ml/kg)	Flexibility	Bench Press	Sit-ups
Excellent	100	54	16	73	1190	51	22	26	36
	95	56	17	83	860	39	21	22	26
	90	59	20	86	820	33	20	18	24
Good	85	60	22	93	725	31	19	14	22
	80	62	24	97	665	30	18	13	20
	75	64	26	100	640	28	18	12	18
Above average	70	66	27	104	610	27	17	11	16
	65	67	28	108	585	26	17	10	15
	60	68	29	114	560	25	16	9	14
Average	55	70	30	117	540	24	15	8	13
	50	71	31	120	525	23	15	6	12
	45	72	32	121	510	22	14	5	11
Below average	40	73	32	123	495	22	13	4	10
	35	75	33	126	480	21	13	3	8
	30	76	34	127	470	20	12	2	6
Poor	25	79	35	129	460	18	11	2	4
	20	80	36	132	425	17	10	1	3
	15	84	37	134	395	17	9	0	2
Very poor	10	88	38	135	370	16	8	0	1
	5	91	40	149	340	15	6	0	0
	0	96	41	151	320	14	2	0	0

(Reprinted with permission from Golding, L. A., Myers, C. R., and Sinning, W. E. (eds.): **Y's Way to Physical Fitness: The Complete Guide to Fitness Testing and Instruction,** 3rd Ed. Champaign, IL, Human Kinetics, 1989.)

Table A-25. Norms and Percentiles by Age Groups and Gender for Predicted Maximal Oxygen Uptake (ml · kg⁻¹ · min⁻¹)

Norms

Age (yrs)	15–19		20–29		30–39		40–49		50–59		60–69	
Gender	M	F	M	F	M	F	M	F	M	F	M	F
Excellent	≥ 60	≥ 43	≥ 57	≥ 40	≥ 48	≥ 37	≥ 42	≥ 35	≥ 38	≥ 30	≥ 30	≥ 25
Above average	58–59	40–42	52–56	37–39	46–47	34–37	40–42	32–34	36–38	27–29	29–30	24–25
Average	54–57	37–39	43–51	35–37	42–45	31–33	37–39	26–31	34–35	25–27	27–28	22–23
Below average	44–53	35–37	40–42	32–34	38–41	29–31	34–37	24–25	31–33	22–25	26–27	20–22
Poor	≤ 43	≤ 34	≤ 40	≤ 31	≤ 37	≤ 29	≤ 33	≤ 23	≤ 30	≤ 21	≤ 26	≤ 19

Percentiles

Age (yrs)	15–19		20–29		30–39		40–49		50–59		60–69	
Gender	M	F	M	F	M	F	M	F	M	F	M	F
95	62	45	59	43	51	39	44	36	40	31	32	26
90	61	43	58	41	50	38	43	35	39	30	31	26
85	60	43	57	40	48	37	42	35	38	30	30	25
80	59	42	56	39	47	37	42	34	38	29	30	25
75	59	41	55	39	47	36	41	33	37	28	29	24
70	58	40	54	38	46	35	40	33	36	28	29	24
65	58	40	52	37	46	34	40	32	36	27	29	24
60	57	39	48	37	45	33	39	31	35	27	28	23
55	57	38	44	36	44	32	38	30	35	26	28	23
50	56	38	43	35	43	32	38	28	34	26	28	22
45	54	37	43	35	42	31	37	26	34	25	27	22
40	52	37	42	34	41	31	37	25	33	25	27	22
35	47	36	42	34	40	30	36	25	33	24	27	21
30	46	35	41	33	39	30	35	24	32	23	27	21
25	44	35	40	32	38	29	34	24	31	22	26	20
20	43	34	40	31	37	29	32	23	28	21	26	20
15	42	34	39	31	36	28	31	22	26	20	25	19
10	41	33	38	30	34	28	30	22	25	19	24	18
5	40	32	37	29	33	27	29	21	24	18	23	17

(Based on data from the Canada Fitness Survey, 1981. Reprinted from **Canadian Standardized Test of Fitness (CSTF) Operations Manual**, 3rd Ed. With the permission of Fitness Canada, Fitness and Amateur Sport Canada, Ottawa, 1986.)

Table A-26. Norms and Percentiles by Age Groups and Gender for Trunk Forward Flexion (cm)

Norms

Age (yrs)	15–19		20–29		30–39		40–49		50–59		60–69	
Gender	M	F	M	F	M	F	M	F	M	F	M	F
Excellent	≥ 39	≥ 43	≥ 40	≥ 41	≥ 38	≥ 41	≥ 35	≥ 38	≥ 35	≥ 39	≥ 33	≥ 35
Above average	34–38	38–42	34–39	37–40	33–37	36–40	29–34	34–37	28–34	33–38	25–32	31–34
Average	29–33	34–37	30–33	33–36	28–32	32–35	24–28	30–33	24–27	30–32	20–24	27–30
Below average	24–28	29–33	25–29	28–32	23–27	27–31	18–23	25–29	16–23	25–29	15–19	23–26
Poor	≤ 23	≤ 28	≤ 24	≤ 27	≤ 22	≤ 26	≤ 17	≤ 24	≤ 15	≤ 24	≤ 14	≤ 23

Percentiles

Age (yrs)	15–19		20–29		30–39		40–49		50–59		60–69	
Gender	M	F	M	F	M	F	M	F	M	F	M	F
95	44	47	44	45	43	45	40	43	41	43	44	40
90	42	44	42	43	40	42	37	40	38	40	35	37
85	39	43	40	41	38	41	35	38	35	39	33	35
80	38	42	38	40	37	39	34	37	32	37	30	34
75	36	41	37	39	35	38	32	36	30	36	28	33
70	35	40	36	38	34	37	30	35	29	35	26	31
65	34	38	34	37	33	36	29	34	28	33	25	31
60	33	37	33	36	32	35	28	33	27	32	24	30
55	31	36	32	35	31	34	26	32	26	31	23	28
50	30	35	31	34	29	33	25	31	25	30	22	28
45	29	34	30	33	28	32	24	30	24	30	20	27
40	28	33	29	32	27	31	23	29	22	29	18	26
35	27	32	27	31	26	30	21	28	20	28	17	25
30	26	31	26	29	24	28	20	26	18	26	16	24
25	24	29	25	28	23	27	18	25	16	25	15	23
20	22	27	23	26	21	25	16	24	15	23	14	23
15	19	25	21	25	20	23	14	22	14	22	13	20
10	17	23	18	22	17	21	12	19	12	19	11	18
5	13	18	14	18	13	16	8	14	7	13	8	13

(Based on data from the Canada Fitness Survey, 1981. Reprinted from **Canadian Standardized Test of Fitness (CSTF) Operations Manual**, 3rd Ed. With the permission of Fitness Canada, Fitness and Amateur Sport Canada, Ottawa, 1986.)

Table A-27. Norms and Percentiles by Age Groups and Gender for Sit-ups (number in 60 seconds)

Norms

Age (yrs)	15–19		20–29		30–39		40–49		50–59		60–69	
Gender	M	F	M	F	M	F	M	F	M	F	M	F
Excellent	≥ 48	≥ 42	≥ 43	≥ 36	≥ 36	≥ 29	≥ 31	≥ 25	≥ 26	≥ 19	≥ 23	≥ 16
Above average	42–47	36–41	37–42	31–35	31–35	24–28	26–30	20–24	22–25	12–18	17–22	12–15
Average	38–41	32–35	33–36	25–30	27–30	20–23	22–25	15–19	18–21	5–11	12–16	4–11
Below average	33–37	27–31	29–32	21–24	22–26	15–19	17–21	7–14	13–17	3–4	7–11	2–3
Poor	≤ 32	≤ 26	≤ 28	≤ 20	≤ 21	≤ 14	≤ 16	≤ 6	≤ 12	≤ 2	≤ 6	≤ 1

Percentiles

Age (yrs)	15–19		20–29		30–39		40–49		50–59		60–69	
Gender	M	F	M	F	M	F	M	F	M	F	M	F
95	53	47	49	43	42	34	36	28	34	26	26	20
90	50	43	45	39	38	31	33	26	28	22	24	18
85	48	42	43	36	36	29	31	25	26	19	23	16
80	46	40	41	34	34	27	30	23	25	17	21	15
75	44	39	40	32	33	26	29	22	24	16	19	14
70	43	37	38	31	32	25	27	21	23	14	18	13
65	42	36	37	31	31	24	26	20	22	12	17	12
60	41	35	36	29	30	23	25	18	21	11	15	10
55	40	34	35	28	29	22	24	17	20	10	15	9
50	39	33	34	27	28	21	23	16	20	7	13	5
45	38	32	33	25	27	20	22	15	18	5	12	4
40	36	31	32	24	26	18	21	13	17	4	11	2
35	35	29	31	23	24	17	20	12	16	3	10	—
30	34	28	30	22	23	16	19	10	15	—	10	—
25	33	27	29	21	22	15	17	7	13	—	7	—
20	32	25	27	19	21	13	16	5	11	—	2	—
15	30	23	26	17	20	11	14	3	10	—	—	—
10	28	21	24	15	17	7	11	—	8	—	—	—
5	23	15	20	11	14	—	6	—	—	—	—	—

(Based on data from the Canada Fitness Survey, 1981. Reprinted from Canadian Standardized Test of Fitness (CSTF) Operations Manual, 3rd Ed. With the permission of Fitness Canada, Fitness and Amateur Sport Canada, Ottawa, 1986.)

Table A–28. Norms and Percentiles by Age Groups and Gender for Push-ups

Norms

Age (yrs)	15–19		20–29		30–39		40–49		50–59		60–69	
Gender	M	F	M	F	M	F	M	F	M	F	M	F
Excellent	≥39	≥33	≥36	≥30	≥30	≥27	≥22	≥24	≥21	≥21	≥18	≥17
Above average	29–38	25–32	29–35	21–29	22–29	20–26	17–21	15–23	13–20	11–20	11–17	12–16
Average	23–28	18–24	22–28	15–20	17–21	13–19	13–16	11–14	10–12	7–10	8–10	5–11
Below average	18–22	12–17	17–21	10–14	12–16	8–12	10–12	5–10	7–9	2–6	5–7	1–4
Poor	≤17	≤11	≤16	≤9	≤11	≤7	≤9	≤4	≤6	≤1	≤4	≤1

Percentiles

Age (yrs)	15–19		20–29		30–39		40–49		50–59		60–69	
Gender	M	F	M	F	M	F	M	F	M	F	M	F
95	50	46	48	37	36	36	30	32	28	30	25	30
90	43	38	41	32	32	31	25	28	24	23	24	25
85	39	33	36	30	30	27	22	24	21	21	18	17
80	35	31	34	26	27	24	21	22	17	17	16	15
75	32	28	32	24	25	22	20	20	15	15	13	13
70	31	26	30	22	24	21	19	18	14	13	11	12
65	29	25	29	21	22	20	17	15	13	11	11	12
60	27	23	27	20	21	17	16	14	11	10	10	10
55	26	21	25	18	20	16	15	13	11	10	10	9
50	24	20	24	16	19	14	13	12	10	9	9	6
45	23	18	22	15	17	13	13	11	10	7	8	5
40	22	16	21	14	16	12	12	10	9	5	7	4
35	21	15	20	13	15	11	11	10	8	4	6	3
30	20	14	18	11	14	10	10	7	7	3	6	2
25	18	12	17	10	12	8	10	5	7	2	5	1
20	16	11	16	9	11	7	8	4	5	1	4	—
15	14	9	14	7	10	6	7	3	5	1	3	—
10	11	6	11	5	8	4	5	2	4	—	2	—
5	8	4	9	2	5	1	4	—	2	—	—	—

(Based on data from the Canada Fitness Survey, 1981. Reprinted from **Canadian Standardized Test of Fitness (CSTF) Operations Manual**, 3rd Ed. With the permission of Fitness Canada, Fitness and Amateur Sport Canada, Ottawa, 1986.)

Table A–29. Percent Fat Estimate for Women: Sum of Triceps, Abdomen, and Suprailium Skinfolds

Sum of Skinfolds (mm)	Age to Last Year								
	18–22	23–27	28–32	33–37	38–42	43–47	48–52	53–57	Over 57
8–12	8.8	9.0	9.2	9.4	9.5	9.7	9.9	10.1	10.3
13–17	10.8	10.9	11.1	11.3	11.5	11.7	11.8	12.0	12.2
18–22	12.6	12.8	13.0	13.2	13.4	13.5	13.7	13.9	14.1
23–27	14.5	14.6	14.8	15.0	15.2	15.4	15.6	15.7	15.9
28–32	16.2	16.4	16.6	16.8	17.0	17.1	17.3	17.5	17.7
33–37	17.9	18.1	18.3	18.5	18.7	18.9	19.0	19.2	19.4
38–42	19.6	19.8	20.0	20.2	20.3	20.5	20.7	20.9	21.1
43–47	21.2	21.4	21.6	21.8	21.9	22.1	22.3	22.5	22.7
48–52	22.8	22.9	23.1	23.3	23.5	23.7	23.8	24.0	24.2
53–57	24.2	24.4	24.6	24.8	25.0	25.2	25.3	25.5	25.7
58–62	25.7	25.9	26.0	26.2	26.4	26.6	26.8	27.0	27.1
63–67	27.1	27.2	27.4	27.6	27.8	28.0	28.2	28.3	28.5
68–72	28.4	28.6	28.7	28.9	29.1	29.3	29.5	29.7	29.8
73–77	29.6	29.8	30.0	30.2	30.4	30.6	30.7	30.9	31.1
78–82	30.9	31.0	31.2	31.4	31.6	31.8	31.9	32.1	32.3
83–87	32.0	32.2	32.4	32.6	32.7	32.9	33.1	33.3	33.5
88–92	33.1	33.3	33.5	33.7	33.8	34.0	34.2	34.4	34.6
93–97	34.1	34.3	34.5	34.7	34.9	35.1	35.2	35.4	35.6
98–102	35.1	35.3	35.5	35.7	35.9	36.0	36.2	36.4	36.6
103–107	36.1	36.2	36.4	36.6	36.8	37.0	37.2	37.3	37.5
108–112	36.9	37.1	37.3	37.5	37.7	37.9	38.0	38.2	38.4
113–117	37.8	37.9	38.1	38.3	39.2	39.4	39.6	39.8	39.2
118–122	38.5	38.7	38.9	39.1	39.4	39.6	39.8	40.0	40.0
123–127	39.2	39.4	39.6	39.8	40.0	40.1	40.3	40.5	40.7
128–132	39.9	40.1	40.2	40.4	40.6	40.8	41.0	41.2	41.3
133–137	40.5	40.7	40.8	41.0	41.2	41.4	41.6	41.7	41.9
138–142	41.0	41.2	41.4	41.6	41.7	41.9	42.1	42.3	42.5
143–147	41.5	41.7	41.9	42.0	42.2	42.4	42.6	42.8	43.0
148–152	41.9	42.1	42.3	42.8	42.6	42.8	43.0	43.2	43.4
153–157	42.3	42.5	42.6	42.8	43.0	43.2	43.4	43.6	43.7
158–162	42.6	42.8	43.0	43.1	43.3	43.5	43.7	43.9	44.1
163–167	42.9	43.0	43.2	43.4	43.6	43.8	44.0	44.1	44.3
168–172	43.1	43.2	43.4	43.6	43.8	44.0	44.2	44.3	44.5
173–177	43.2	43.4	43.6	43.8	43.9	44.1	44.3	44.5	44.7
178–182	43.3	43.5	43.7	43.8	44.0	44.2	44.4	44.6	44.8

(From Jackson, A. S., and Pollock, M. L.: Practical assessment of body composition. **Phys. Sportsmed.** 13:76–90, 1985. Reprinted by permission of *The Physician and Sportsmedicine,* Copyright McGraw-Hill, Inc.)

Table A–30. Percent Fat Estimate for Men: Sum of Triceps, Chest, and
Subscapular Skinfolds

Sum of Skinfolds (mm)	Age to Last Year							
	Under 22	*23–27*	*28–32*	*33–37*	*38–42*	*43–47*	*48–52*	*53–57*	*Over 57*
8–10	1.5	2.0	2.5	3.1	3.6	4.1	4.6	5.1	5.6
11–13	3.0	3.5	4.0	4.5	5.1	5.6	6.1	6.6	7.1
14–16	4.5	5.0	5.5	6.0	6.5	7.0	7.6	8.1	8.6
17–19	5.9	6.4	6.9	7.4	8.0	8.5	9.0	9.5	10.0
20–22	7.3	7.8	8.3	8.8	9.4	9.9	10.4	10.9	11.4
23–25	8.6	9.2	9.7	10.2	10.7	11.2	11.8	12.3	12.8
26–28	10.0	10.5	11.0	11.5	12.1	12.6	13.1	13.6	14.2
29–31	11.2	11.8	12.3	12.8	13.4	13.9	14.4	14.9	15.5
32–34	12.5	13.0	13.5	14.1	14.6	15.1	15.7	16.2	16.7
35–37	13.7	14.2	14.8	15.3	15.8	16.4	16.9	17.4	18.0
38–40	14.9	15.4	15.9	16.5	17.0	17.6	18.1	18.6	19.2
41–43	16.0	16.6	17.1	17.6	18.2	18.7	19.3	19.8	20.3
44–46	17.1	17.7	18.2	18.7	19.3	19.8	20.4	20.9	21.5
47–49	18.2	18.7	19.3	19.8	20.4	20.9	21.4	22.0	22.5
50–52	19.2	19.7	20.3	20.8	21.4	21.9	22.5	23.0	23.6
53–55	20.2	20.7	21.3	21.8	22.4	22.9	23.5	24.0	24.6
56–58	21.1	21.7	22.2	22.8	23.3	23.9	24.4	25.0	25.5
59–61	22.0	22.6	23.1	23.7	24.2	24.8	25.3	25.9	26.5
62–64	22.9	23.4	24.0	24.5	25.1	25.7	26.2	26.8	27.3
65–67	23.7	24.3	24.8	25.4	25.9	26.5	27.1	27.6	28.2
68–70	24.5	25.0	25.6	26.2	26.7	27.3	27.8	28.4	29.0
71–73	25.2	25.8	26.3	26.9	27.5	28.0	28.6	29.1	29.7
74–76	25.9	26.5	27.0	27.6	28.2	28.7	29.3	29.9	30.4
77–79	26.6	27.1	27.7	28.2	28.8	29.4	29.9	30.5	31.1
80–82	27.2	27.7	28.3	28.9	29.4	30.0	30.6	31.1	31.7
83–85	27.7	28.3	28.8	29.4	30.0	30.5	31.1	31.7	32.3
86–88	28.2	28.8	29.4	29.9	30.5	31.1	31.6	32.2	32.8
89–91	28.7	29.3	29.8	30.4	31.0	31.5	32.1	32.7	33.3
92–94	29.1	29.7	30.3	30.8	31.4	32.0	32.6	33.1	33.4
95–97	29.5	30.1	30.6	31.2	31.8	32.4	32.9	33.5	34.1
98–100	29.8	30.4	31.0	31.6	32.1	32.7	33.3	33.9	34.4
101–103	30.1	30.7	31.3	31.8	32.4	33.0	33.6	34.1	34.7
104–106	30.4	30.9	31.5	32.1	32.7	33.2	33.8	34.4	35.0
107–109	30.6	31.1	31.7	32.3	32.9	33.4	34.0	34.6	35.2
110–112	30.7	31.3	31.9	32.4	33.0	33.6	34.2	34.7	35.3
113–115	30.8	31.4	32.0	32.5	33.1	33.7	34.3	34.9	35.4
116–118	30.9	31.5	32.0	32.6	33.2	33.8	34.3	34.9	35.5

(From Jackson, A. S., and Pollock, M. L.: Practical assessment of body composition. **Phys. Sportsmed.** 13:76–90, 1985. Reprinted by permission of *The Physician and Sportsmedicine,* Copyright McGraw-Hill, Inc.)

Table A–31. Estimation of Target Weight for Men*

| % Fat | \
Weight (pounds) | | | | | | | | | | | | | | | | | | | | | | | | |
|---|---|---|---|---|---|---|---|---|---|---|---|---|---|---|---|---|---|---|---|---|---|---|---|---|---|
| | 120 | 125 | 130 | 135 | 140 | 145 | 150 | 155 | 160 | 165 | 170 | 175 | 180 | 185 | 190 | 195 | 200 | 205 | 210 | 215 | 220 | 225 | 230 | 235 | 240 |
| 16 | 120 | 125 | 130 | 135 | 140 | 145 | 150 | 155 | 160 | 165 | 170 | 175 | 180 | 185 | 190 | 195 | 200 | 205 | 210 | 215 | 220 | 225 | 230 | 235 | 240 |
| 18 | 117 | 122 | 127 | 132 | 137 | 142 | 146 | 151 | 156 | 161 | 166 | 171 | 176 | 181 | 186 | 190 | 195 | 200 | 205 | 210 | 215 | 220 | 225 | 229 | 234 |
| 20 | 114 | 119 | 124 | 129 | 133 | 138 | 143 | 148 | 152 | 157 | 162 | 167 | 171 | 176 | 181 | 186 | 190 | 195 | 200 | 205 | 210 | 214 | 219 | 224 | 229 |
| 22 | 111 | 116 | 121 | 125 | 130 | 135 | 139 | 144 | 149 | 153 | 158 | 162 | 167 | 172 | 176 | 181 | 186 | 190 | 195 | 200 | 204 | 209 | 214 | 218 | 223 |
| 24 | 109 | 113 | 118 | 122 | 127 | 131 | 136 | 140 | 145 | 149 | 154 | 158 | 163 | 167 | 172 | 176 | 181 | 186 | 190 | 195 | 199 | 204 | 208 | 213 | 217 |
| 26 | 106 | 110 | 115 | 119 | 123 | 128 | 132 | 137 | 141 | 145 | 150 | 154 | 159 | 163 | 167 | 172 | 176 | 181 | 185 | 189 | 194 | 198 | 203 | 207 | 211 |
| 28 | 103 | 107 | 111 | 116 | 120 | 124 | 129 | 133 | 137 | 141 | 146 | 150 | 154 | 159 | 163 | 167 | 171 | 176 | 180 | 184 | 189 | 193 | 197 | 201 | 208 |
| 30 | 100 | 104 | 108 | 113 | 117 | 121 | 125 | 129 | 133 | 137 | 142 | 146 | 150 | 154 | 158 | 162 | 167 | 171 | 175 | 179 | 183 | 188 | 192 | 196 | 200 |
| 32 | 97 | 101 | 105 | 109 | 113 | 117 | 121 | 125 | 130 | 134 | 138 | 142 | 146 | 150 | 154 | 158 | 162 | 166 | 170 | 174 | 178 | 182 | 186 | 190 | 194 |
| 34 | 94 | 98 | 102 | 106 | 110 | 114 | 118 | 122 | 126 | 130 | 134 | 137 | 141 | 145 | 149 | 153 | 157 | 161 | 165 | 169 | 173 | 177 | 181 | 185 | 189 |
| 36 | 91 | 95 | 99 | 103 | 107 | 110 | 114 | 118 | 122 | 126 | 130 | 133 | 137 | 141 | 145 | 149 | 152 | 156 | 160 | 164 | 168 | 171 | 175 | 179 | 183 |
| 38 | 89 | 92 | 96 | 100 | 103 | 107 | 111 | 114 | 118 | 122 | 125 | 129 | 133 | 137 | 140 | 144 | 148 | 151 | 155 | 159 | 162 | 166 | 170 | 174 | 177 |
| 40 | 86 | 89 | 93 | 96 | 100 | 104 | 107 | 111 | 114 | 118 | 121 | 125 | 129 | 132 | 136 | 139 | 143 | 146 | 150 | 154 | 157 | 161 | 164 | 168 | 173 |

*Target weight is based on 16 percent fat. To determine target weight, find present weight at the top of the table and then descend vertically to horizontal row corresponding to percentage of fat. See Chapter 6 (body composition) for equation to determine target weight.

(Reprinted with permission from Golding, L. A., Myers, C. R., and Sinning, W. E. (eds.): **The Y's Way to Physical Fitness: The Complete Guide to Fitness Testing and Instruction,** 3rd Ed. Champaign, IL, Human Kinetics, 1989.)

Table A–32. Estimation of Target Weight for Women*

% Fat	\multicolumn{19}{c}{Weight (pounds)}

% Fat	105	110	115	120	125	130	135	140	145	150	155	160	165	170	175	180	185	190	195
24	104	109	114	118	123	128	133	138	143	148	153	158	163	168	173	178	183	188	192
25	102	107	112	117	122	127	131	136	141	146	151	156	161	166	170	175	180	185	190
26	101	106	111	115	120	125	130	135	139	144	149	154	159	163	168	173	178	183	187
27	100	104	109	114	119	123	128	133	137	142	147	152	156	161	166	171	175	180	185
28	98	103	108	112	117	122	126	131	136	140	145	150	154	159	164	168	173	178	182
29	97	101	106	111	115	120	124	129	134	138	143	148	152	157	161	166	171	175	180
30	95	100	105	109	114	118	123	127	132	136	141	145	150	155	159	164	168	173	177
31	94	99	103	108	112	116	121	125	130	134	139	144	149	152	157	161	166	170	175
32	93	97	102	106	110	115	119	124	129	132	137	141	146	150	155	159	163	168	172
33	91	96	100	104	109	113	117	122	126	131	135	139	144	148	152	157	161	165	170
34	90	94	99	103	107	111	116	120	124	129	133	137	141	146	150	154	159	163	167
35	89	93	97	101	106	110	114	118	122	127	131	135	139	144	148	152	156	160	165
36	87	91	96	100	104	108	112	116	121	125	129	133	137	141	145	150	154	158	162
37	86	90	94	98	102	106	110	115	119	123	127	131	135	139	143	147	151	155	160
38	85	89	93	97	101	105	109	113	117	121	125	129	133	137	141	145	149	153	157
39	83	87	91	95	99	103	107	111	115	119	123	127	131	135	139	143	147	151	154
40	82	86	90	94	97	101	105	109	113	117	121	125	129	132	136	140	144	148	152

*Target weight is based on 23 percent fat. To determine target weight, find present weight at the top of the table and then descend vertically to horizontal row corresponding to percentage of fat. See Chapter 6 (body composition) for equation to determine target weight.

(Reprinted with permission from Golding, L. A., Myers, C. R., and Sinning, W. E. (eds.): **The Y's Way to Physical Fitness: The Complete Guide to Fitness Testing and Instruction**, 3rd Ed. Champaign, IL, Human Kinetics, 1989.)

APPENDIX B

Additional Information and Forms Used in Cardiac Rehabilitation Programs

---

**EMERGENCY PHYSICIAN'S ORDERS FOR
INPATIENT AND OUTPATIENT CARDIAC REHABILITATION**

Emergency Protocol for Unstable Angina, Serious Arrhythmias or Cardiac Arrest:
1) Stop exercise.
2) Start and maintain oxygen therapy by nasal cannula or mask.

THEN IF:

  1) Angina

   A. Nitroglycerin gr 1/150 prn and monitor blood pressure.
   B. Obtain 12 lead ECG STAT.
  2) Symptomatic Bradycardia

   A. Start intravenous 500 cc D_5W and keep open.
   B. Give atropine 0.5 to 1.0 mg IV bolus.
  3) Ventricular Dysrhythmias

   Serious Ventricular Arrhythmias

   A. Start intravenous 500 cc D_5W and keep open.
   B. For uncontrolled and/or symptomatic PVC's, give lidocaine 100 mg
      IV STAT. May repeat with 50 mg every 5 minutes for a total dose of
      250 mg.
   C. Begin lidocaine drip with 1 gram in 250 cc D_5W at 2 mg/minute (range
      1–4 mg/minute as needed).
   Ventricular Tachycardia–Ventricular Fibrillation

   A. Defibrillate with 300–400 watt-seconds when life threatening.
  4) Cardiac Arrest

   A. CPR.
   B. Sodium bicarbonate 1 amp IV following defibrillation.

  NOTIFY M.D. IMMEDIATELY AFTER ABOVE ACTION HAS BEEN TAKEN

Signature of Physician: _____

Date: _____

Figure B–1. Emergency physician's orders for cardiac rehabilitation. (Courtesy of Cardiac Rehabilitation Program, Cardiovascular Disease Section, Mount Sinai Medical Center, Milwaukee, WI.)

INPATIENT MEDICAL EVALUATION

Patient's Name: _____ Age: _____ Date: _____

Attending Physician: _____ Cardiologist: _____ Surgeon: _____

Specific Cardiac Diagnoses: _____

_____

_____ Surgery: Type_____Date: _____

_____ MI: Type and Date: _____ _____

_____ CHF   _____

_____ Other
      (describe): _____

Pertinent Medical History: _____   Risk Factors: _____

_____   _____

_____   _____

_____   _____

Nuclear Studies, Cath Data, etc.: _____

_____

_____

_____

Medications and Dose: _____

            _____

            _____

Allergies: _____

Drug Reactions: _____

Physical Exam: _____

Weight: _____ Height: _____

Resting Heart Rate (range): _____

Resting Systolic Blood Pressure (range): _____

Resting Diastolic Blood Pressure (range): _____

Temperature: _____

Lab Results: Hct_____ Hgb_____ K+_____

Chest X-ray: _____

ECG (most recent): _____

CPK_____ MB_____% Others: _____

Complications post-op: _____

_____

_____

Additional Comments: _____

_____

            Completed by: _____

Figure B–2. Inpatient medical evaluation. (Courtesy of Cardiac Rehabilitation Program, Cardiovascular Disease Section, Mount Sinai Medical Center, Milwaukee, WI.)

694

INPATIENT EXERCISE RECORD—INPATIENT EXERCISE CENTER

Name _____ Age _____ Sex _____ Surgeon _____

Address _____ Cardiologist _____

street _____ city _____ state _____ zip _____ Date of Surgery/MI _____

Exercise
TM = Treadmill
BI = Bicycle
ST = Stairs
PT = Physical Therapy
OT = Other (specify)

ECG Changes
1 = ST-T Depression ($\geq$ 1 mm)
2 = ST-T Elevation ($\geq$ 1 mm)
3 = Unifocal PVC (indicate #/min)
4 = Multifocal PVC (indicate #/min)
5 = SVT
6 = V Tach
7 = Other (specify)

Signs and Symptoms
A = Chest pain and discomfort
B = Faintness, syncope, dizziness
C = Fatigue
D = Dyspnea
E = Hypertension
F = Hypotension
G = Pallor
H = Other (specify)

Body Composition
Axilla _____ mm
Triceps _____ mm
Suprailium _____ mm
% Fat _____
Ideal Wt _____ lb

Date	Weight (lb/kg)	Exer	mph, rpm	Workload Resist	Duration	Heart Rate Rest	Heart Rate Exer	Blood Pressure Rest	Blood Pressure Imm Post-Ex	Blood Pressure 5' Post-Ex	RPE	Comments/Signature (ECG changes, signs, symptoms, drugs, etc)

(Revised 2/1/81)

Figure B–3. Inpatient exercise record for an inpatient exercise center. (Courtesy of Cardiac Rehabilitation Program, Cardiovascular Disease Section, Mount Sinai Medical Center, Milwaukee, WI.)

695

Conversion Table for Upper Limit/Target Heart Rate

beats/10 sec		beats/min	beats/10 sec		beats/min	beats/10 sec		beats/min
9	=	54	15	=	90	21	=	126
10	=	60	16	=	96	22	=	132
11	=	66	17	=	102	23	=	138
12	=	72	18	=	108	24	=	144
13	=	78	19	=	114	25	=	150
14	=	84	20	=	120	26	=	156

Perceived Exertion Scale

6
7 Very, Very Light
8
9 Very Light
10
11 Fairly Light
12
13 Somewhat Hard
14
15 Hard
16
17 Very Hard
18
19 Very, Very Hard
20

MOUNT SINAI ✡ MEDICAL CENTER
Cardiac Rehabilitation
950 North 12th Street
Milwaukee, Wisconsin
(414) 289-8040

Revised 2/20/81

ACTIVITY LOG
FOR

_____

MOUNT SINAI

MILWAUKEE

"The journey of a thousand miles
starts with a single step"

Upper Limit/Target HR _____

Date	Distance	Duration	Pre HR	Mid HR	End HR	Perceived Exertion	Comments

Figure B–4. Activity log. (Courtesy of Cardiac Rehabilitation Program, Cardiovascular Disease Section, Mount Sinai Medical Center, Milwaukee, WI.)

INPATIENT PROGRESS REPORT

Dear Dr. _____ :

    The following report is a summary of your patient, _____ 's, progress in the Inpatient Cardiac Rehabilitation Program, which he/she entered on _____ .

Age:

Date of MI:

Date of Surgery:

Predischarge low-level Graded Exercise Test   Date:

    See enclosed report.

Exercise Data:

    Started walking on treadmill for _____ minutes at _____ mph 0% grade on _____ . Upon discharge was able to walk at _____ mph 0% grade for _____ minutes and climb _____ stairs.

ECG Changes and Problems: _____

_____

_____

_____

_____

_____

Recommendations: _____

_____

_____

_____

_____

_____   _____

Program Director   Medical Director

_____

Inpatient Program Coordinator

Figure B–5. Inpatient progress report. (Courtesy of Cardiac Rehabilitation Program, Cardiovascular Disease Section, Mount Sinai Medical Center, Milwaukee, WI.)

OUTPATIENT REFERRAL FORM

Patient's Name: _____ Date: _____

           Last   First   Middle

Address: _____ Age: _____ Phone: _____

_____ Cardiac Surgery (Type & Date): _____

_____ MI (Type & Date): _____

_____ CHF: _____

_____ Post MI/Surgery Complications: _____

_____

Medical Hx: _____

_____

_____

Angina: _____ Date of Onset: _____ Stable: _____ Unstable: _____

    Precipitated By: _____

    Therapy: _____

Hypertension: _____ Date of Onset: _____ Therapy: _____

Arrhythmias (Type): _____

    Date(s): _____ Therapy: _____

Cardiac Catheterization (most recent, post incident/surgery): Date: _____

    Cardiologist: _____ Location: _____

    Coronary Angiography (patency of grafts if post surgical): _____

_____

    Ventricular Function: _____ Ejection Fraction: _____

Nuclear Cardiology: _____

    Rest & Exercise Dynamics: _____ Date: _____

    Resting Ejection Fraction: _____ Resting Wall Motion: _____

    Exercise Ejection Fraction: _____ Exercise Wall Motion: _____

MI Scan: _____ Date: _____ Neg ☐   Pos ☐   Equiv ☐

    Positive Area: _____

Exercise Tolerance Test: Please enclose complete report and ECG.

    Yes ☐   No ☐   Date: _____

    If it is outdated (past 3 months), may this patient be tested: Yes ☐   No ☐

    If not, when? _____ Will you schedule the test?   Yes ☐   No ☐

    Shall we schedule and perform the test here at M.S.M.C.?   Yes ☐   No ☐

Risk Factors for Coronary Heart Disease: (please check those which apply to this patient)

    ☐ Smoking   ☐ Hypertension   ☐ Family History   ☐ Obesity

    ☐ Diabetes   ☐ Hyperlipidemia, Please Specify: ☐ Cholesterol   ☐ Triglycerides

Allergies: _____

Additional medical or orthopedic problems which may alter program participation (i.e.,

        insulin-dependent diabetes, claudication, COPD, asthma, prosthesis, psychiatric

        problems, etc.): _____

        _____

        _____

```
┌─────────────────────────────────────────────────────────────────────┐
│              OUTPATIENT REFERRAL FORM (CONTINUED)                     │
│  Present Medications (date and dosage):                              │
│                                                                       │
│  _____    _____    _____              │
│  _____    _____    _____              │
│  _____    _____    _____              │
│  _____    _____    _____              │
│                                                                       │
│  Has patient been participating in an exercise program:   □ Yes   □ No│
│       If yes, please describe:_____        │
│                                                                       │
│  I recommend the above-named patient to participate in Mount Sinai   │
│  Medical Center's Outpatient Cardiac Rehabilitation Program.         │
│                                                                       │
│  _____    _____         │
│  Date                       Signature of Referring Physician         │
│                                                                       │
│  Name of Physician: _____        │
│  Address: _____        │
│  _____    Phone: _____         │
│                                                                       │
│  _____    _____         │
│  Date                       Signature of Medical Director            │
└─────────────────────────────────────────────────────────────────────┘
```

Figure B–6. Outpatient referral form. (Courtesy of Cardiac Rehabilitation Program, Cardiovascular Disease Section, Mount Sinai Medical Center, Milwaukee, WI.)

INFORMED CONSENT FOR OUTPATIENT EXERCISE REHABILITATION

I voluntarily consent to participate in a medically supervised exercise rehabilitation program in conjunction with the Mount Sinai Medical Center Cardiac Rehabilitation Program which has been prescribed for me by my physician, Doctor _____. This program is part of my treatment to hasten improvement in my cardiovascular function.

Before I enter the exercise phase of the outpatient rehabilitation program, I will have had a clinical evaluation within the last three months which will include a medical history questionnaire, a physical examination, laboratory tests, a chest X-ray, a resting electrocardiogram, measurements of resting heart rate and blood pressure, and a graded exercise tolerance test. The purpose of this evaluation is to detect any condition which would indicate that I should not participate in a medically supervised exercise program and aid in exercise prescription.

The program will follow an exercise prescription prepared by the medical and program directors of the Cardiac Rehabilitation Program in conjunction with the personal physician and will be carefully monitored by the program coordinator and a coronary care nurse. The exercise rehabilitation program will consist of physical therapy, flexibility exercise, and endurance activity, e.g., walking, stationary cycling, stair-climbing, arm pedaling, and jogging as tolerated. The amount of exercise will be regulated on the basis of my functional capacity.

The exercise activities are designed to place a graduated increased work load on the cardiovascular system, thus improving its function. I understand that my heart rate and electrocardiogram will be monitored continuously by telemetry prior to, during, and at least 10 minutes post-exercise in order to detect abnormal responses to the exercise. In addition, my blood pressure will be measured before and following exercise. However, I realize that the response of the cardiovascular system to exercise cannot be predicted with complete accuracy and, consequently, there is a risk of certain changes occurring during or following the exercise. These changes include disorders of heart beats, abnormal blood pressure responses, and, in rare instances, heart attack or cardiac arrest. Proper care in selection and supervision of patients and proper exercise prescription and monitoring provide appropriate precautionary measures to reduce or eliminate such problems. Before starting the program, I will be instructed as to the signs and symptoms that will alert me to stop or slow down my activities. Also, I will be observed by trained personnel who will be alert to changes which would suggest that I modify my exercise. Furthermore, trained medical personnel, emergency equipment, and supplies for my safety will be present for all exercise sessions.

The benefits to me of an exercise program are the enhancement of my recovery from surgery or heart attack, improvement in cardiovascular function in order to perform daily activities, observation of daily activities for life-endangering signs and symptoms, and the scientific assessment of exercise rehabilitation as therapy for heart disease. The information which is obtained during the laboratory evaluations and exercise sessions of this program will be treated as privileged and confidential and will not be released to any unauthorized nonmedical person without my expressed written consent. The information obtained, however, may be used for a statistical or scientific purpose with my right of privacy retained. I also approve of periodic progress reports being sent to my physician of data relating to my laboratory evaluations and exercise sessions.

I have read and understand the preceding information. In addition, the program and its benefits and risks have been discussed with me by the medical or program director of the Cardiac Rehabilitation Program and any questions which have arisen or occurred to me have been answered to my satisfaction. If at any time during my program of rheabilitation I have any additional questions regarding the exercises or procedures in which I am involved, I may freely go to the medical or program directors or program coordinator with my questions. Further, I am guaranteed the right to withdraw from the program at any time.

Date of Signature: _____

Patient: _____

Witness: _____

Medical or Program Director: _____

Figure B–7. Informed consent. (Courtesy of Cardiac Rehabilitation Program, Cardiovascular Disease Section, Mount Sinai Medical Center, Milwaukee, WI.)

OUTPATIENT EXERCISE RECORD

Name: _____

GXT
Date: _____
☐ LL   ☐ SL
RHR: _____
MHR: _____
METS: _____
THR: _____
M.D. Comments: _____

Exercise Codes

TM = Treadmill
AE = Arm Ergometer
BI = Stationary Bicycle
AD = Air Dyne
RE = Rowing Ergometer
SR = Stretching
OT = Other, Specify: _____

Date	Wt (lb)	Resting		Exer Code	Workload			Duration	Exercise			Post		Comments
		HR	B/P		mph, rpm	resist			HR	BP	RPE	HR	BP	

Figure B–8. Outpatient exercise record. (Courtesy of Cardiac Rehabilitation Program, Cardiovascular Disease Section, Mount Sinai Medical Center, Milwaukee, WI.)

DATA RECORD—OUTPATIENT PROGRAM

Name _____ Age _____ Cardiologist _____ Surgeon _____

MI _____ Surgery _____ Phase II Entry Date _____

Smoking   Obesity   Hypertension   Cholesterol   Heredity   Diet: _____

Medical History: _____

_____

Phase I: _____

I. Stress Test Data

Date				
☐ LL ☐ SL	☐ LL ☐ SL	☐ LL ☐ SL	☐ LL ☐ SL	☐ LL ☐ SL
Double Product				
RHR				
MHR				
METS				
THR				
Results				
Time Mph-Grade				

III. Tests

Holter Monitor				
Echo				
Spirometry				
Psychological				

Allergies: _____

_____

V. Patient Education

	Assess	Int.	R.F.	Ed. #1	Ed. #2
Date					

II. Nuclear Cardiology Data

Date				
R EF				
Wall Motion				
Exer EF				
Wall Motion				

MI Scan

Date _____   Pre Pos ☐ Neg ☐ Equiv ☐

Positive Area _____

Date _____   Post Pos ☐ Neg ☐ Equiv ☐

Positive Area _____

Cardiac Cath

Date _____: _____

_____

Grafts _____

Date _____: _____

_____

Grafts _____

IV. Body Composition

Date				
Sum				
Fat %				
Weight/Ht.				
Ideal Wt.				

Figure B–9. Data record for an outpatient program. (Courtesy of Cardiac Rehabilitation Program, Cardiovascular Disease Section, Mount Sinai Medical Center, Milwaukee, WI.)

OUTPATIENT PROGRESS REPORT

Date: _____

Dear Dr. _____ :

The following report is a summary of your patient, _____ 's,
progress in the Outpatient Cardiac Rehabilitation Program, which he/she entered on

_____ .

Age: _____   MI (Type & Date): _____

Surgery (Type & Date): _____

Other (please specify): _____

Graded Exercise Test (GXT)	Graded Exercise Test (GXT)
Date: _____	Date: _____
☐ Low Level GXT	☐ Low Level GXT
☐ Symptom-Limited GXT	☐ Symptom-Limited GXT
Standing Resting Heart Rate: _____	Standing Resting Heart Rate: _____
Maximum Heart Rate: _____	Maximum Heart Rate: _____
METs: _____	METs: _____
Results: _____	Results: _____
Double Product (at 5 METs): _____	Double Product (at 5 METs): _____

Nuclear Dynamics	Nuclear Dynamics
Date: _____	Date: _____
Resting E.F.: _____	Resting E.F.: _____
Resting Wall Motion: _____	Resting Wall Motion: _____
Exercise E.F.: _____	Exercise E.F.: _____
Exercise Wall Motion: _____	Exercise Wall Motion: _____

Exercise Data

Entrance Week #1 Dates: _____	Final Week # _____ Dates: _____
Body Weight (lb): _____	Body Weight (lb): _____
Percent Fat (%):* _____	Percent Fat (%)* _____
Target Heart Rate:† _____	Target Heart Rate:† _____

Week #1	Final Week
Activity: _____	Activity: _____
MET level: _____	MET level: _____
Duration: _____	Duration: _____
Workload: _____	Workload: _____

Illustration continued on following page

OUTPATIENT PROGRESS REPORT (CONTINUED)

Exercise Data (continued)

HR Achieved: _____   HR Achieved: _____

Perceived Exertion: _____   Perceived Exertion: _____

Total Calories/Session: _____   Total Calories/Session: _____

Stretching/Wt. Training: _____   Stretching/Wt. Training: _____

Attendance: _____

ECG Changes and Problems: _____

_____

_____

_____

_____

Summary: _____

_____

_____

_____

_____

Recommendations: _____

_____

_____

_____

_____

_____   _____
Program Director   Medical Director

_____
Coordinator, Outpatient Program

Figure B–10. Outpatient progress report.

*Less than 19% fat is recommended for men, and less than 23% is recommended for women.

†Formula used in calculating Target Heart Rate from Symptom-Limited GXT: (Max HR − Standing RHR) × Percent + Standing RHR. The percentage may increase, as tolerated, as the patient progresses in the program (70%→75%→80%).

(Courtesy of Cardiac Rehabilitation Program, Cardiovascular Disease Section, Mount Sinai Medical Center, Milwaukee, WI.)

Table B–1. Emergency Cart—Recommended Equipment and Supplies for Hospital-Based Programs

Top
Life-Pak (monitor/defibrillator)
Saline pads
Electrode gel
Airway

Side
Cardiac board
Clipboard:
  Cart content list
  Resuscitation record
  Emergency protocol
Oxygen tank
Suction
Back-up drug box

First Drawer
(2) Medium airways
Laryngoscope with curved blade
(2) Extra laryngoscope batteries
(1) Extra laryngoscope bulb
Endotracheal tubes:
  (1) #6
  (1) #7
  (1) #8
  (1) #9
McGill forceps and stylet
(1) 10 ml syringe without needle
(1) Hemostat with rubber ends
(1) Oxygen mask
(1) Oxygen cannula
(1) Oxygen extension tubing
(1) Suction connecting tubing
(1) Oxygen flowmeter (on tank)
(1) Suction connecting tubing
(2) Suction kits
(1) Yankauer suction tube
(1) Nasogastric tube
(1) Lubafax—small tube
(1) 60 ml Toomey syringe
(4) Arterial blood gas kits
(1) Flashlight

Second Drawer
Syringes with needles:
  (4) TB
  (2) 3 ml
  (6) 10 ml
  (2) 30 ml syringes without needle
Extra needles:
  (2) 18 gauge
  (2) 21 gauge
  (2) Intracardiac needles
(6) Jelco IV catheters—2″—18 guage
(2) Intercath 8″—19 gauge
(2) Subclavian 12″—16 gauge
(2) IV catheter plugs
(2) Dual injection sites
Band-Aids
(4) Tourniquets
Alcohol wipes
Sepps
(1) 30 ml sterile water
(1) 30 ml sterile saline
Adhesive tape:
  (2) 1″
  (2) 2″
Spinal needles—18 gauge
Scalpel

Third Drawer

NaHCO$_3$ (44.6 or 50 mEq/50 ml)	5 syringes
Epinephrine (1:10,000; 1 mg/10 ml prefilled syringe)	2 syringes
Epinephrine (1:1000; 1 mg/ml amp)	4 ampules
Atropine SO$_4$ (1 mg/ml; gr 1/60	4 ampules
Isuprel (1 mg/5 ml amp)	2 ampules
Valium (10 mg/2 ml syringe)	2 syringes
Lidocaine (40 mg/ml; 1 g 25 ml vial)	2 vials
Lidocaine (100 mg/5 ml syringe)	3 syringes
Pronestyl (100 mg/ml; 10 ml vial)	2 vials
Levophed (1 mg/1 ml; 4 ml amp)	2 ampules
Dopamine (200 mg/5 ml vial)	2 ampules
Calcium Cl (1 g/10 ml amp)	2 ampules
Dextrose (50% 50 ml syringe)	1 syringe
Bretylium (500 mg/10 ml ampules)	2 ampules

Fourth Drawer

NaHCO$_3$ (44.5 or 50 mEq/50 ml)	5 syringes
Epinephrine (1:10,000; 1 mg/10 ml prefilled syringe)	3 syringes
(6) 4 × 4's	
(4) Sterile towels	

Fifth Drawer
(4) 250 cc D5W
(2) 250 cc NS
(2) 500 cc D5NS
(2) Regular IV administration set
(3) Mini-drip
(2) IV extension tubing
CVP manometer (McGraw)
Prep Tray:
  (2) Novocaine/xylocaine amps
  (2) 000 silk without needle
  (2) 000 silk on curved needle
  (1) Bottle iodine liquid
  Betadine ointment
  Disposable razor

Bottom of Cart
Venous access/pneumothorax tray
Ambu bag with mask and O$_2$ tubing
Surgeon's gloves:
  (2) Size 7½
  (2) Size 8
  (2) Size 8½
Normal saline (sterile) 1000 ml
Oxygen humidifier
Chest tube (28 Fr/16″)

(List compiled and recommended by the American College of Sports Medicine, 1 Virginia Avenue, Indianapolis, IN. Published with permission.)

Table B–2. Emergency Cart—Recommended Equipment and Supplies for
Community-Based Programs

Equipment	Supplies
1. Defibrillator—monitor with ECG electrodes—defibrillator paddles, or portable DC defibrillator and portable ECG monitor	1. Sodium bicarbonate IV
	2. Catecholamine agents
	Epinephrine IV
	Isoproterenol IV
2. Airways—nasopharyngeal and oral (endotracheal desirable)	Dobutamine IV
	3. Atropine sulfate
3. Face mask and Robert Shaw valve	4. Antiarrhythmic agents
4. Oxygen	Lidocaine IV
5. Suction apparatus	Procainamide IV
6. Syringes	Propranolol IV/oral
7. Intravenous sets	5. Morphine sulfate
8. Intravenous stand	6. Calcium chloride
9. Adhesive tape	7. Vasoactive agent
10. Laryngoscope (desirable)	Norepinephrine
	8. Corticosteroids
	Methylprednisolone sodium succinate
	Dexamethasone phosphate
	9. Digoxine IV/oral
	10. Lasix IV
	11. Dextrose 5% in water
	12. Nitroglycerin tablets
	13. Amyl nitrite pearls

(Reprinted with permission from American College of Sports Medicine: **Guidelines for Graded Exercise Testing and Exercise Prescription,** 2nd Ed. Philadelphia, Lea & Febiger, 1980.)

APPENDIX C

American College of Sports Medicine Position Stand on the Prevention of Thermal Injuries During Distance Running*

Purpose of the Position Stand

1. To alert sponsors of distance-running events to potentially serious health hazards during distance running—especially thermal injury.
2. To advise sponsors to consult local weather history and plan events at times when the environmental heat stress would most likely be acceptable.
3. To encourage sponsors to identify the environmental heat stress existing on the day of a race and communicate this to the participants.
4. To educate participants regarding thermal injury susceptibility and prevention.
5. To inform sponsors of preventive actions which may reduce the frequency and severity of this type of injury.

   This position stand replaces that of *Prevention of Heat Injury During Distance Running*, published by the American College of Sports Medicine in 1975. It has been expanded to consider thermal

---

*Copyright American College of Sports Medicine 1985: Position Stand, The prevention of thermal injuries during distance running. **Med. Sci. Sports Exerc.** 19:529–533, 1987.

problems which may affect the general community of joggers, fun runners, and elite athletes who participate in distance-running events. Although hyperthermia is still the most common serious problem encountered in North American fun runs and races, hypothermia can be a problem for slow runners in long races such as the marathon, in cold and/or wet environmental conditions or following races when blood glucose is low and the body's temperature regulatory mechanism is impaired.

Because the physiological responses to exercise and environmental stress vary among participants, strict compliance with the recommendations, while helpful, will not guarantee complete protection from thermal illness. The general guidelines in this position stand do not constitute definitive medical advice, which should be sought from a physician for specific cases. Nevertheless, adherence to these recommendations should help to minimize the incidence of thermal injury.

POSITION STAND

It is the position of the American College of Sports Medicine that the following RECOMMENDATIONS be employed by directors of distance runs or community fun runs.

1. Medical Director

A medical director knowledgeable in exercise physiology and sports medicine should coordinate the preventive and therapeutic aspects of the running event and work closely with the race director.

2. Race Organization

a) Races should be organized to avoid the hottest summer months and the hottest part of the day. As there are great regional variations in environmental conditions, the local weather history will be most helpful in scheduling an event to avoid times when an unacceptable level of heat stress is likely to prevail. Organizers should be cautious of unseasonably hot days in the early spring, as entrants will almost certainly not be heat acclimatized.

b) The environmental heat stress prediction for the day should be obtained from the meteorological service. It can be measured as wet bulb globe temperature (WBGT) (see Appendix I), which is a temperature/humidity/radiation index.[1] If WBGT is above 28°C (82°F), consideration should be given to rescheduling or delaying the race until safer conditions prevail. If below 28°C, participants may be alerted to the degree of heat stress by using color-coded flags at the start of the race and at key positions along the course (Appendix II).[26]

c) All summer events should be scheduled for the early morning, ideally before 8:00 a.m., or in the evening after 6:00 p.m., to minimize solar radiation.

d) An adequate supply of water should be available before the race and every 2–3 km during the race. Runners should be encouraged to consume 100–200 ml at each station.

e) Race officials should be educated as to the warning signs of an impending collapse. Each official should wear an identifiable arm band or badge and should warn runners to stop if they appear to be in difficulty.

f) Adequate traffic and crowd control must be maintained at all times.

g) There should be a ready source of radio communications from various points on the course to a central organizing point to coordinate responses to emergencies.

3. Medical Support

a) *Medical Organization and Responsibility:*
The Medical Director should alert local hospitals and ambulance services to the event and should make prior arrangements with medical personnel for the care of casualties, especially those suffering from heat injury. The mere fact that an entrant signs a waiver in no way absolves the organizers of moral and/or legal responsibility. Medical personnel supervising races should have the authority to evaluate, examine, and/or stop a runner who displays the symptoms and signs of impending heat injury, or who appears to be mentally and/or physically out of control for any other reason.

b) *Medical Facilities:*
   i. Medical support staff and facilities should be available at the race site.
   ii. The facilities should be staffed with personnel capable of instituting immediate and appropriate resuscitation measures. Apart from the routine resuscitation equipment, ice packs and fans for cooling are required.

  iii. Persons trained in first aid, appropriately identified with an arm band, badge, etc., should be stationed along the course to warn runners to stop if they exhibit signs of impending heat injury.

  iv. Ambulances or vans with accompanying medical personnel should be available along the course.

  v. Although the emphasis in this stand has been on the management of hyperthermia, on cold, wet, and windy days, athletes may be chilled and require "space blankets," blankets, and warm drinks at the finish to prevent or treat hypothermia.[23, 45]

4. Competitor Education

The education of fun runners has increased greatly in recent years, but race organizers must not assume that all participants are well informed or prepared. Distributing guidelines at the pre-registration, publicity in the press and holding clinics/seminars before runs are valuable.

The following persons are particularly prone to heat illness: the obese,[3, 17, 43] unfit,[13, 29, 39, 43] dehydrated,[6, 14, 31, 37, 38, 47] those unacclimatized to the heat,[20, 43] those with a previous history of heat stroke,[36, 43] and anyone who runs while ill.[41] Children perspire less than adults and have a lower heat tolerance.[2] Based on the above information, all participants should be advised of the following.

a) Adequate training and fitness are important for full enjoyment of the run and also to prevent heat-related injuries.[13, 28, 29, 39]

b) Prior training in the heat will promote heat acclimatization and thereby reduce the risk of heat injury. It is wise to do as much training as possible at the time of day at which the race will be held.[20]

c) Fluid consumption before and during the race will reduce the risk of heat injury, particularly in longer runs such as the marathon.[6, 14, 47]

d) Illness prior to or at the time of the event should preclude competition.[41]

e) Participants should be advised of the early symptoms of heat injury. These include clumsiness, stumbling, excessive sweating (and also cessation of sweating), headache, nausea, dizziness, apathy, and any gradual impairment of consciousness.[42]

f) Participants should be advised to choose a comfortable speed and not to run faster than conditions warrant.[18, 33]

g) Participants are advised to run with a partner, each being responsible for the other's well-being.[33]

BACKGROUND FOR POSITION STAND

There has been an exponential rise in the number of fun runs and races in recent years and, as would be expected, a similar increase in the number of running-related injuries. Minor injuries such as bruises, blisters and musculoskeletal injuries are most common.[41, 45] Myocardial infarction or cardiac arrest is, fortunately, very rare and occurs almost exclusively in patients with symptomatic heart disease.[44] Hypoglycemia may be seen occasionally in normal runners[11] and has been observed following marathons[21] and shorter fun runs.[41]

The most serious injuries in fun runs and races are related to problems of thermoregulation. In the shorter races, 10 km (6.2 miles) or less, hyperthermia with the attendant problems of heat exhaustion and heat syncope dominates, even on relatively cool days.[4, 5, 10, 15, 16, 18, 27, 41] In longer races, heat problems are common on warm or hot days,[31] but on moderate to cold days, hypothermia may be a real risk to some participants.[23]

Thermoregulation and Hyperthermia. Fun runners may experience hyperthermia or hypothermia, depending on the environmental conditions and clothing worn. The adequately clothed runner is capable of withstanding a wide range of environmental temperatures. Hyperthermia is the potential problem in warm and hot weather, when the body's rate of heat production is greater than its ability to dissipate this heat.[1] In cold weather, scanty clothing may provide inadequate protection from the environment and hypothermia may develop, particularly towards the end of a long race when running speed and, therefore, heat production, are reduced.

During intense exercise, heat production in contracting muscles is 15–20 times that of basal metabolism and is sufficient to raise body core temperature in an average size individual by 1°C every 5 min if no temperature-regulating mechanisms were activated.[25] With increased heat production, thermal receptors in the hypothalamus sense the increased body temperature and respond with an increased cutaneous circulation; thus, the excess heat is transferred to the skin surface to be dissipated by physical means, primarily the evaporation of sweat.[9] The precise quantitative relationships in heat transfer are beyond the scope of this position stand, but are well reviewed elsewhere.[24, 25]

When the rate of heat production exceeds that of heat loss for a sufficient period of time, thermal injury will occur. In long races, sweat loss can be significant and result in a total body water deficit of 6–10% of body weight.[47] Such dehydration will subsequently reduce sweating and predispose the runner to hyperthermia, heat stroke, heat exhaustion, and muscle cramps.[47] For a given level of dehydration, children have a greater increase in core temperature than do adults.[2] Rectal temperatures have been reported above 40.6°C after races and fun runs[7, 22, 31, 35] and as high as 42–43°C in fun run participants who have collapsed.[32, 34, 41, 42]

Fluid ingestion before and during prolonged running will minimize dehydration (and reduce the rate of increase in body core temperature).[7, 14] However, in fun runs of less than 10 km, hyperthermia may occur in the absence of significant dehydration.[41] Runners should avoid consuming large quantities of highly concentrated sugar solution during runs, as this may result in a decrease in gastric emptying.[8, 12]

Thermoregulation and Hypothermia. Heat can be lost readily from the body when the rate of heat production is exceeded by heat loss.[46] Even on moderately cool days, if the pace slows and/or if weather conditions become cooler en route, hypothermia may ensue.[23] Several deaths have been reported from hypothermia during fun runs in mountain environments.[30, 40] Hypothermia is common in inexperienced marathon runners who frequently run the second half of the race much more slowly than the first half. Such runners may be able to maintain core temperature initially, but with the slow pace of the second half, especially on cool, wet, or windy days, hypothermia can develop.[23]

Early symptoms and signs of hypothermia include shivering, euphoria, and an appearance of intoxication. As core temperature continues to fall, shivering may stop, and lethargy and muscular weakness may occur with disorientation, hallucinations, and often a combative nature. If core temperature falls below 30°C, the victim may lose consciousness.

Organizers of distance races and fun runs and their medical support staff should anticipate the medical problems and be capable of responding to significant numbers of hyperthermic and/or hypothermic runners. Thermal injury can be minimized with appropriate education of participants and with adequate facilities, supplies, and support staff.

Appendix I
Measurement of Environmental Heat Stress

Ambient temperature is only one component of environmental heat stress; others are humidity, wind velocity, and radiant heat. Therefore, measurement of ambient temperature, dry bulb alone, is inadequate. The most useful and widely applied approach is wet bulb globe temperature (WBGT).

$$WBGT = (0.7 \text{ Twb}) + (0.2 \text{ Tg}) + (0.1 \text{ Tdb}),$$

where Twb = temperature (wet bulb thermometer), Tg = temperature (black globe thermometer), and Tdb = temperature (dry bulb thermometer).

The importance of wet bulb temperature can be readily appreciated, as it accounts for 70% of the index, whereas dry bulb temperature accounts for only 10%. A simple portable heat stress monitor which gives direct WBGT in degrees C or degrees F to monitor conditions during fun runs has proven useful.[19]

Alternatively, if a means for readily assessing WBGT is not available from wet bulb, globe, and dry bulb temperatures, one can use the following equation.[48]

$$WBGT = (0.567 \text{ Tdb}) + (0.393 \text{ Pa}) + 3.94,$$

where Tdb = temperature (dry bulb thermometer) and Pa = environmental water vapor pressure. These environmental variables should be readily available from local weather or radio stations.

Instruments to measure WBGT are available commercially. Additional information may be obtained from the American College of Sports Medicine.

Appendix II
Use of Color-Coded Flags to Indicate the Risk of Thermal Stress*

1. A RED FLAG: High Risk: When WBGT is 23–28°C (73–82°F). This signal would indicate that all runners should be aware that heat injury is possible and any person particularly sensitive to heat or humidity should probably not run.

---

*This scale is determined for runners clad in running shorts, shoes and a T-shirt. In warmer weather, the less clothing the better. For males, wearing no shirt or a mesh top is better than wearing a T-shirt because the surface for evaporation is increased. However, in areas where radiant heat is excessive, a light top may be helpful.

2. AN AMBER FLAG: Moderate Risk: When WBGT is 18–23°C (65–73°F).

It should be remembered that the air temperature, probably humidity, and almost certainly the radiant heat at the beginning of the race will increase during the course of the race if conducted in the morning or early afternoon.

3. A GREEN FLAG: Low Risk: When WGBT is below 18°C (65°F). This in no way guarantees that heat injury will not occur, but indicates only that the risk is low.

4. A WHITE FLAG: Low Risk for hyperthermia, but possible risk for hypothermia: When WBGT is below 10°C (50°F).

Hypothermia may occur, especially in slow runners in long races, and in wet and windy conditions.

Appendix III
Road Race Checklist

Medical Personnel

1. Have aid personnel available if the race is 10 km (6.2 miles) or longer, and run in warm or cold weather.
2. Recruit back-up personnel from existing emergency medical services (police, fire rescue, emergency medical service).
3. Notify local hospitals of the time and place of the road race.

Aid Stations

1. Provide major aid station at the finish point which is cordoned off from public access.
2. Equip the major aid station with the following supplies:

   - tent
   - cots
   - bath towels
   - water in large containers
   - ice in bag or ice chest or quick-cold packs
   - hose with spray nozzle
   - tables for medical supplies and equipment
   - stethoscopes
   - blood pressure cuffs
   - rectal thermometers or meters (range up to 43°C)
   - dressings
   - blankets
   - aluminum thermal sheets ("space blankets")

- elastic bandages
- splints
- skin disinfectants
- intravenous fluids (supervision by a physician is required)

3. Position aid stations along the route at 4 km (2.5 mile) intervals for races over 10 km and at the halfway point for shorter races.
4. Stock each aid station with enough fluid (cool water is the optimum) for each runner to have 300–360 ml (10–12 ounces) at each aid station. A margin of 25% additional cups should be available to account for spillage and double usage.

Table C–1. Equipment Needed at Aid Stations and the Field Hospital (per 1000 runners)

Aid Stations	
No.	*Item*
	ice in small plastic bags or quick-cold packs
5	stretchers (10 at 10 km and beyond)
5	blankets (10 at 10 km and beyond)
6 each	6 inch and 4 inch elastic bandages
½ case	4 × 4 inch gauze pads
½ case	1½ inch tape
½ case	surgical soap
	small instrument kits
	adhesive strips
	moleskin
½ case	petroleum jelly
2 each	inflatable arm and leg splints
	athletic trainer's kit

Field Hospital	
No.	*Item*
10	stretchers
4	sawhorses
10–20	blankets (depending on environmental conditions)
10	intravenous set-ups
2 each	inflatable arm and leg splints
2 cases	1½ inch tape
2 cases each	elastic bandages (2, 4, and 6 inches)
2 cases	sheet wadding
	underwrap
2 cases	4 × 4 inch gauze pads
	adhesive strips
	moleskin
½ case	surgical soap
2	oxygen tanks with regulators and masks
2	ECG monitors with defibrillators
	ice in small plastic bags
	small instrument kits

(Adapted from Noble, H. B., and Bachman, D.: Medical aspects of distance race planning. **Phys. Sportsmed.** 7:78–84, 1979.)

Communications/Surveillance

1. Set up communication between the medical personnel and the major aid station.
2. Arrange for a radio-equipped car or van to follow the race course, and provide radio contact with the director.

Instructions to Runners

1. Apprise the race participants of potential medical problems in advance of the race so precautions may be followed.
2. Advise the race director to announce the following information by loudspeaker immediately prior to the race:

   • the flag color; the risks for hyperthermia and/or hypothermia
   • location of aid stations and type of fluid available
   • reinforcement of warm weather or cold weather self-care

3. Advise the race participants to print their names, addresses, and any medical problems on the back of the registration number.

Appendix IV
Medical Stations
General Guidelines

Staff for Large Races

1. Physician, podiatrist, nurse or EMT, a team of 3 per 1000 runners. Double or triple this number at the finish area.
2. One ambulance per 3000 runners at finish area; one cruising vehicle.
3. One physician to act as triage officer at finish.

Water

Estimate 1 liter (0.26 gallon) per runner per 16 km (10 miles), or roughly, per 60–90 min running time, and depending on number of stations.

For 10 km, the above rule is still recommended.

Cups = (number of entrants × number of stations)
         + 25% additional per station
     = (2 × number of entrants) extra at finish area

Double this total if the course is out and back. In cold weather, an equivalent amount of warm drinks should be available.

References

1. Adolph, E. I. *Physiology of Man in the Desert*. New York: Interscience, 1947, pp. 5–43.
2. Bar-Or, O. Climate and the exercising child—a review. *Int. J. Sports Med.* 1:53–65, 1980.
3. Bar-Or, O., H. M. Lundegren, and E. R. Buskirk. Heat tolerance of exercising lean and obese women. *J. Appl. Physiol.* 26:403–409, 1969.
4. Buskirk, E. R., P. F. Iampietro, and D. E. Bass. Work performance after dehydration: effects of physical conditioning and heat acclimatization. *J. Appl. Physiol.* 12:189–194, 1958.
5. Clowes, G. H. A., Jr. and T. F. O'Donnell, Jr. Heat stroke. *N. Engl. J. Med.* 291:564–567, 1974.
6. Costill, D. L., R. Cote, E. Miller, T. Miller, and S. Wynder. Water and electrolyte replacement during days of work in the heat. *Aviat. Space Environ. Med.* 46:795–800, 1970.
7. Costill, D. L., W. F. Kammer, and A. Fisher. Fluid ingestion during distance running. *Arch. Environ. Health* 21:520–525, 1970.
8. Costill, D. L. and B. Saltin. Factors limiting gastric emptying during rest and exercise. *J. Appl. Physiol.* 37:679–683, 1974.
9. Ellis, F. P., A. N. Exton-Smith, K. G. Foster, and J. S. Weiner. Eccrine sweating and mortality during heat waves in very young and very old persons. *Isr. J. Med. Sci.* 12:815–817, 1976.
10. England, A. C., III, D. W. Fraser, A. W. Hightower, et al. Preventing severe heat injury in runners: suggestions from the 1979 Peachtree Road Race experience. *Ann. Intern. Med.* 97:196–201, 1982.
11. Felig, P., A. Cherif, A. Minagawa, and J. Wahren. Hypoglycemia during prolonged exercise in normal men. *N. Engl. J. Med.* 306:895–900, 1982.
12. Fordtran, J. A. and B. Saltin. Gastric emptying and intestinal absorption during prolonged severe exercise. *J. Appl. Physiol.* 23:331–335, 1967.
13. Gisolfi, C. V. and J. Cohen. Relationships among training, heat acclimation and heat tolerance in men and women: the controversy revisited. *Med. Sci. Sports* 11:56–59, 1979.
14. Gisolfi, C. V. and J. R. Copping. Thermal effects of prolonged treadmill exercise in the heat. *Med. Sci. Sports* 6:108–113, 1974.
15. Hanson, P. G. and S. W. Zimmerman. Exertional heatstroke in novice runners. *JAMA* 242:154–157, 1979.
16. Hart, L. E., B. P. Egier, A. G. Shimizu, P. J. Tandan, and J. R. Sutton. Exertional heat stroke: the runner's nemesis. *Can. Med. Assoc. J.* 122:1144–1150, 1980.
17. Haymes, E. M., R. J. McCormick, and E. R. Buskirk. Heat tolerance of exercising lean and obese prepubertal boys. *J. Appl. Physiol.* 39:457–461, 1975.
18. Hughson, R. L., H. J. Green, M. E. Houston, J. A. Thomson, D. R. MacLean, and J. R. Sutton. Heat injuries in Canadian mass participation runs. *Can. Med. Assoc. J.* 122:1141–1144, 1980.
19. Hughson, R. L., L. A. Standl, and J. M. Mackie. Monitoring road racing in the heat. *Phys. Sportsmed.* 11(5):94–105, 1983.
20. Knochel, J. P. Environmental heat illness: an eclectic review. *Arch. Intern. Med.* 133:841–864, 1974.
21. Levine, S. A., B. Gordon, and C. L. Derick. Some changes in the chemical constituents of the blood following a marathon race. *JAMA* 82:1778–1779, 1924.
22. Maron, M. B., J. A. Wagner, and S. M. Horvath. Thermoregulatory responses during competitive distance running. *J. Appl. Physiol.* 42:909–914, 1977.
23. Maughan, R. J., I. M. Light, P. H. Whiting, and J. D. B. Miller. Hypothermia, hyperkalemia, and marathon running. *Lancet* II:1336, 1982.
24. Nadel, E. R. Control of sweating rate while exercising in the heat. *Med. Sci. Sports* 11:31–35, 1979.
25. Nadel, E. R., C. B. Wenger, M. F. Roberts, J. A. J. Stolwijk, and E. Cafarelli.

Physiological defenses against hyperthermia of exercise. *Ann. NY Acad. Sci.* 301:98–109, 1977.

26. Noble, H. B. and D. Bachman. Medical aspects of distance race planning. *Phys. Sportsmed.* 7(6):78–84, 1979.
27. O'Donnell, T. J., Jr. Acute heatstroke. Epidemiologic, biochemical, renal and coagulation studies. *JAMA* 234:824–828, 1975.
28. Pandolf, K. B., R. L. Burse, and R. F. Goldman. Role of physical fitness in heat acclimatization, decay and reinduction. *Ergonomics* 20:399–408, 1977.
29. Piwonka, R. W., S. Robinson, V. L. Gay, and R. S. Manalis. Preacclimatization of men to heat by training. *J. Appl. Physiol.* 20:379–384, 1965.
30. Pugh, L. G. C. E. Cold stress and muscular exercise with special reference to accidental hypothermia. *Br. Med. J.* 2:333–337, 1967.
31. Pugh, L. G. C. E., J. L. Corbett, and R. H. Johnson. Rectal temperatures, weight losses and sweat rates in marathon running. *J. Appl. Physiol.* 23:347–352, 1967.
32. Richards, D., R. Richards, P. J. Schofield, V. Ross, and J. R. Sutton. Management of heat exhaustion in Sydney's *The Sun* City-to-Surf fun runners. *Med. J. Aust.* 2:457–461, 1979.
33. Richards, R., D. Richards, P. J. Schofield, V. Ross, and J. R. Sutton. Reducing the hazards in Sydney's *The Sun* City-to-Surf fun runs, 1971 to 1979. *Med. J. Aust.* 2:453–457, 1979.
34. Richards, R., D. Richards, P. J. Schofield, V. Ross, and J. R. Sutton. Organization of *The Sun* City-to-Surf fun run, Sydney, 1979. *Med. J. Aust.* 2:470–474, 1979.
35. Robinson, S., S. L. Wiley, L. G. Boudurant and S. Mamlin, Jr. Temperature regulation of men following heatstroke. *Isr. J. Med. Sci.* 12:786–795, 1976.
36. Shapiro, Y., A. Magazanik, R. Udassin, G. Ben-Baruch, E. Shvartz, and Y. Shoenfeld. Heat tolerance in former heatstroke patients. *Ann. Intern. Med.* 90:913–916, 1979.
37. Shibolet, S., R. Coll, T. Gilat, and E. Sohar. Heatstroke: its clinical picture and mechanism in 36 cases. *Q. J. Med.* 36:525–547, 1967.
38. Shibolet, S., M. C. Lancaster, and Y. Danon. Heat stroke: a review. *Aviat. Space Environ. Med.* 47:280–301, 1976.
39. Shvartz, E., Y. Shapiro, A. Magazanik, et al. Heat acclimation, physical fitness, and responses to exercise in temperate and hot environments. *J. Appl. Physiol.* 43:678–683, 1977.
40. Sutton, J. Community jogging vs. arduous racing. *N. Engl. J. Med.* 286:951, 1972.
41. Sutton, J., M. J. Coleman, A. P. Millar, L. Lazarus, and P. Russo. The medical problems of mass participation in athletic competition. The "City-to-Surf " race. *Med. J. Aust.* 2:127–133, 1972.
42. Sutton, J. R. Heat illness. In: *Sports Medicine,* R. H. Strauss (Ed.). Philadelphia: W. B. Saunders, 1984, pp. 307–322.
43. Sutton, J. R. and O. Bar-Or. Thermal illness in fun running. *Am. Heart J.* 100:778–781, 1980.
44. Thompson, P. D., M. P. Stern, P. Williams, K. Duncan, W. L. Haskell, and P. D. Wood. Death during jogging or running. A study of 18 cases. *JAMA* 242:1265–1267, 1979.
45. Williams, R. S., D. D. Schocken, M. Morey, and F. P. Koisch. Medical aspects of competitive distance running. *Postgrad. Med.* 70:41–51, 1981.
46. Winslow, C. E. A., L. P. Herrington, and A. P. Gagge. Physiological reactions of the human body to various atmospheric humidities. *Am. J. Physiol.* 120:288–299, 1937.
47. Wyndham, C. H. and N. B. Strydom. The danger of inadequate water intake during marathon running. *S. Afr. Med. J.* 43:893–896, 1969.
48. Yaglou, C. P. and D. Minard. Control of heat casualties at military training centers. *AMA Arch. Ind. Health* 16:302–305, 1957.

Index

Note: Page numbers in *italics* refer to illustrations; page numbers followed by t refer to tables.